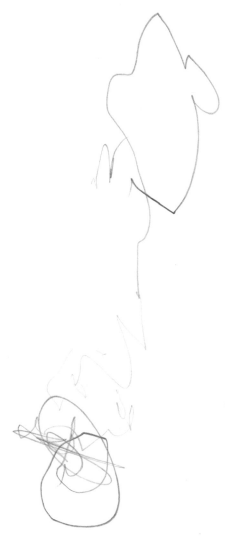

D1567525

ULTRASOUND IN GYNECOLOGY

SECOND EDITION

ULTRASOUND IN GYNECOLOGY

ILAN E. TIMOR-TRITSCH, MD

Professor of Clinical Obstetrics and Gynecology
Department of Obstetrics and Gynecology
Director of Division of Obstetric/Gynecologic Ultrasound
New York University School of Medicine
New York, New York

STEVEN R. GOLDSTEIN, MD

Professor of Obstetrics and Gynecology
Department of Obstetrics and Gynecology
Director of Gynecologic Ultrasound
Co-Director of Bone Densitometry
New York University School of Medicine
New York, New York

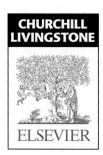

CHURCHILL
LIVINGSTONE

ELSEVIER

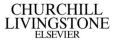

1600 John F. Kennedy Blvd.
Ste 1800
Philadelphia, PA 19103-2899

ULTRASOUND IN GYNECOLOGY

ISBN-13: 978-0-443-06630-6
ISBN-10: 0-443-06630-2

Notice

Knowledge and best practice in this field are constantly changing. As new research and experience broaden our knowledge, changes in practice, treatment and drug therapy may become necessary or appropriate. Readers are advised to check the most current information provided (i) on procedures featured or (ii) by the manufacturer of each product to be administered, to verify the recommended dose or formula, the method and duration of administration, and contraindications. It is the responsibility of the practitioner, relying on his or her own experience and knowledge of the patient, to make diagnoses, to determine dosages and the best treatment for each individual patient, and to take all appropriate safety precautions. To the fullest extent of the law, neither the Publisher nor the Editors assume any liability for any injury and/or damage to persons or property arising out or related to any use of the material contained in this book.

The Publisher

Library of Congress Cataloging-in-Publication Data
Timor-Tritsch, Ilan E.
  Ultrasound in gynecology / Ilan E. Timor-Tritsch, Steven R. Goldstein.—2nd ed.
    p. ; cm.
  Goldstein's name appears first on earlier edition.
  Includes bibliographical references and index.
  ISBN 0-443-06630-2
  1. Generative organs, Female—Ultrasonic imaging. 2. Ultrasonics in obstetrics. I. Goldstein, Steven
R. II. Title.
  [DNLM: 1. Genital Diseases, Female—ultrasonography. 2. Pregnancy. 3. Ultrasonography—methods.
WP 141 T585u 2007]
  RG107.5.U4G65 2007
  618.1′07543—dc22   2006040303

Acquisitions Editor: Meghan McAteer
Developmental Editor: Ryan Creed
Publishing Services Manager: Tina Rebane
Project Manager: Amy Norwitz
Design Direction: Ellen Zanolle

Printed in China

Last digit is the print number: 9 8 7 6 5 4 3 2 1

To our patients, who educate us.

ILAN E. TIMOR-TRITSCH, MD

This book is dedicated to my brother, Howard S. Goldstein, MD, who has supported me literally since my first footsteps and is my trailblazer, my sounding board, and overall the nicest guy I know!

STEVEN R. GOLDSTEIN, MD

Contributors

Leeber Cohen, MD
Associate Professor
Department of Obstetrics and Gynecology
Division of Obstetric and Gynecologic Ultrasound
Northwestern University Medical School
Staff Sonologist
Prentice Women's Hospital
Northwestern Memorial Hospital
Chicago, Illinois
Transvaginal Sonography and Ovarian Cancer

David A. Fishman, MD
Professor and Director
Gynecologic Oncology, Cancer Prevention, and Early
   Detection
New York University Cancer Institute
Department of Obstetrics and Gynecology
New York University Medical Center
New York, New York
Transvaginal Sonography and Ovarian Cancer

Steven R. Goldstein, MD
Professor of Obstetrics and Gynecology
Department of Obstetrics and Gynecology
Director of Gynecologic Ultrasound
Co-Director of Bone Densitometry
New York University School of Medicine
New York, New York
*Ultrasound in Gynecology: Development and Continuing
   Evolution*
*Menopausal Dilemmas: How Ultrasound Has Changed
   Clinical Management*
Early Pregnancy
Pregnancy Failure
Sonohysterography
Ultrasound-Enhanced Bimanual Examination
Pearls and Pitfalls of Transvaginal Sonography

Lawrence Grunfeld, MD
Associate Clinical Professor
Department of Obstetrics and Gynecology
The Mount Sinai Medical Center
New York, New York
Infertility

Davor Jurkovic, MD, MRCOG
Consultant Gynaecologist
Kings College Hospital
London, England
Congenital Uterine Anomalies

Faye C. Laing, MD
Professor of Radiology
Harvard Medical School
Brigham and Women's Hospital
Boston, Massachusetts
Ectopic Pregnancy

Jodi P. Lerner, MD
Associate Clinical Professor of Obstetrics and Gynecology
Columbia University College of Physicians and Surgeons
Associate Attending
New York Presbyterian Hospital
New York, New York
Ultrasound-Guided Procedures in Gynecology

Ana Monteagudo, MD
Professor of Obstetrics and Gynecology
New York University School of Medicine
Director of Obstetrical and Gynecological Ultrasound
Bellevue Hospital Center
New York, New York
Ultrasound-Guided Procedures in Gynecology
Three-Dimensional Ultrasound in Gynecology
Differential Diagnosis of Inflammatory Diseases of the Pelvis

David B. Peisner, MD
Staff Perinatologist
Atlantic Maternal-Fetal Medicine
Morristown, New Jersey
Applied Physics: Selecting and Adjusting the Equipment
Instrumentation, Modality Selection, and Documentation

Rehan Salim, MD, MRCOG
Research Fellow
Kings College Hospital
London, England
Congenital Uterine Anomalies

Benjamin Sandler, MD
Assistant Clinical Professor
Mount Sinai School of Medicine
Attending Physician
Mount Sinai Hospital
New York, New York
Infertility

Dirk Timmerman, MD
Professor in Obstetrics-Gynaecology
University Hospitals
Leuven, Belgium
Adenomyosis

Ilan E. Timor-Tritsch
Professor of Clinical Obstetrics and Gynecology
Department of Obstetrics and Gynecology
Director of Division of Obstetric/Gynecologic Ultrasound
New York University School of Medicine
New York, New York
Conducting the Gynecologic Ultrasound Examination
Relevant Pelvic Anatomy
Adnexal Masses
Lower Urinary Tract
Early Pregnancy
Color Doppler Mapping in Gynecology
Three-Dimensional Ultrasound in Gynecology
Differential Diagnosis of Inflammatory Diseases of the Pelvis

Foreword

I was flattered and a bit astonished to be asked to write a foreword to the second edition of this marvelous book. The reason for my surprise is that I am a perinatologist and was only reluctantly drawn into gynecologic imaging. On the other hand, it was the editors, Drs. Ilan E. Timor-Tritsch and Steven R. Goldstein, who inspired me to be so drawn. Put simply, they are in love with their subject, and their energy and enthusiasm for gynecologic ultrasound are infectious. Each has a special ability to render the most complex sonographic image sensible and to leave you ready and eager for the next case. In this book, that enthusiasm and clarity of thought are marshaled to inspire the reader to perform gynecologic scans with growing confidence and increasing competence. They have selected outstanding contributors with proven ability to edify and clarify. The chapters build on each other in a logical and almost seamless manner, though each can also stand alone.

Ultrasound in Gynecology, 2nd edition, begins by reminding the reader why it is that gynecologists are uniquely qualified to perform gynecological ultrasound—who else is as well versed in pelvic anatomy and pathology? Chapters 2 and 3 provide a fascinating and practical primer on the physics of gynecologic scanning with excellent trouble-shooting tips. Chapter 4 reviews the basics of gynecologic scanning, and Chapter 5 stands out as a veritable tour de force of pelvic sonographic anatomy. Chapter 6 covers the topic of adenomyosis, which, beyond its importance in the work-up of menorrhagia and pelvic pain, is likely to play an increasingly important role in the next few years as a source of infertility. Chapter 7 covers müllerian duct defects, making good use of 3D imaging techniques. Chapter 8 is a truly outstanding review of the sonographic diagnosis of adnexal pathology, while Chapters 9 and 10 provide practical tips on the use of gynecologic scanning in managing menopause and urinary incontinence, respectively. Chapters 11 through 13 cover early pregnancy, its failure, and the detection of ectopic pregnancies, respectively, and provide many useful clinical pearls for managing patients. Chapter 14 provides tips on the use of ultrasound in the work-up of infertile patients. Chapters 15, 16, 17, and 19 are technically oriented discussions of sonohysterography, ultrasound-guided procedures, color mapping, and 3D imaging, respectively. Chapters 18 and 21 provide useful information on the detection of ovarian cancer and pelvic inflammatory disease, respectively. Chapter 20 describes the adjunctive role of ultrasound used with bimanual examination, and Chapter 22 reveals an array of helpful hints and potential pitfalls to gynecologic scanning.

This marvelous text is a must for all who employ gynecologic ultrasound in their offices. However, it really should be read by every gynecologist, as it provides the reader with an appreciation of the enormous utility of gynecologic ultrasound in improving clinical management.

Charles J. Lockwood, MD
The Anita O'Keefe Young Professor and Chair
Obstetrics, Gynecology, and Reproductive Sciences
Yale University School of Medicine
Chief, Obstetrics and Gynecology
Yale–New Haven Hospital
New Haven, Connecticut

Foreword to the First Edition

I have long been an admirer of Steve Goldstein and Ilan Timor-Tritsch, and therefore I accepted with alacrity when invited to write the foreword to *Ultrasound in Gynecology*. Writing a "forward" seemed apt to me because that is precisely the word I would ascribe to their efforts in teaching and research in sonography. Ilan Timor-Tritsch has been a major investigator in ultrasound from its inception. He has been a leading proponent of new advances in sonography and has led the way in transvaginal sonography. Steven Goldstein has promoted new and unique applications of sonography. He has always advocated that the sonogram be an adjunct to the physical pelvic examination. These two educators have been outstanding in moving the science and practice of sonography forward.

This book deals with gynecologic sonography. It has three chapters covering pregnancy, but it is really devoted to gynecology. A well written and well illustrated book, it is informal in style and draws upon the experience of the authors. They offer opinions and provide practical information in an efficient manner. For example, the book offers two unique appendix sections entitled Trouble-Shooting Guide for Chapter 2 on applied physics and Chapter 3, which covers instrumentation. These guides provide the reader the nuts and bolts of operating the equipment. There is even a chapter devoted to conducting the sonography examination. This text provides the physics, anatomic information, and practical advice to benefit readers of every level. The chapters on adnexal masses, ovarian cancer screening, and color flow Doppler offer practical clinical information for all practitioners. The illustrations are excellent. There are line drawings to complement the sonograms when appropriate.

Today ultrasonography has become an integral part of gynecology. *Ultrasound in Gynecology* is an excellent source of practical information on ultrasonography as it pertains to gynecology. It provides a reference source, a "how to" manual, practice guidelines, and a look to the future, all in one volume.

John T. Queenan, MD
Chairman
Department of Obstetrics and Gynecology
Georgetown University Medical Center
Washington, DC

Preface

We were among the first to advocate strongly for the widespread—in fact, routine—use of transvaginal ultrasound for gynecologic patients. We believe it can, and should, be part of the overall gynecologic examination. Ilan said in 1987, "The transvaginal probe will be as common as the speculum itself." In those early days we were on the fringe of a new movement. Since that time, all bimanual examinations in our private practices have been ultrasound enhanced, and all attendings in the Faculty Practice Suites at New York University Medical Center have access to transvaginal ultrasound in an exam-room setting so that they can perform an ultrasound evaluation *themselves* at the time of the examination. These physicians make liberal use of consultative ultrasound when the physical findings are not totally clear. Our residents have vaginal probe ultrasound in the clinic, in the emergency room, in the operating room, and, of course, on labor and delivery. As we predicted, there is now quality equipment that is to the traditional ultrasound machine what the laptop (or maybe even the PDA) is to a desktop computer.

The field of gynecologic ultrasound has it own learning curve, just as individuals have a learning curve. The first edition of *Ultrasound in Gynecology* attempted to bring state-of-the-art gynecologic ultrasound knowledge to practicing clinicians, imagers, or sonographers. However, the fast pace of advancement in sonography in general and in Ob/Gyn sonography in particular made the first edition of this book outdated in many aspects and incomplete in others. We knew that it was time to incorporate our new experiences and knowledge in an updated second edition. However, we had wondered whether in the cyber age, when information is exchanged in electronic form and when articles and books are available at the click of the computer mouse, there was a need for another book. At conferences, meetings, and courses we were increasingly asked if and when we would offer the second edition of our book. This encouraged our own view that a printed text with representative images of gynecologic pathology is still not totally obsolete. Our text is, as far as we know, the only available comprehensive text dedicated to gynecologic ultrasound. So we went to work and expanded the existing text, updating it with new images obtained with the newest high-resolution ultrasound machines. Our chief concerns continue to be early pregnancy (the bridge between obstetrics and gynecology), menopause, ovarian masses, sonohysterography, invasive puncture procedures, and descriptions of normal anatomy, with an emphasis on correlating physiologic changes with the images obtained. In this second edition we add the concept of "color as morphology"; the refinement of saline infusion sonohysterography; the uniqueness of tamoxifen; newer delineation of tubal disease, adenomyosis, ectopic pregnancy, and uterine malformations; and ovarian cancer screening. As residents of a three-dimensional world, imaging specialists and practitioners are increasingly preferring to view the pelvic organs in three dimensions. Hence, we included a detailed chapter dealing with the constantly and rapidly increasing use of three-dimensional ultrasound in gynecology.

Gynecologic ultrasound cannot be separated from gynecology. It is an integral part of day-to-day, hour-to-hour gynecologic patient care. Gynecology has been and continues to be transformed by transvaginal ultrasound. This new edition brings that transformation up-to-date.

Steven R. Goldstein, MD
Ilan E. Timor-Tritsch, MD

Preface to the First Edition

The practice of gynecology today is very different from that of previous decades. There is an increasing trend toward less surgery in general and more minimally invasive procedures, which are more beneficial to the patient and more cost-effective for the hospital. We now have more medical management of disease. A large portion of the change in gynecology is due to the introduction and better understanding of gynecologic ultrasound.

The task of the modern gynecologist is to accurately characterize the postmenopausal adnexa and the endometrial findings. Endometriomas have to be reliably distinguished from hemorrhagic corpora lutea or from possible neoplasia. The number of diagnostic curettages and invasive endometrial procedures can be diminished by using transvaginal ultrasound and, more recently, fluid-enhanced sonohysterography. Pregnancy has to be diagnosed early and followed more consistently than was previously thought necessary. If pregnancy failure ensues, this can be anticipated before spontaneous passage. The diagnosis of ectopic pregnancy is expected to return to the gynecologist's hands by enabling its reliable diagnosis in the office when the patient presents. The practice of infertility treatment has changed remarkably as a result of using ultrasound images created in the office. An increasing number of ultrasound-guided puncture procedures can be used to avoid more complicated and cumbersome surgical procedures. Using ultrasound in the emergency room or as part of an overall bimanual examination not only allows an assessment of objective anatomic information, but also allows the gynecologist to correlate between ovarian function (or lack thereof) and the endometrial response.

When we stop to reflect on the path that ultrasound has followed in gynecology, we realize that the vaginal probe, and the detail it affords, has not only created many new applications but also enabled their efficient use in the field of gynecology.

Ultrasound has enabled a vast amount of new gynecologic data in the form of journal articles or presentations at national and international meetings. This has created the need for a comprehensive text dealing with this subject, and a book, such as this one, has naturally evolved. One trip to the medical bookstore reveals many volumes on obstetrical ultrasound and others that deal with ultrasound in obstetrics and gynecology, but invariably these are almost entirely obstetrics. There has been no dedicated text that embraces the subject of ultrasonography in gynecology alone until now.

Clearly the practice of gynecology is being continuously transformed, and the role of ultrasound in this transformation is immense. We chronicle it in the chapters that follow.

Steven R. Goldstein, MD
Illan E. Timor-Tritsch, MD

Acknowledgments

Time flies! It seems only last year that I expressed my thanks to persons without whom a text like this could not have been possible. First and foremost, my gratitude goes out to the more than 240,000 patients scanned at Bellevue Hospital Center and at Tisch Hospital in the 11 years since the first edition of our book was published. They are our real teachers, continuously enriching our knowledge. The editors and our contributing authors take that knowledge and experience and bring it to our readers, who in turn apply the teaching to their practice. In this way the practitioners can "pay back" the patients who provided us with our knowledge by healing them faster and better.

I have to thank our contributors, who took the time to share their knowledge and expertise and updated their own chapters or wrote new ones. Thanks also to our sonographers, who provided the "material" base of this book: Ellena Avizova, Ran Dong, Wendy Hua Huang Feng, Tova Eisenberger, Irina Labovskaya, Susan Monda, Ana Pastor, Grace Pineda, Rosalba Santos, Irina Strok, and Tatiana Tsymbal.

Special thanks to Steve Goldstein, who is always there for me, providing input, help, encouragement, and superb clinical correlations to our ultrasound observations. I could not imagine this book's being edited without his enormous cooperation. Thanks also goes to Ana Monteagudo, a maternal-fetal medicine specialist who became a seasoned gynecologic imaging specialist and not only contributed countless cases for my chapters, but also carried the clinical burden of covering our ultrasound units when I needed it.

All chapters of the book were typed, arranged, and corrected by my office manager, Christonia Joseph. Her help was invaluable.

The editorial office of Elsevier deserves praise because the cooperation, copy editing, and artwork processing was professional, effective, and always friendly.

Ilan E. Timor-Tritsch, MD

My favorite part of writing a book is writing the acknowledgments. This is my chance to reflect on the people I want to thank for enabling me to have performed this time-consuming but also rewarding task. I first want to thank anyone (and there have been quite a few) who has come up to me at a conference, or after a lecture, or at Grand Rounds and thanked me for what I have said, written, or taught. The appreciation shown to me by so many practitioners for the clinical observations that I have made and espoused never ceases to astonish me. You have no idea how much this means and how it further energizes and galvanizes me. I want to thank (posthumously) Gordon W. Douglas, MD, whose initial skepticism in my academic commitment caused me to become an overachiever in order to prove him wrong; Robert F. Porges, MD, and Charles J. Lockwood, MD, past chairmen at New York University School of Medicine and now friends who let me ride the wave; John P. Curtin, MD, my current chairman, who has stepped up to the plate and allowed me to continue my efforts; Victor Douek, MD, Andy Gardner, MD, and especially Gary Mucciolo, MD, whose clinical coverage is so crucial to my academic success; Jon R. Snyder, MD, and Lila Nachtigal, MD, for just being there, always; Bruce K. Young, MD, for continued mentorship and counsel; my staff, Christine Sweeney, Lily Gjidija, Ivanka Zajac, and Jennifer Friele, for always pointing me in the right direction; and Penny Franco, my assistant, for putting up and keeping up with me. I want to thank Ilan Timor-Tritsch and Ana Monteagudo, whose presence at New York University these last 6 years has been a wonderful boost to me and my beloved institution. Their commitment and enthusiasm for ultrasound as well as their friendship have kept me going. I want to thank my brother, Howard S. Goldstein, MD, who has always been so supportive and taught me most of what I learned growing up; my children, Phoebe and Luke, who teach me more about myself every day; but mostly I want to acknowledge my wife, Kathy Clement Dillon Goldstein, because it was not until I married her that I settled down and had the presence of mind to accomplish all the things that I have.

To all of you who have done so much for me, I thank you.

Steven R. Goldstein, MD

Contents

Development of Ultrasound

Chapter 1

Ultrasound in Gynecology: Development and Continuing Evolution

Steven R. Goldstein

Earlier linear array ultrasound equipment was adequate for measuring biparietal diameter (BPD), placental localization, and presentation. As equipment and its resolution have improved, the amount and quality of information have virtually exploded. More scans are performed. Virtually every postgraduate ultrasound course has a talk or a panel discussion concerning whether the time for routine obstetric scanning has arrived. The National Institutes of Health (NIH) consensus panel in 1984 thought that there was not enough information available to recommend routine ultrasound screening. More recently, studies by Eik-Nes et al.[1] and the Helsinki Ultrasound Trial[2] indicated that routine obstetric screening may indeed be of benefit. The RADIUS (Routine Antenatal Diagnostic Imaging with Ultrasound) study[3] in the United States generated much controversy over this issue.

Changing Expectations

In the early developmental stages of obstetric ultrasound, limited information was relatively easily obtained, and expectations were correspondingly modest. As instrumentation became increasingly sophisticated, those clinicians whose equipment, talent, and commitment did not evolve hid behind the excuse of the level I/level II differentiation (i.e., "we don't do level II here").[4] Recognizing this problem, the American College of Radiology, the American Institute of Ultrasound in Medicine (AIUM),[5] and the American College of Obstetricians and Gynecologists (ACOG)[6] adopted guidelines for a "standard obstetric ultrasound examination" that set the standard for all obstetric ultrasound examinations. Later, the guidelines for the standard obstetric examination were updated and revised to include even more information (e.g., four-chamber view of the heart outflow tracts, all extremities).[7,8] *Consultative* examinations for difficult cases—to identify the particular abnormality—are sought based on the ability of the examiner to recognize the *normal* and thus to realize that what he or she is seeing is deviating from normal.

It is a curious paradox that the use of ultrasound by obstetrician-gynecologists evolved in the way that it did, with their assumption of responsibility for imaging the complex anatomy of the fetus but not of the pelvis itself. Early real-time equipment allowed very crude assessment of very limited information. A typical early study consisted of little more than BPD, placental localization, and fetal presentation. It was not very difficult to perform. Hundreds of physicians and many office assistants, nurses, secretaries, and others took short courses and began to "scan." Thus, in those days, performing the mid-trimester obstetric ultrasound examination seemed appropriate for the obstetric clinician—after all, the fetus was the patient. Gynecologic scanning of the pelvis, however, initially with static arms and then with real-time sector scans, was more complex. Such cases were generally reserved for the hospital-based ultrasound laboratory or the radiologist's office. Hence, a "rule-out ectopic" scan was routinely sent to a radiologist.

At an ultrasound postgraduate course, I heard a prominent radiologist lecture on hydrocephalus in utero. In the course of his talk, he commented, "In our residencies we are taught that ventriculomegaly begins in the occipital horn." That comment struck a nerve. Obstetrician-gynecologists do not do a 4- to 6-month rotation in neuroradiology in their residency, nor are they trained in neuroanatomy or cardiac anatomy. The assumption that they should be the ones to do cross-sectional anatomic images of a multitude of organ systems is not reasonable merely because the subject is a fetus; rather, it is simply the way clinical practice evolved.

While obstetrician-gynecologists receive no specialized training in neuroanatomy and cardiology, they do spend several months studying gynecologic pathology, cutting open uteri and ovarian tumors and examining virtually every type of pathologic process found in the pelvis. In practice, obstetrician-gynecologists examine the pelvis daily and operate in the pelvis. It is therefore reasonable that they should perform imaging in the pelvis.

Pressures on the Clinician

It is this very paradox that places real pressures on the clinician who has not been warned of or prepared for the explosion in ultrasound capability. This pressure comes from increased sophistication of equipment and results in increased time required to do a good job, increased patient expectations, and increased liability.

Clinicians accustomed to performing obstetric scans as part of their practice have come to anticipate the revenue that scanning brings. The clinician who feels uncomfortable with the expanded expectations of the guidelines also feels the financial pressure that results from giving up performing obstetric ultrasound. In addition, there is the pressure of patient expectations—consider the patient who in her past pregnancies had an ultrasound performed by the clinician or staff in the office. How does the clinician now explain why he or she no longer performs obstetric ultrasound?

The point is not that primary obstetric clinicians should not be performing obstetric ultrasound, but rather that if they do, they must upgrade their skills, their knowledge, and their equipment—in other words, their commitment. This means following the spirit and the letter of the guidelines (and now the expanded guidelines). Persons performing obstetric ultrasound should be comfortable with a four-chamber view of the heart; understand more intracranial anatomy than simply a midline echo; and be able to find the cord insertion at both ends. Clinicians who are unwilling to make this commitment no longer belong in the business of performing obstetric ultrasound.

The Role of the Sonographer

Many clinicians, owing to lack of training, interest, or commitment, have hired others (previously called *technicians*, better referred to as *sonographers*) to perform ultrasound studies. Initially, many of these persons were nurses, office managers, or secretaries who took short courses at universities in preparation for performing obstetric ultrasound. However, a growing number of obstetric sonographers are receiving high-quality training (some through accredited schools or, increasingly, through on-the-job training in major university ultrasound laboratories), as evidenced by the ever-increasing number of registered diagnostic medical sonographers (RDMSs), now greater than 45,000 since the inception of the American Registry of Diagnostic Medical Sonographers in 1975. These individuals have met eligibility requirements and passed a rigorous test in obstetric-gynecologic ultrasound as well as ultrasound physics that certifies a standard of competency. Often they are employed by physicians who know little about obstetric ultrasound themselves but merely sign off on the study performed by the sonographer. Although RDMSs are competent and are preferable to sonographers who have not passed the registry examination, they are only one part of the team of health care professionals meant to work with trained physicians, and should not replace them.

The Physician as Sonologist

Once skills such as fetal monitoring and laparoscopy have been incorporated into residency training, all graduating residents will become part of the solution rather than part of the problem. For physicians already in practice, postgraduate courses will have to fill the training need. Such courses are offered by organizations such as ACOG and AIUM and various universities and institutions. Each physician will learn sonography at his or her own pace; during that learning curve, the patient may still be triaged according to the physician's method of practice. Once the physician becomes comfortable with the information derived from the vaginal probe examination, he or she can begin to bring it into the overall clinical management. In 1996, the AIUM established the voluntary accreditation of ultrasound practices in the United States and Canada.[9] Accreditation by the AIUM is provided for practices rather than individuals. Ultrasound practices seeking AIUM accreditation must show evidence of the physician's training in sonography, credentialing of sonographers performing ultrasound examinations, continuing medical education (CME) for physicians and sonographers, and the presence of protocols and procedures to ensure proper and safe practice of sonography. Practices also submit four case studies for each specified area of accreditation (Obstetrics, Gynecology, or both). These case studies are evaluated by independent reviewers according to established criteria that conform to the minimum standards and guidelines for ultrasound practices as developed by the AIUM.[10,11] Currently over 1000 practices have achieved ultrasound accreditation. Accreditation is offered for 3 years, after which practices must apply for reaccreditation.

Practices that had received ultrasound accreditation were studied and found able to improve the scores of their case studies and to improve their compliance with published minimum standards and guidelines for the performance of obstetric and gynecologic ultrasound examinations when reevaluated 3 years after the initial applications.[12] This improvement should translate into enhanced quality of ultrasound practice.

Admittedly, the equipment will add cost for the practitioner, although as the technology has become more refined, dedicated examination room devices have become available at markedly decreased prices that may soon make a machine in every examination room a reality. However, obstetrician-gynecologists cannot routinely examine all patients with sonography and yet charge them at the rate the system now allows. Ideally, the global fee will be raised enough to reflect the true cost of administering such an ultrasound-enhanced bimanual examination.

New Technologies

The Doppler principle allows quantitative assessment of resistance to blood flow. Color flow mapping provides a rapid, easy method of determining where to place the Doppler gate to perform such spectral analysis. Color power Doppler has the additional advantage of being nondirectional. Whereas the exact role of resistance to blood flow in gynecology remains unestablished, the presence or absence of blood flow, something I refer to as "color as morphology," can often add valuable information to constructing a differential diagnosis. Blood vessels, especially dilated veins, often appear cystic on two-dimensional, gray-scale sonography. The presence of flow can usually distinguish cystic structures from vascular structures. In addition, old blood, such as in an endometrioma, would not be expected to yield any flow and can help corroborate a diagnosis suspected morphologically.

Three-dimensional (3D) scanning also has the ability to revolutionize sonography. Although examiners currently re-create 3D anatomy in their mind's eye, the ability to construct the "z plane" has important ramifications, especially in the area of uterine malfunctions, where 3D scanning can show the serosal and endometrial surfaces simultaneously, as if one were doing laparoscopy and hysteroscopy at the same time. Perhaps more important, 3D technology may affect the manner in which scanning is performed. All the information may be obtained in a matter of moments. The reconstruction and interpretation can then be performed off-line without the need for the patient to be present. This may have ramifications for the role of the sonographer, especially as image acquisition becomes more and more like the "auto-focus" capability found in 35-mm and digital cameras. Furthermore, having all of the information stored after acquisition allows for easy digital transmission for referral and consultation. In the future, the entire process of image acquisition and interpretation may be very different from what we do today.

Conclusion

The use of pelvic imaging with vaginal ultrasound by the office practitioner offers tremendous assets. Often, diagnoses can be made on the spot, allowing more timely therapy or, in the case of normal findings, relieving patient anxieties. It saves time for both the physician and the patient. In the past, with transabdominal scanning, patients often had to be rescheduled because time constraints would not permit waiting for the bladder to fill. Vaginal scanning in the office has reduced the need to refer patients elsewhere (except for consultation), which in turn reduces the errors that inevitably accompany the transmission of information from one source to another. Patients uniformly prefer vaginal scanning over the discomfort of a full-bladder transabdominal approach. Patients also can better understand their care; the pictures generated on the screen are very helpful in communicating the pathologic process to the patient.

Gynecologic scanning with the vaginal probe should not be reserved solely for the imaging specialist. It allows for instant confirmation of the primary obstetrician-gynecologist's findings at the time of the pelvic examination.

REFERENCES

1. Eik-Nes SH, Okland O, Aure JC, Ulstein M: Ultrasound screening in pregnancy: A randomised controlled trial. Lancet 1988;2:585-588.
2. Saari-Kemppainen A, Karjalainen O, Ylostalo P, Heinonen O: Ultrasound screening and perinatal mortality: Controlled trial of systematic one-stage screening in pregnancy. The Helsinki Ultrasound Trial. Lancet 1990;336:387-391.
3. LeFevre ML, Bain RP, Ewigman BG, et al: A randomized trial of prenatal ultrasonographic screening: Impact on maternal management and outcome. RADIUS (Routine Antenatal Diagnostic Imaging with Ultrasound) Study Group. Am J Obstet Gynecol 1993;169:483-489.
4. Filly RA: Level 1, level 2, level 3 obstetric sonography: I'll see your level and raise you one. Radiology 1989;172:312.
5. American Institute of Ultrasound in Medicine: Official Guidelines and Statements on Obstetrical Ultrasound. Rockville, Md, American Institute of Ultrasound in Medicine, 1985, p 1.
6. American College of Obstetricians and Gynecologists: Ultrasound in Pregnancy Technical Bulletin 116. Washington, DC, American College of Obstetricians and Gynecologists, 1986.
7. American Institute of Ultrasound in Medicine: Standards and Guidelines for Performance of Antepartum Obstetrical Examination. Rockville, Md, American Institute of Ultrasound in Medicine, 1990.
8. American Institute of Ultrasound in Medicine: Standards and Guidelines for Performance of the Antepartum Obstetrical Examination, 2nd ed. Rockville, Md, American Institute of Ultrasound in Medicine, 1994.
9. Arger PH: Letter from the president: Update on the Ultrasound Practice Accreditation Commission. AIUMs Reporter 1996;12:1.
10. American Institute of Ultrasound in Medicine: AIUM Practice Guidelines for the Performance of an Antepartum Obstetric Ultrasound Examination. Laurel, Md, American Institute of Ultrasound in Medicine, 2003. Available at www.aium.org/provider/standards/obstetrical.pdf.
11. American Institute of Ultrasound in Medicine: Guidelines for Performance of the Ultrasound Examination of the Female Pelvis. Laurel, Md, American Institute of Ultrasound in Medicine, 1995. Available at www.aium.org/provider/standards/pelvis.pdf.
12. Abuhamad AZ, Benacerraf BR, Woletz P, Burke BL: The accreditation of ultrasound practices: Impact on compliance with minimum performance guidelines. J Ultrasound Med 2004;23:1023-1029.

SECTION II

Scanning Techniques and Instrumentation

After more than 30 years of using transabdominal sonography and nearly 20 years of using transvaginal sonography, several points regarding gynecologic ultrasound scanning are evident.

The first point is that although transabdominal scanning of the female pelvis was an important step in differentiating a normal from an abnormal pelvic finding, transvaginal sonography has the unique ability to refine the diagnosis.

The second point is that because of the clarity and resolution of transvaginal sonography images, ultrasound findings have a greater immediate impact on practicing obstetricians and gynecologists in the office to clarify the diagnosis while they examine the patient. Improved imaging also enables the specialized ultrasound laboratories to refine their diagnostic abilities and apply more sophisticated modalities, such as color and power Doppler flow studies and specific real-time ultrasound-guided puncture procedures. More recently, the introduction of three-dimensional gray-scale and color Doppler applications for transvaginal probes has further enhanced the diagnostic as well as therapeutic capabilities of gynecologic ultrasound.

Finally, it is clear that sonography of the female reproductive organs shows promise in screening for ovarian cancer. Screening for ovarian cancer is now the most important goal in this field, and the process is still in the research stages. There is little doubt, however, that in the future we will determine how best to use this diagnostic modality to screen, first, high-risk, and later perhaps low-risk populations for ovarian cancer.

Chapter 2

Applied Physics: Selecting and Adjusting the Equipment

David B. Peisner

Ultrasound machines are better than ever before. As with point-and-shoot cameras, the operator does not have to be a physicist to obtain good images with today's machines. However, some patients have unusual findings or are difficult to study. In these cases, the automatic features of an ultrasound machine may not present the sonographer with a diagnostic-quality image. For the same reason that a sunset picture is almost impossible to take with an automatic camera, a deep cystic structure with irregular walls in an obese patient will not image well on automatic settings.

To obtain a good image, the operator has to know how to use *all* of the settings of an ultrasound machine, and there are many concepts that form the basis for adjusting the various settings. While this chapter uses the theories of physics to explain concepts, the bulk of the chapter consists of hints and rationales for adjusting the machine controls to produce and improve images.

A good image, a clear M-mode graph, or a good Doppler tracing can make patient diagnosis and management easy. To supplement the text, this chapter includes a trouble-shooting guide for fixing poorly displayed images.

Important Choices in Obtaining a Good Image

When a scan is performed, the sonographer usually selects various options and then adjusts the controls to optimize the image. This assumes that the machine and image recording equipment have already been properly adjusted (discussed in Chapter 3). Although many machine functions are automated, the selections and adjustments discussed in this chapter are important because they can transform a mediocre image into a spectacular image.

The actual image is produced by bouncing sound waves at high frequencies (2 to 9 MHz or 2,000,000 to 9,000,000 cycles/second). The sound waves are transmitted by crystals in the probe that are electrically stimulated. The sound information bounces off the organs and other tissue, and the returning waves are detected by the crystals in the probe. Because the strength of the echoes from body structures varies with the density of those structures, the ultrasound machine can translate the returning sound energy into a visual representation of the organs and tissue.

Many factors can influence image quality. Basically, the detail of the image improves with higher-frequency sound waves with short pulse lengths and narrowly focused beams. The image also improves with varying methods of image processing. This is the physics of sonography. The following sections discuss the clinical application of this physics in producing a good image.

Selecting the Appropriate Equipment

Ultrasound Machine

Today, there is little physics involved in choosing an ultrasound machine. Most machines are versatile, offering a variety of probe and imaging options. However, older machines may be more limited. An examination may be more appropriate on one machine than on another. One machine may produce excellent pictures for abdominal scans and poor pictures in the transvaginal mode, and vice versa. This may be influenced by the type of probe, transducer architecture (the size of the probe, the shape of the imaging surface, and the shape of the crystals within the probe), pulse length, penetrating ability, image processing, display quality, and many other factors. One machine may produce a better image of a structure of interest than another machine. As an example, some older machines had huge probes that could scan a large part of the body at once. If there is a large tumor that needs to be visualized all at once, the older machine would make the best choice.

Summary. An ultrasound machine (unless it is one of the versatile—and more expensive—machines) should be chosen based on its ability to see a certain structure as well as resolve images (length of pulse, frequency, transducer architecture, number of crystals, ability to focus the beam) and based on its penetrating power. If the image quality cannot be improved because of machine limitations, another machine should be considered.

Probe

The physics of probe selection pertains to choosing a modality (mechanical or electronic), the type of image (linear, curvilinear, or sector), the physical style of the probe, and the frequency.

Modality

A mechanical probe has the advantage of producing a refined ultrasound beam with minimal side lobe distortion (artifacts). Many mechanical probes also have a feature that allows the image sector to be shifted off axis, thus allowing the probe literally to peer around a corner (e.g., under the symphysis pubis or out into the lateral adnexum). However, these probes usually have a fixed focus and limited M-mode and Doppler capabilities, *and* they require increased maintenance to maintain correct fluid levels.

Virtually all probes are now electronic; electronic processing has evolved to overcome side lobe distortion, and improved probe crystal development has allowed smaller and more versatile transducers. The electronic probes also avoid the maintenance problems of maintaining fluid levels in mechanical probes.

> **Physics.** The probes contain fluid because ultrasound waves do not travel through air more than a few millimeters without losing energy.

Type of Image

The image type of most probes today is curvilinear as opposed to linear or sector. The reason involves physics and electronics. Whereas a linear probe is simple because all of the ultrasound transducers (crystals) are lined up to send and receive their pulses one by one in a row, the probe is large. On the other hand, an electronic sector probe is complicated because it consists of a crystal array that is tightly packed, and it is more difficult to manufacture.

> **Physics.** The electronic sector probe sends and receives pulses at varying angles by exciting the transducers somewhat out of sequence. This is called a *phased array*. The resulting beam travels into the tissue at an angle rather than straight from the transducer. This is electronically more complicated and also may produce artifacts known as *side lobes*.

The compromise solution is the curvilinear probe, which is basically a linear array with a curved shape to produce an image showing a lot of tissue with a probe that is not too large or complicated.

Probe Style

Obviously, the style of the probe will depend on the type of image needed, and for external transducers the choice may be subjective. However, virtually all transvaginal probes by necessity are sector probes (either mechanical or phased arrays) or tight curvilinear arrays. The mechanical probe is advantageous because the sector can be steered off the axis of the probe to explore the sides of the pelvis with virtually no change in image quality. Because of side lobe distortion artifact, electronic probes cannot do this easily. Some companies have addressed this problem by designing probes that are bent and direct their sector off the axis of the probe. However, this may require the sonographer to twist the probe to see the other side of the pelvis. This feature—the shape of the probe—then becomes a personal preference of the sonographer. Some do not mind the twisting, but others (including my department) prefer the end-firing probes because it is easier to orient the images and requires less manipulation of the probe to scan the entire pelvis.

Frequency

Finally, a higher-frequency probe will produce a more detailed image, but the depth of penetration is less.

> **Physics.** High-frequency waves on a lake caused by a small stone dropped into it do not travel far. However, a large water displacement with low frequency, such as that caused by an undersea earthquake, can cause the wave to travel for thousands of miles. Because it is usually necessary only to see organs that are located a few centimeters from the probe, a higher frequency is usually appropriate.

A probe should be selected that has the highest frequency that can penetrate the depth to be studied. Because some probes work at multiple frequencies, the sonographer may need fewer probes. However, the choice of a probe should not be compromised. The wrong-frequency probe may produce images that are not of diagnostic quality.

Summary. Electronic curvilinear probes have the most versatility, and their frequency should be chosen to produce the best image of the structure to be examined. The physical shape of the probe is mostly a matter of personal preference.

Selecting Ultrasound Machine Settings

Depth of the Scan

Some physics is involved in selecting the depth of scan. Obviously, the depth must be chosen to include the organs being studied. However, less depth on the screen makes the interesting part of the image larger. For the same reason, zooming (see under Optimizing the Image of the Structures Being Studied, later) is used to increase the size of the structure of interest, if possible. Both depth selection and zooming improve the visualization of this structure.

> **Physics.** Internally, the machine has only a certain number of pixels, the spots that make up a picture, to create an image. When the image is small, fewer pixels are used. If a small image is enlarged with the zoom feature, a small number of pixels may make the image look grainy and some image detail may be lost. However, if the depth of the scan is decreased, the structure of interest will be larger on the screen and will use more pixels internally in the machine. If the image is enlarged in this way, more detail may be visible. It is only when the limits of resolution based on ultrasound frequency and focus limitations are reached that image quality will not improve with increased screen size, regardless of the method used to enlarge it.

Summary. The structure of interest should be imaged at as shallow a depth as possible, until image quality stops improving because of physical limitations.

Power Level (If Possible)

It is important to understand the difference between power level and gain. *Power level* refers to the amount of energy produced by the transducer. *Gain* refers to the amount of amplification of the returning sound waves. If it is possible to control the power output (not available on all machines), the quality of the image can be adjusted. Intuitively, it might seem that more power is better, and in fact more power may be necessary when very deep structures are imaged in an obese patient. However, increasing the power may produce artifacts.

Physics. Increased power may transmit enough energy to cause some tissue interfaces to produce secondary vibrations. This causes an artifact known as *ring-down*. When a cyst is visualized at high power, the edge of the cyst nearest the transducer may appear blurry as the fluid–solid interface vibrates (see Fig. 2A–20). Also, higher power levels may cause some of the sound energy to bounce back and forth within a cyst, resulting in another artifact known as *reverberation*. Familiar examples of excessive power artifacts from nonsonographic contexts include increasing the volume of a stereo system beyond the speakers' rating, resulting in distorted sound; taking a photograph in light that is too bright, resulting in a washed-out image on the film; and turning the brightness setting on a television screen too high, causing bright objects to appear to "bloom" or expand.

If the power is too low, the image on the screen may be faint or contain additional noise artifacts that resemble snow.

Physics. Less power means a weaker returning signal. A weak signal will be mixed with the electronic noise inherent in any equipment, and the result is a degraded image or "snow." The situation is analogous to trying to receive a weak station on a television: the brightness can be turned up, but the picture will still contain snow. To get a better picture, the transmitter power needs to be increased.

The same holds true for an ultrasound image. If the power output is too low, the gain and other controls can be adjusted but the image will still have lots of graininess (snow).

Summary. Use enough power to avoid an image with "snow." Avoid using too much power, which might cause artifacts.

Frequency (If Possible)

Frequency was briefly discussed in the probe section. If frequency can be chosen independently on the machine being used, two facts are important: higher frequency improves image detail, and high-frequency beams do not penetrate into the body well. Therefore, the sonographer should use the highest frequency possible that penetrates to the structure he or she wishes to image.

Physics. Because sound travels at a relatively constant speed in tissue, higher-frequency waves have a shorter distance between each sound wave. The shorter the wavelength, the smaller the structure that can be visualized. Because the amount of detail that can be seen relates to the wavelength, smaller objects can be seen more clearly with higher-frequency sound waves. However, higher-frequency waves do not penetrate as well as lower-frequency waves because the intervening tissue takes a greater percentage of the energy out of the signal for each centimeter of penetration. Although analogies from other physical systems to help understand these facts are a little more difficult to grasp, one of the easiest to understand is a visual comparison between the appearance of a specimen under an electron microscope and a light microscope. Much more detail of the specimen is seen using electron microscopy because the frequency of the imaging waves is higher. With higher frequency, the "ons" and "offs" (i.e., the details of the

image) happen more quickly (or in the visual case, are closer together), and thus the image, whether visual or sonic, has more detail. Detail also relates to penetration. If higher-frequency waves pass through something with detail (closely spaced features), these detailed structures will interfere with the waves and decrease them, while lower-frequency waves will pass. The easiest way to understand this is through a sonic example. When you listen to music, the sound is good if there are no intervening structures. If there is a wall (with closely spaced objects such as wood fibers or plaster) in the way, the sound will be muffled because only the low-frequency sounds will get through. High-frequency sounds do not penetrate as well.

Harmonic Imaging (If Possible)

Harmonic imaging is an application of changing the frequency. However, in some machines, it is possible to use several frequencies at once to visualize a structure. When an ultrasound beam is transmitted, the reflections contain more than a single frequency. Analyzing only one frequency (which is the way most machines work) provides a satisfactory image. However, the image quality improves if more frequencies are analyzed. The trade-off is in processing speed. If multiple frequencies are analyzed and processed for the same image, it will take longer to form the image than if a single frequency was used. The benefit is a sharper image. Thus, if more detail is required and other settings are not successful in achieving satisfactory resolution, harmonic imaging can be used.

Physics. The best way to understand harmonic imaging is once again through a combination of sonic and visual phenomena. The creation of additional frequencies from an ultrasound beam is analogous to striking a bell. A metal bell can be struck with a single blow (frequency), but it will vibrate at several frequencies: the dominant frequency, which is the musical note you hear, and other frequencies at lower volume, which give the bell its character. In this way, a single structure can create multiple frequencies. To understand how this phenomenon can improve an image, consider a visual scene. If you look at the scene through a red filter, you will visualize the scene at a single frequency. However, some portions of the scene will not have as much detail because of the lack of visual information from the other frequencies (e.g., blue, green). However, if you analyze all frequencies (i.e., colors) from the visual scene, the image will appear sharper.

Selecting the Image
Overall Gain

To produce a satisfactory image, the machine controls must be adjusted properly. The concept of gain was introduced earlier, under Power Level. In this case, the adjustment controls the amount of amplification of the returning signal from the tissue. The primary rationale behind gain adjustment is mostly practical; gain is basically an overall brightness control. However, there are interactions between some controls of the machine, and it is important to understand the purpose of each control and its underlying physics. The most obvious set of controls that interact with the gain control is the time–gain adjustments. Because of limitations in the display screen as well as the human eye, there are both upper and lower limits to how bright an image can be. This is a physics concept. The practical consequence is that the gain control must be adjusted to produce a good image. When it is set properly, the rest of the controls can be easily adjusted. However, if it is not set properly, other controls may not work properly. For example, if the gain control is too low, the sonographer may not be able to use the time–gain controls to improve visualization of some parts of the image.

Therefore, for best results, the time–gain controls and any other fine-tuning controls should be set to their middle range and the gain adjusted first. With the gain optimally adjusted, there is plenty of range of adjustment for the other controls. Note that the monitor (cathode ray screen or flat panel [e.g., liquid crystal] display) must be properly adjusted *before* any machine controls are adjusted (see Chapter 3). If the monitor is not set properly, an image may appear adequate on the screen but will not be stored properly, and future retrieval of that image will be flawed.

Summary. Adjust the overall gain for a reasonable image first and adjust the finer aspects of the image later.

Dynamic Range

Different structures are best seen using different settings of the ultrasound machine. Dynamic range is one of the best examples of this. Cystic structures with smooth walls are best imaged with low dynamic range, and solid tumors require high dynamic range.

> **Physics.** The important part of a cystic structure is the interface between solid and liquid, which is best visualized on a high-contrast image. This means the fewer the gray levels, the better, and the corresponding translation for dynamic range is "less." However, subtle tissue differences are important if a solid tumor is being imaged. More gray levels are necessary to show this, and the corresponding translation for dynamic range is "more." The best analogy to the dynamic range is a comparison between a photocopy machine and a camera. The photocopy machine copies only black or white—nothing between—with low dynamic range and sharp edges. However, a camera with black-and-white film will record various shades of gray, providing more dynamic range, and subtle differences in the texture of a structure can be seen.

If fetal cardiac chambers are being studied, it is important to see the edge of the chambers—gray zones are less important, whereas sharp edges (black and white) are desirable. Therefore, less dynamic range is useful for studying these structures. However, if tissue characterization is important, such as with a solid ovarian mass, then many shades of gray (increased dynamic range) will improve the detail of the image. This means that the dynamic range must be increased. In simple terms, dynamic range represents the range of shades of gray that are displayed.

Summary. Less dynamic range for cystic structures and greater dynamic range for solid objects should be chosen.

Time–Gain Curve

The time–gain curve is so named because of the physics behind the reception of ultrasound signals. However, the important point to grasp about these controls is that they are essentially fine gain controls for portions of the image—generally horizontal strips of the picture. Just as a graphic equalizer controls the volume (or gain) of only a portion of the sound coming from a stereo system, the time–gain controls control the brightness (or gain) of only a portion of the picture. Once the overall gain is set (see under Overall Gain,

earlier), these controls permit fine-tuning of the picture's brightness.

> **Physics.** When the ultrasound beam is transmitted into tissue, it takes longer for the sound energy to return from deeper structures. In view of this, the machine can increase or decrease the brightness of the picture from selected depths by merely applying the selected setting on the time–gain curve to the ultrasound energy that returns at a specific time after it was transmitted.

Time–gain curves are necessary because the ultrasound machine does not know anything about the tissue that is being imaged. If there are many cystic structures close to the transducer, the ultrasound beams will pass through them easily and will have more power as they bounce off the deeper structures. Returning to the transducer, these more powerful beams will create a structure that appears to be brighter than expected. The time–gain adjustments can selectively correct this problem.

Summary. The time–gain curve adjustments are used to selectively correct bands of brightness or darkness on the image.

Focal Zone

If the focal zone is not near the structure of interest, the image may be blurry.

> **Physics.** Waves, both sound and light, spread out as they travel. To obtain a good image, the waves can be directed to converge at one point before they spread out again. If an interesting structure is located at this convergence point, the reflection of the waves from this point will carry more detail. If the instrument is a camera, the object on the film will be sharp. If the instrument is an ultrasound machine, the structure on the screen will have more detail if the sound waves converge at this structure.

If the probe is mechanical, the focus is usually fixed at a tissue depth that is likely to give good images most of the time. The identical concept applies to a fixed-focus camera that produces reasonably good pictures most of the time. However, if one can focus the beam, pictures can be improved in many cases.

The key concept for focal zone is an understanding that image quality is better at the focal zone depth. As seen in Figure 2–1, an ultrasound beam is not razor-thin but actually has some width. In the case of a linear probe (shown in the drawing), the beam starts out wide, focuses to a narrow (but not zero) width at the focal zone, and then starts to spread again. Unlike a laser beam, whose light waves are essentially parallel, ultrasound beams spread out like waves on a lake. Better probes do well at approximating a thin beam with a sharp focus, but all ultrasound transducers have the same problem of spreading beams. When a beam that is *not* precise bounces off an irregular surface, the resulting image may show artifacts (Fig. 2–2). In this drawing, the irregular surface is a sphere. The beam is spreading out as it passes through and reflects off the surfaces. Because part of the beam is reflected off the sides of the sphere (ignoring refraction artifact for now), there will be partial reflections along the borders (top and bottom) of the sphere. Thus, these borders are not distinct in the final image. If the beam is thinner (in the focal range), this artifact disappears and the image becomes sharper.

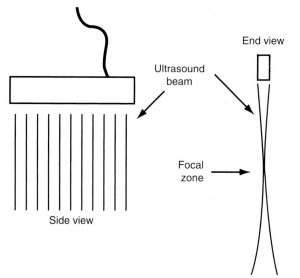

Figure 2–1. An ultrasound beam is not razor-thin but has width. As shown, with the linear probe, the beam starts out wide, focuses to a narrow width at the focal zone, and then begins to spread again.

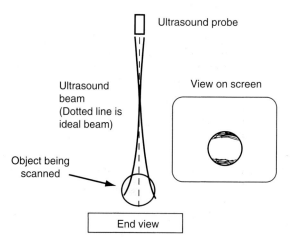

Figure 2–2. When a beam that is not precise bounces off an irregular surface, the resulting image may have an artifact. In this figure, the irregular surface is a sphere, and as the beam passes through, it spreads out and reflects off the surfaces. If the beam is thinner and in focal range, this artifact disappears and the image becomes sharper. In this example there is an artifact at the top and bottom of the image because of the additional echoes from the edge of the wide ultrasound beam.

In the case of electronic probes, some appear to focus in multiple zones simultaneously. However, this is an electronic trick. The probe can focus in only one zone at a time, but the machine combines several scans with several focal zones into a single detailed image. Because it takes several scans to produce a single image, the image frame rate will decrease.

Summary. Select a focal zone that is in the vicinity of the structure being studied. If it is a large structure and the probe is electronic, multiple focal zones can be used at the expense of frame rate.

Adjusting for a Spectacular Image

Optimizing the Image of the Structures Being Studied

Horizontal Positioning

A physical principle of the ultrasound medium dictates that horizontal structures will reflect ultrasound beams back to the transducer better than vertical structures. Therefore, the first concept involves turning and rotating the probe to bring as much of the structure being studied into as horizontal a position as possible.

> **Physics.** If the reflection of sound is stronger, the image will have less electronic noise (or snow), as was described under Power Level. Thus, similar to the problem of seeing detail on a sign that is parallel to the road as opposed to a sign that is perpendicular to the road, the challenge in sonography is to move the patient or probe to orient the imaged structure as perpendicular to the ultrasound beam as possible.

Zooming

Zooming is essentially identical to the physical concept discussed earlier under Depth of the Scan. The only difference is that image enlargement is effected by selecting a portion of the image instead of the global depth of the image. Once the image is enlarged, it will be displayed by more pixels (dots) on the screen, and more detail may be present. An additional point about zooming is that there are two ways to zoom. In the first way, the ultrasound machine puts the entire image in storage but displays only a portion of it. In this case, the amount of zooming can be changed even when the image is frozen, but the number of pixels that comprise the structure may be less. The other way of zooming takes only a portion of the returning ultrasound energy but converts that portion into an entire image, resulting in more pixels for the structure than with the first way of zooming.

Reducing Artifact

The final important concept of image optimization is the reduction of artifact. Nature can be cruel, and the presence of unwanted reverberations, reflections, and refractions may change an image dramatically. There are several considerations.

First (as was discussed earlier under Power Level), the artifact of ring-down may cause unwanted horizontal lines across the image in cystic structures below a solid interface.

> **Physics.** The lines are caused by increased power in the near fields. A strong ultrasound signal may cause secondary vibrations of the solid–liquid interface. As these extra vibrations continue to return to the ultrasound machine, the electronics is fooled into displaying more (artifact) echoes below the solid–liquid interface. As the power of the ultrasound beam decreases, this artifact disappears.

To get rid of these lines, the operator should merely pull the probe away from the structure a bit, or apply less power.

Another type of artifact is reverberation. An example of this is an image of a pelvis with an intrauterine device (IUD) in the uterus. If the device is parallel to the transducer (and perpendicular to the ultrasound beam), a ghost image of the IUD may appear at twice the depth of the actual IUD.

> **Physics.** If a solid structure is parallel to the transducer and the power level is high enough, a portion of the ultrasound

signal may bounce back and forth between the transducer and the solid object (e.g., an IUD) several times while the remainder of the ultrasound signal travels to the depths of the tissue and back again. After bouncing, some of the signal will arrive at the same time as the ultrasound reflections from deeper tissue. This fools the electronics of the machine into producing a ghost image.

To prevent a ghost image, the patient or probe should be moved to avoid a parallel orientation of the object to the probe, but one should beware of reflection artifacts, as described later.

If the pelvis contains both cystic and solid objects, a refraction artifact may be possible. This occurs when there is a solid object below a liquid–solid interface that is not parallel to the probe. In this case, the solid object may be distorted. Another example is the apparent visualization of two gestational sacs in early pregnancy when the probe is held at a certain angle. In other views, there is only one sac. The appearance of two sacs is caused by refraction of some of the ultrasound beam through the mother's rectus muscle, which acts like an acoustic lens and refracts the beam passing through it.

> **Physics.** Refractions are best compared with the appearance of an object seen at the bottom of a swimming pool. Physical laws describe the phenomenon in which light or sound bends when it crosses a solid–liquid or liquid–gas interface. Thus, if one looks in a pool at an angle and tries to reach in to grab the object at the bottom, the object will be at a different location from where one reaches because the path of the light beams from the object to the eye is bent by the air–liquid interface.

If the solid and cystic objects are at similar depths in the pelvis, a solid object that has an oblique surface with respect to the ultrasound transducer may cause a reflection artifact. A structure such as a cyst nearby may be duplicated because of secondary reflections from the solid structure. This is particularly accentuated by a solid structure such as an IUD that is imaged at an angle.

> **Physics.** As in the case of the reverberation artifact, the solid structure causes some of the ultrasound beam to reflect off its surface, but this time it travels in a different direction, bounces off something, and then returns. Because this "something" is probably imaged by the ultrasound machine directly, the additional reflections will cause a ghost image somewhere on the screen.

Summary. To prevent reflection and refraction artifacts, the image should be oriented to avoid certain angles or perpendicular orientation of solid–liquid interfaces. Also, reducing the power output may decrease these artifacts slightly.

Selecting the Postprocessing Curve

The postprocessing curve is an additional tool that can be used for fine-tuning the gray levels in an image.

> **Physics.** The human eye does not perceive light levels in a uniform fashion. Specifically, doubling the amount of light present does not necessarily mean that one sees an object as twice as bright. Therefore (without going into the technical details), the ability to change the postprocessing curve allows the sonographer to change the way the machine produces gray levels to improve the image, compensating for the imprecise interpretation of light levels by the human eye. Basically, the machine can change the amount of gray displayed at a certain returning energy level.

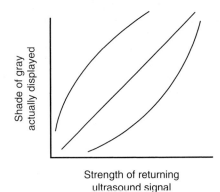

Examples of Postprocessing Curves

Figure 2–3. The ideal relationship between the shade of gray actually displayed and the strength of the returning ultrasound signal is shown here as a diagonal line. However, the human eye is not a precise instrument, and it is sometimes useful to skew this relationship. The curves in the graph depict how more or fewer shades of gray can be obtained for a particular signal range.

Although the concept is important, the details are not—the sonographer chooses a curve that maximizes image quality.

If the sonographer is studying a particular type of tissue, a more technical explanation of postprocessing curves may be useful. This is because tissue characterization depends on gray-scale differentiation of the ultrasound signal. It is obviously important to get more detail by displaying many levels of gray. (Some displays may use only 16 or 32 levels, whereas others may use 64 or 128.) However, not all gray areas are alike. There are not just 32 or 128 grays! The visual spectrum is continuous, and there is an infinite number of possible shades, but the ultrasound machine can display only a fixed number of shades. Therefore, the following problem arises: which shade of gray should be displayed for a particular signal strength that is received by the machine? Logically, it might seem that if a returning signal from one structure is twice as strong as the signal from a second structure, the pixel on the screen from the first structure should be twice as bright as the pixel from the second structure. In Figure 2–3, this relationship is depicted as a diagonal line on the graph. However, as mentioned previously, the human eye is not a precise instrument, and it is sometimes useful to skew this relationship. As depicted by the curves in this graph, more (or sometimes fewer) shades of gray can be shown for a particular signal range. By adjusting the number of grays available for a particular signal range, certain types of tissue characterization may be enhanced. Because the choice of the shades of gray versus the signal strength can be represented by a curve on a graph, this adjustment is called the *postprocessing curve*.

Image Averaging

Because an ultrasound beam is fairly weak, there is some noise (or snow) in the best of images. Image averaging may reduce this problem.

> **Physics.** An image will not change from frame to frame, whereas the noise (snow) is random and will change. Therefore, if several frames are averaged, the snow will tend to be canceled, leaving an improved image.

Because this average must be calculated on several frames (usually adjustable), it should not be surprising that the frame rate may decrease when image averaging is turned on. If the processing is done on a moving average basis, the frame rate may not decrease. For static structures, this is not a problem, but for moving objects such as the fetal heart, averaging is always a problem because the complete cardiac cycle occurs in half a second or less. If the frame rate is slowed to four or five frames per second, the heart may appear as a constant blur because it is moving so fast. To visualize more detail, the frame rate must be faster.

Summary. Image averaging should be used only for structures that are not moving.

Adjusting Three-Dimensional Ultrasound Images

Three-dimensional (3D) ultrasound has become much more common in the last 6 years. Although it is best suited for structures floating in a liquid (i.e., the fetus), it can also be used in gynecology. If there is a cystic structure, the walls can be examined in three dimensions. However, for solid tissue, 3D imaging is useful in situations where transducer movement is limited, such as transvaginal sonography.

Volume

The first step in obtaining a 3D image is to scan a volume of tissue. Unlike two-dimensional (2D) ultrasound, which looks at a slice of the anatomy, the 3D scan stores numerous slices (usually more than 100) from one side of a structure to the other side of the structure. This set of consecutive slices comprises a volume of the anatomy. When it is stored in the ultrasound machine, the computer in the machine can rearrange the 2D pixels in any plane to obtain slices of anatomy for display that would be impossible to obtain from a transducer outside the body.

> **Physics.** When 3D ultrasound is used, a volume of tissue (e.g., cubic, trapezoidal, or cone-shaped selection) is stored in the machine. What you see on the screen is either a slice from one part of that volume or a composite view of a series of solid–fluid interfaces. The latter is used to view the details of the wall of a cyst (or fetus). However, if the original selection of the volume does not include the entire structure, a portion of it will appear to be amputated.

Summary. Make sure the entire structure is stored in the selected volume before 3D processing is done.

Threshold

Threshold is adjusted when a representation of a 3D image is viewed in two dimensions. A good example of a representation of a 3D image that is viewed in two dimensions is the rendering of the surface of the fetal face. This usually occurs when a solid object, such as a cyst wall or a fetus, is bathed in fluid. In this case, the entire surface of the cyst wall is visualized from a different viewpoint to see more detail. Rather than cut a single slice through a cyst, 3D ultrasound allows a sonographer to view the entire inner surface of a cyst as if he or she were standing at the edge of the cyst and could actually look at its surface, looking through the fluid within the cyst. In reality, the machine is instructed to ignore echoes from the fluid so that the surface of the cyst wall can be rendered (drawn on the screen).

> **Physics.** This principle is similar to that discussed previously under Selecting the Postprocessing Curve. However, in this case, the curve is cut off sharply at lower energy levels, so that structures responsible for these weak echoes (i.e., fluid) are not imaged. However, if the threshold is increased, some of the weaker ultrasound echoes from the structure of interest, which would normally be rendered as light gray, will disappear if the threshold selection is set to make that signal invisible. As a result, there will appear to be a hole in the structure of interest.

Summary. Select a threshold that makes fluid, but not the structure of interest, invisible.

Adjusting Doppler Studies

Angle of Probe

Because Doppler studies investigate the movement of objects (usually blood cells), it is important that the probe be placed so that the movement can be detected. This simple concept concerns the orientation of the probe to obtain a Doppler signal. If the blood cells are moving away from or toward the transducer, the movement can be detected. However, if the blood cells are moving perpendicular to the transducer, the ultrasound beam is not affected by the movement. Therefore, the best angle for the probe is one that shows the vessels as vertical on the screen. However, most machines are sensitive enough that most angles other than directly perpendicular will allow detection of motion. Obviously, a vessel with minimal or slow blood flow must be oriented more vertically to the probe for the machine to detect flow than would be the case with a large artery with fast-moving blood.

Summary. If flow is suspected, the probe should be turned so the vessel is oriented more vertically on the screen to see if flow actually exists.

Size of the Color Image

When color is displayed, the machine calculates a frequency shift for the returning ultrasound beam for every pixel on the screen. Because this takes an enormous amount of computation, even at modern computing speeds, the speed of image generation on the screen slows if the size of the color area is increased. Although it is physically possible to increase the frame rate, the sheer number of calculations per second—hundreds of millions—has forced compromises on ultrasound manufacturers. Perhaps the ideal solution would be to put more computers in the machines so that the calculations could be done faster, increasing the frame rate. However, manufacturers have chosen a middle road, providing sufficient computational power to make the color image update rapidly when the area is small, but more slowly if the color image is large.

Summary. Until computers and machines get less expensive, the size of the color image must be as small as possible to capture a useful image at a reasonable rate.

Gate Size for Waveform Studies

When a vessel is studied, the gate selects where the flow is studied. If it is in the wrong location, the flow measurement may not be correct.

Physics. When a waveform is displayed, it originates from a sample that is chosen on the screen. This is called a *gate*, and all motion within the gate is recorded. If the gate is small, it may be difficult to detect flow if the gate is positioned just outside of the vessel. However, if the gate is too large, it may pick up more than one vessel if there are multiple vessels next to each other. Even more confusing is the graph that is generated if two vessels with flow in opposite directions are recorded at the same time.

Summary. A gate should be selected that is as small as possible and still able to display the flow in the vessel.

Doppler Gain

Doppler gain adjustment is essentially a volume control. As with ultrasound images, it is important to adjust the gain so the Doppler graph is bright enough.

Velocity Range

Flow in a vessel may be fast or slow. When flow is measured, the sonographer must be able to guess approximately how fast the flow is and choose a velocity range to show the flow. If the velocity range is too high, the Doppler display may be tiny. If color is being displayed, not much may show if blood flow is slow. If the velocity range is too low, the graph will overflow the top (and wrap around the bottom—an artifact known as *aliasing*). If color is being displayed, one color will seem to change into another in the middle of the vessel (another example of the aliasing artifact).

Physics. The mechanism of aliasing depends on how often the movement of the structure is sampled. If sampling is infrequent, the result may be artifact. A good example is a movie of a rotating wagon wheel. This rotation will be faithfully displayed if the frame rate of the movie is fast enough (i.e., the movement is sampled often). However, if the frames are infrequent, the spokes of the wheel may appear to be turning backward because of a sampling error.

Although the physics is complicated, the concept is simple: the velocity range that produces a graph that does not overflow on the top or bottom should be chosen. If color is being displayed (and the flow is nonturbulent), a velocity range should be chosen so that the color of a vessel does not change in the middle.

Baseline

Normally, the ultrasound machine can show flow in both directions (or both colors). However, if the flow is always in the same direction, the baseline can be shifted from the middle of the velocity range to allow the graph or the color more range for the direction of flow being displayed. Again, the physics is complicated, but in practice the sonographer should adjust this control to show as much graph (or color) as possible.

Angle of Vessel

Correction for the angle of vessel (or vessels) is a simple concept that is useful only if the actual flow measurement of

a vessel is required. Because virtually all Doppler studies depend on ratios, actual flow measurements in a vessel are almost always unnecessary. When a ratio is calculated, one flow measurement is divided by another flow measurement, and a methodology error (such as measuring the vessel at an angle) is usually canceled. If an actual flow (milliliters per minute) must be determined, the angle of the vessel must be known.

Physics. The Doppler frequency shift of the returning ultrasound signal is what the machine uses to calculate the actual flow. Because this shift changes as the angle between the vessel and the probe changes, the actual flow can be calculated only if this angle is known. Fortunately, most Doppler machines have a control that allows the angle to be superimposed on the vessel for this purpose.

Summary. For precise flow measurements, the angle of the vessel must be entered (usually by matching the graphics on the gate to the vessel) to calculate an exact flow within the vessel.

Variance Display

Because most blood vessel flow has little turbulence, a simple color display of red and blue for two directions of flow is adequate. However, if blood flow is turbulent (near a stenosis or other malformation), the blood flow may vary tremendously from one point to the next. This can be displayed in some ultrasound machines by adding varying amounts of yellow (depending on the amount of turbulence) to the red or blue colors to yield shades of orange or green. In machines that can do this, it is usually an option that can be switched on and off. However, it is useful only if some sort of obstruction or stenosis is being studied.

Conclusion

When an ultrasound study is performed, it is important to know a little bit of physics. If the concepts behind choosing a particular power level, frequency, focal zone, or image processing format are understood, it becomes easy to obtain great images. A practical understanding of the ultrasound medium, not requiring actual calculations, will allow this technology to be used to its fullest extent.

BIBLIOGRAPHY

Burke RK, Fine RA: Basic physical principles of ultrasonography for the practicing clinician. Infertil Reprod Med Clin North Am 1991;2:643.

Fleischer AC, Romero R, Manning FA, et al (eds): The Principles and Practice of Ultrasonography in Obstetrics and Gynecology, 4th ed. East Norwalk, Conn, Appleton & Lange, 1991.

Kremkau FW (ed): Doppler Ultrasound Principles and Instruments. Philadelphia, WB Saunders, 1990.

Timor-Tritsch IE, Rottem S (eds): Transvaginal Sonography, 2nd ed. New York, Elsevier, 1991.

Trouble-shooting Guide

This section serves a purpose similar to that of the remaining chapters of this book: providing examples of images that the sonographer can compare with images he or she has obtained but cannot identify with certainty. But in this section, the images in question are of poor diagnostic quality. The goal is to figure out what is wrong.

In this section, various images are classified by visual topics. If one encounters a technical problem while scanning a patient, the solution will be found here. In many cases the normal image is placed alongside the problem image to emphasize the technical differences.

Image Is Too Dark

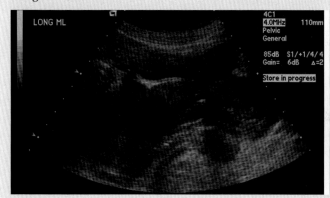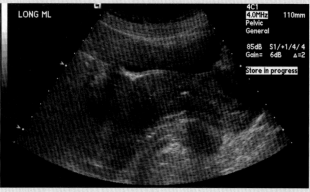

Figure 2A–1

A normal image is on the right. The same image is on the left, but the display is too dark. Notice the dark letters, compared with the letters in the image on the right—this is a clue that the problem is the monitor and not the ultrasound machine settings. (See Chapter 3 for more information about adjusting output devices.)

Solution: Readjust the display.

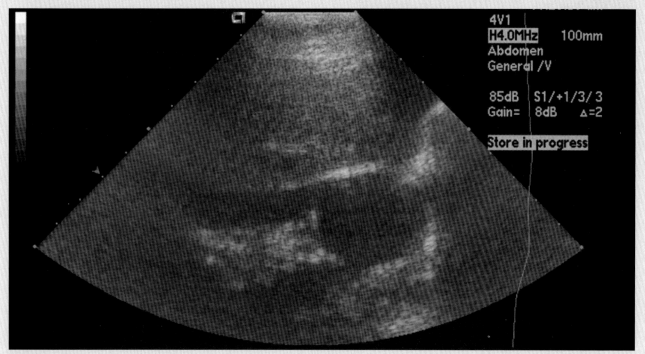

Figure 2A–2

In this image (and most of the rest in this section, except as noted), assume that the display is set properly. However, here the power output is too low to provide enough echoes for the machine to produce an image. Note that the gain is actually set fairly high, yet the image is still dark. Therefore, this is a good example of an image that cannot be corrected with gain or postprocessing because the echoes are just not there.

Solution: Increase the power output. (Many machines no longer have a power setting. Therefore, if the deeper parts of the image are dark because of a lack of echoes, the problem is probably that the frequency is wrong [see Fig. 2A–4].)

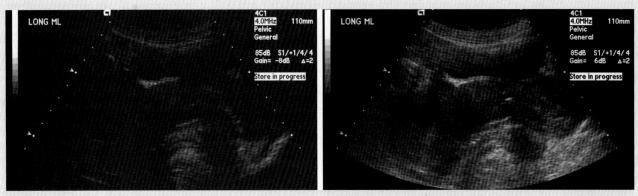

Figure 2A–3

The overall gain is set too low in the image on the left. The normal image is on the right. One might be tempted to use the time–gain slide controls to improve the image. However, it might be harder to fine-tune the image if one or more of the slide controls is already at its maximum setting. Note that the letters on the display are bright and the gray scale is seen well. This indicates that the problem is an ultrasound setting and not a display problem (compare with Fig. 2A–1).

Solution: Increase the gain control.

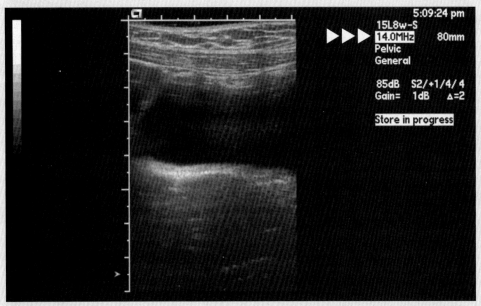

Figure 2A–4

The lower half of this image is too dark, even with time–gain control compensation. The problem is that the probe is the wrong frequency *(arrowheads)*. Higher-frequency ultrasound does not penetrate well, and the resulting image from deep structures is dark, regardless of the settings on the machine.

Solution: Change to a probe with a lower frequency.

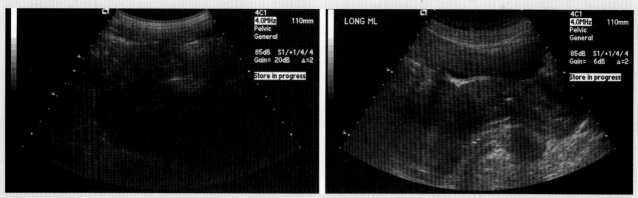

Figure 2A–5

Everything is dark in the image on the left, although the settings appear to be appropriate. The problem is a lack of coupling gel on the skin. Ultrasound waves do not travel well through air, and even though the probe is touching the skin, there is still a small amount of air, sufficient to degrade the image.

Solution: Use more gel.

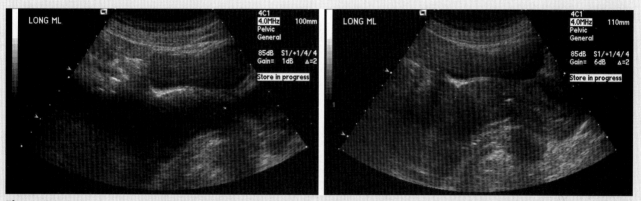

Figure 2A–6

A dark, curving streak is seen in the middle of the image on the left because the time–gain controls are not set properly. These fine-tuning controls permit adjustment of individual horizontal strips of the image. There is a small amount of overlap, but for the most part, each control corresponds to one horizontal or curving section of the image. In this image, one of the controls is at its minimum point.

Solution: Adjust the appropriate time–gain control.

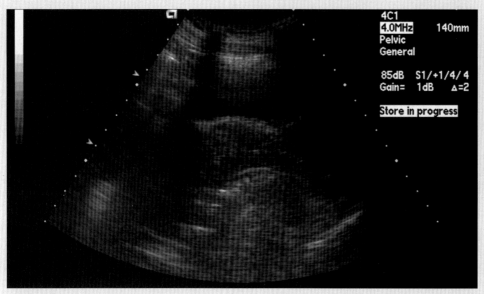

Figure 2A–7

This image has dark streaks that are close to vertical. There are several possibilities: there are spots on the skin where gel is missing and the signal is not getting through; there is something between the probe and the skin (for abdominal scans, the umbilicus almost always causes this type of image because of the air that is usually trapped in its depths); or there is a probe problem. (See Chapter 3 for more information on solving this image problem.)

 Solution: Move the probe. If the image improves, then check for gel or an obstruction. If the image does not improve, check the probe.

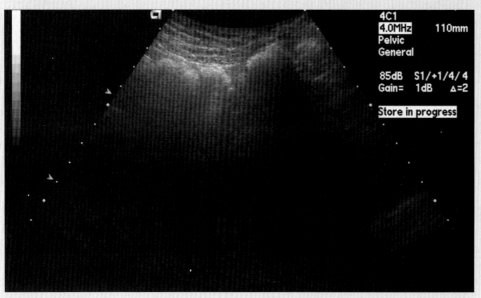

Figure 2A–8

The bottom half of this image is dark because of what is in the near field. In this case, the air in the intestines totally blocks ultrasound waves, and the rest of the image is dark. The giveaway is the very bright echo from the air in the near field.

 Solution: Move the probe to avoid the gas, or have the patient turn so the gas will move to a different location.

Image Is Too Light

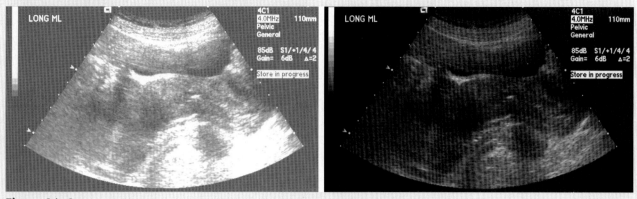

Figure 2A–9

The image on the left is actually a good image, but the display is too bright. Note that the black areas in the left image are not black, and the letters are also brighter and a little fuzzy. Both of these findings are clues that the display and not the ultrasound machine is the problem. (See Chapter 3 for more information about adjusting output devices.)

Solution: Readjust the display.

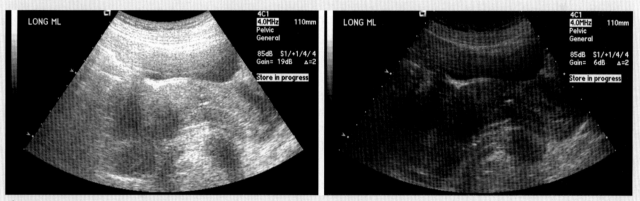

Figure 2A–10

The overall gain is set too high in the image on the left. Note that the letters in the normal image on the right have the same brightness as those in the bad image on the left. This is a clue that the problem is the ultrasound settings and not the display. One might be tempted to use the time–gain slide controls to improve the image. However, it might be harder to fine-tune the image if one or more of the slide controls is moved to its minimum setting.

Solution: Decrease the gain control.

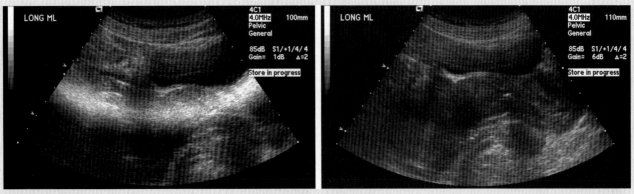

Figure 2A–11

A bright, curving streak is seen in the image on the left because the time–gain controls are not set properly. These fine-tuning controls permit adjustment of individual horizontal strips of the image. There is a small amount of overlap, but for the most part, each control corresponds to one horizontal or curving section of the image. In this image, one of the controls is at its maximum point.

Solution: Adjust the appropriate time–gain control.

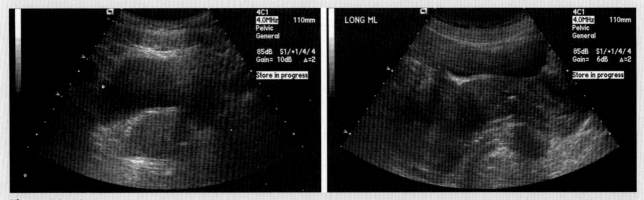

Figure 2A–12

The image on the left has a bright vertical streak in the middle. There are several possibilities: there are areas on the skin where gel is missing and the signal is not getting through, *and the sonographer has increased the gain to compensate;* there is something between the probe and the skin, *and the sonographer has increased the gain to compensate;* there is a probe problem, *and the sonographer has increased the gain to compensate.*

Solution: Move the probe and adjust the gain setting. If the image improves, check for gel or an obstruction. If the image does not improve, check the probe.

Image Is "Blurry" or "Fuzzy" or "Looks Funny"

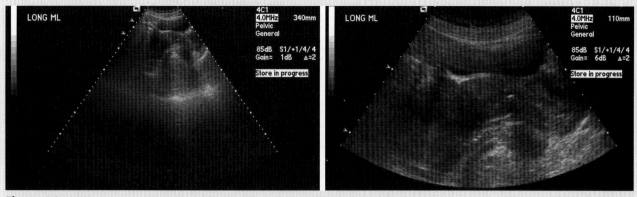

Figure 2A–13

The sonographer is studying something in the near field, but the depth is so great in the image on the left that the structure appears small, with little detail. Compare with the normal image on the right.

Solution: Decrease the depth to increase the size and detail of the image.

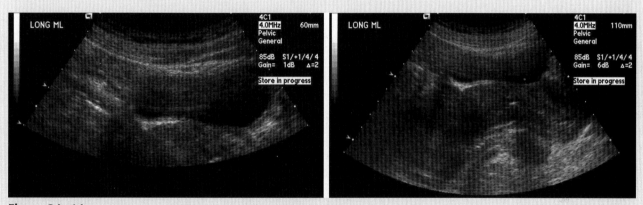

Figure 2A–14

The sonographer is studying something in the near field, but the depth is so shallow that part of the structure (uterus) is missing in the image on the left. Compare with the normal image on the right.

Solution: Increase the depth to see the whole image.

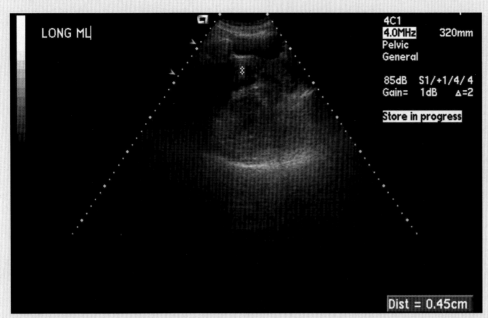

Figure 2A–15

The sonographer is studying a small object, but detail is lacking. There are two ways to increase detail: the depth can be decreased or the zooming feature can be used. If the object is at great depth, the best solution is the zooming feature.
  Solution: Use the zooming feature to increase the size of the structure.

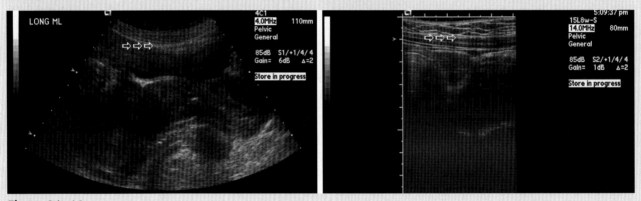

Figure 2A–16

These two images demonstrate the effect of frequency. In looking at shallow structures *(arrows),* note that detail is lacking in the low-frequency image on the left compared with the high-frequency image on the right. Because a higher frequency increases resolution, the highest frequency that will penetrate to this depth should be used.
  Solution: Use a higher-frequency probe to study shallow structures.

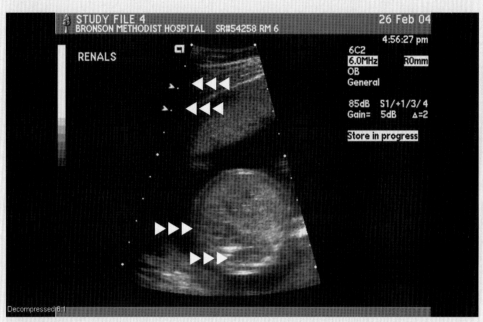

Figure 2A–17

A higher-frequency probe was used at the correct settings, but the important part of the image is still fuzzy. In this case, the focal zone *(left-pointing arrowheads)* is far from the image of interest, fetal kidneys *(right-pointing arrowheads)*. Because the ultrasound beam is wide at the area of interest, detail is lost.

Solution: Move the focal point down. On some machines, multiple focal zones may be used to improve the image even more.

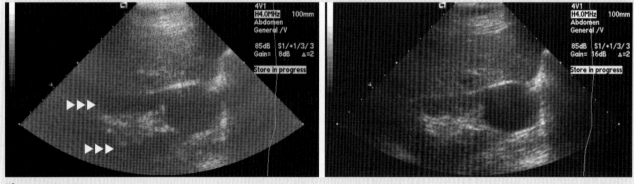

Figure 2A–18

The image on the left has "snow" in it, which is caused by too little power. In this case, there is sufficient power to produce a bright image, but not enough to show detail (note that much of the kidney detail is absent *[arrowheads]*). In addition, there is electronic noise because the ultrasound signal is low. Compare with the same image on the right, in which the transmitted power is increased.

Solution: Increase the transmitted power.

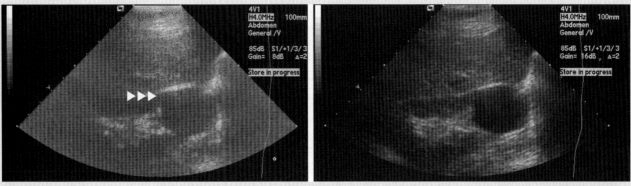

Figure 2A–19

The image on the left has some blurring of detail even though the gain and time–gain control settings are correct. In this case, the transmitted power is too high for this study. Just as too much light can cause a photograph to be distorted, too much ultrasound power can degrade an image. Notice the ring-down in this kidney cyst *(arrowheads)*. Compare with the image on the right, in which the transmitted power is lower.

Solution: Decrease the transmitted power for near-field studies.

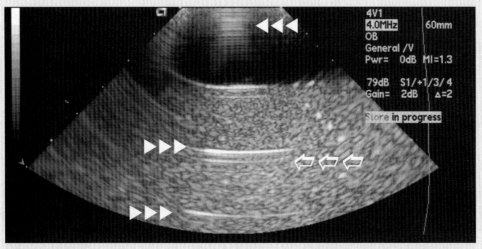

Figure 2A–20

This image was produced on an ultrasound phantom with a layer of water on top. Notice the ring-down in the water at the top of the image *(left-pointing arrowheads)*. This image also shows reverberation from the water–phantom interface *(right-pointing arrowheads)*. In addition, the power is high enough that there is ring-down from the reverberations *(arrows)*. (See under Power Level for a complete discussion.)

Solution: Decrease the power to reduce the ring-down and rotate the probe so there are no surfaces parallel to the probe to produce reverberations. Finally, move the probe so that the structure of interest is farther away to reduce ring-down further.

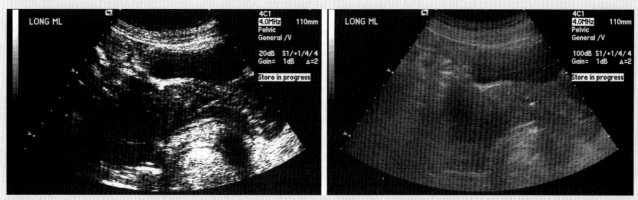

Figure 2A–21

The image on the left looks like one from a first-generation ultrasound machine because the structures are either black or white, with very little gray scale. The problem is lack of dynamic range. The image on the right has normal dynamic range.
Solution: Increase the dynamic range.

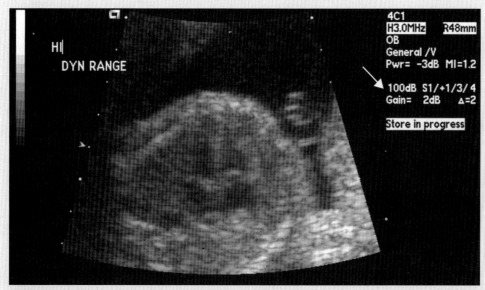

Figure 2A–22

In this image of the fetal heart, the borders of the ventricle are not as clear as possible. The problem is too much dynamic range *(arrow)*. To see liquid–solid interfaces well, the number of grays in the image should be decreased by adjusting the dynamic range.
Solution: Decrease the dynamic range.

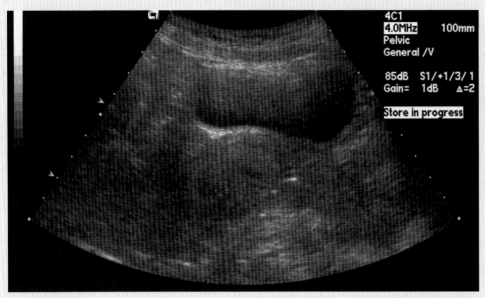

Figure 2A–23

This image looks a bit strange. There is no question that it is a uterus, but the detail is not quite right. The reason is that the postprocessing curve is set improperly. This curve is useful for viewing certain kinds of tissue, but the image will appear unusual if the wrong curve is used.

Solution: Use another postprocessing curve.

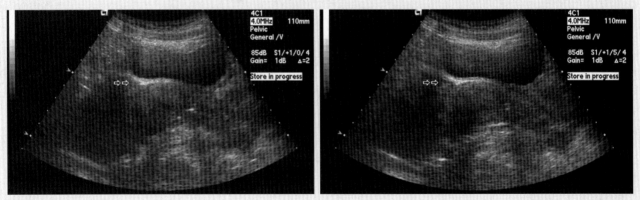

Figure 2A–24

These two images demonstrate image averaging (also called *persistence* in some systems). The right image has maximum persistence and the left image has none. When there is no persistence, the amount of noise (snow) in the image is greater and detail is less. Note that the ovary *(arrows)* can be seen in the right image but not in the left image.

Solution: Increase image averaging to see more detail.

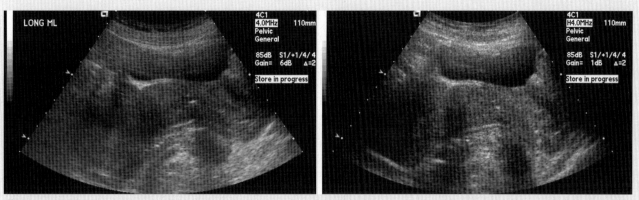

Figure 2A–25

The display on the right uses harmonic imaging; the one on the left does not. In this case, the difference is subtle, but note that the tissue characterization on the right has more detail than on the left.

Solution: For greater detail, turn on harmonic imaging (see text).

Doppler Graph Is Poor

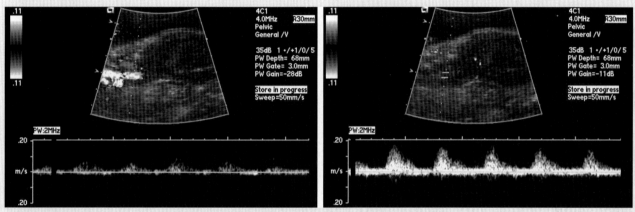

Figure 2A–26

The gate is positioned properly, but the graph on the left is weak. A normal Doppler graph is shown on the right. The problem is lack of Doppler gain. On most machines, this is a separate control, which means that the image may be perfect but the graph poor.

Solution: Increase the Doppler gain.

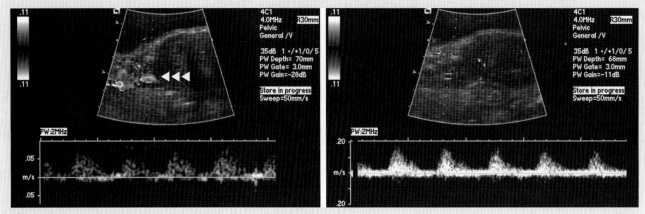

Figure 2A–27

The settings are correct in the image on the left, but the graph is still weak. The problem here is the orientation of the vessel with relation to the probe *(arrowheads)*. If the vessel is parallel to the surface of the probe, little fluid motion can be detected. On the right, the probe has been rotated slightly and the graph is much better.

Solution: Move (rotate) the probe or move the patient to make the vessel appear at an angle on the screen.

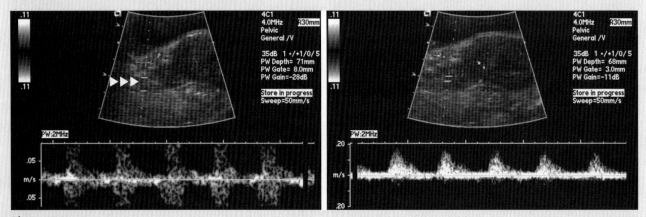

Figure 2A–28

The graph on the left is confusing. The pattern suggests that there are two different vessels with flow in opposite directions. In this case, the problem is a gate that is too large *(arrowheads)*. If it covers more than one vessel, the tracing will represent a combination of all the vessels. The image on the right is the same tissue with a smaller gate and the graph of a single vessel.

Solution: Decrease the gate size.

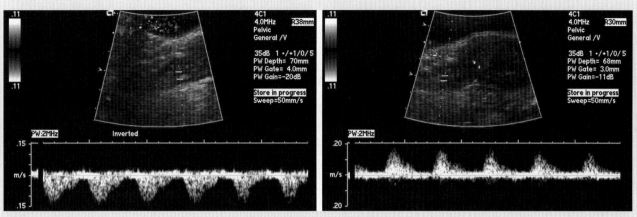

Figure 2A–29

The graph on the left is upside down. This happens because blood may be flowing in any direction. If it is flowing away from the transducer, the graph is plotted below the baseline. To see a graph that is above the baseline, invert the graph.

Solution: Press the invert button for Doppler graphs that are upside down.

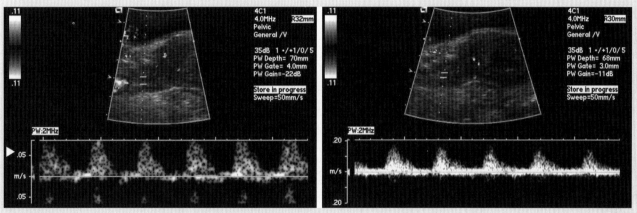

Figure 2A–30

The graph on the left is overflowing the top and wrapping around to the bottom (aliasing). The problem is too much velocity range. In this case, the flow in the vessel is very fast, but the setting on the machine is too low *(arrowhead),* and the sampling rate is causing a display error. The correct display is on the right.

Solution: Increase the velocity range if the Doppler display is aliasing.

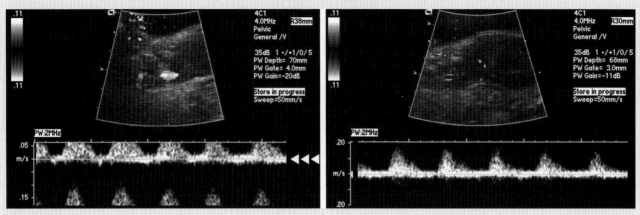

Figure 2A–31

The velocity ranges are adequate for both of these images, but the Doppler graph is aliasing in the left image. This has happened because the baseline is too high *(arrowheads)*. On the right, the baseline is dropped to display a normal graph.

Solution: Move the baseline down (or up) to display the Doppler graph correctly if the velocity range is not quite right.

Chapter 3

Instrumentation, Modality Selection, and Documentation

David B. Peisner

Whereas Chapter 2 discusses techniques for maximizing the appearance of ultrasound images, this chapter discusses the instrumentation itself. Some of the topics relate to scanning, and some relate to factors that might not have been considered before the purchase of a machine. Also, concepts of documentation and calibration of the equipment, display, and recording devices are discussed.

Machine Characteristics

Physical specifications are often overlooked but may be important for several reasons. First, sonography may be used for procedures outside the ultrasound suite. Therefore, the dimensions and weight of the machine will be factors if the machine is to be moved. A smaller machine is obviously easier to manipulate in an operating room or around beds in a patient's room. Although even the heaviest machines can be moved, some weigh several hundred pounds, and this should be considered if the machine may be moved frequently. Finally, a machine that is inconvenient to move may be more prone to damage.

The length and storage facilities of cables relate directly to machine longevity and reliability. The length of the power cord determines how mobile the machine can be, and the length of the probe cables can be a limiting factor in a procedure. Some machines have a place to store cords and cables, and some do not. For a machine with many probes, a camera, and a video recorder, the number of loose cables may create problems. If the cables are short or inconvenient to store, the users of the machine may bend or coil the cables in unusual ways that may subject them to premature failure. The better machines have sturdy hooks or other systems to manage the many cables that are usually attached.

Characteristics such as electrical power become important for practical reasons. For example, voltage requirements are usually not a major problem because manufacturers are aware of differing specifications in various countries. However, the amount of power that a machine requires (measured in watts) may be important. In a room with many machines, a larger machine may overload the electrical system and cause a power failure. Careful planning can avoid this problem.

Similarly, the environmental requirements of the machine may be a consideration. Because all electronic machines generate heat, the elimination of heat should be considered. A large machine may produce a significant amount of heat, sometimes as much as a space heater, which may raise the temperature of the examination room. The key issue is planning. If the amount of air conditioning is planned ahead of time, some patient (and sonographer) comfort problems can be avoided. Furthermore, some machines have fans and some do not. Those that do may produce a significant amount of noise and may have filters that require frequent cleaning. Although filters may be inconvenient to use, they may prolong the life of the machine. Finally, most machines operate in a variety of temperature and humidity conditions. However, for use in some parts of the world, such as the tropics, the operating requirements of a machine should be verified before the machine is purchased.

A seemingly mundane option is the space on the cart or machine for storing equipment and supplies. Some machines have space for gel bottles. Many clinics use a gel warmer, and a designated place on the machine for this is useful. Most machines have a place for a camera or video recorder. However, additional space (shelves or other compartments) can be helpful for storing supplies, charts, probes, and so forth. One should not forget the possibility of adding more equipment or options to a machine. If extra shelves or compartments are provided when a machine is purchased, the addition of a computer or other equipment will be much easier in the future.

The number of probe receptacles may affect the daily operation of the machine. For example, some machines allow many probes to be plugged in simultaneously, which allows them to be selected from the console. (Most machines have protective mechanisms if a probe is unplugged with the power turned on.) Machines with a single receptacle force the user to plug and unplug the probes whenever a different probe is desired, which can cause damage to the connector or its receptacle if the probe connector is inserted crookedly. Finally, it can be difficult to insert a big plug if the receptacle is near the floor or not on the front panel or at the rear of the machine. Therefore, a machine with probe selection controlled from a switch or keyboard is preferable.

Other connectors on the machine may be important. A clinic may use both a recorder and another camera or instant printer. Some may wish to have an auxiliary monitor (a spare computer monitor works nicely) connected to allow the patient (or others) to observe the examination. All these require connections that may not be present on some scanners. Also, some machines may provide connectors for other signals such as Doppler, electrocardiogram, or remote control of the auxiliary equipment. Planning for other devices helps determine the proper machine to obtain.

The location and size of the monitor are simple but important factors. Although virtually all modern machines produce good ultrasound pictures, a picture on a small screen may be difficult to see if the operator is far away from the machine. Furthermore, some monitors are fixed in their cabinets and do not swivel. This can be a factor if the operator is moving around the patient. All of these depend to some degree on operator preference but nevertheless should be considered when a machine is chosen.

Transducers

The number and type of transducers vary widely among manufacturers. Some characteristics do not apply to transvaginal probes. For example, linear transducers exist for abdominal and transrectal but (usually) not for transvaginal sonography, in which the probes produce sector images. The different types of sector probes are mechanical, phased array, and curvilinear.

Mechanical Sector Transducer

The mechanical sector transducer consists of a rotating or oscillating (back-and-forth) crystal (or crystals) in an oil bath. This method is the simplest way of scanning and allows the widest field of view. The field of view is dependent on the movement of the crystal and is limited only by the mechanical characteristics of the transducer motor and shape of the handle. In some machines, fields of view approaching 240 degrees or more are possible.

There are several disadvantages to a mechanical sector transducer. First, whereas a real-time image requires a moving transducer, the use of other modalities such as M-mode and Doppler requires a fixed transducer. M-mode and Doppler can be used on a limited basis by moving the probe to get an image and stopping it to get the M-mode or Doppler data, but the image will be jerky. The second disadvantage is maintenance. Mechanical parts wear out, and the oil in the probe must be replaced occasionally. If any air gets into the mechanism, the bubble in the probe will produce shadowing in the image. If this occurs, the examination can be interrupted while additional oil is added to the probe. The third disadvantage of the mechanical sector transducer is inherent noise in the near field. This is not a problem in the abdomen, but with transvaginal sonography, some pelvic structures may lie within 1 cm of the transducer. However, the problem can be solved by slightly withdrawing the probe from the vagina to move the structure away from the near field.

The transducer of a mechanical probe consists of a few crystals (sometimes just one) that are attached to the mechanism that wobbles or rotates them. Early machines consisted of transducers that focused at a fixed point. Another variation was a probe with several transducers, each of which focused at a different point, allowing the user to select a focal point for a particular examination. Newer machines incorporate a technology known as *annular arrays*. An annular array is a transducer that consists of concentric circular crystals as opposed to the single circular crystal used in the past. Each annulus (literally, "ring") has a different focal zone that can be used with the other annuli to focus at different tissue depths. When these crystals are rotated or wobbled, the user can select one or more of them for different focal zones, even though the probe is mechanical.

Phased Array Sector Transducer

A phased array sector transducer consists of a fixed array of crystals that are tightly packed into a very small space. These crystals are sequentially triggered in a complicated scheme to aim the ultrasound beam in a sector. Although this methodology requires no moving parts, it is electronically more difficult to process. In the past these machines were more expensive, but today the cost differential is small. The most pressing consideration with this technology is the problem of side lobe artifacts. These cause structures to be distorted at the edge of the sector because of the mathematical problem of steering some of the beams at an angle other than perpendicular to the surface of the transducer, but modern processing algorithms have eliminated most of this problem. The advantage of such a probe lies in its small size, which may be important in menopausal patients or patients with strictures. Because there are no mechanical parts, these transducers are usually the smallest of the various transducers. The sector of this probe can be steered to the side of the pelvis like the mechanical probe. However, the amount of deviation of the sector is limited compared with a mechanical probe, and its use is more prone to artifacts. Phased array options have excellent near-field noise characteristics.

Curvilinear Sector Transducer

The curvilinear sector transducer consists of an array of crystals that are arranged along a curved end of the probe. Because the beam from each crystal exits perpendicularly from the transducer surface, the curvature of the probe end yields a sector image from this array. There are two advantages to this method. First, side lobe artifacts are less of a problem than for phased array probes; second, this arrangement is electronically simpler than the phased array. However, the field of view of a curvilinear probe is fixed, whereas that of a phased array may be variable. Curvilinear sector transducers have excellent near-field noise characteristics. Modern techniques for fabricating crystals have made it possible to obtain multiple focal zones. The differences in image quality between a phased array and curvilinear transducer are minimal, and individual user preferences may be a more important factor in the choice of a probe.

Other Probe Criteria

Dimensions

When a probe is selected, physical dimensions may be important. One of the most significant is the shape of the handle. Because sonographers may scan for a long period, the handle of the probe should be comfortable. In transvaginal sonography, some probes have bent ("broken") handles and some have straight handles. Probes with bent handles may be easier to manipulate if the patient is not on a gynecologic table. However, a transverse view of the lateral portions of the adnexa is difficult to obtain with this type of probe unless the probe is turned around for opposite sides of the pelvis. When the probe is rotated, the operator must then invert the image on the screen to maintain proper orientation—an inconvenience. Probes with straight handles are easier to aim and do not have to be rotated when the adnexa are examined. Finally, weight and dimensions of the transducer may make a difference for some operators. Mechanical probes are generally somewhat heavier and larger than the electronic ones. They may also vibrate slightly during operation.

Miscellaneous

Some probes have machine controls mounted in the probe body. These may allow the operator to freeze the picture or operate other machine functions. Some probes have attachable biopsy or needle guides that allow ultrasound-guided puncture procedures, including follicle retrievals, drainage of cysts, and pregnancy terminations. Specially designed probe covers are available for some machines used for such procedures. When a probe cover is not available, placing a surgical glove over the end of a variety of both transabdominal and transvaginal transducers usually works well and is inexpensive.

Probe Frequency, Focal Zone, Power Output, and Field of View

After a probe type and mechanism are chosen, there are several other characteristics of a probe that affect image quality. In some cases, only one choice is available for a particular probe, but in other cases, many options are available. This will vary by manufacturer and must be determined before a new probe is obtained. The characteristics include probe frequency, focal zone, power output, and field of view.

Probe Frequency. The frequency used for transvaginal sonography is higher than for transabdominal sonography, usually ranging from 5 to 7.5 MHz for various probes. Some probes may be capable of scanning at multiple frequencies, sometimes simultaneously. This feature is a major advantage because there is no need to exchange the probe during an examination if the operator wants to improve the image by changing the frequency. When multiple frequencies are combined with multiple focal zones, the ability to visualize important details in the pelvis improves dramatically. Harmonic imaging and averaging may further improve the image. As the frequency increases, the resolution of the image also increases, but the depth of penetration decreases (see Chapter 2).

Focal Zone. Another consideration is the focal zone of the probe. Mechanical probes usually have fixed focal zones whose depth depends on the frequency of the probe. Lower-frequency probes have a deeper focal zone. However, some mechanical probes with annular array transducers (see earlier) may be able to focus at more than one depth. Non-mechanical transducers may also have fixed focal zones or may have multiple zones. As with frequency, some probes may be capable of multiple focal zones simultaneously in the same scan.

Power Output. The power output of each probe varies by manufacturer. In general, probes comply with American Institute of Ultrasound in Medicine (AIUM) guidelines. One exception in which power outputs may be increased is Doppler flow applications. In this case, the operator should determine whether the power output of the probe is within the clinical guidelines for a particular application. Most modern machines offer a control for power selections. (Remember that power output selection is *not* the same as gain selection—see Chapter 2.)

Field of View. The field of view is one of the most important concepts in transvaginal and transabdominal sonography. The sector displayed is measured in degrees, based on a circle of 360 degrees; a quarter circle displays just 90 degrees. In sonography, an examination may be severely limited if the field of view of the sector is less than 90 degrees because the relationships between nearby structures may be difficult to establish. However, a narrow field of view may be used in certain cases in which a high frame rate is desired. The update rate on the screen slows as the sector size increases, and this may compromise the examination of a moving object such as a small heart in an early pregnancy.

There are two important characteristics of the field of view. The first characteristic is the absolute width of the field, described previously and measured in degrees of a circle. A probe with a larger field of view will be able to visualize more of a large organ, such as a uterus with myomas. The second characteristic is steerable fields of view in some probes. For example, a probe may have a field of view of 120 degrees. If this is symmetric with respect to the end of the probe, the field of view will be 60 degrees on each side of the imaginary line extending from the end of the transducer. However, for ovaries that are located laterally in the pelvis, examination may be difficult with some probes, especially if the patient has limited thigh mobility. For this reason, some probes and machines allow their fields of view to be shifted from the midline of the probe. Another development is the ability to scan in a plane perpendicular to the original scan plane, sometimes simultaneously. If available, this can give the sonographer additional flexibility in the examination.

Penetration, Resolution, Contrast Resolution, Frame Rate, and Invasive Procedure Options

Probe and machine specifications related to penetration, resolution (both axial and lateral), contrast resolution, frame rate, and the ability to add a biopsy guide should be considered before committing to a purchase or lease agreement. Unfortunately, not all specifications are easily available from the manufacturers.

Penetration. Although all machines transmit beams within AIUM guidelines, some machines may penetrate deeper than others at a similar power setting. This is because penetration depends not only on the power of the ultrasound beam the transducer produces but also on the geometry and sensitivity of the crystals as well as the quality of the receiving electronics.

Resolution. Resolution is an important factor because this characteristic essentially defines how much detail can be seen in an image. If a linear probe is used, lateral resolution depends on the frequency and focal zone of the ultrasound beam. If either a sector or curvilinear probe is used, lateral resolution also depends on the depth of the image. (Lateral resolution gets worse with deeper structures as the ultrasound beam spreads out in the sector format.) Thus, deeper structures are not as clear as more superficial structures. Resolution also depends on the number of crystals in the probe and the machine's ability to sharpen the image using mathematical techniques. Resolution may also increase with different focusing techniques. The vertical resolution depends primarily on the pulse length and purity, which can vary by manufacturer. Because an ultrasound image is produced by sending out a short pulse and then listening to reflections, a shorter pulse will be able to "see" smaller objects. Note that horizontal and vertical resolution are specified separately because they depend on different factors in the probes and machine electronics.

Contrast Resolution. Contrast resolution is a measure of how well the probe and machine can differentiate structures of slightly different echogenicity. If the contrast resolution is very high, structures with only slightly different echogenicity will appear as separate images on the screen. If contrast resolution is low, these structures may not be differentiated on the screen. Although this specification is not often provided by manufacturers, it can be estimated by looking at the number of gray levels the machine uses. If this number is high, the contrast resolution should be good. If this number is low, the contrast resolution will be less, and it may be more difficult to distinguish a placenta from the uterine wall. Note that most machines use either 128 or 256 gray levels. However, many actually display only 16 or 32 on the screen or image. The grays that are actually displayed can be changed with the post-processing controls. Nevertheless, the sonographer should carefully evaluate image quality with this factor in mind when choosing a machine.

Frame Rate. During the examination, the frame rate or number of images displayed per second on the monitor may be a factor. Most machines display an image at 20 to 30 frames/second, which is adequate. However, the frame rate is different for each probe. If various zoom features, multiple focal zones, M-mode, or Doppler is used, the frame rate may decrease dramatically. Consequently, a fetal heart that may be beating 150 times/minute (2.5 times/second) may be difficult to visualize if the frame rate is only 5/second. Note that this specification directly relates to the quality of the machine's electronics. Because ultrasound machines are essentially computers (they contain chips like those in personal computers), it is not surprising that newer models with faster electronics can update the screen more quickly than older models. Also note that the machine software can sometimes be upgraded, which might also affect the frame rate.

Invasive Procedure Options. Laboratories that do invasive procedures under ultrasound guidance will need biopsy guide options. This usually consists of a device that attaches to the probe to guide a needle or other device into the body. The manufacturer usually provides a software package to display a guide on the screen and depict the path that the needle will take as it is inserted. For some biopsy guides, a spring-loaded option may be available. This device propels a needle rapidly to a preset depth along a path defined on the screen by software. Although this does not differ in principle from a freehand approach for introducing a needle into a pelvic structure, the rapidity of needle introduction by this device avoids much of the organ movement that may make the freehand technique inaccurate. It also greatly reduces the need for analgesia.

For other procedures, some companies now manufacture a rotating transducer that fits in a narrow catheter, allowing the entire transducer to be inserted deep into the body. Although this is primarily used in blood vessels, other locations may be suitable for future applications of this very small probe.

Probe Calibration and Maintenance

Every ultrasound probe is different, so an ultrasound machine performs internal adjustments, usually automatically, to modify performance to obtain a good image. Also, the measurements that are displayed on the screen from one point to another need to be accurate. Although the calibration adjustments cannot be performed by the sonographer, a calibration check can be done. Specifically, it is important periodically to test every ultrasound probe on an accurately measured phantom to check image quality as well as measurement accuracy. If the measurements displayed on the screen do not match the phantom, a service technician should be called.

Image quality is another area the sonographer can check. Although it will usually be obvious during an actual scan if a probe is not performing well, there are some techniques that can be used to determine whether the probe is scanning optimally. For linear or curvilinear probes, the transducer crystals are lined up and can be individually tested by placing a small amount of gel on the probe and taking a thin key (e.g., from your key ring) and sliding it along the probe. If all the transducer crystals are operating, a vertical line will be seen moving smoothly from one side of the screen to the other. If any of the crystals are bad, the line will seem to move in a jerky fashion in the vicinity of the bad crystal. In the case of sector probes (which generate the image by different means), the probe can be placed on the phantom and rotated so that one of the reflections moves from one edge of the sector to the other. In this case, the reflections depend on many transducers, so the effect may not be as dramatic if there is one bad crystal. Nevertheless, as the probe is rotated, the brightness of the reflection on the screen should not vary.

Finally, in the case of mechanical probes, the fluid in the probe should not have any air bubbles in it. An air bubble will severely degrade the image, and if the bubble is large enough, the image may flicker. The sonographer often can add additional fluid to the probe to displace the air bubble.

User Interface

The physical features of machine operation are often called the *user interface*. This consists of both the data input system (transducers, keyboard, joystick, or trackball and their physical characteristics) and the data processing system (software for manipulating images and characters). There is a considerable amount of variability from machine to machine and also variability in operator preference. The interface should be chosen by the person who will operate the machine.

When selecting an image, the sonographer tries to obtain as good an image as possible before making the final adjustments. Selection of an image is a part of the user interface. Newer machines can store many images because of advances in microelectronics. As the images are being displayed, the machine stores the last several frames in its memory. If the sonographer freezes the image but notices that a better image was being displayed just a split second before the "freeze" was activated, most modern machines allow the user to play back the most recent images from memory. This allows selection of the best possible image. Of all the components of the user interface, playback of previous images is one of the most useful newer developments. However, every machine is different, and some machines have faster electronics than others. A slow machine may take several seconds to start playing back its image memory, whereas another machine will display past images almost instantaneously.

Most machines have controls only on the console. However, some have detachable control panels or keyboards. Some have auxiliary keyboards, and a few have true remote controls to allow the sonographer to stand some distance from the machine. This can be advantageous if one is doing a transvaginal examination on an obese patient. A hand-held control may be much easier to manipulate. Some machines may even be operated primarily from a mouse. Finally, some machines have limited remote control capability on the transducers themselves.

A foot pedal may be available for some machines, allowing the operator to freeze the screen, take pictures, or operate a video recorder. During a transvaginal ultrasound examination, a foot pedal may be helpful when the sonographer is holding the probe with one hand and manipulating the organs through the abdominal wall with the other hand.

The keyboard has many variations. Some have true typewriter-style keys. Others are membrane keyboards, such as those found on a calculator, and there are touch-sensitive pads, such as those found in elevators. All have advantages and disadvantages. True typewriter keys are usually the easiest to use but may be the most prone to breakage owing to mechanical failure or dust (flexible plastic keyboard covers may help). Membrane keyboards are the least expensive to produce, are often found on inexpensive machines, and are impervious to dust. However, they may be difficult to operate because of the limited travel of the keys themselves. Finally, the touch-sensitive keys are the most rugged because they have no moving parts and are also impervious to dust. Again, they may be difficult to operate because of their lack of motion. Another problem with some keyboards is their size. Smaller machines often have smaller keyboards, and this may impede the sonographer's typing. Whatever keyboard is chosen, the "best" one is the one that suits the personal preference of the sonographer.

When an ultrasound machine is turned on, it usually has the correct date and time on the screen. This clock is usually run by an internal battery. One minor consideration is whether this battery can be replaced by the operator. Battery life is another feature. Usually, user-replaceable batteries last only 1 or 2 years but are easy to replace. A non–user-replaceable battery may last as long as 10 years but may be expensive to replace if the machine is not covered by a service contract. Finally, some machines may contain an energy storage device that keeps the clock running without a battery. Although these devices are reliable, they may not work for more than a few days if the machine is left unplugged.

Most recent machines feature alternative forms of data input. These include a joystick, trackball, mouse, touch screen, barcode wand, and others. A joystick is usually an acceleration device. When the operator pushes the stick to one side, the cursor (spot on the screen) moves in that direction. When the stick is released, the cursor stops moving. Some joysticks may be position devices, in which the position of the cursor depends on the physical location of the stick. This type of operation may be more difficult to use because of inaccuracies in stick movement. The trackball and mouse are also position devices but may be easier to use because a more pronounced movement of the device is necessary to produce a certain movement on the screen. Both are similarly easy to use. The mouse requires a flat surface on the machine to operate but is easy to service if it stops working. The trackball takes less space on the console but may be more difficult to service if it fails. In my experience, trackballs rarely fail and consequently are the preferred device. The touch screen allows the operator to point his or her finger at the screen to make a choice rather than using a trackball or joystick to point electronically at the screen. Finally, a barcode wand may be used in some situations to "read" patient information. Although I have not seen this feature in ultrasound machines, it is available in some laboratory equipment and is mentioned here for completeness. As more and more offices convert to picture archiving on computers and electronic medical records, barcode wands may appear in ultrasound installations. Another type of patient identification is RFID—radiofrequency identification. There is much discussion in the literature about this technology in medical applications and it could theoretically be used in ultrasound machines.

The operation of the machine is usually controlled from a keyboard or from a separate set of keys or switches on the console. Some machines use menus or choices displayed on the monitor. Other machines have dedicated keys or switches for major functions. If keys are used, these may be labeled with the function (e.g., "FREEZE") or may have an international symbol. In sonography, however, there is no international standard for machine symbols, and consequently these can be confusing. Other machines may use a combination of keys from the keyboard to control some functions. These work well but may not be readily obvious from either the keyboard or the monitor screen. The best systems, in my opinion, are either the dedicated keys with word labels or the screens with menus.

It is difficult to go into great detail about machine operation in a generic sense because the operations of the various features are so different. There are, however, several features that may be advantageous.

One of the most important features for transvaginal sonography is a variable zoom that allows a structure to be moved on the screen after the zoom is engaged. In other words, once the zoomed image is on the screen, the operator often will move the probe to get a slightly better view. When this happens, the structure of interest may move from the screen. If the zoomed area can also be moved without displaying the entire image again, the examination can be continued without waiting for the machine to reset itself. Some machines may allow the zoomed image to move even after the image is frozen. This feature greatly improves the efficiency of high-resolution transvaginal sonography.

Another important aspect of machine operation is software speed. A potential user of a machine should try the various features to see how long the machine takes to turn a feature on or off and how fast the cursor moves in response to a joystick or trackball. Because all ultrasound machines are basically modified computers, some processors are faster than others, and this can determine how fast the machine will react to a particular command from the operator. In some cases, the boot-up process of the internal computer may take several minutes, which can adversely affect the efficiency of mobile operations.

Modality Selection

Current modalities for ultrasound machines include B-mode (gray-scale image), M-mode (motion), Doppler (flow studies at a single point), color Doppler (flow studies covering an area of the image), and power Doppler. Three-dimensional (3D) imaging has also become common. Three-dimensional imaging involves storing many (dozens to hundreds) two-dimensional (2D) images and calculating a 3D view. These machines are used to display meaningful structures by extracting what is important (e.g., the boundary of the structure) and discarding what is not. For example, when we look at a person, we see only the boundary (skin and clothes)—we do not see inside. The computer must do the same thing, and this can take a long time for each image. A 3D machine can also create a two-dimensional image of a structure that would not be possible with standard probes. One example is an axial image from a transvaginal probe.

M-mode and Doppler Ultrasound

Two modalities that complement real-time sonography are M-mode and Doppler. An M-mode ultrasound scan is obtained to view the movements of a structure along an imaginary line that is placed on the screen by the sonographer. This line is placed exactly on top of the structure that is being investigated. The line, which directly determines the size of the M-mode tracing, should be as short as possible while still covering the structure being examined. Many machines that offer M-mode images allow the length and location of the line to be changed. However, some allow only limited changes. This is another area that may not be well described in a machine's specifications. The various gain controls of the machine can usually produce an excellent tracing that displays the information of interest. However, the sweep speed of the M-mode tracing may not be adjustable on some machines. A faster speed may be useful for examining the structure of a fetal heart, whereas a slower speed may be better for studying fetal breathing.

Doppler ultrasound is usually performed to study blood flow. This modality was discussed extensively in Chapter 2. However, an important feature of this modality is that it requires a stronger ultrasound beam, and the sonographer must pay attention to this when using Doppler in certain situations. In some cases, the manufacturers state clearly that the transmitted power is greater than 100 mW/cm². If the power

levels are high, most machines provide a low-power setting at the expense of image quality.

Color Doppler

Color Doppler is one of the most exciting developments in sonography. For most scans, color is useful for locating blood vessels. The production of color-coded information involves a tremendous amount of electronic processing in the ultrasound machine. Although much of the technique was described in Chapter 2, there are a few additional important points. First, color will not reveal all blood vessels. This is because blood cells reflect ultrasound energy rather poorly, and a fairly large amount of blood is needed to register flow on the screen. Therefore, although other chapters in this book describe the usefulness of measuring blood flow in various tumors, some tumors may not have measurable flow. A second point concerns perseverance. Although this book describes the measurement of flow in various organs and tumors, the location of this flow, even with a good machine, may be difficult to ascertain and require more time than one would think. Finally, it must be emphasized that flow, whether displayed in color or in graph form, can be detected only if the vessel is not parallel to the probe surface.

Power Doppler

Power Doppler is similar to color Doppler except that the color image reflects the power or strength of moving objects (usually blood cells), without regard to direction of flow. Because direction is not displayed, it is immune to aliasing.

Scanning Route Selection

All modalities can be used for both transabdominal and transvaginal sonography. However, the choice of scanning route depends more on the purpose of the scan than on the type of modality. Each route has its advantages and limitations.

Transabdominal Sonography

Transabdominal scanning was the first to be developed. Its advantages include relative comfort for the patient (although a full bladder for certain types of examinations may cause some discomfort), a wide variety of probes, ability to move the probe in all directions, ability to scan large fetuses or large pelvic tumors, ability to scan other organs such as the kidneys, liver, gallbladder, and spleen, and increased depth of penetration of most probes.

The primary limitation of transabdominal scanning is decreased resolution, which has several causes. First, the frequency of abdominal probes is usually lower than that of most transvaginal probes. Because higher-frequency probes have better resolution, the high-frequency transvaginal probe produces a better image of the same structure viewed transabdominally. Second, transabdominal scanning is done through the abdominal wall, which contains fat, tendons, and muscle. All three of these structures act as sonic lenses to distort the ultrasound image. Consequently, a transabdominal image at one frequency will *always* be poorer than a transvaginal image of the same structure at the same frequency. The best analogy for this is a comparison of an earth-based telescope with a space telescope: because of the lack of an intervening substance (air), the space telescope produces better images. Third, the relatively greater distance to the organs being studied further decreases the resolution of the image of these structures. Fourth, transabdominal scanning of deep pelvic organs is limited if the bladder is empty. Without the distended bladder as contrast, intestines fill the pelvis and literally hide the pelvic organs. Fifth, loops of bowel may contain air, which totally blocks a view of deeper structures.

Transvaginal Sonography

The primary advantage of transvaginal sonography is the marked increase in resolution. The proximity of the probe to the pelvic organs allows the use of a high-frequency probe, which provides details in the submillimeter range. Although this technique requires insertion of the probe into the vagina, the procedure is no more uncomfortable than obtaining a Pap smear. In addition, because this examination is performed with an empty bladder, it may be more comfortable for some patients than a transabdominal scan with a full bladder. Three other advantages are unique to the transvaginal probe. The first is the ability to touch the pelvic organs with the probe to test for pain. Because the probe is literally only 1 cm or less from the organs, this is an excellent method to determine the source of some types of pelvic pain. Another advantage is the ability to move the pelvic organs with the probe to see if they slide easily. If they do not, adhesions may be diagnosed. A final advantage also involves the proximity of the probe to the organs. It is sometimes necessary to image organs at a different depth to reduce various artifacts such as ring-down or reverberation. The transvaginal probe can be pulled out of or pushed into the vagina to adjust the depth of the organs on the screen—a unique advantage in sonography.

The limitations of transvaginal sonography concern penetration and mobility. Because the transvaginal probe is a high-frequency probe, its depth of penetration is limited. This means that large myomatous uteri or a fetus greater than 14 to 16 weeks' gestation cannot be easily scanned. The second disadvantage is lack of mobility. Because of the confines of the introitus, the probe cannot be moved in all dimensions, and some views of organs may be limited.

Documentation

This discussion consists of two parts. The first is technical and describes calibration and adjustment of the equipment, including recording devices. The second discussion includes some of the medical-legal aspects of documenting an ultrasound examination. The reader is also directed to the end of the chapter, where a trouble-shooting guide presents various images that relate to adjusting the equipment.

Technical Factors

Before an examination is performed, the imaging equipment, including monitors, printers, and recorders, should be adjusted and synchronized. This means that an image presented in one medium should look identical to an image presented in another medium. When the sonographer reviews an image, problems may arise if a stored image looks different from the image that was on the screen at the time of the examination.

Adjusting an Image

The following is a suggested method for adjusting the display screen:

1. The brightness and contrast are adjusted to make the background black and the brightest color completely white.
2. If there is any "blooming" or enlarging of bright objects, the brightness should be decreased until that artifact disappears.
3. The contrast is adjusted to see all levels of gray in the display distinctly.
4. The brightness is readjusted as necessary to maintain a black background and bright white for the whitest areas on the screen.
5. Steps 3 and 4 are repeated as necessary until there is no further improvement to the image.

When the display has been properly adjusted, the camera or printer should be adjusted in the same manner to make the image on the hard copy identical to the image on the screen. Once the controls are set, they should not be further adjusted. Only machine gain, power, postprocessing, and so forth should be adjusted to improve image quality and avoid losing image synchronization. Most video recorders have an automatic level control that is quite effective; it normally does not require adjustment.

Recording an Image

Recording an image is perhaps the second most important part of the ultrasound examination, after obtaining the image itself. There are basically three main types of archiving: hard copy (paper and film), analog video (tape or possibly disk), and computer (digital) storage. Each of these will be presented in a general way. However, the different types of equipment are beyond the scope of this chapter and are best investigated by the individual practitioner after a methodology is chosen. The one factor that is fairly standard among all the modalities, regardless of the system, is that image capture is usually performed by pressing a button or stepping on a foot pedal.

Hard Copy. The oldest type of archiving is hard copy. The various types include a Polaroid picture of the ultrasound screen, images on x-ray film, thermal images (a development in the past 15 years, partly as a result of the maturing facsimile [fax] industry), images on slides, and images on a laser printer (black and white as well as color). There are advantages and disadvantages to a hard-copy system. The advantages include immediate and rapid evaluation of the images, excellent image resolution, and ease of comparison with a previous examination. In the previous edition of this book, a claim was made that only hard-copy images from different examinations could be placed side by side for comparison. However, with the advent of modern computerized archiving systems, this claim is no longer true. The disadvantages of hard-copy archiving include cost (a color image can cost $1.00 per copy), difficulty in making copies after the examination is concluded (often requiring the services of a photographic studio), and increased personnel time (processing of x-ray film often takes several minutes per patient). Nevertheless, despite its disadvantages, the hard-copy alternative is a tried-and-true methodology for maintaining images.

Analog Video. Attaching a video cassette recorder to an ultrasound machine is easy and inexpensive, and it allows recording the real-time aspects of an examination. It is also easy to copy the images. Although an entire day's examinations may be recorded on a single cassette, locating a specific examination may be difficult. Because the tape may need to be rewound and then forwarded to the correct spot, a specific image may take a significant amount of time to locate. On the other hand, if a single patient is assigned to a single cassette, storage space will fill up rapidly. Although some higher-end video systems record on a magnetic disk, they usually are not used in medical settings, and thus analog video recording is usually done only on video cassette.

Digital Storage. Computer storage, also called *picture archiving computer systems* (PACS), uses an electronic method to digitize the analog image from the ultrasound machine or, in some machines, extract a digital image directly and store it in the computer. The advantages include almost immediate retrieval, good resolution, and ease of copying the image to a hard-copy device. Most machines can transmit the image in digital format. As computer storage becomes more prevalent (and less expensive), this digital interface will become the primary image storage mechanism. If real-time images are needed for future review, a DVD (digital versatile disk) is an excellent and cost-effective means of storing these data.

The primary disadvantage of PACS is cost. The research and development process for the software (computer programs) to run these systems is expensive. Although the actual equipment and technology are not expensive (about $1000 to $5000 per ultrasound machine, depending on the system, and $5000 to tens of thousands of dollars for the actual computer storage), the cost of the software is high. As programming techniques improve and systems evolve, the cost of these systems will drop as rapidly as the costs of computers themselves. At that point, the biggest cost of the system will be maintenance.

The incremental cost of storing images on a computer is low. A CD can store several thousand images and costs less than $1. Whereas an optical CD used to cost as much as $100, the cost of storage has dropped to less than $.01 per image. Ultimately, PACS will be the equipment of choice, and other hard image systems will disappear, just as static ultrasound systems have disappeared in favor of real-time systems. This transformation will likely occur within a few years of the publication of this edition.

Medical-Legal Issues

There are many components to good documentation of an examination. Some of them may seem trivial, but in the medical-legal world, both lawyers and doctors have many examples of charts in which some of the following precepts were not followed, and problems resulted. Good documentation of an ultrasound examination involves the following:

- Document all of the findings.
- Document what is seen.
- Document the date (and time) of the findings.
- Avoid adjectives.
- Label the images.
- Make hard copies.
- Do a complete examination.
- Write legibly.
- Do not argue in the chart.
- Follow Rosen's Rules.
- Use the correct machine.

Document All of the Findings. When the patient's scan is finished and the information is fresh in the sonographer's mind, the findings should be written or dictated immediately. The findings need to be recorded anyway, and it will be much faster to record the information immediately after the examination when it is remembered most vividly.

Second, notes should be taken during an examination because important facts may occur to the sonographer during a complex scan that might not be remembered later. An ultrasound scan is a dynamic process, and not all of the images may be recorded (unless everything is videotaped). Because some images are better than others, a good description of the findings can help compensate for certain recorded images that may not be as clear as some of those seen during the scan.

Document What Is Seen. When a sonographer performs an examination, it is easy to draw conclusions based on what is visualized. However, the patient's care provider (physician or otherwise), not the sonographer, should be the one to make the diagnosis in most cases. Making a wrong diagnosis can create considerable difficulty for the sonographer. If the sonographer merely describes all the structures that are visualized during the examination, other clinicians can then use this information to diagnose the patient's problem.

Sonographers should avoid describing something they think they see. For example, if the fetal head cannot be clearly visualized, one should state "the fetal head could not be visualized owing to its position" rather than "the fetus appeared to be normal within the limits of the examination." Although both statements are basically correct, the second may imply that the sonographer saw more than he or she actually did.

Document the Date (and Time) of the Findings. In medicine, timing can be crucial. There is no question that a scan for fetal gestational age must be properly dated to provide the correct information to the obstetrician. Similarly, the evaluation of infertility requires precise measurements of follicular size and endometrial thickness correlated to the dating of the patient's menstrual cycle. Consequently, all ultrasound machines today superimpose the date and usually the time on every image. The job of the sonographer is to make sure that the date and time are correct and match the date and time in the report that is sent to the physician.

Avoid Adjectives. Words such as *inadvertent* should be banished from medical reports. If this word is used, it can be construed as "mistake." In documenting a curettage performed under ultrasound guidance, the physician may describe a perforation during the procedure with the following: "When Dr. Jones was curetting the right horn of the bicornuate uterus, he inadvertently perforated the fundus medial to the tube insertion." Although everyone knows that Dr. Jones had good intentions, someone else (a lawyer or juror) may interpret the word *inadvertently* as "carelessly" or "incompetently." In this case, *inadvertently* can be omitted from the report without changing its meaning and may avoid medical-legal problems later.

In general, adjectives are an unnecessary part of a medical report. When a cyst is described, just give its dimensions. It is unnecessary to state that it is "massive" or "huge." The size of a structure may mean one thing for one patient and something else for another patient.

Label the Images. All structures should be labeled. When a scan is ongoing, it is usually easy to identify the various structures on the screen. However, when scans are reviewed retrospectively, it may be difficult to determine what structures are in a particular view. Furthermore, if the sonographer who performed the scan is not available to interpret the images later, lack of labels can make interpretation of the examination practically impossible. Complete labeling of images may prolong the examination slightly but will save time later and make interpretation easier.

Make Hard Copies. If images are recorded, it is easy to prove what was seen in the context of subsequent controversy. If the images are not recorded, it is as if the situation in question had not occurred at all. Just as videotape is now revealing situations in police and government work that previously "did not occur," the liberal use of pictures in sonography can help avoid problems by properly recording all portions of the examination. One can imagine what would happen if a sonographer scanned a patient and found a fetal death but did not take any pictures. Later, if the patient claimed that the fetus was alive when she went to the physician's office, medical-legal difficulties might occur if the sonographer could not document what was found in the examination.

Do a Complete Examination. In a brief examination, the sonographer might image only the area of interest and not look at all the structures in the pelvis. However, in the presence of an ill-defined intrauterine sac, for instance, it is possible to have a coexisting ectopic pregnancy in the adnexum. If a complete examination is performed, this will not be missed.

A good way to ensure that a complete examination is performed is always to perform a pelvic ultrasound examination in the same order. Whether the uterus is examined first and the adnexa last, or vice versa, is unimportant. However, the fact that all organs were examined (or a documented attempt was made to examine them) may be significant in retrospect.

Similarly, an obstetric scan should include a survey of the entire fetus. Occasionally a patient may present for a routine scan and the complete examination finds an unexpected problem. Some ultrasound facilities have a policy of doing a complete anatomic survey with biometry if the patient has not been scanned within approximately 3 weeks, even if the reason for the scan is as simple as checking the amniotic fluid volume.

Write Legibly. If later the sonographer cannot read his or her report of the examination, it is almost as bad as not writing the report at all. If the report is barely legible, the extra time it takes to read it probably outweighs the slight increase in time for preparation of a legible report in the first place.

Do Not Argue in the Chart. Sometimes clinicians do not agree. However, they should argue behind closed doors and not in the chart. If there is a permanent record of arguments in the chart, an outside party may use this argument as a basis for a lawsuit. If one opinion is not appropriate, it may be used as a basis for a malpractice lawsuit. In particular, if someone writes that a particular diagnosis or procedure is "wrong" or "risky," the medical-legal problems will be more serious if a complication occurs, even if the complication is a known risk ahead of time. If a group of physicians must argue on paper, this should be done on scraps of paper that are not permanent parts of the chart (e.g., message pads). Once the message has been read, the note can be discarded. However, in general, it is best not to use written notes at all but instead to talk with one's colleagues, so a case can be completely discussed and the consensus opinion then written in the chart.

Follow Rosen's Rules. Mortimer Rosen, the former chairman of the Department of Obstetrics and Gynecology at Columbia University College of Physicians and Surgeons in New York, promoted the following statements related to medicine and law:

1. If you practice good obstetrics and have a good outcome, you will not be sued.
2. If you practice bad obstetrics but have a good outcome, you will not be sued.
3. If you practice good obstetrics but have a bad outcome, you may be sued.
4. If you practice bad obstetrics and have a bad outcome, you may be sued (and probably should be sued—Dr. Rosen's comment).

His conclusion was that if a lawsuit is going to be started, it will be because of the outcome. The quality of a practice, according to these rules, has little influence on whether a lawsuit will be filed. Therefore, one may as well practice good obstetrics (and sonography) because it makes sense, and if there is a bad outcome it will be easier to defend it if the practice meets the standard of care. In terms of sonography, sound practice involves good documentation of examinations in addition to comprehensive scanning: a little planning and attention to detail now may avoid larger problems in the future.

Use the Correct Machine. Some machines are better suited to certain tasks than others. Some probes are better than others for certain examinations. To document a finding properly, the patient should be examined on the appropriate machine. If the machine is not appropriate, do not let the patient leave the ultrasound suite without examining her on another machine. In some cases, the best diagnosis may be made if the patient is scanned on different machines to obtain multiple views of the same structure. A good analogy of this is the documentation of the *Challenger* space shuttle accident in 1986. All the cameras showed the shuttle exploding, but *different* selected cameras revealed gases escaping on the launch pad and, later, fire coming out of one of the solid rocket joints. All the cameras were technically good, but because of different kinds of specialization, some were better suited than others to reveal a specific aspect of the investigation. This concept also holds for medical examinations.

Trouble-shooting Guide

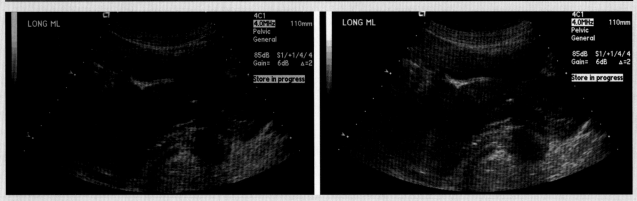

Figure 3A–1

The image on the left is dark because the brightness is too low. Part of the gray scale is missing, and the image itself is too dark. A clue to this problem is the fact that the letters (which are normally bright) are also dark on the left but are brighter in the normal image on the right.

Solution: Increase the display brightness until the entire gray scale is seen.

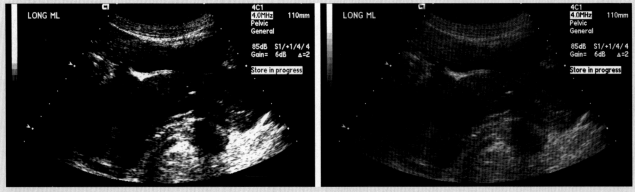

Figure 3A–2

The image on the left seems dark, and the problem is too much contrast. Note that the letters are quite bright, but the gray scale contains only a few levels of gray. In fact, an image with too much contrast can be too dark, just right (see Fig. 3A–7), or too bright (see Fig. 3A–5), depending on where the brightness level is set. In this case, the contrast is too high but the brightness is also low.

Solution: Decrease the contrast to allow more gray levels to be seen and then adjust the brightness. (Note that on some machines, the contrast and brightness controls will interact with each other, and multiple adjustments may be required to get them right, as noted in the text.)

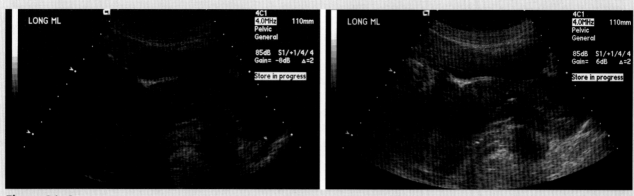

Figure 3A–3

The image on the left is too dark because the gain on the ultrasound machine is too low. Note that the brightness of the letters is normal and that the entire gray scale is visible (compare with Fig. 3A–1). What may have happened here is that the sonographer turned up the brightness on the screen so much that the gain had to be decreased to get a reasonable picture. This makes it difficult to make a good hard copy because the range of the printer may not be as good as the range displayable on the screen.

Solution: Make sure the display is set properly with bright letters and the entire gray scale, *then* adjust the ultrasound gain to obtain a pleasing image, and *then* adjust the printer settings so the image matches the screen.

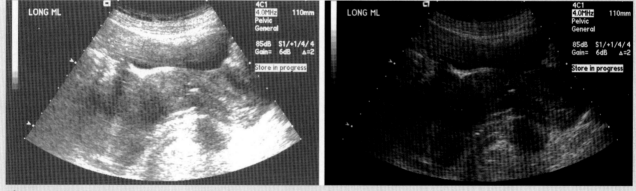

Figure 3A–4

The image on the left is too bright because the brightness is set too high. Almost all the gray scale is visible, but the image overall is too bright. A key to this is the fact that the background, which should normally be jet black, is gray in this image.

Solution: Decrease the brightness until the background is black.

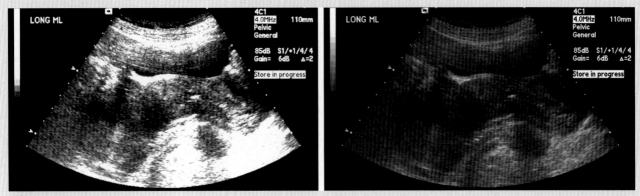

Figure 3A–5

The image on the left seems bright, but the problem here is too much contrast (compare with Figs. 3A–2 and 3A–7). The key points are that the letters are quite bright but the gray scale contains few levels of gray. In this case, the brightness of the display has also been increased.

Solution: Decrease the contrast to allow more gray levels to be seen, then adjust the brightness, ultrasound machine settings, and finally the printer controls to obtain good images. (Note that on some machines, the contrast and brightness controls will interact with each other, and multiple adjustments may be required to get them right, as noted in the text.)

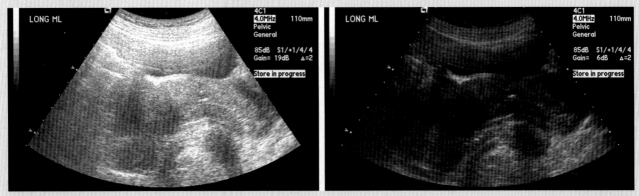

Figure 3A–6

The image on the left is too bright because the gain on the ultrasound machine is too high. Note that the brightness of the letters is normal and the entire gray scale is visible and is identical to that in the normal image on the right (compare with Figs. 3A–1 and 3A–3). What may have happened here is that the sonographer turned down the brightness on the screen so much that the gain had to be increased to get a reasonable picture. This makes it difficult to make a good hard copy because the range of the printer may not be as good as the range displayable on the screen.

Solution: Increase the screen controls and decrease the gain on the ultrasound machine, then adjust the printer controls to match the screen.

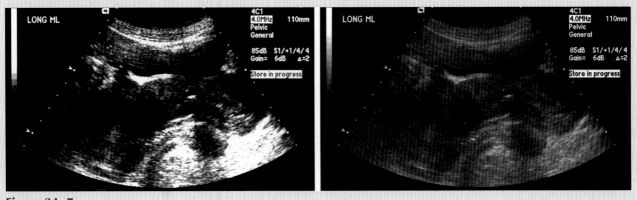

Figure 3A–7

The image on the left consists mostly of black and white, with very little gray. The problem is that the contrast setting is too high. The key observation here is that the gray scale at the side of the image has very little actual gray; it is mostly black or white.

Solution: Adjust the contrast to allow all the levels of gray to be seen. If shades of gray cannot be seen, some image information may have been lost.

Chapter 4

Conducting the Gynecologic Ultrasound Examination

Ilan E. Timor-Tritsch

This chapter will equip the sonologist (a physician trained in ultrasound) and sonographer (an ultrasound technician) with the necessary information for obtaining the best results in scanning the female pelvis. The first part of the chapter deals with issues pertinent to beginners in imaging the female pelvis. We have attempted to provide a concise and practical summary of the main technical aspects, and the reader is referred to some of the detailed resources available.[1-6]

Preparation and Equipment

Examination Table

Most gynecologic and obstetric patients are examined and scanned on a gynecologic table. Such a table is equipped with a foot rest for the lithotomy position, which facilitates transvaginal scanning. An extendable leg support is also available for transabdominal ultrasound scanning in the supine position. On a flat examination table, using a transvaginal probe would be rather cumbersome, indeed almost impossible, unless the pelvis is elevated, which would enable the probe handle to be tilted backward.

Some recent examination tables have been fitted with swinging arms to support the placement of a colposcope and to accommodate a smaller type of ultrasound machine.

Patient Preparation: Empty Bladder versus Full Bladder

Because of their physical properties, transabdominal and transvaginal probes are different.[7-12] The choice of scanning method depends on the goal of scanning. The status of the patient's bladder should also be considered. It is easier to empty the urinary bladder than to fill it—an important point to consider before sending the patient to the toilet to empty her bladder.

The transabdominal probe enables a panoramic view of the pelvis, showing anatomic interrelationships and possible pathologic findings. It is equipped with crystals that emit lower-frequency ultrasound, which penetrates deep into the pelvis. With this probe, a full bladder is needed to displace interposing bowel loops; consequently, a full bladder also displaces the pelvic organs even farther away from the face of the transducer. However, a full bladder does provide a convenient acoustic window into the pelvis.

The transvaginal probe, however, is placed close to the pelvic organs and therefore does not need to penetrate more than 7 to 10 cm to image a smaller section of the pelvic organs. Usually the bowel does not interfere with transvaginal sonography. A full bladder would displace the pelvic organs by interposing itself between the transducer tip and pelvic organs, at times pushing the region of interest beyond the effective focal range of the vaginal probe. Hence, transvaginal sonography is usually performed with a completely or mostly empty urinary bladder.

In most laboratories, if the patient is being seen for the first time, transabdominal sonography (with a full bladder) is performed before transvaginal scanning. This avoids the problem of having to fill the bladder if an unsatisfactory transvaginal image is obtained.

For the same reason, a patient suspected of having an ectopic pregnancy should undergo transabdominal sonography before transvaginal sonography, and the patient should not be allowed to drink at all in anticipation of possible surgery. If the bladder is empty, however, transvaginal sonography is performed first, and usually by the end of this examination enough urine will have trickled into the bladder to enable transabdominal sonography.

Some distention of the bladder may be useful when scanning patients with a severely anteflexed uterus. The bladder elevates or straightens the uterus, as is desirable for performing chorionic villus sampling. Some urine in the bladder is helpful when imaging a low-lying placenta or placenta previa, as well as for performing transvaginal cervical studies.[13-19] In these cases, the "lower corner" of the bladder serves as the marker of the anterior cervical lip. Benacerraf and colleagues clearly question whether a full bladder is still needed for a comprehensive ultrasound examination.[18,19]

Pelvic Examination and Patient Education

Patients sent to specialized ultrasound laboratories usually do not receive a routine pelvic examination there; these laboratories are guided by the information provided by the obstetrician-gynecologist. Before a patient is scanned in the gynecologist's office or emergency department, however, a detailed and thorough pelvic examination is done to provide the examiner with general information; if the patient has a palpable abnormality, it can be investigated closely using sonography. A vaginal examination performed before or perhaps after the ultrasound examination will help correlate the findings with the image obtained. This pelvic palpatory examination is even more useful if there is a discrepancy between the obtained image and the expected image.

Informing the patient about the kind of examination she is about to undergo is important. Information can be conveyed to the patient in three ways. Probably the best way is for the patient to be informed by the gynecologist, during the bimanual pelvic examination or in the gynecologist's office, about a sonographic examination she will need to undergo. At this time, the words *transabdominal* and *transvaginal* should be explained. Another way is for the patient to be provided with printed material, readily available in most countries. The third and probably least satisfactory way is for the patient to be informed about scanning when she is about to be seated on the examination table for the scanning procedure. At this time patients cannot ask many questions, and in our experience most patients who refuse a transvaginal scan do so in this context. If transvaginal examination is to be performed, the operator should point out the similarity between the vaginal transducer and the familiar vaginal speculum and explain that the procedure resembles a Pap test, which the patient has probably experienced before. The patient should be reassured that the probe is small; it is helpful to show her the probe. Some laboratories allow the patient to insert the probe into her vagina.

It is anticipated that in the near future all women will have some familiarity with customary ultrasound examinations and scanning routes. In fact, in most cases it is currently unnecessary to explain the technicalities involved in transabdominal sonography, as this procedure is familiar.

Equipment and Transducers

A detailed explanation of the equipment and the available transducers is found in Chapter 3. Here, a more clinically oriented discussion of the use of the equipment and transducers is provided.

It is important to prepare and program the equipment before the examination begins. This is especially important when a transvaginal scan is planned. The patient's identification data, the date of her last menstrual period, and other pertinent observations should be typed using the keyboard. Recording devices such as the video cassette recorder, different cameras, or printers should be switched to a position that enables their immediate operation. It is helpful to have a foot switch to freeze the screen and then take hard copies of the desired images. This is crucial for transvaginal sonography because the operator needs both hands, one to manipulate the probe and the other to manipulate the pelvic content through the abdominal wall.

Transabdominal probes are usually used uncovered; however, transvaginal probes are inserted in a protective sheath.[20] This can be a commercially available condom or the digit of a surgical rubber glove (which does not need to be sterile). Condoms are very thin, however, and they have slight imperfections and may rupture; therefore, based on our expe-

rience, if a higher degree of protection from infection is desired, the slightly thicker layer provided by the digit of a surgical rubber glove should be considered. Amis et al.[21] assessed condoms as probe covers for transvaginal sonography. They showed that condoms have a low rate of perforation and that disinfecting the probes with isopropyl alcohol wipes further reduces the risk of contamination. Ultrasound coupling gel must be placed inside the protective cover to enable smooth passage of the sound waves from the transducer to the pelvic organs. Recently, individually packaged thin plastic covers have become available. These are provided with an adequate amount of coupling gel inside the cover.

It was postulated that use of common ultrasound coupling gels for lubricating vaginal transducers has a negative effect on sperm penetration, so it has been suggested that patients undergoing insemination immediately after transvaginal examination should avoid the use of these gels.[22] At or close to mid-cycle, the cervix produces plenty of mucus to enable a good coupling between the transducer and vagina; it is also possible to perform the scan using normal saline.

Cleaning the probes is important. Transabdominal and transvaginal probes should be wiped of the gel first, after which an alcohol spray or alcohol sponge may be used to clean the probe thoroughly. In the United States, to obtain accreditation, an ultrasound facility must be compliant with the guidelines for cleaning and preparing endocavitary transducers between patients (see the Appendix of this book for a copy of this document). However, if other disinfectants are anticipated, it is wise to contact the probe manufacturer to ask about safe and effective cleaning and disinfecting methods. A practical method is to insert the probe in a disinfecting solution at the end of an examination, and by the time the next patient is ready for examination, sufficient time has elapsed to enable a complete cleaning of the probe. Odwin et al.[23] have provided some guidelines for the different solutions available to disinfect probes.

Techniques

Techniques for Transabdominal and Transvaginal Scanning

The different kinds of probes used in transabdominal and transvaginal scanning are discussed in Chapter 3, and the characteristics of these two techniques are compared in Table 4–1.

The use of transabdominal probes is straightforward. The clinician may use a 3.5- or a 5-MHz probe. The linear or curved two-dimensional (2D) or three-dimensional (3D) transducer array probes provide a wider scanning field, whereas the sector probes are usually designed to enable a narrower scanning angle, thereby producing higher-resolution pictures. The motion of the probe on the abdominal wall and the scanning plane is obvious to the scanner, and hence orientation is usually not a problem with transabdominal sonography.

Because scanning with the transvaginal probe is somewhat more complicated, a more detailed description of its use is provided. As described in Chapter 3, transvaginal probes can be 2D or 3D, electronic or mechanical probes provided with one fixed or several variable focuses. They normally operate at frequencies of 5 to 7.5 MHz (or higher) and can provide variable scanning angles that are steered mechanically or elec-

Table 4–1	Capabilities, Advantages, and Disadvantages of Transabdominal Sonography versus Transvaginal Sonography	
	Transabdominal Sonography	**Transvaginal Sonography**
Urinary bladder	Does not always require a full bladder	Requires an empty bladder
Best transducer frequencies (MHz)	3.5-5	5-9
Picture resolution and clarity	Lower	Higher
Ability to scan obese patients	Lower	Higher
Ability to scan in case of obstructed vagina or contraindication to transvaginal sonography	Possible, although resolution may be low	Low or none Transrectal scanning is a good alternative
Ability to guide punctures	Adequate Depends on skill	High because of high resolution Automated puncture device can be used
Ability to use on first days after abdominal surgery	Low	High
Quality of images under matched conditions	Lower	Higher

Data modified from Kossoff G, Griffith KA, Dixon CE: Is the quality of transvaginal images superior to transabdominal ones under matched conditions? Ultrasound Obstet Gynecol 1991;1:29-35.

tronically. Recently a new set of ultrasound probes was developed. These apply a 2D array of a large number of crystals. Such an electronic transducer is able to acquire an entire volume within a short time, thus enabling a true real-time 3D as well as a 4D rendering. The transabdominal version of such a transducer is already in clinical use.

Although different probes vary somewhat in shape, the following maneuvers apply to all:

1. *Pushing/pulling the entire probe.* This movement brings the tip of the probe closer to the region of interest and places it in the probe's focal length. A pushing and pulling motion of the probe can be used to elicit one of the dynamic tests performed with the probe: the "sliding organ sign."[2] If the organs seen on the monitor slide freely by each other and the pelvic wall, it is a good indication that no pelvic adhesions are present. If the organs do not change position relative to each other or the pelvic wall, pelvic adhesions are suspected.
2. *Tilting or angling the shaft.* This is done by moving the probe handle to point the tip in any direction in the pelvis, a movement similar to that used in the digital pelvic examination (imagine that there is a forward-looking eye on the tip of the examining finger).
3. *Rotating the probe around its axis.* This allows 360-degree scanning of the entire pelvis in all longitudinal planes.
4. *Automated volume acquisition.* More recent probes designed for 3D ultrasound are usually equipped with a mechanical motor that moves the transducer at constant speeds to acquire the volume. Electronic 3D transvaginal probles are also in wide use. The operator holds the probe steady, targeting the region of interest, while the probe automatically acquires the volume.
5. *Testing for pain.* Touching and gently pushing on any pelvic organ or structure in the probe's reach while constantly watching the screen allows localization of pain.
6. *Combining the transvaginal ultrasound examination and the bimanual examination.* To do this, the examiner places his or her free hand on the patient's abdomen while operating the vaginal probe with the other. Combining the two examinations confers several advantages; organs can be moved in and out of the "visual" field of the transvaginal probe. Of course, foot pedals are essen-

tial to operate the image freeze control and hard-copy device.

Scanning Routine

A methodical scanning routine should be followed. Regardless of whether the scanning is done transabdominally or transvaginally, the sonologist or sonographer should systematically scan the organs one after another and should not be distracted by obvious findings to neglect more subtle but important pathologic processes.

In transabdominal sonography, usually the first organ to be scanned is the uterus, followed by the adnexa and ending with the cervix and cul-de-sac. However, with transvaginal sonography, following a routine is even more important.[24] The following order is suggested:

1. First, the cervix should be scanned in the sagittal and coronal planes. In most cases, the distance from the internal os to the external os can be measured in the sagittal plane. A picture of the area of the internal os should be taken.
2. At the same time, the urinary bladder, which is in close anatomic proximity to the cervix, should also be examined in the sagittal plane and the transverse or coronal plane.
3. By advancing the probe, the sonographer can locate and scrutinize the uterus.
4. The next target is the adnexal area. While scanning the adnexa, the sonographer can evaluate the ovaries and the fallopian tubes and can detect and describe any possible masses.
5. The cul-de-sac is scanned next. This area of the pelvis is sometimes neglected, but it is of the utmost importance to scan it carefully. The cul-de-sac should be evaluated for the presence of fluid and possible contents such as the ovary or fallopian tube, or different pathologic structures.

Other locations and structures as well as suspected pathologic processes can be addressed once the examiner has formed a general impression about the pelvic contents.

It is important to use the greatest possible magnification that still enables orientation as well as recognition of organs and their pathology. Magnification does not usually alter the resolution of high-frequency probes.

Orientation of Transabdominal and Transvaginal Probes

Orientation for transabdominal probes is simple. The patient's right side on a coronal scan is placed on the left side of the monitor, whereas the left side of the anatomy is seen on the right side of the screen picture. This is much like the conventional orientation used in radiology. On the sagittal scan, the direction toward the patient's head (cephalad) is displayed on the left side of the monitor or the picture. The direction toward the patient's feet (caudad) is displayed on the right side of the sagittal transabdominal plane.

Transvaginal sonography is different because the images are created with the probe orientated perpendicularly. Moreover, the control board of an ultrasound machine is provided with a "left/right" orientation touch control as well as an "image-invert" switch. If there was a universal way to display ultrasound pictures, these controls would be redundant. However, sonologists from different countries display sonograms according to different rules.[25] An explanation of how transvaginal ultrasound images are displayed is important for an understanding of on-screen image orientation.

In the United States, transvaginal images are displayed as follows:

- If a fetus is scanned, the left and right sides are determined according to the position of the fetal stomach and the fetal heart. The examination should always be complemented with transabdominal sonography.
- On the longitudinal plane, the bladder appears on the upper left side of the screen, with the external cervical os pointing to the right side of the screen. With an anteverted uterus, the fundus appears on the left side of the picture below the urinary bladder (see Fig. 5–20). The fundus points toward the opposite side of the bladder if a retroverted uterus is scanned (see Figs. 5–9 and 5–20).
- On the cross-section of the pelvis (coronal plane), the patient's right ovary is seen on the left side of the screen, as on a radiographic image in the coronal plane.

In some countries, as well by some individuals, it is thought more logical to display the picture with the apex pointing down. While it would be desirable to have a uniform display convention worldwide, this is unlikely to occur soon.[26] Some sonologists think that displaying transvaginal sonograms with the apex pointing to the bottom of the picture and displaying transabdominal sonograms with the apex at the top permits an immediate distinction regarding the scanning route. However, others are used to displaying *all* ultrasound pictures with the apex toward the top of the picture. Therefore, it is crucial to label every image for easier evaluation.

Images produced by transvaginal sonography do not generally correspond to the normal anatomic planes. In a patient in the supine position, the vagina is directed upward and slightly backward within the pelvis itself, and it is also tilted at an angle of 30 degrees to the longitudinal axis of the body. In the coronal plane, there is no difference between pictures obtained by transvaginal sonography and those generated by transabdominal sonography. However, the sagittal plane will be displayed "rotated" 90 degrees counterclockwise.

Dodson and Deter[27] suggested the use of transverse and anteroposterior planes only in transvaginal sonography.

A better approach to orientation within the pelvis is to pay attention to the target organ rather than the anatomic pelvic planes[27,28]; this is called *organ-oriented scanning*. There are good reasons for this approach:

- Because of the short distance between the tip of the probe and the target area, the focused image usually contains only one organ or sometimes only a fragment of the organ.
- The plane of the probe changes constantly as the operator moves it. Using this technique, the sonologist or sonographer can search for each specific organ and then display it at his or her convenience. For this reason, it is practical to refer to the longitudinal axis of the scanned organ (i.e., the uterus or the ovary) instead of using the orientation of the conventional scanning planes with the known pelvic coordinates. This is termed *organ-oriented scanning.*[28]

Choice of Procedure

Transvaginal versus Transabdominal Sonography

The two major scanning routes to evaluate the female pelvis (i.e., the transabdominal and transvaginal routes) complement each other in obtaining the diagnosis. However, there are very few diagnoses that cannot be fully established by using transvaginal sonography alone. The transvaginal probe, which uses higher frequencies, provides images of pelvic organs with superior resolution. Because the vaginal transducer is placed close to the pelvic structures, less ultrasound penetration is required, so higher frequencies can be used to obtain higher-resolution images of pelvic organs (Fig. 4–1). It is possible to use frequencies of up to 7.5 MHz in a vaginal probe, whereas transabdominal sonography is limited to 5-MHz probes at the most. The lower frequency of the abdominal probes alone is sufficient to limit their resolution.[12] Another advantage of transvaginal over transabdominal sonography is that it can be performed with an empty bladder. Patients prefer the procedure because they do not have to wait for the scan with an unpleasantly full bladder. Obese patients can also be scanned with a higher yield of diagnostic-quality pictures. Transvaginal puncture procedures, such as drainage of pelvic fluid, culdocentesis, treatment of different kinds of ectopic gestations, and puncture of ovarian cysts, can be performed. A needle guide attached to the vaginal probe facilitates accurate needle placement in these cases (see Chapter 16 for a full discussion of puncture procedures).

Under matched conditions, vaginal probes perform better than abdominal probes because of the different tissue characteristics each probe encounters.[29]

Transrectal Sonography

As discussed previously, transvaginal sonography provides clear images of the region of interest, provided that the target organ is within the reach (i.e., the focal range) of the vaginal probe and that the probe can be placed near the organ in question. There are a few situations in which transvaginal sonography is disadvantageous. Among these are extreme obesity, agenesis of the vagina, a virginal introitus, and fear of introducing infection, as in the case of premature rupture of the membranes. In such cases, introducing a commercially avail-

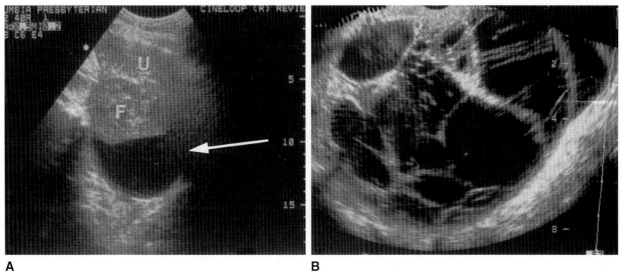

A   **B**

Figure 4–1. Use of transabdominal (**A**) and transvaginal (**B**) probes. The cyst *(arrow)* under the uterus (U) and a posterior fibroid (F) show no detail using the transabdominal scan. The 5- to 9-MHz vaginal probe displays the fine-mesh septa because of its proximity and high resolution.

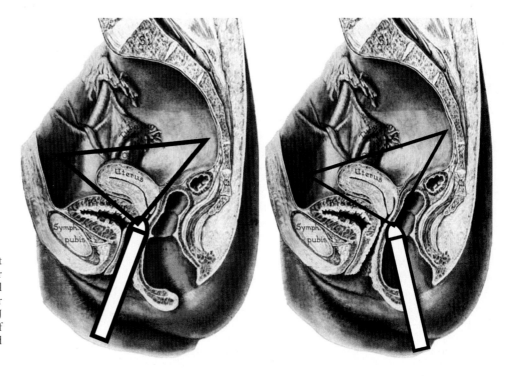

Figure 4–2. The vantage point of the tip of the probe is similar for transvaginal and transrectal scanning modes, providing similar angles of view. (From Romanes GJ [ed]: Cunningham's Textbook of Anatomy, 11th ed. Oxford, Oxford University Press, 1972, p 518.)

able, properly covered vaginal probe through the anal sphincter into the rectum is a reasonable alternative for imaging pelvic structures (Fig. 4–2).

Transrectal scanning (TRS) was used in a variety of clinical situations.[30-33] We used TRS in 42 patients with absolute or relative contraindications to transvaginal sonography,[34] comparing it with transabdominal sonography in the same patient.

All scans were completed without significant discomfort or complaints. TRS was clearly superior to transabdominal sonography in 31 cases. In nine cases transabdominal sonography yielded some clinical information, but TRS yielded better images.

Only in one case was transabdominal sonography similar in quality to TRS. In a similar article, Wachsberg[35] reinforced the value of TRS of the female internal reproductive tract to complement (and at times replace) transabdominal sonography.

REFERENCES

1. Fleischer AC, Romero R, Manning FA, et al: The Principle and the Practice of Ultrasonography in Obstetrics and Gynecology, 4th ed. East Norwalk, Conn, Appleton & Lange, 1991.
2. Timor-Tritsch IE, Rottem S (eds): Transvaginal Sonography, 2nd ed. New York, Chapman & Hall, 1991.
3. Goldstein SR: Endovaginal Sonography, 2nd ed. New York, Wiley-Liss, 1991.

4. Sabbagha RE: Diagnostic Ultrasound Applied to Obstetrics and Gynecology, 3rd ed. Philadelphia, JB Lippincott, 1994.
5. Chervenak FA, Isaacson GC, Campbell S: Ultrasound in Obstetrics and Gynecology. Boston, Little, Brown, 1993.
6. Nyberg DA, Hill LM, Böhm-Velez M, Mendelson EB: Transvaginal Ultrasound. St. Louis, Mosby-Yearbook, 1992.
7. Timor-Tritsch IE, Rottem S, Thaler I: Review of TVS ultrasonography: A description with clinical application. Ultrasound Q 1988;6:1-34.
8. Tessler FN, Schiller VL, Perrella RR, et al: TAS versus endovaginal pelvic sonography: Prospective study. Radiology 1980;170:553-556.
9. Timor-Tritsch IE, Bar-Yam Y, Elgali S, Rottem S: The technique of TVS sonography with the use of 6.5 MHz probe. Am J Obstet Gynecol 1988;158:1019-1024.
10. Coleman BG, Arger PH, Grumbach K, et al: TVS and TAS sonography: Prospective comparison. Radiology 1988;168:639-643.
11. Mendelson EB, Böhm-Velez M, Joseph N, Neiman HL: Gynecologic imaging: Comparison of TAS and TVS sonography. Radiology 1988;166:321-324.
12. Lavery MJ, Benson CB: Transvaginal versus transabdominal ultrasound. In Timor-Tritsch IE, Rottem S (eds): Transvaginal Sonography, 2nd ed. New York, Chapman & Hall, 1991, p 77.
13. Confino E, Mayden KL, Giglia RV, et al: Pitfalls in sonographic imaging of the incompetent uterine cervix. Acta Obstet Gynecol Scand 1986;65:593-597.
14. Varma TR, Patel RH, Pillari U: Ultrasonic assessment of cervix in normal pregnancy. Acta Obstet Gynecol Scand 1986;65:229-233.
15. Zemlyn S: The effect of the urinary bladder in obstetrical sonography. Radiology 1978;169:169-175.
16. Mason G: Ultrasound assessment of the cervix: The bladder effect, abstracted. In Proceedings of the British Medical Ultrasound Society Meeting, December 1989.
17. Persutte WH, Lenke RR: Maternal urinary bladder filling for middle and late trimester ultrasound: Is it really necessary? J Ultrasound Med 1998;7:207-209.
18. Benacerraf BR, Shipp TD, Bromley B: Is a full bladder still necessary for pelvic sonography? J Ultrasound Med 2000;19:237-241.
19. Benacerraf BR: Filling of the bladder for pelvic sonograms: An ancient form of torture. J Ultrasound Med 2003;22:239-241.
20. Jimenez R, Duff P: Sheathing of the endovaginal ultrasound probe: Is it adequate? Infect Dis Obstet Gynecol 1993;1:37-39.
21. Amis R, Ruddy M, Kibbler CC, et al: Assessment of condoms as probe covers for transvaginal sonography. J Clin Ultrasound 2000;28:295-298.
22. Schwimmer SR, Rothman CM, Lebovic J, Oye DM: The effect of ultrasound coupling gels on sperm motility in vitro. Fertil Steril 1989;42:946-947.
23. Odwin CS, Fleischer AC, Kepple DT: Probe covers and disinfectants for transvaginal transducers. J Diagn Med Sonogr 1990;6:130-135.
24. Zimmer EZ, Timor-Tritsch IE, Rottem S: The technique of transvaginal sonography. In Timor-Tritsch IE, Rottem S (eds): Transvaginal Sonography, 2nd ed. New York, Chapman & Hall, 1991, p 61.
25. Bernaschek G, Deutinger J: Current status of vaginosonography: A worldwide inquiry. Ultrasound Obstet Gynecol 1992;2:352-356.
26. Timor-Tritsch IE: Standardization of ultrasonographic images: Let's all talk the same language! Ultrasound Obstet Gynecol 1992;2:311-312.
27. Dodson MG, Deter RL: Definition of anatomical planes for use in transvaginal sonography. J Clin Ultrasound 1990;18:239-242.
28. Rottem S, Thaler I, Goldstein SR, et al: Transvaginal sonographic technique: Targeted organ scanning without resorting to "planes." J Clin Ultrasound 1990;18:243-247.
29. Kossoff G, Griffith KA, Dixon CE: Is the quality of transvaginal images superior to transabdominal ones under matched conditions? Ultrasound Obstet Gynecol 1991;1:29-35.
30. Kushnir O, Garde K, Blankstein J: Rectal sonography for diagnosing hematocolpometra: A case report. J Reprod Med 1997;42:519-520.
31. Anguenot JL, Ibecheole V, Salvat J, Campana A: Hematocolpos secondary to imperforate hymen: Contribution of transrectal echography. Acta Obstet Gynecol Scand 2000;79:614-615.
32. Fedele L, Portuese A, Bianchi S, et al: Transrectal ultrasonography in the assessment of congenital vaginal canalization defects. Hum Reprod 1999;14:359-362.
33. Lopez-Rasines G, Abascal F, Calabia A, et al: Transrectal sonography in the assessment of vaginal pathology: A preliminary study. J Clin Ultrasound 1998;26:353-356.
34. Timor-Tritsch IE, Monteagudo A, Rebarber A, et al: Transrectal scanning: An alternative when transvaginal scanning is not feasible. Ultrasound Obstet Gynecol 2003;21:473-479.
35. Wachsberg RH: Transrectal ultrasound for problem solving after transvaginal ultrasonography of the female internal reproductive tract. J Ultrasound Med 2003;22:1349-1356.

SECTION III

General Gynecology

Some ultrasound examinations are performed in the office or emergency department setting and some in designated ultrasound laboratories. This book aims to be descriptive enough to appeal to those who need guidance in their offices but also sufficiently detailed to appeal to those working in specialized ultrasound units. The first audience is addressed by the complete presentation of the normal ultrasound pelvic anatomy (Chapter 5), as such images are usually those encountered by the practicing obstetrician-gynecologist. The second audience is served by the discussion of the pathologic findings as well as by the ample literature reference base provided for those interested in pursuing a specific topic.

Chapter 5

Relevant Pelvic Anatomy

Ilan E. Timor-Tritsch

Chapter 5 addresses the cervix, uterus, and cul-de-sac, presenting their normal and abnormal ultrasound aspects. Examination of the normal fallopian tube and ovary is included as well. However, the pathologic aspects of the adnexa on sonography are dealt with in Chapter 8.

For background material on ultrasound applications in obstetrics and gynecology, the reader is referred to several textbooks on the subject.[1-6]

Cervix

Normal Anatomy and Ultrasound Orientation

Although the cervix can be scanned in the sagittal and coronal planes, in the great majority of cases the sagittal midline view provides the necessary information. On an image in this orientation, the tip of the probe is almost touching the anterior lip of the cervix (Fig. 5–1). The bladder should be seen just above it. The internal os is on the right side of the cervical canal. The cervical canal is sometimes difficult to image throughout its entire length. However, only if the canal is visualized from the internal os all the way to the external os in an anteverted uterus (on the right side of the image) can the image be described as perfect. The cervical canal lies at (or nearly at) a 90-degree angle to the axis of the vagina and, hence, of the vaginal probe. Images in the coronal plane, usually seen best with three-dimensional (3D) ultrasound, can provide important information concerning uterine malformations by allowing the examiner to detect and follow the directions of the cervical canals for a correct diagnosis (Fig. 5–2; and see Fig. 5–36).

The length of the cervix is measured from the internal to the external os (Fig. 5–3). Because cervical length is an important measurement primarily in the context of pregnancy, the database for ultrasound cervical measurements was acquired from pregnant patients. The normal cervical length in pregnancy is 4 ± 1 cm.[7-17] It is important not to include the vaginal wall in the measurement (see Fig. 5–1). This error occurs when the uterus is anteverted, in which position the posterior vaginal wall lies at a right angle to the cervical canal and is closely apposed to the cervix. Although not as important clinically, cervical width and dilation can also be measured.

Based on personal experience, measurement of cervical length in a nonpregnant uterus is difficult to perform and probably inaccurate because of the uncertain location of the internal os. However, cervical length in the nonpregnant state is probably similar to that in normal first-trimester pregnancy. The only published study dealing with measurement of the nonpregnant cervix is that of Jackson et al.,[18] who report cervical length measurements of 38 ± 8 mm.

The cervical glands parallel the echogenic changes of the endometrium quite closely; however, during mid-cycle, these glands excrete anechoic mucus that fills and outlines the cervical canal (Fig. 5–4). Cervical canal mucus can also be seen in pregnancy (Fig. 5–5).

Clinical Applications of Cervical Sonography

Transvaginal sonography (TVS) of the cervix is technically easy to perform in the office or emergency department, as well as in delivery and labor suites. It can be performed in a few minutes, more quickly than any other routine ultrasound procedure. It is easily learned and taught, so that residents and practitioners without the backup of an ultrasound laboratory can use it, provided they have a vaginal probe. The procedure is well tolerated by all patients. It is particularly useful in patients who are obese and have cervices that are hard to reach, or in those who fear a painful bimanual examination.

Cervical sonography is performed mainly in pregnancy. In the 1990s, it was developed into a powerful tool for assessing the pregnancy status. Cervical ultrasound is extensively used to predict preterm labor and delivery in singletons[19-44] and in twins.[45] However, because this text is geared toward gynecologic imaging, no detailed account of these articles is given here.

The boundary between gynecologic and obstetric scanning of the cervix is blurred, especially during the first trimester of pregnancy. Therefore, the images presented in this chapter include examples of both pregnant and nonpregnant women.

Pathologic Conditions

Nabothian Cysts

The most common pathologic process of the cervix detected by sonography is the finding of dilated, thin-walled, anechoic, inclusion cysts called *nabothian cysts*. They can be of various sizes (Fig. 5–6). It is important to identify them as such without confusing them with other cervical or adnexal lesions.

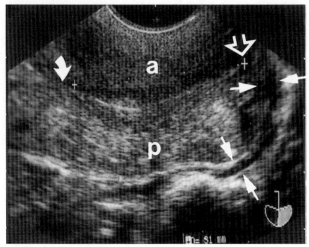

Figure 5–1. Sagittal view of a normal cervix. The cervical canal measures 3.1 cm from the internal os *(curved solid arrow)* to the external os *(open arrow)*. The vaginal wall thickness *(opposing arrows)* should not be included in the measurement of the cervical length. a, anterior lip; p, posterior lip.

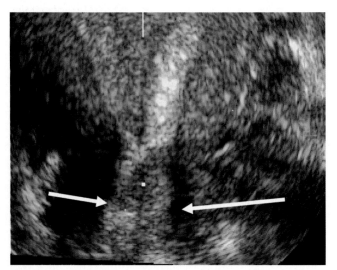

Figure 5–2. Three-dimensional image of the cervix *(between the arrows)*, which should be obtained in every work-up of patients with suspected uterine anomalies (see also Fig. 5–36).

Vaginal Bleeding

A significant pathologic condition of the cervix is vaginal bleeding in the first trimester of the pregnancy in which a subchorionic hematoma or blood collection is seen in the area of the internal os. This is promptly recognized on TVS. If vaginal bleeding is present but there is a detectable embryonic or fetal heartbeat and a firmly attached placenta, with some concealed fluid collection in the area of the internal os, the patient may be reassured. After drainage of such blood clots close to the cervix, the outcome is generally good (Fig. 5–7).

Cervical Malignancy

Although sonography is not a first-line tool for the diagnosis of cervical malignancy, it is important that the examiner

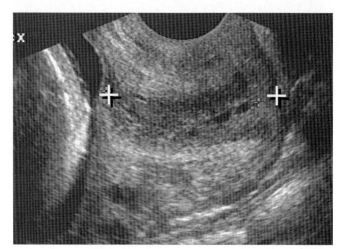

Figure 5–3. Technique of measuring the cervix. Only the closed cervical canal length should be reported.

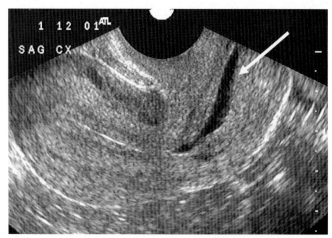

Figure 5–4. At mid-cycle the cervical glands excrete mucus, which appears as an anechoic stripe in the cervical canal *(arrow)*.

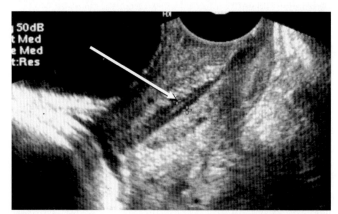

Figure 5–5. The mucus content of the cervical canal is visualized in pregnancy *(arrow)*. This could be the mucus plug referred to by clinicians.

suspect or recognize this lesion if it is encountered on the ultrasound image. The transvaginal sonography picture of cervical cancer consists of an unusually bulky and large cervix, relative difficulty in locating a normal and straight cervical canal, and a cervical width greater than 4 cm.

Cervical Pregnancy

A rare pathologic process of the cervix is cervical pregnancy (Fig. 5–8A and B). In the presence of a positive pregnancy test, an empty uterus with a thick, hyperechoic decidual reaction, an otherwise normal pelvis, and a dilated, barrel-shaped cervix containing a live embryo are necessary to establish the diagnosis of cervical pregnancy.[46] Sometimes concomitant intrauterine and cervical pregnancies are seen (Fig. 5–8C). This presents a significant management problem, one usually solved by puncture injection and reduction of the cervical embryo.[47] A large body of literature addresses the ultrasound

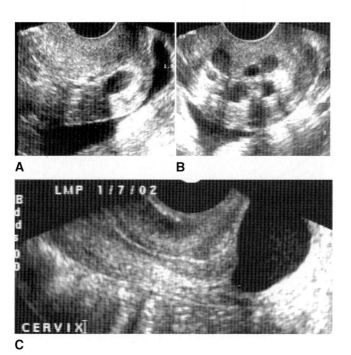

Figure 5–6. Images of the cervix containing a single (**A**) or multiple (**B**) nabothian cysts. Some can be relatively large, occupying most of the cervix (**C**).

diagnosis of cervical pregnancy; as with most pelvic lesions, TVS is the best diagnostic tool. A full discussion of the diagnosis and treatment of cervical pregnancy is provided in Chapter 13.

Related to cervical pregnancy is a gestation implanted in the scar of a previous cesarean section. This is often referred to as a *pregnancy in the scar* and by definition is not a classic cervical pregnancy (Fig. 5–9). In the nonpregnant state, the scar or niche left by a cesarean section can be clearly identified by ultrasound[48] (Fig. 5–10).

Cervical Insufficiency

Probably the most important clinical application of cervical sonography is prediction of cervical insufficiency, a subject dealt with extensively in the sonography literature. In the nonpregnant patient, the cervical canal ends cranially in the area of the internal os. The normal internal os in pregnancy is T-shaped on a sagittal image[32] (Fig. 5–11A). If this area assumes a V or a Y shape or becomes ballooned or U-shaped, it is considered pathologic and may predict cervical incompetence or preterm delivery (PTD) (Fig. 5–11B and C). Early diagnosis of cervical insufficiency is extremely important because the placement of cerclage seems to yield better results when done earlier rather than when bulging of the membranes or extreme dilation has already started. Technically, it is easy to visualize and evaluate cervical sutures by TVS (Fig. 5–12).

The ultrasound diagnosis of cervical insufficiency has been based on measuring the dilation of the internal os or the cervical length. Brook et al.[21] considered cervical insufficiency to be present if the diameter of the internal os was greater than 1.9 cm. Podobnik et al.[13] submitted patients for cerclage if their cervical length was less than 3.4 cm at 15 to 19 weeks' gestation. Ayers and colleagues[12] considered any cervical length less than 4 cm as abnormal. Andersen et al.[35] evaluated patients who had a clinical history of cervical insufficiency and compared them with a control group of patients without cervical insufficiency. The mean cervical length in the study group was shorter than that of the control group, 34.5 mm versus 41 mm, respectively. In another study, Andersen and

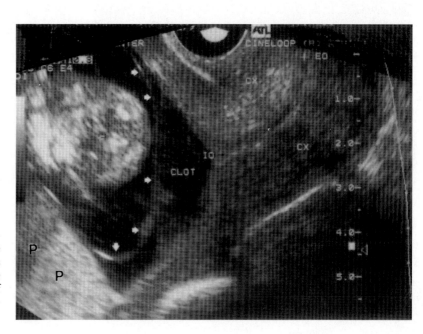

Figure 5–7. Sagittal view of a patient who complained of slight bleeding at 16 weeks' gestation. The cervix (CX) appears normal; however, a clot appears to push away the membranes (*arrowheads*) from the area of the internal os (IO). There is no dilation of the cervical canal or the external os (EO). The placenta (P) is not detached.

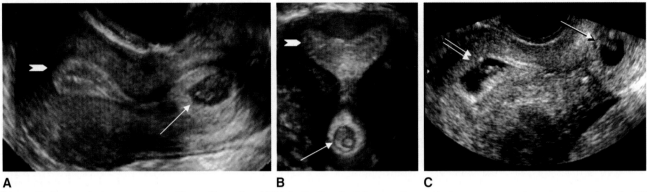

Figure 5–8. Cervical pregnancy. **A,** Three-dimensional "thick slice" sagittal image of a cervical pregnancy at 6 postmenstrual weeks. The *solid arrow* demonstrates the empty uterine cavity with decidual reaction. The *long arrow* points to the cervical gestation. **B,** The same cervical pregnancy on a coronal section. **C,** Heterotopic pregnancy. The *double arrow* indicates the live intrauterine pregnancy; the *single arrow* points to the cervical gestation.

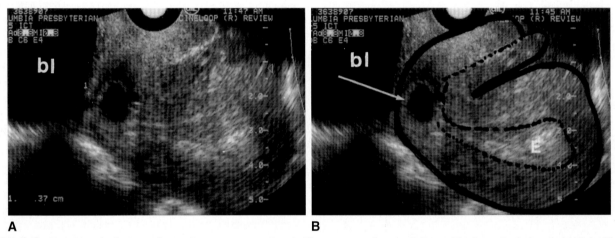

Figure 5–9. Pregnancy in the scar of a previous cesarean section. **A,** The retroverted uterus is imaged in the sagittal plane behind the bladder (bl). **B,** A drawing is superimposed on the same image for greater clarity. The *arrow* indicates the gestational sac.

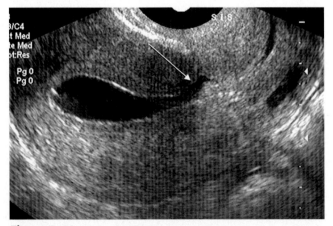

Figure 5–10. A nonpregnant uterus in which saline infusion sonohysterography highlights a filling defect or niche *(arrow).*

Ansbacher[49] suggested that cervical length alone was an inadequate screening criterion for cervical insufficiency. They suggested that in addition to measuring length, the internal cervical os should be examined. If funneling or early herniation of the amniotic sac is seen, the diagnosis of cervical insuf-

ficiency can be made with higher confidence. Based on the literature, then, certain conclusions can be drawn. The shorter the cervix, the greater the risk of PTD.[45,50-53] Although the detection of funneling was thought to contribute to the prediction of PTD, it does not seem to contribute significantly to diagnostic power.[40,43]

A cervix less than 20 mm in length has a likelihood ratio of 8 to predict labor before 32 weeks[54] and a likelihood ratio of 18 to predict PTD before 36 weeks.[53] A cervix measuring less than 25 mm any time during the second trimester increases the likelihood of PTD by a factor of 3.[44,55] A cervical length less than 25 mm measured at 16 to 18 weeks' gestation increases the risk of PTD before 34 weeks with a likelihood ratio of 9.5.[44] Both transabdominal sonography and TVS have been used to follow patients after placement of cervical sutures or other treatment of cervical insufficiency.[30,31] Cerclages have also been placed under transrectal sonographic guidance.[56]

The literature is replete with articles on the use of cervical sutures to prevent PTD.[57-60] A complete review is beyond the scope of this chapter, although one study deserves special attention because it is a randomized, controlled trial.[60] Rozenberg et al.[61] reviewed the literature dealing with TVS examination of the cervix in asymptomatic women with regard to

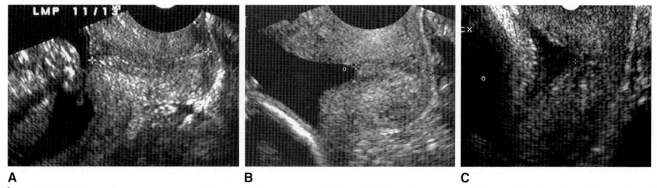

Figure 5–11. The various appearances of the cervix in pregnancy. **A,** Normal T-shaped appearance of an uneffaced cervix with normal canal length. **B,** U-shaped shorter cervix. **C,** V-shaped or funneled effaced cervix.

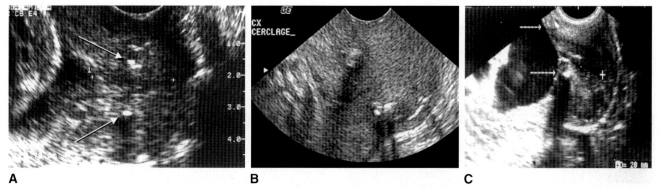

Figure 5–12. Cervical sutures imaged by transvaginal sonography, sagittal views. **A,** The *arrows* indicate the correctly placed McDonald cervical sutures. **B,** The appearance of the Shirodkar suture. **C,** In spite of the cerclage, the cervix is in the process of being effaced and shortened. The cerclage barely keeps the cervix closed. The *arrows* point to the effaced length of the cervix.

placement of cerclages. They concluded that TVS clearly demonstrates that cerclage leads to a measurable increase in cervical length, which may have contributed to the success of this procedure in reducing PTD. They also evaluated the benefit of measuring the length of the cervix above the cerclage and the risk of PTD, and found that the shorter the cervix above the cerclage, the larger the risk for PTD. They concluded that although there are no prospective, randomized studies in a general population assessing the placement of cerclages in asymptomatic women, there seems to be a benefit to performing cerclage rather than continuing with expectant management in cases where ultrasound shows evidence of cervical incompetence in asymptomatic women. Sonography can reduce the indication for cerclage in cases in which the diagnosis is uncertain as well as help identify symptomatic women who are at high risk for PTD. However, Rozenberg et al.[61] show that a clear benefit for cerclage based on ultrasound indications has not yet been demonstrated.

Measuring the Cervix in Early Pregnancy

TVS has been done to measure the cervix in the first trimester to predict PTD in high-risk patients. Berghella and colleagues[62] concluded that a cervical length of less than 25 mm rarely is seen before 14 weeks' gestation even in high-risk patients who later experience PTD. In these patients, cervical changes predictive of PTD develop mostly after 14 weeks. Conoscenti et al.[63] also concluded that TVS measurement of the cervix at 14 weeks to predict PTD is not a reliable screen-

ing procedure. Carvalho and associates[64] observed a spontaneous shortening of the cervix from the first to the second trimester of pregnancy. This shortening was more rapid in women who deliver prematurely and who had a history of PTD. Shalev et al.[65] claimed that TVS performed between 5 and 15 weeks' gestation can determine the location of the internal os using the urinary bladder as a reference, which may be useful for those who wish to make longitudinal measurements of the cervix at early gestational ages.

Other Cervical Evaluations

A TVS evaluation of the cervix in cases of spontaneous or induced mid-trimester abortion is easy to obtain (Figs. 5–13 and 5–14) and provides an objective "progress report" on the patient's clinical status.

Cervical polyps are better seen on a speculum examination of the cervix; however, if they are encountered on TVS, they can be identified by a vessel arising from the cervix (Fig. 5–15). The importance of detecting the feeding vessel is shown in the case presented in Figure 5–16. Even though the polyp was located in the cervix in this patient, who was 13 weeks' pregnant, the feeding vessel was traced back to the posterior wall of the uterus. The correct diagnosis is therefore prolapsed endometrial polyp.

A diagnosis of a cervical fibroid (Fig. 5–17) may become important if termination of the pregnancy or delivery is considered, because it may impede delivery or cervical dilation owing to its location. Cervical fibroids can be recognized by three characteristic features: they have a spheric shape, their texture appears similar to that of the surrounding cervical tissues, and the vascular supply on color Doppler appears as a circular pattern on the surface of the fibroid (Fig. 5–18).

Three-dimensional ultrasound has been used recently in imaging the cervix.[66-70] This technique makes it easy and convenient to scroll through the acquired 3D volume or to position the cervix optimally to evaluate the placement of a cerclage or determine the location of a cervical pregnancy.

Uterus

Normal Anatomy and Ultrasound Orientation

The uterus is the largest midline structure in the female pelvis. Because of its location, it is used as a reference for scanning the adnexa and the cul-de-sac.

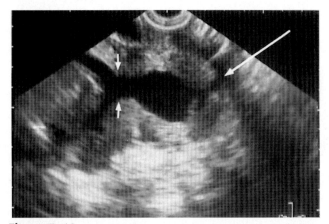

Figure 5–13. Sagittal view of the cervix in a patient undergoing second-trimester medical abortion. The distinct ballooning of the cervical-canal was observed several hours after the intra-amniotic injection of prostaglandin. The external os *(long arrow)* is not yet dilated, and the internal os is still recognizable *(small arrows)*.

The orientation of the uterine image on TVS is fairly complicated. With two-dimensional (2D) transabdominal or transvaginal sonography, the uterus is usually imaged in two major scanning planes, sagittal and transverse. Scans in the sagittal plane can show the cervix, the body of the uterus, the fundus, the endometrial cavity, and the cervical canal on the same image. Obtaining an image in the transverse plane depends on the orientation of the uterus. Transverse sections are possible if the uterus is in frank anteversion, anteflexion, or retroversion. The uterus may be in an axial position during the late postmenopausal period. In this case, the axis of the transvaginal probe is aligned with the axis of the uterus, which enables a coronal section to be obtained, displaying the endometrial cavity as a triangle. This view can be obtained easily with 3D ultrasound by rotating the uterus to the desired position. Bimanual manipulation of the uterus, with or without a full bladder, permits different degrees of this axial or coronal section of the uterus to be obtained even if 2D ultrasound is used.

On the sagittal TVS image, the fundus of the anteverted uterus will be on the same side of the image as the urinary bladder, if the bladder is seen and included in the picture (i.e., the left upper corner; Fig. 5–19A). Conversely, if the uterus is retroflexed, the fundus on a sagittal image will be displayed on the right side of the picture, the side opposite the urinary bladder (Fig. 5–20). The sonographer should remember that, by consensus, the bladder is imaged on the left upper side of the picture in sagittal scans. On transverse sections, the right side of the uterus is displayed on the left side of the picture (Fig. 5–19B). Unfortunately, not all sonographers follow these conventions for image orientation in displaying the cervix and uterus; therefore, care should be exercised when reading publications dealing with sonography of these organs.

The uterine size by sonography depends on the patient's age and parity as well as menopausal status.[71-73] Normal uterine sizes for the nulliparous, parous, and postmenopausal woman are listed in Table 5–1.

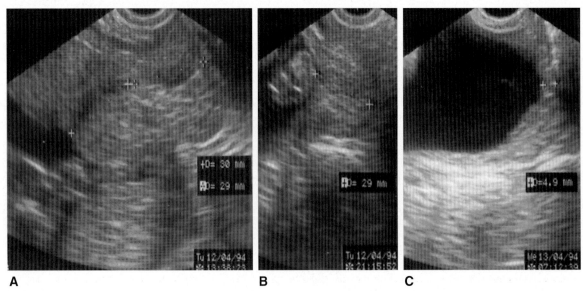

A   **B**   **C**

Figure 5–14. Serial sagittal views of the cervix in patient undergoing medical abortion at 20 weeks' gestation. **A,** Before intra-amniotic prostaglandin injection, the cervix measures 5.9 cm in length. **B,** Seven hours and 45 minutes later, the cervix measures 2.9 cm. **C,** The next morning, about 17 hours and 45 minutes after the injection, the cervix is almost completely effaced and measures 4.9 mm. The fetus was aborted 5 hours later.

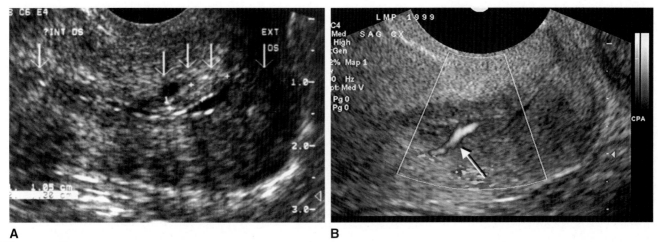

Figure 5–15. Cervical polyps on sagittal views. **A,** With scant fluid around it, a small cervical polyp is evident *(arrows).* **B,** The vascular pedicle of the same polyp *(arrow)* enhanced by power Doppler.

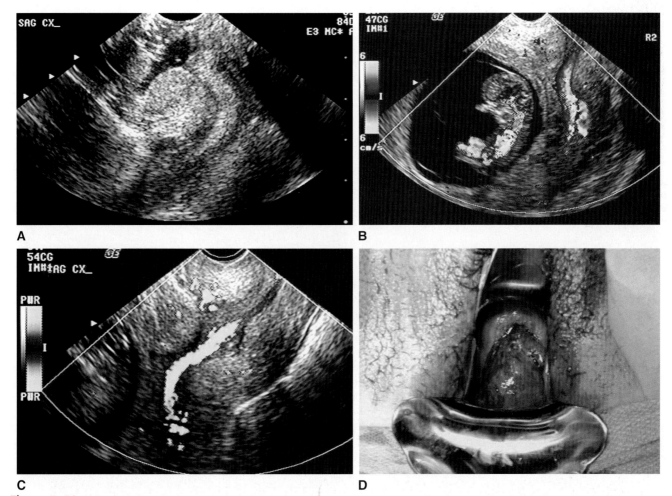

Figure 5–16. An endometrial polyp prolapsing through the cervix in a patient in early pregnancy. **A,** Gray-scale appearance of the polyp in the cervix. **B,** Color Doppler highlights the vessel leading to the polyp. The fetus in the uterine cavity is also seen. **C,** Power Doppler clearly shows the pedicle extending from the posterior uterine wall to the polyp. **D,** The appearance of the polyp protruding from the external cervical os.

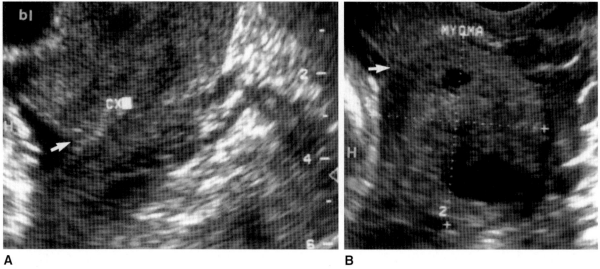

Figure 5–17. Cervical fibroid in 16-week pregnancy. **A,** Midsagittal view showing the fetal head (H) and the internal os *(arrow)* of the cervix (cx). **B,** Fibroid measuring 4 × 3.6 cm.

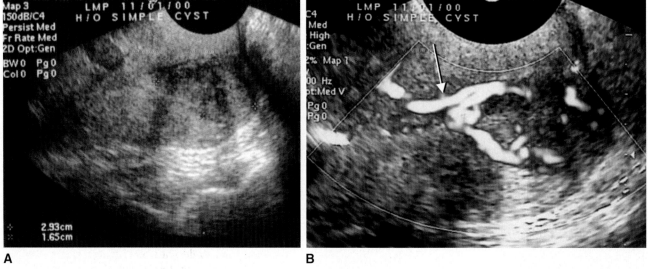

Figure 5–18. A submucous fibroid prolapsing through the cervical canal. **A,** Gray-scale image of the myoma. **B,** Power Doppler displays the typical circular vascular pattern of fibroids *(arrow)*.

On real-time sonography, especially when performed using the transvaginal probe, uterine contractions will be evident; in addition, Birnholtz[74] in 1984 described the detection of subendometrial contractions. Subendometrial contractions are best seen using a technique applied by deVries et al.,[75] Lyons et al.,[76] and Abramowicz and Archer,[77] which consists of recording the contractions on a video cassette recorder and playing them back using the recorder's fast-forward feature. During ovulation, the contractions are directed toward the fundus; as menstruation approaches, their direction changes toward the cervix. These groups also found a correlation between estrogen and progesterone levels and the frequency of these contractions. Other reports[78-83] have addressed contractility of the nonpregnant uterus as a function of the menstrual cycle and during embryo transfer. The real importance of subendometrial contractions has yet to be elucidated.

When describing the normal anatomy of the uterus, one should include the ultrasound image of the uterine vascular supply and its venous drainage.[84,85] Although it is possible to detect the vascular supply of the uterus on gray-scale sonography, it is easier to assess uterine perfusion by using duplex Doppler or color Doppler of the uterine arteries. Color Doppler interrogation of the uterus highlights the arcuate vessels (Fig. 5–21A); it is easy to see a sonolucent circular structure at the outer third of the myometrium, which represents the arcuate arteries and veins (Fig. 5–21B). These arteries may calcify and present a typical picture in postmenopausal patients. One should be familiar with the echogenic ring created by the strong echoes arising from partially calcified arcuate arteries (Fig. 5–21C). This ring corresponds to the location of the sonolucent structure indicating the arcuate vessels during the reproductive years.

Table 5–1	Uterine Size				
	Length (cm)	Width (cm)	Anteroposterior (cm)	Volume (mL)	Cervix–Corpus Ratio
Adult (nulliparous)	6-8	3-5	3-5	30-40	1:2
Adult (parous)	8-10	5-6	5-6	60-80	1:2
Postmenopausal	3-5	2-3	2-3	14-17	1:1

From Warwick W (ed): Gray's Anatomy. Edinburgh, Churchill Livingstone, 1973, with permission.

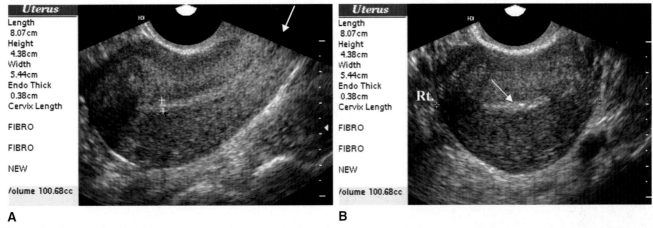

Figure 5–19. Orientation of the uterus on the basic scan. **A,** Sagittal view of an anteverted uterus with the cervix pointing toward the upper right corner of the image *(arrow)*. Note how the thickness of the endometrial stripe is measured. **B,** Transverse section of the same uterus. The *arrow* points to the endometrial stripe. The right side of the uterus should appear on the left side of the picture, like the coronal image orientation used in radiology.

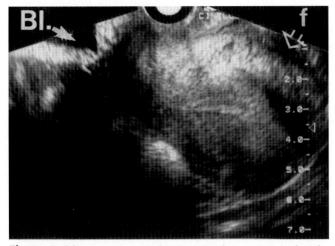

Figure 5–20. Sagittal view of a retroverted uterus. Note that the uterine fundus (f) points toward the right of the picture and up to the opposite side of the bladder (Bl).

Endometrium

With TVS, it has long been obvious that the appearance of the endometrium changes throughout the menstrual cycle.[86-93] During the phase preceding ovulation, the endometrium has a multilayered appearance with an inner hypoechoic and an outer echoic layer (see Fig. 5–19). In the secretory phase, the endometrium's thickness increases to between 8 and 14 mm, and it becomes more echoic (Fig. 5–22). The increased echogenicity is probably the result of the tortuous endometrial glands, which generate echogenic interfaces. The thickness of the myometrium should be measured in the sagittal plane and should include both endometrial layers (i.e., the measurement is taken from the anterior myometrial–endometrial interface to the posterior endometrial–myometrial interface; see Fig. 5–19A).

Grunfeld and colleagues[91] introduced the concept of patterns I through III to describe the ultrasound appearance of the endometrium during the menstrual cycle. Pattern I consists of the three-layered endometrium. Pattern II, which is observed at or near ovulation, still depicts the three layers, but the hyperechoic layer is much thinner. Pattern III is consistent with the secretory phase of the cycle and is characterized by complete echogenicity of the functional and basal layers of the endometrium. The authors suggested that this echogenicity stems from a stromal edema. Gonen et al.[92,93] showed that the thickness of the endometrium on day 8 was significantly less in women who conceived as opposed to those who did not (3.3 mm vs. 5.9 mm, respectively). They also showed that endometrial thickness or growth between day 8 of the cycle and the peak of luteinizing hormone secretion was significantly greater in those patients who conceived than in those who did not (5.5 mm vs. 2.5 mm, on average). This group recorded no subsequent pregnancies when the endometrium was less than 6 mm thick on the day of ovulation. The presence on TVS of a three-layered endometrium with a thickness of at least 6 mm on the day of ovulation was predictive of conception. Also, the presence of a three-layered endometrium on the day of ovulation was associated with a positive predictive

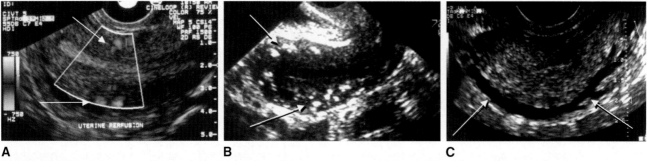

A   **B**   **C**

Figure 5–21. The arcuate vessels of the uterus. **A,** Color Doppler appearance. The *arrows* indicate the typical location of these vessels at the outer third of the myometrium on this sagittal view. **B,** Sagittal view of the uterus in an elderly patient. Hyperechoic signals *(arrows)* are seen along the arcuate vessels. This is probably caused by the calcified walls of the arteries *(arrows)*. **C,** Arcuate vessels *(arrows)* on a transverse view in a woman in her reproductive years.

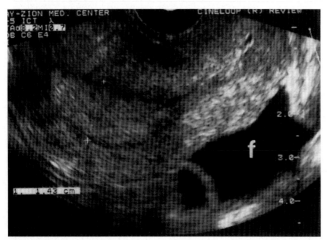

Figure 5–22. Sagittal view of the uterus 2 to 3 days postovulation. The hyperechoic endometrium measures 1.43 cm in thickness. Some fluid (f) is present in the cul-de-sac.

value for pregnancy of 50%, whereas the premature appearance of a hyperechoic pattern at the time of ovulation had a negative predictive value of 100%. Pierson[94] also concludes that women with a heterogeneous endometrial lining less than 6 mm thick will rarely conceive.

After menopause, the endometrium becomes thinner. This is considered a normal evolution. However, this is also the age when some women elect to use hormone replacement therapy. Numerous studies have evaluated the potential associations between endometrial pattern, thickness, or vascular flow in the postmenopausal endometrium on hormone replacement and endometrial malignancy. This topic is discussed in depth in Chapters 9 and 15.

Endometrial Pathologic Conditions

TVS is the tool of choice for evaluating pathologic processes of the endometrium. The clear picture of the endometrium obtained in sagittal as well as coronal planes in the anteverted or retroverted uterus results from the fact that sound waves encounter the endometrium at a right angle; hence, the interfaces are clear. In elderly patients in whom the uterus is small and may lie parallel to the axis of the pelvis as well as the sound waves, the endometrium may not be imaged with such clarity.

Normal endometrial thickness and appearance across the menstrual cycle are discussed in the previous section. As noted, sonography reliably depicts the actual thickness of the endometrium.[86-88] The endometrium should be evaluated at every visit to the gynecologist, provided a transvaginal probe is available. Endometrial imaging assumes particular importance in two specific contexts. The first situation is for follow-up of dynamic endometrial changes as a function of hormonal influences in patients followed or treated for infertility (see Chapter 14 for a detailed discussion). The second clinical situation is in the postmenopausal patient with metrorrhagia or undergoing hormone replacement therapy, a subject discussed more broadly in Chapter 9. In this situation, endometrial thickness and the interface or boundaries between the myometrium and the endometrium are carefully scrutinized.

In evaluating patients with uterine bleeding disorders, it is important to know if the patient is premenopausal or postmenopausal. In the premenopausal period, endometrial thickness varies from 4 to 8 mm in the follicular phase and from 7 to 14 mm in the secretory phase.[95,96] Patients on oral contraceptives show a very thin endometrium.

Doppler flow velocity measurements, both in the normal and in the abnormal endometrium, across the natural menstrual cycle, were performed by Scholtes et al.,[97] Bourne,[98] and Sladkevicius and coworkers.[99] Steer and colleagues[100] believe that measuring the resistance to flow during the cycle can predict the success of fertilized ovum implantation.

Additional studies were conducted to establish the value[101-107] or lack thereof[108] of color Doppler flow evaluation of the subendometrial layers for predicting embryo receptivity and success of conception. The results are contradictory, leaving this issue open for improved studies.

The goals of evaluation are different during the postmenopausal period. Management depends in part on whether the patient is symptomatic and whether hormone replacement therapy is being given. Most studies have been dedicated to finding a cut-off point of endometrial thickness to guide the gynecologist in managing the patient with potential endometrial malignancy. Granberg et al.[109] set the cut-off point for detection of endometrial pathology as a thickness of 5 mm or more, and they reported an 87% positive predictive value for detection of significant disease. Varner and associates[110] and Goldstein and colleagues[111] also identified 5 mm as the cut-off point, below which no cases of endometrial cancer, polyps, or hyperplasia were detected. Others had different cut-off points[112] or strategies for staging endometrial cancer.[113] Fleischer et al.[114] were able to detect the depth of invasion of the cancer into the endometrium and myometrium. Smith-Bindman and colleagues[115] proposed that in a postmenopausal woman without vaginal bleeding, if the endometrial thickness is greater than 11 mm, a biopsy should be considered because the risk of cancer is 6.7%, whereas if it measures 11 mm or less, a biopsy is not needed because the risk of cancer is extremely low. The reader is directed to other articles of interest, including a special Dutch Study in Postmenopausal Bleeding,[116] among the references.[117-122]

Recently, endometrial blood flow mapping using power Doppler TVS has been done in perimenopausal women with bleeding and a thickened endometrium.[123,124]

Color-coded flow studies have also been suggested[125,126] to evaluate the probability of endometrial cancer.

Pathologic Conditions

In addition to lesions affecting the most important structure in the uterine cavity (i.e., the endometrium), pathologic findings of the uterus that should have their ultrasound appearance described include intracavitary fluid, adhesions, polyps, tiny or medium-sized fibroids bulging into the cavity, and foreign bodies.

Intracavitary Fluid

Intracavitary fluid, the most common pathologic finding, involves a small amount of fluid seen in the uterine cavity on the first days of menstrual flow.

The sonographer should consider pregnancy-related fluid accumulations in the uterus, and pregnancy should be suspected and ruled out. The findings can range from a normal pregnancy with an intact and healthy gestational sac to an early pregnancy failure in which no or very few extraembryonic structures are seen in the uterine cavity. Another example of pathologic intracavitary fluid collection related to pregnancy is the pseudogestational sac of the ectopic gestation. This is discussed in more detail in Chapters 11 and 12.

Various degrees of cervical obstruction, mostly in the postmenopausal years, can give rise to intracavitary fluid. When intracavitary fluid is found, endometrial cancer should be considered first. However, a well-delineated and thin endometrial lining is usually not pathognomonic of endometrial cancer[127-135] (Fig. 5–23). Rarely, varying amounts of intracavitary fluid are detected, mostly at the time of menarche. The most worrisome manifestation of this condition is the occurrence of a fluid collection behind an imperforate hymen. In this case, a good history as well as a transabdominal or transperitoneal scan will clarify the situation.

Most important, intracavitary fluid can be the sign of an active endometrial cancer in the presence of thick, irregular endometrium or loss of the endometrial–myometrial interface.[136-142] In such cases, known as *pyometra*, the fluid collection is caused by endometrial or even cervical carcinoma, in which some obstruction prevents the fluid from draining.[128,129,133]

Adhesions

This entity is known as *Asherman's syndrome*.[142,143] Sonography shows endometrial irregularities that appear as mildly echogenic, sometimes sonolucent bridges between the opposing walls of the myometrium (Fig. 5–24). They are better

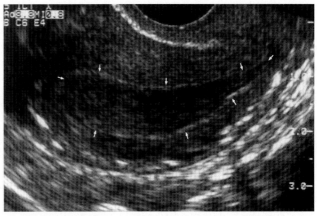

Figure 5–23. Pyometra in a postmenopausal patient. The cavity (outlined by *small arrows*) is filled with weakly echogenic fluid. The endometrial lining is smooth and thin; however, no cancer was detected in the pathologic specimen.

observed with artificial distention of the uterine cavity using fluid,[144,145] or simply by scanning the patient in the secretory phase of the cycle when endometrial echogenicity serves as a natural contrast to the myometrium. The best tool to diagnose this entity (or rule it out), however, is saline infusion sonohysterography (SIS).

Polyps

Polyps may be small or extremely large, filling the intracavitary space. They typically have a slightly higher echogenicity than the endometrium itself or the myometrium (Fig. 5–25A and B). However, their changes in echogenicity during the menstrual cycle are due to the changing echogenicity of the endometrium that covers them.

The differential diagnosis of endocavitary polyps can be difficult because it is not easy to distinguish between a polyp and a submucous fibroid (see also under Leiomyomas, later). As a rule, the polyp is oval or fusiform, it is slightly more echogenic than the surrounding myometrium (or a fibroid), and its main feeding vessel divides into several smaller branches within the polyp (Fig. 5–26). The submucous fibroid, however, is spheric (round on 2D ultrasound), its echotexture matches that of the adjacent myometrium, and its feeding vessel supplies the surface of the fibroid in a circular pattern (Fig. 5–27). If the patient is scanned during the late secretory phase of the cycle, submucous fibroids can be distinguished by their lower echogenicity and distal shadowing.

Sometimes, fluid present in the uterine cavity can delineate a polyp.[142] Injection of fluid into the cavity (i.e., sonohysterography; Fig. 5–25D–F) can increase the chances of an accurate diagnosis.[143-145] Goldstein et al.[146,147] found some correlation between blood flow indices, including resistance and flow velocity, and the histologic nature of polyps; hence, color Doppler evaluation of polyps can provide information about their origin and vascular supply (Fig. 5–28). Sometimes the presence of endometrial polyps can be diagnosed without injection of saline into the cavity, simply by applying color or power Doppler: the feeding vessel "lights up," marking the site and the stalk of the polyp (Fig. 5–29). The technique, evaluation, and clinical value of sonohysterography are discussed in Chapter 15.

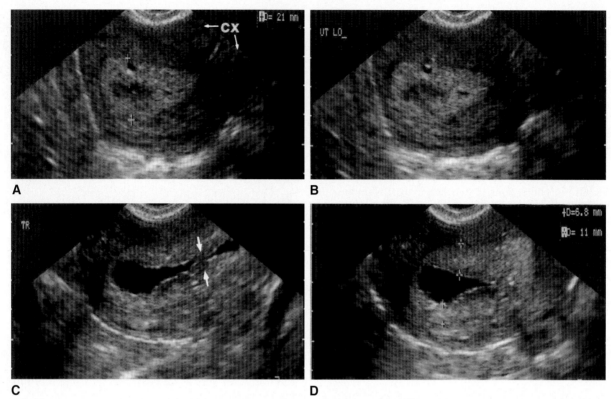

Figure 5–24. Asherman's syndrome. **A** and **B,** Sagittal views of the uterus in the secretory phase of the cycle (CX, cervix). The endometrium is 21 mm thick and is irregular in shape. **C** and **D,** Sonohysterography. A permanent synechia *(arrows)* between the walls of the cavity is seen.

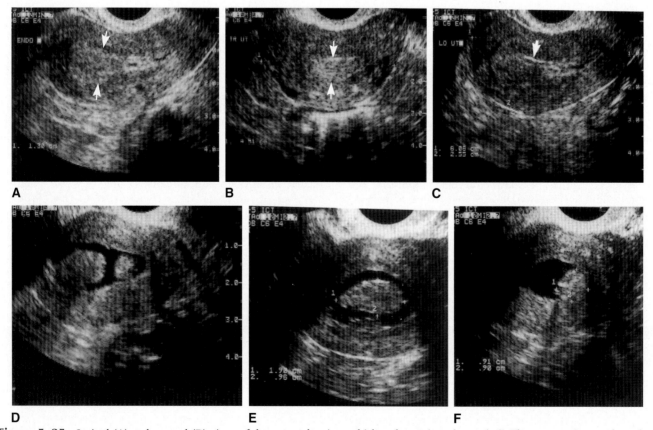

Figure 5–25. Sagittal (**A**) and coronal (**B**) views of the uterus showing a thick endometrium *(arrows)*. **C,** The *arrow* points to the polyp. **D** through **F,** Sonohysterography revealed the true identity of the lesion: two endometrial polyps.

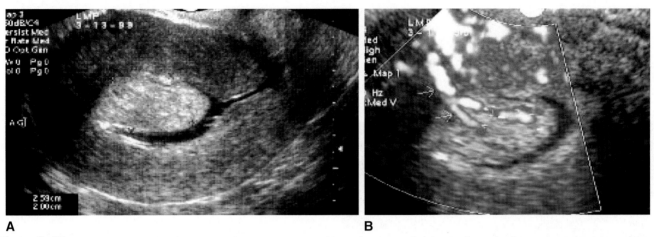

A   **B**

Figure 5–26. Recognizing a polyp by sonographic criteria using saline infusion sonohysterography and color or power Doppler. **A,** Gray-scale appearance. The fusiform or oval polyp is more hyperechoic than the myometrium. **B,** Power Doppler demonstrates typical branching of the feeding vessel *(arrows)* of this fundal polyp.

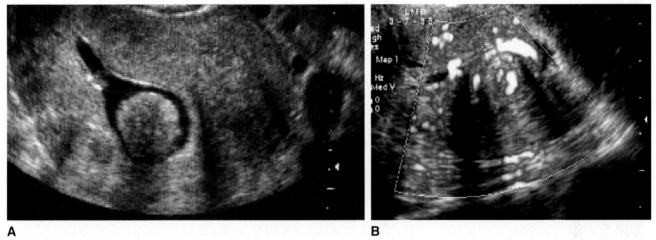

A   **B**

Figure 5–27. Recognizing a submucous fibroid by sonographic criteria using saline infusion sonohysterography and color or power Doppler. **A,** Gray-scale appearance of the round (spheric on three-dimensional ultrasound) posterior wall submucous fibroid. **B,** Power Doppler shows the typical circular pattern of vessels running on the surface of the fibroid.

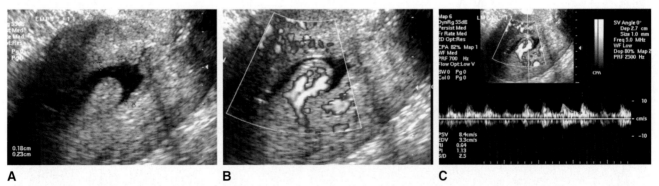

A   **B**   **C**

Figure 5–28. Studying the vascular supply of endometrial polyps after saline infusion sonohysterography. **A,** Gray-scale appearance of the polyp. **B,** Power Doppler enhancement of the vessel in the posterior wall pedicle. **C,** Doppler velocity waveform analysis.

Occasionally, a peculiar pattern in the uterine central area is seen in scans of patients receiving tamoxifen therapy for breast cancer[148] (Fig. 5–30). These findings may be misdiagnosed as endometrial polyps unless SIS is performed, which will reveal their true nature. Such patterns most probably reflect subendometrial changes consistent with adenomyosis

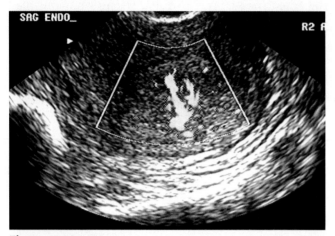

Figure 5–29. Vascular supply of a polyp. The feeding vessel originates from the posterior wall of the uterine cavity.

(see Chapter 6). Flow studies may show a low resistance to flow.

Intrauterine Foreign Bodies

The most common foreign body introduced into the intrauterine cavity is the intrauterine contraceptive device (IUD). These devices appear as highly reflective echogenic interfaces (Fig. 5–31). They are better visualized with TVS than by transabdominal sonography, although they can be recognized on transabdominal scans by their specific shape, shadowing, or reverberation echoes.[144,145] Often, the string of the IUD cannot be located during a speculum examination of the patient. In this case, TVS may be the most important tool for locating the "lost" IUD.[1-3,85,149-152] It is useful to know the exact shape of the lost IUD to be able to recognize it swiftly during the ultrasound evaluation. Three-dimensional ultrasound may be better able to define the type of device (Fig. 5–32). The possible concomitant existence of an IUD and pregnancy also has to be considered and recognized.

Congenital Anomalies of the Uterus

Two-dimensional TVS and transabdominal sonography can accurately determine the presence of various types of congenital uterine anomalies (Fig. 5–33). The American Fertility

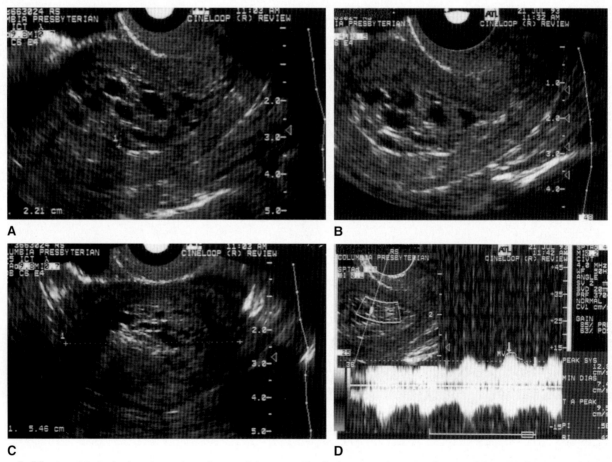

A   **B**

C   **D**

Figure 5–30. **A** and **B,** Sagittal sections of a patient receiving tamoxifen for breast cancer. In **A,** the size of the central uterine echo is 2.2 cm. Note the thick appearance of what seems to be the endometrial cavity, with multiple sonolucent structures. **C,** Transverse section. **D,** Color-flow Doppler velocity measurement of the feeding artery shows a pulsatility index of 0.51 and a resistance index of 0.41. Histopathologic evidence of cancer was not found in this case.

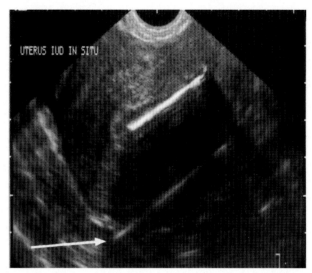

Figure 5–31. Sagittal view of the uterus with an intrauterine contraceptive device (IUD). Shadowing is seen behind the device. A reverberation artifact of the IUD also can be seen *(arrow)*.

Society's classification of uterine anomalies into seven groups should be used as a guideline for the work-up of such patients.[153] For both transabdominal and transvaginal scanning, knowledge of the possible anomalies is important so the clinician can mentally visualize the image obtained in both the coronal and sagittal planes.

The advantages and disadvantages of transabdominal sonography versus TVS for imaging various kinds of uterine anomalies are discussed in the literature. Whichever method is chosen, it is important that the scanning be performed in the progestative (secretory) phase of the cycle, when the hyperechoic endometrium provides good contrast to outline the shape of the uterine cavity[154-164] (Fig. 5–34).

The introduction of 3D ultrasound revolutionized the ultrasound work-up of uterine anomalies by finally making it possible to image the "elusive" coronal plane of the uterus. With or without SIS (Fig. 5–35), the shape of the uterine cavity and cervix, as well as the fundal contours, can be seen. A reliable diagnosis can then be established, making the contrast hysterosalpingogram redundant. Chapter 19 provides a detailed discussion of the use of 3D ultrasound in the work-up of uterine pathologic processes.

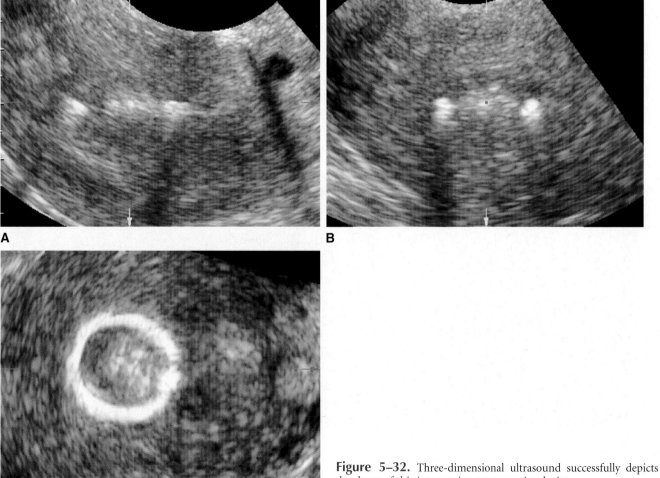

A

B

C

Figure 5–32. Three-dimensional ultrasound successfully depicts the shape of this intrauterine contraceptive device.

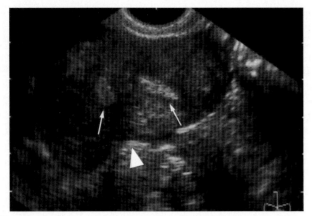

Figure 5–33. Coronal view of a bicornuate uterus. The two endometria *(arrows)* in the secretory phase of the cycle and the discrete notch between the cornua *(arrowhead)* are depicted.

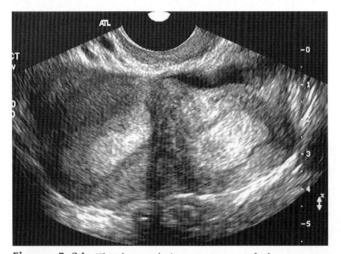

Figure 5–34. The hyperechoic appearance of the secretory endometrium can be used as a natural contrast to diagnose uterine anomalies on two-dimensional ultrasound.

Leiomyomas

Leiomyomas, or fibroids, are the most common tumors of the female patient. They are also the most common cause of uterine enlargement. These benign tumors arise from the smooth muscle covering of the intramyometrial and arcuate vessels as well as from the soft connecting tissue. They can be classified according to their location, such as fundal, subserosal, pedunculated (Fig. 5–36), submucous (see Fig. 5–27), intramural (Fig. 5–37), and cervical (see Fig. 5–17). Depending on the location, they may or may not cause clinical signs and symptoms. They are hormone dependent and therefore grow to significant sizes in the reproductive years. Ultrasound attributes of leiomyomas include distortion of the outer uterine contours, occasional poor sound transmission, pressure deformity of the endometrium, and, if they are dense, distal shadowing. If they are calcified, hyperechoic foci may appear, causing significant distal shadowing (Fig. 5–38). Cystic degeneration may also be a complication of a large fibroid (Fig. 5–39).

TVS is the scanning route of choice when the uterine volume is relatively small and the focal range of the higher-frequency vaginal probe can accommodate all the fibroids within the uterus. Frequently, however, only the combination of transabdominal and the transvaginal routes will permit complete imaging of an unusually large fibroid uterus. It is clear, however, that ultrasound is the easiest and least expensive modality to diagnose uterine fibroids.

Submucous fibroids should be diagnosed using TVS (enhanced by color or power Doppler and 3D ultrasound) and SIS (Fig. 5–40) before a more invasive diagnostic hysteroscopy is performed.[165] If submucous fibroids are diagnosed, the degree of endometrial cavity distortion must be established. This is important mainly for patients followed and treated for infertility and in regard to possible mechanical disturbances within the endometrial cavity.

The ultrasound differential diagnosis of pedunculated uterine fibroids includes adnexal or ovarian masses and fibroids, to name the most common ones. A submucous

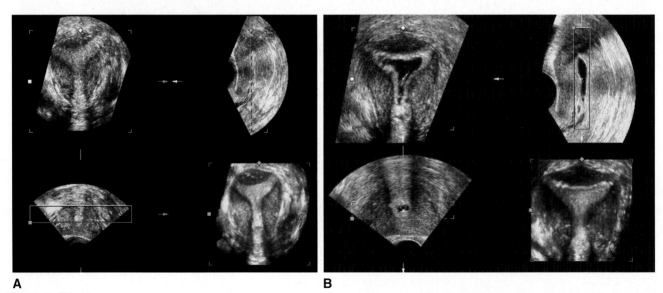

A   **B**

Figure 5–35. Three-dimensional evaluation of suspected uterine malformations. The clinical value of displaying the uterus in the coronal plane (box A) cannot be overemphasized. **A,** Orthogonal display of a normal uterus. The rendered thick-slice image of the uterus in the coronal plane is seen in box D. **B,** Orthogonal display of saline infusion hysterosonography enhances the normal uterine cavity.

fibroid may be misdiagnosed as an endometrial polyp, retained blood, or retained products of conception within the uterine cavity. A molar pregnancy usually resembles a cluster of grapes, with sonolucent cystic structures of different sizes (Fig. 5–41). These cystic structures can become quite large (Fig. 5–42). Three-dimensional power Doppler evaluation of molar pregnancies shows significant vascularization (Fig. 5–43). Figure 5–44 depicts a mass on the left side of the urethra of a patient previously diagnosed with a molar pregnancy. The appearance could be mistaken for a fibroid. The diagnosis in this case was metastatic choriocarcinoma.

Adenomyosis

Adenomyosis, a fairly common condition involving the uterus, usually is characterized by diffuse uterine enlargement,

numerous microcysts of different sizes, and multiple shadows that give a "rain-in-the-forest" appearance (Fig. 5–45). Its ultrasound diagnosis is difficult, and Popp et al.[166] suggested puncture biopsy of the uterus to establish the correct diagnosis in such cases (see Chapter 15). Sometimes, multiple tiny sonolucencies in the myometrium appear. Chapter 6 provides an in-depth discussion of adenomyosis.

Fallopian Tubes

Normal Anatomy

Because the normal fallopian tube is a very poor sonic reflector, is tortuous, and lacks clear interfaces, it is very difficult to image sonographically and hence is imaged only rarely. Even the diseased tube often cannot be imaged with sufficient clarity by transabdominal sonography. If the goal is to obtain good-quality ultrasound images of the fallopian tubes, the first choice would be to use a high-frequency transvaginal probe.[1-6,167-169]

A healthy fallopian tube can be imaged only if some contrasting fluid surrounds it (Fig. 5–46). Intrapelvic fluid that may help outline a normal fallopian tube may be present after ovulation, at or just after mid-cycle, so scanning should be done at that time. The proximal end of the tube can be imaged by TVS for approximately 1 or 2 cm after it leaves the cornual area.

Pathologic Conditions

Pathologic conditions, such as neoplastic, vascular, infectious, or other conditions, can produce blood, ascitic fluid, pus, or other fluids that provide contrast. The tool of choice for diagnosis is the vaginal probe. Disease in the tube is relatively easy to detect, as is discussed in more detail in Chapter 21.

Text continued on p. 74

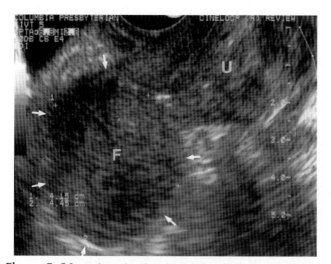

Figure 5–36. Pedunculated, right-sided uterine fibroid *(arrows)*. F, fibroid; U, uterus.

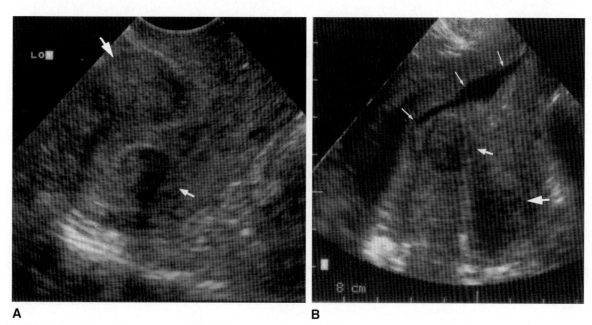

A   **B**

Figure 5–37. Two sections of a uterus containing discrete intramural fibroids *(arrows)*. **A,** These fibroids measure between 1.5 and 2 cm. Shadowing is seen behind each of them. **B,** Instillation of fluid into the cavity *(thin arrows)* highlights the slight bulging of one of the small fibroids into the uterine cavity *(small arrows)*.

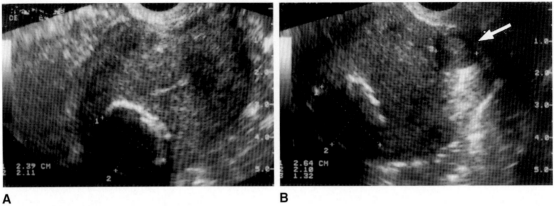

Figure 5–38. Sagittal (**A**) and coronal (**B**) views of a fibroid with hyperechoic outline (calcification?) measuring 2.4 × 2.1 × 2.6 cm. A small, 1.3-cm noncalcified fibroid also is shown *(arrow).*

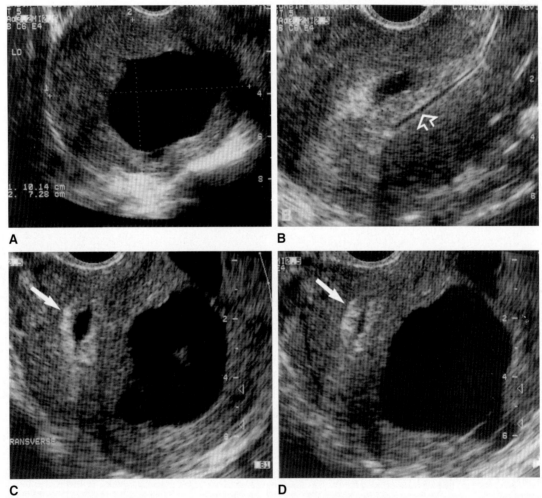

Figure 5–39. Serial views of a large posterior fibroid showing sonolucent core (degeneration?). **A,** The degenerating fibroid. **B,** The relation of the fibroid to the cavity was studied by injecting fluid into the cavity through the catheter *(open arrow).* **C** and **D,** Fluid distends the cavity *(arrows)* and shows that the fibroid is about 1 cm remote from the cavity.

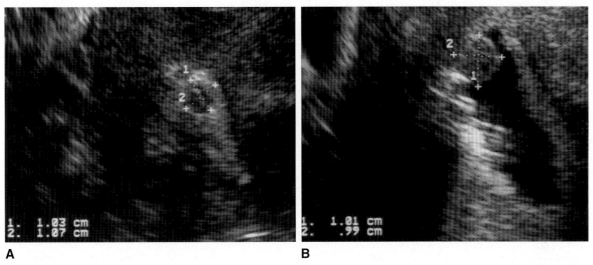

A   **B**

Figure 5–40. Submucous fibroid. **A,** Hyperechoic endometrium in the secretory phase serves as a good contrast to the small 1 × 1-cm sonolucent submucous fibroid. **B,** The same submucous fibroid is shown enhanced by instillation of a small amount of fluid into the cavity. These tiny fibroids may not cause shadowing behind them; therefore, at times it is difficult to recognize them without special sonohysterographic studies. Hysteroscopy was confirmatory.

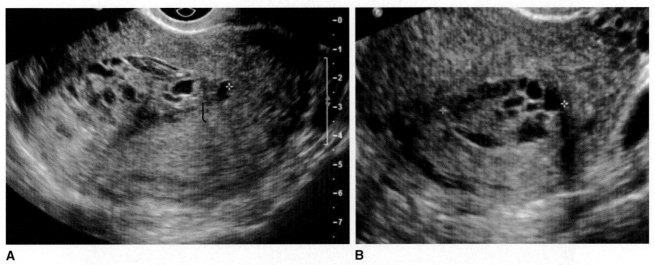

A   **B**

Figure 5–41. Sagittal (**A**) and transverse (**B**) views of early molar pregnancy with typical multiple cystic appearance.

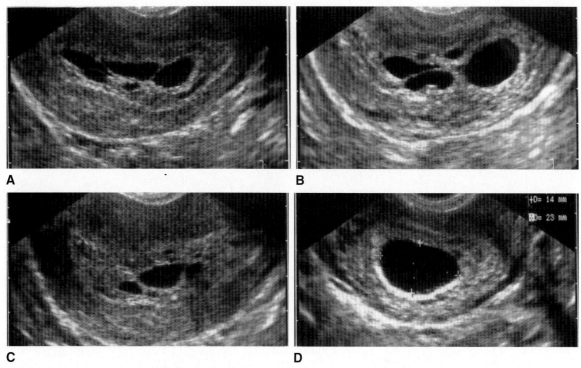

Figure 5–42. **A** through **D,** Four serial coronal views of the uterus in a patient with molar pregnancy of 10 weeks' gestation and a human chorionic gonadotropin level of 60,000 mIU/mL (IRP). Note the cystic structures of various sizes from 1 or 2 mm to a larger 14 × 23-mm space, creating the false impression of an intrauterine pregnancy. Histologic study revealed only molar tissue.

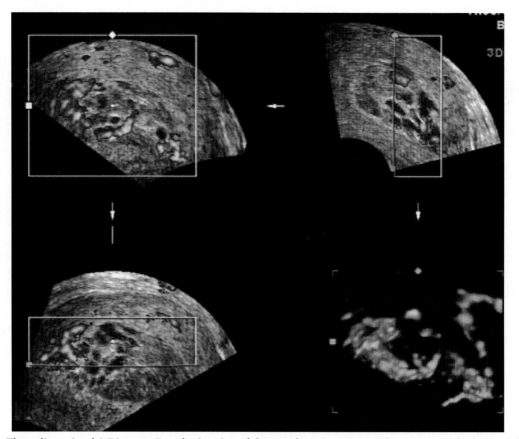

Figure 5–43. Three-dimensional (3D) power Doppler imaging of the vascular pattern in a molar pregnancy (orthogonal display). Box D shows the rendering of the 3D power Doppler angiogram of the vascular supply.

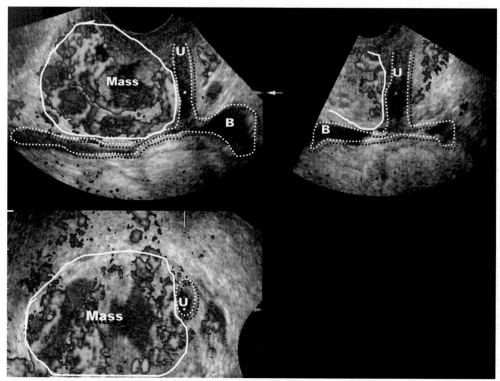

Figure 5–44. Three-dimensional power Doppler display of a right paraurethral mass in a patient with metastatic choriocarcinoma. B, bladder; U, urethra.

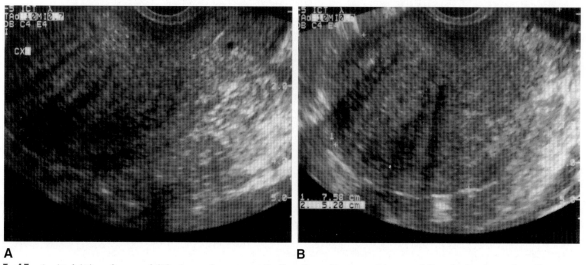

A   **B**

Figure 5–45. Sagittal (**A**) and coronal (**B**) views of a symmetrically enlarged uterus with several fine shadowings of small structures in the myometrium. The clinical and histopathologic findings were consistent with adenomyosis.

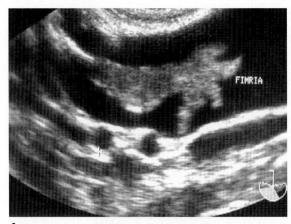

Figure 5–46. The normal fallopian tube. **A,** Free pelvic fluid surrounding the fimbrial end of a normal tube. **B,** Normal fallopian tube (F) and fimbriae float in the sonolucent fluid of a peritoneal inclusion cyst. The peritoneal inclusion cyst is defined by two features: its walls are the pelvic side walls *(arrows)*, and thin adhesions are visible *(arrowheads)*. CDS, cul-de-sac; OV, ovary.

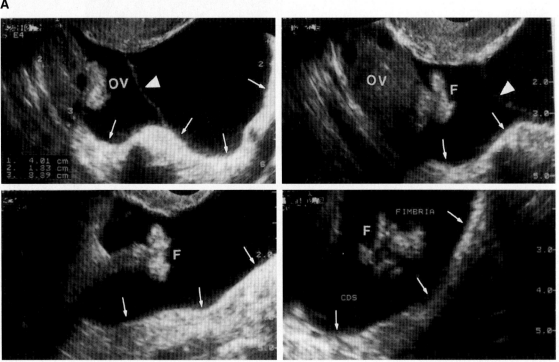

Tubal Patency

Hysterosalpingography is the gold standard for evaluating tubal patency.[169-171] It involves injection of an ultrasound contrast material and observing its passage through the tubes by TVS. The contrast material is visible during its passage through the tubal lumen or spilling out the fimbrial end. Among the ultrasound contrast materials used, the simplest is normal saline.[169-171] However, specific contrast materials such as Albunex[172] (Molecular Biosystems, San Diego, Calif) and Echovist-450 (Schering AG, Berlin, Germany) also have been developed.[173-178] When the results using ultrasound contrast materials are compared with those obtained by laparoscopic chromoperturbation (injection of dye through the cervix to observe its tubal passage by laparoscopy), 50% to 85% agreement is reported in the literature.[179]

The 1990s saw the development of gray-scale as well as color Doppler evaluation of tubal patency. Color-flow studies of tubal patency, which is based on Doppler evaluation of the fimbrial area, also have been reported[178-182]; correlation of these results with hysterosalpingography and chromopertubation under laparoscopic control is as high as 93%. Testing fallopian tube patency as an office-based procedure also has been advocated.[181] Nevertheless, ultrasound evaluation of fallopian tube patency is still in the research state.

Ovary

Normal Anatomy and Sonography

One of the most important tasks of gynecologic sonography is imaging the ovaries. Scanning of the ovaries is important to the endocrinologist, infertility specialist, general gynecologic practitioner, and gynecologic oncologist. Transabdominal sonography provides the examiner with a panoramic view and the exact relationships between the adnexal organs, uterus, and cul-de-sac. Using transabdominal sonography, Goswamy et al.[183] were able to see the ovary in 99% of their postmenopausal patients. However, because of transabdominal scanning's relatively low resolution, discerning fine detail of a normal or pathologic ovary is almost impossible. Therefore, the tool of choice to image the female pelvis in general and the adnexa in particular is the transvaginal probe equipped with a high-frequency transducer. Even with TVS, locating the ovaries can be a time-consuming procedure. Once they are identified, however, high-resolution capability permits detection of minute structures (<1 to 2 mm) in the ovarian stroma and their interrogation by color-flow Doppler studies.

Using TVS, Rodriguez and colleagues,[184] scanning 52 menopausal women, could see the ovaries in 81%. Sassone et al.,[185] scanning 143 women between 20 and 85 years of age, were able to see the ovaries with a frequency of 76%. Gollub and associates[186] were successful in imaging the ovaries in post-menopausal women in 64% of cases. Holbert[187] detected one or both ovaries in 65% of postmenopausal women scanned.

The normal ovary is relatively easy to detect in the reproductive years. Follicles or the corpus luteum serves as ultrasound markers. The transvaginal probe should be directed toward the side walls of the pelvis. The normal-sized ovary in a patient without previous surgery or pelvic inflammatory disease will be found overlying the hypogastric vein in most cases (Fig. 5–47). The examiner's free hand should be placed on the patient's abdomen to apply pressure and manipulate the ovary into the vaginal probe's field of view, much like a bimanual pelvic examination. The examination should begin with TVS, performed with an empty bladder, reserving the transabdominal scan in the event any unanswered questions remain after TVS.[188]

If intrapelvic fluid is present, the ovaries are easily visualized by TVS (Fig. 5–48). It is more difficult to image the ovaries in the postmenopausal patient because the ovaries are smaller and devoid of follicles, and there is a decreased amount of pelvic fluid to provide an acoustic interphase. In this case, peristalsis of the surrounding small bowel may help outline the static, usually hypoechoic and shrunken ovary.

It should be remembered that follicles are normal physiologic structures in the ovary during the reproductive years. They should be called *follicles*, not "follicular cysts" or "ovarian cysts," which would imply a pathologic process. They can be easily and concisely differentiated from structures that are nonphysiologic components of the ovary. When they are large, the term *unruptured follicles* may be appropriate.[189]

There is no consensus regarding under what circumstances an ovarian pathologic process can be ruled out. One view holds that a scan can be deemed normal only if the ovary was imaged and appears normal. The opposing view, however, requires the use of a transvaginal probe and its high resolution, which would detect the presence of even a small lesion. Therefore, if TVS examination of the pelvis is negative by such a high-resolution probe, there is sound reason to believe that no tumor or pathologic process is present.

Ultrasound evaluation of the ovaries in the context of infertility is discussed in detail in Chapter 14. Hyperstimulated ovaries are easily located because of their large number of follicles. Occasionally, even the cumulus oophorus is visible (Fig. 5–49).

If a patient has undergone hysterectomy, the ovaries are more difficult to see because of the presence of bowel, which fills the space left by the removal of the uterus. It is important in this case to displace the bowel loops by placing a hand on the abdomen (see also Chapter 4). Bowel peristalsis also helps to differentiate between moveable structures in the pelvis and the static ovary, which will quietly stand out.

An important point to consider is when to scan for ovarian problems. In the reproductive years, it is recommended that the ovarian scan be performed before mid-cycle. This is to avoid the presence of the corpus luteum, which adds volume to the ovary and may mislead even the most experienced sonologist with its potentially bizarre appearance. If flow measurements are contemplated, they also need to be done during the first part of the menstrual cycle and certainly before the appearance of the corpus luteum. However, if there are important clinical indications for performing the scan, the examination should not be postponed. We usually advise our referring providers to ask for evaluation of ovarian (and endometrial) problems between days 5 and 9 of the cycle. If it is impossible to date the cycle because of hysterectomy, we usually rescan the ovaries exactly 14 days after the first scan to ensure that at least one of the two scans was performed before ovulation occurred. The smaller postmenopausal ovaries are somewhat harder to detect, so TVS should always be used for their imaging.[183]

The size of the normal ovary varies with the time in the menstrual cycle as well as with the patient's age (more specifically, with her hormonal status). Usually, the volume of the ovary is calculated by multiplying its longest diameter by the two additional diameters lying in the planes at right angles to it ($A \times B \times C$), and dividing by 2 (grossly, the formula for the

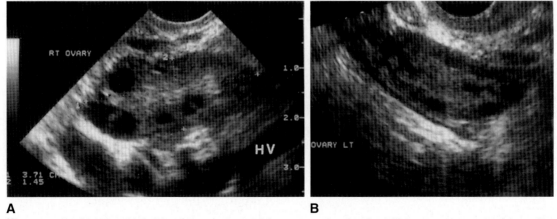

A   **B**

Figure 5–47. Normal right (**A**) and left (**B**) ovaries on day 7 of the menstrual cycle. The follicles serve as sonographic markers during the woman's reproductive years. HV, hypogastric vein.

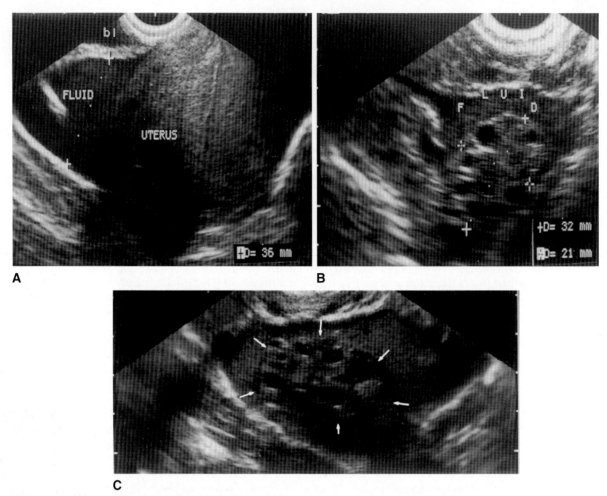

Figure 5–48. Pelvic fluid with low-level echogenicity (blood). **A,** Sagittal view shows fluid anteriorly between the uterus and the bladder (bl). **B** and **C,** The fluid serves as good contrast to highlight the normal-size ovary *(arrows)*.

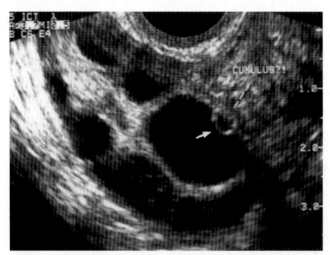

Figure 5–49. The hormonally stimulated right ovary with several follicles. In the largest one, a structure may be consistent with a cumulus oophorus *(arrow)*.

Table 5–2	Ovarian Volumes in Menopause	
Study	**Mean Volume (cm³)**	**Range (cm³)**
Goswamy et al.[183] (transabdominal)	3.6	0.8-6.4
Granberg and Wikland[188] (transvaginal)	1.3	0.7-1.9
Rodriguez et al.[184]	1.8	0.8-4.7
Pavlik et al.[194]	—	8 (upper limit)
McCarthy et al.[132]	—	2.5 (upper limit)

volume of an ovoid). Before ovulation, the ovary measures 5.1 ± 3.1 cm³. After ovulation, it measures 3.2 ± 1.7 cm³. TVS measurements of ovarian volumes are slightly lower than those obtained transabdominally,[184] which may be due to more precise measurements on higher-resolution scans. Volumes in the menopause are shown in Table 5–2.

Recently, a dedicated 3D ultrasound software program became available for measuring ovarian volume. Figure 5–50 demonstrates the volume measurement of a polycystic ovary using this software.

Corpus Luteum and Its Variants

The ultrasound image of the corpus luteum changes from day to day as it reflects the processes of bleeding, clot formation,

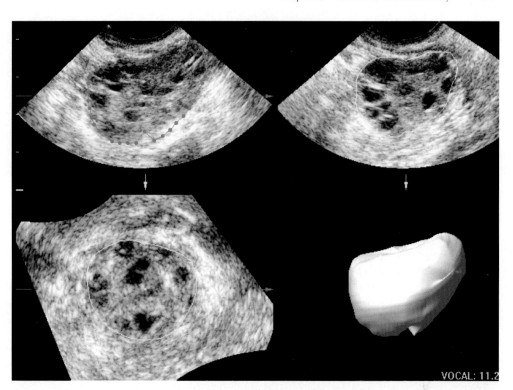

Figure 5–50. Three-dimensional display of an ovary. Using the GE Kretz (Zipf, Austria) Virtual Organ Computer-aided Analysis (VOCAL) software program, its volume and contour (*yellow lines*) can be calculated—in this case, volume is 11.2 cm³.

retraction, and reabsorption of blood. It assumes the most bizarre internal structures imaginable. One of the many "faces" of the corpus luteum is depicted in Figure 5–51. The clot may appear as an echogenic or an anechoic structure, a cavernous or an irregularly echogenic area with multilocularity, an echogenic core with spikes branching out of the center to the periphery, or even a fine, meshlike texture. It can mimic a pathologic process, such as an ectopic gestation, neoplasia, or a degenerated fibroid. The image can be interpreted correctly, however, by identifying normal ovarian tissue around the structure, scanning during the early follicular phase of the cycle, and evaluating the blood flow pattern by using power or color Doppler (Fig. 5–52). Knowledge of the exact time in the cycle is imperative. Sometimes, in the nonpregnant state, the corpus luteum may persist, grow, and form a corpus luteum cyst. The cyst may rupture, making the TVS diagnosis extremely difficult. Also, a small, 2- to 4-mm hyperechoic structure may be seen in the ovary of a woman in her reproductive years (Fig. 5–53). This is consistent with the involuted remnant of a corpus luteum (corpus albicans) and may persist for several cycles. If such a structure persists for more than three or four cycles, the diagnosis is most probably a benign ovarian teratoma, although a degree of shadowing should be expected in this case.

A word about terminology is appropriate here: a normal-sized corpus luteum (2 to 3 cm) should *never* be called a "corpus luteum cyst"; rather, it should be called simply a *corpus luteum* or *hemorrhagic corpus luteum,* avoiding the unnecessary word "cyst." It should be described in terms of the day of the patient's cycle and its content, wall structure, and typical peripheral circular blood flow pattern. If a follicle or a corpus luteum is called a "cyst" (these are the two most common examples of this misnomer), the patient will refer to it as a pathologic finding, misleading herself and each subsequent physician taking her gynecologic history. When a

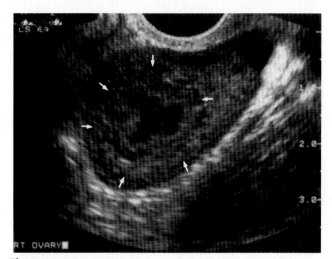

Figure 5–51. Corpus luteum (*arrows*) amid the ovary. The crenated internal edges of the cystic structure are clearly seen.

corpus luteum is labeled a "cyst," patients may be subjected to other, more expensive and unnecessary imaging tests and even to a potentially harmful surgical procedure.[188] Only if the corpus luteum exceeds 4 to 5 cm is there some justification for describing it as a cyst. In this case, the term *hemorrhagic corpus luteum cyst* may be used.[187,188]

On duplex Doppler flow velocity studies, a low-impedance-velocity waveform for the ovarian blood supply is almost always typical of the luteal phase of the menstrual cycle.[99] This waveform results from the extensive neovascularization and temporary angiogenesis around the corpus luteum, which are probably developing to carry the products of the corpus luteum into the menstrual circulation. Such prominent diastolic flow is typical for the duration of the corpus luteum. Hence, if the resistance and pulsatility indices of a corpus

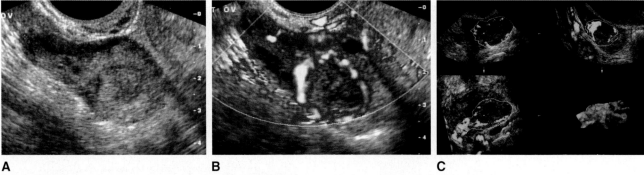

A   **B**   **C**

Figure 5–52. Three different sonographic approaches for correctly diagnosing the presence of a corpus luteum. **A,** Gray-scale appearance. (Note that there are endless sonographic variants and appearances of corpora lutea.) **B,** Power (or color) Doppler depicts the circular flow pattern typical of a fresh corpus luteum. **C,** Three-dimensional (3D) power Doppler angiogram with rendering of the vasculature around and within the corpus luteum. Box D contains the 3D angiographic rendering of the vessels in and leading to (and from) the structure.

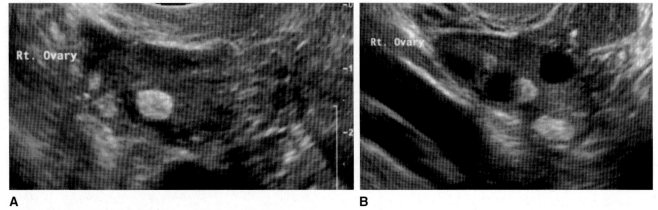

A   **B**

Figure 5–53. The hyperechoic nodule on this normal ovary represents the remnant of an "old" corpus luteum on its way to becoming a corpus albicans. **A,** Coronal section. **B,** Longitudinal section.

luteum need to be differentiated from those typical for ovarian cancer, the patient should be reexamined on the first days of the next menstrual cycle. The rationale for scheduling patients for ovarian scanning before ovulation is therefore twofold: first, to avoid confusing the low resistance and pulsatility indices associated with a corpus luteum in the luteal phase of the cycle with the flow characteristics associated with ovarian cancer; and second, to avoid confusing the morphologic features of the cancerous ovary with those of the corpus luteum.

Some clinicians make a distinction between the corpus luteum and a hemorrhagic corpus luteum cyst (Figs. 5–54 and 5–55). Those who diagnose hemorrhagic cysts agree that these do, in fact, result from the "basic" corpus luteum. However, the ultrasound picture is that of a cystic mass with low-level echoes, although it can also simulate a solid mass with slightly hypoechoic content.[190-192] When the clot in the cyst retracts, the ultrasound appearance can vary widely. I consider the hemorrhagic corpus luteum cyst to be a variant of the corpus luteum; the only differences between the two may be size (i.e., the corpus luteum is somewhat larger) and certain clinical implications.

Cul-de-sac

The space above the peritoneal recess covering the posterior aspect of the uterus and the anterior aspect of the rectum is called the *pouch of Douglas* or the *cul-de-sac*. The cul-de-sac, which is a potential space, may contain clear fluid, blood, pus, and occasionally organs or parts of organs with or without adhesions. Scrutinizing the cul-de-sac is one of the most important parts of pelvic imaging. The cul-de-sac can also be used to drain fluid, and it may serve as a passage through which to obtain puncture biopsies of the ovaries, uterus, and fallopian tubes.

The cul-de-sac can be imaged in the sagittal plane as well as the coronal or transverse plane if the probe is pointed in an extreme posterior direction. A moderate amount of pressure exerted on the cervix will move the uterus into the sagittal plane; normally, free displacement of the uterus over adjacent tissues should be observed. Adhesions, if present, can be observed and described using this technique. For a patient in the lithotomy position, the probe should point nearly in the direction of the floor. Free fluid usually collects in this space and is easily seen even in small amounts. Some fluid may be present immediately after ovulation (if no fluid was seen previously in the cul-de-sac); however, even in nonovulating women, some pelvic fluid may be present.[193] Large amounts of fluid, as with ascites or profuse bleeding, will not be missed even by the novice sonographer or sonologist.

Any amount of fluid in the cul-de-sac should be measured and included in the report. Its echogenicity, such as clear, specular, mixed, or containing floating structures, should be described (Figs. 5–56 to 5–60). An approximation of the

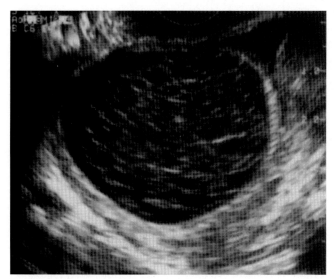

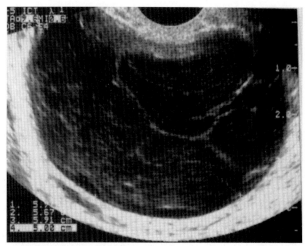

Figure 5–55. This cystic structure measures 5.7 × 5.6 × 5.9 cm and was scanned in the follicular phase of the cycle. It is probably a hemorrhagic corpus luteum cyst.

Figure 5–54. Hemorrhagic corpus luteum 3 weeks after the menstrual period. It measures 4.5 × 3.9 × 3.8 cm and is filled with speckles of low-level echogenicity.

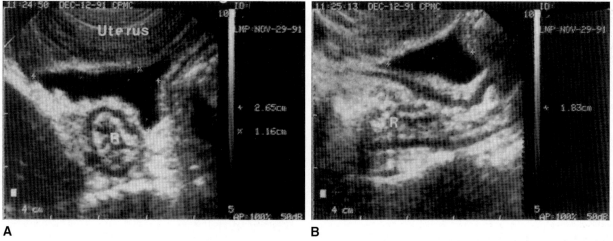

A   B

Figure 5–56. A small amount of free fluid in the cul-de-sac below the uterus and above the rectum (R) is visible on coronal (**A**) and sagittal (**B**) views. The amount of fluid is approximately 2.8 mL.

volume is obtained by measuring the fluid pocket in its three largest dimensions on two planes and using the well-known formula (A × B × C) × 0.5. For example, the approximate amount of fluid in the patient in Figure 5–56 is (2.65 × 1.16 × 1.83) × 0.5 = 2.8 mL. Only very rarely is it necessary to puncture this space and extract fluid for a diagnosis, but if this is required, a TVS-directed puncture procedure should be used instead of blind needle insertion. Finally, when writing up the clinical evaluation, it is important to place the appearance of fluid in the cul-de-sac in the context of the patient's history for the observation to be clinically useful.

The following structures can be seen in the cul-de-sac with or without the presence of pelvic fluid:

- Bowel, which can be recognized by peristalsis and its specular content (see Fig. 5–59)
- A fallopian tube, which can be difficult to discern if it is normal and not surrounded by fluid; however, it is easily diagnosed if it is pathologic and filled with fluid or its wall

is thickened or it is floating in fluid (see Figs. 5–45, 5–46, and 5–57)
- Ovaries, which occasionally fall behind the uterus into the cul-de-sac and can be diagnosed by their appearance (see Fig. 5–58)
- Various adnexal masses (i.e., if fluid is present in the cul-de-sac, the side wall of the pelvis may reveal projections or seedings of tumor originating from different abdominal sites)

Peritoneal inclusion cysts are simply loculated pelvic fluid. Their "walls" are the adjacent organs or the lesser pelvic wall. They are usually present after surgery or as a result of pelvic inflammatory disease. They may show filmy adhesions extending between the bowel, uterus, ovaries, and pelvic wall, and the diagnosis is made based on the patient's history and typical ultrasound findings (see Figs. 5–57 and 5–58).

At times, infected fluid is present in the cul-de-sac. Figure 5–60 shows a moderate amount of fluid in a patient with tuberculosis. The picture is similar in other types of infections.

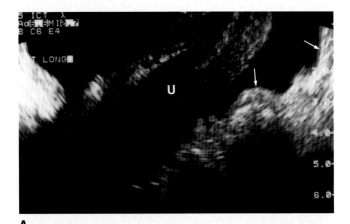

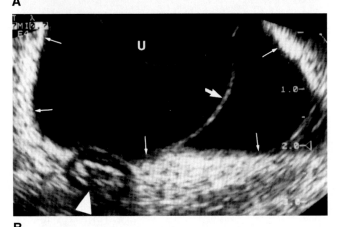

Figure 5–57. **A** and **B,** Two views of a pelvic peritoneal inclusion cyst. The two diagnostic features of this localized fluid collection are present: the boundaries of the fluid are the side walls of the pelvis *(thin arrows),* and thin, filmy adhesions are visible within the sonolucent fluid *(thick arrow).* The *arrowhead* indicates the rectum. U, uterus.

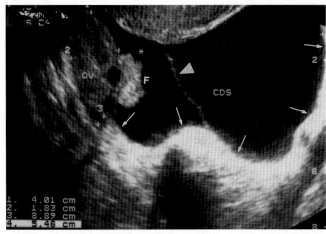

Figure 5–58. Peritoneal inclusion cyst defined by two features: its walls are the pelvic side walls *(arrows)* and there are thin adhesions *(arrowhead).* The normal fallopian tube (F) and fimbriae and ovary (OV) float in the sonolucent fluid. CDS, color Doppler study.

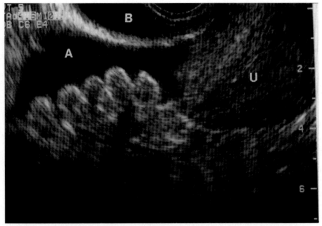

Figure 5–59. Small bowel loops float in ascites (A) above the uterus (U) and the bladder (B).

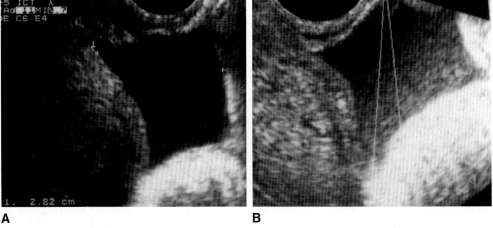

Figure 5–60. **A,** A small amount of fluid with diffuse, low-level echogenicity is seen in the cul-de-sac. The image in part **B** was obtained with increased gain to highlight the floating particulate matter. Laparoscopy revealed a serosanguineous fluid with cellular debris. Special stains were positive for tuberculosis bacilli.

Often, the fluid provides a detailed outline of almost all internal reproductive organs as well as their supportive ligaments (Fig. 5–61).

If one suspects a larger amount of free fluid in the pelvis, a longitudinal transabdominal scan should be performed in the anterior axillary line overlying the liver and the right kidney (Fig. 5–62). The presence of fluid in the space between the kidney and the liver (Morison's pouch) is a sensitive marker of a fluid collection exceeding 200 to 300 mL in a patient in the supine position.

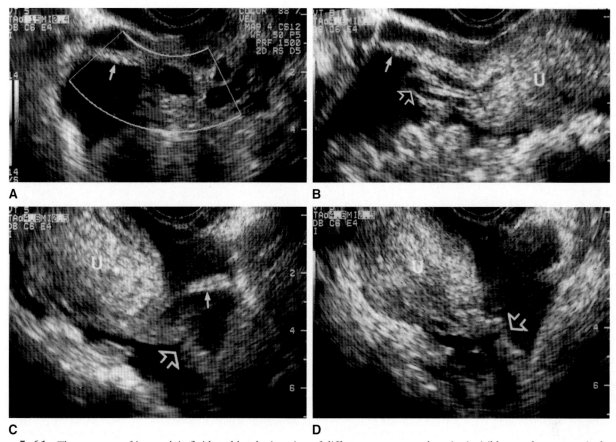

Figure 5–61. The presence of intrapelvic fluid enables the imaging of different structures otherwise invisible even by transvaginal sonography. **A** and **B,** On the right side, the right round ligament *(arrow)* and the fallopian tube *(open arrow)* are seen emerging from the uterine cornua (U). **C** and **D,** On the left side, the left round ligament *(arrow)* and the fallopian tube *(open arrow)* are seen originating from the uterus (U).

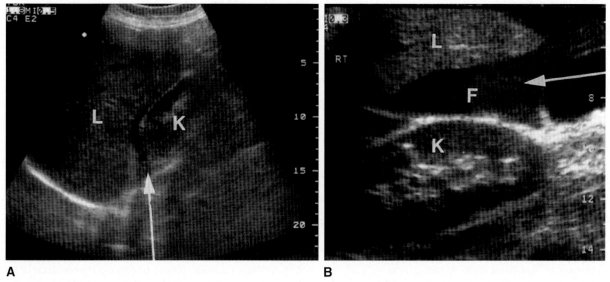

Figure 5–62. Morison's pouch *(arrow)* between the liver (L) and the right kidney (K). **A,** No fluid is seen. **B,** Fluid (F) is seen in the space.

REFERENCES

1. Fleischer AC, Romero R, Manning FA, et al: The Principle and the Practice of Ultrasonography in Obstetrics and Gynecology, 4th ed. East Norwalk, Conn, Appleton & Lange, 1991.
2. Timor-Tritsch IE, Rottem S: Transvaginal Sonography, 2nd ed. New York, Chapman & Hall, 1991.
3. Goldstein SR: Endovaginal Sonography, 2nd ed. New York, Wiley-Liss, 1991.
4. Sabbagha RE: Diagnostic Ultrasound Applied to Obstetrics and Gynecology, 3rd ed. Philadelphia, JB Lippincott, 1994.
5. Chervenak FA, Isaacson GC, Campbell S: Ultrasound in Obstetrics and Gynecology. Boston, Little, Brown, 1993.
6. Nyberg DA, Hill LM, Böhm-Velez M, Mendelson EB: Transvaginal Ultrasound. St. Louis, Mosby-Yearbook, 1992.
7. Varma TR, Patel RH, Pillai U: Ultrasonic assessment of cervix in normal pregnancy. Acta Obstet Gynecol Scand 1986;65:229-233.
8. Zemlyn S: The effect of the urinary bladder in obstetrical sonography. Radiology 1978;169:169-175.
9. Paterson-Brown S, Fisk NM, Rodeck CH, Rodeck E: Preinduction cervical assessment by Bishop's score and transvaginal ultrasound. Eur J Obstet Gynecol Reprod Biol 1991;40:17-23.
10. Bowie JD, Andreotti RF, Rosenberg EL: Sonographic appearance of the uterine cervix in pregnancy: The vertical cervix. Am J Radiol 1983;138:737-740.
11. Varma TR, Patel RH, Pillai U: Ultrasonic assessment of cervix in "at risk" patients. Acta Obstet Gynecol Scand 1986;65:147-152.
12. Ayers J, DeGrood R, Compton A, et al: Sonographic evaluation of the cervical length in pregnancy: Diagnosis and management of preterm cervical effacement in patients at risk for premature delivery. Obstet Gynecol 1988;71:939-944.
13. Podobnik M, Bulic M, Smiljanic N, et al: Ultrasonography in the detection of cervical incompetency. J Clin Ultrasound 1988;13:383-391.
14. Kushnir O, Vigil DA, Izquierdo L, et al: Vaginal sonographic assessment of cervical length changes during normal pregnancy. Am J Obstet Gynecol 1990;162:991-993.
15. Andersen HF: Transabdominal and transvaginal sonography of the uterine cervix during pregnancy. J Clin Ultrasound 1991;19:77-82.
16. Murakawa H, Utumi T, Hasegawa I, et al: Evaluation of threatened preterm delivery by transvaginal ultrasonographic measurement of cervical length. Obstet Gynecol 1993;82:829-832.
17. Smith CV, Anderson JC, Matamoros A, Rayburn WF: Transvaginal sonography of cervical width and length during pregnancy. J Ultrasound Med 1992;11:465-467.
18. Jackson GM, Ludmir J, Bader TJ: The accuracy of digital examination and ultrasound in the evaluation of cervical length. Obstet Gynecol 1992;79:214-218.
19. Bernstine RL, Lee SH, Crawford WL, et al: Sonographic evaluation of the incompetent cervix. J Clin Ultrasound 1981;9: 417-420.
20. Redford DHA, Nicol BD, Willman BK: Diagnosis by real time ultrasound of hourglass herniation of the fetal membranes. Br J Obstet Gynaecol 1981;88:73-75.
21. Brook I, Feingold M, Schwartz A: Ultrasonography in the diagnosis of cervical incompetence in pregnancy: A new diagnostic approach. Br J Obstet Gynaecol 1981;88:640-643.
22. Fried A: Bulging amnion in premature labor: Spectrum of sonographic findings. Am J Radiol 1981;136:181-185.
23. Vaalamo P, Kivikoski A: The incompetent cervix during pregnancy diagnosed by ultrasound. Acta Obstet Gynecol Scand 1983;62:19.
24. Feingold M, Brook I, Zakut H: Detection of cervical incompetence by ultrasound. Acta Obstet Gynecol Scand 1984;63:407.
25. Confino E, Mayden KL, Giglia RV, et al: Pitfalls in sonographic imaging of the incompetent uterine cervix. Acta Obstet Gynecol Scand 1986;65:593-597.
26. Michaels WH, Montgomery C, Karo J, et al: Ultrasound differentiation of the competent from the incompetent cervix: Prevention of preterm delivery. Am J Obstet Gynecol 1986;154:537-546.
27. Ludmir J: Sonographic detection of cervical incompetence. Clin Obstet Gynecol 1988;31:101-109.
28. Parulekar S, Kiwi R: Dynamic incompetent cervix uteri: Sonographic observations. J Ultrasound Med 1988;7:481-485.
29. Soneck JD, Iams JD, Blumenfeld M, et al: Measurement of cervical length in pregnancy: Comparison between vaginal ultrasonography and digital examination. Obstet Gynecol 1990;76:172-175.
30. Raner J, Davis Harrigan JT: Improving the outcome of cerclage by sonographic follow-up. J Ultrasound Med 1990;9:275-278.
31. Quinn MJ: Vaginal ultrasound and cervical cerclage: A prospective study. Ultrasound Obstet Gynecol 1992;2:410-416.
32. Brown JE, Thiema GA, Shah DM, et al: Transabdominal and transvaginal endosonography: Evaluation of the cervix and lower uterine segment in pregnancy. Am J Obstet Gynecol 1986;155:721-726.
33. Boozarjomehri F, Timor-Tritsch IE, Chao CR, Fox HE: Transvaginal sonographic evaluation of the cervix in labor: Presence of cervical wedging is associated with shorter duration of induced labor. Am J Obstet Gynecol 1994;171:1081-1087.
34. Bartolucci L, Hill W, Katz M, et al: Ultrasonography in preterm labor. Am J Obstet Gynecol 1984;149:52-56.
35. Andersen HF, Nugent CE, Wanty SD, et al: Prediction of risk for preterm delivery by ultrasonographic measurement of cervical length. Am J Obstet Gynecol 1990;163:589-593.
36. Stubbs TM, Van Dorsten P, Miller MC: The preterm cervix and preterm labor: Relative risk, predictive values and change over time. Am J Obstet Gynecol 1986;155:829-834.
37. Papiernik E, Bonyer J, Collin D, et al: Precocious cervical ripening and preterm labor. Obstet Gynecol 1986;67:238-242.
38. Okitsu O, Mimura X, Nakayama T, Aono T: Early prediction of preterm delivery by transvaginal ultrasonography. Ultrasound Obstet Gynecol 1992;2:402-409.
39. Gomez R, Galasso M, Romero R, et al: Sonographic examination of the uterine cervix is a better predictor of the likelihood of preterm delivery than digital examination of the cervix in preterm labor with intact membranes. Am J Obstet Gynecol 1994;171:956-964.
40. Guzman ER, Rosenberg JC, Houlihan C, et al: A new method using vaginal ultrasound and transfundal pressure to evaluate the asymptomatic incompetent cervix. Obstet Gynecol 1994;83:248-252.
41. Romero R, Gomez R, Sepulveda W: Editorial: The uterine cervix, ultrasound and prematurity. Ultrasound Obstet Gynecol 1992;2:385-388.
42. Iams JD, Goldenberg RL, Mercer BM, et al. The preterm prediction study: Can low-risk women destined for spontaneous preterm birth be identified? Am J Obstet Gynecol 2001;184:652-655.
43. Berghella V, Kuhlman K, Weiner S, et al: Cervical funneling: Sonographic criteria predictive of preterm delivery. Ultrasound Obstet Gynecol 1997;10:161-166.
44. Owen J, Yost N, Berghella V, et al: Mid-trimester endovaginal sonography in women at high risk for spontaneous preterm birth. JAMA 2001;286:1340-1348.
45. Souka AP, Heath V, Flint S, et al: Cervical length at 23 weeks in twins in predicting spontaneous preterm delivery. Obstet Gynecol 1999;94:450-454.
46. Timor-Tritsch IE, Monteagudo A, Mandeville EO, et al: Successful management of viable cervical pregnancy by local injection of methotrexate guided by transvaginal sonography. Am J Obstet Gynecol 1994;170:737-739.
47. Monteagudo A, Tarricone NJ, Timor-Tritsch IE, et al: Successful transvaginal ultrasound-guided puncture and injection of a cervical pregnancy in a patient with simultaneous intrauterine pregnancy and a history of a previous cervical pregnancy. Ultrasound Obstet Gynecol 1006;8:381-386.
48. Monteagudo A, Carreno C, Timor-Tritsch IE: Saline infusion sonohysterography in nonpregnant women with previous cesarean delivery: The "niche" in the scar. J Ultrasound Med 2001;20:1105-1115.
49. Andersen HF, Ansbacher R: Ultrasound: A new approach to the evaluation of cervical ripening. Semin Perinatol 1991;15:140-148.
50. Taipale P, Hiilesmaa V: Sonographic measurement of uterine cervix at 18-22 weeks' gestation and the risk of preterm delivery. Obstet Gynecol 1998;92:902-907.
51. Heath VC, Southall TR, Souka AP, et al: Cervical length at 23 weeks of gestation: Relation to demographic characteristics and previous obstetric history. Ultrasound Obstet Gynecol 1998;12:304-311.
52. Iams JD, Goldenberg RL, Mercer BM: The preterm prediction study: Recurrence risk of spontaneous preterm birth. Am J Obstet Gynecol 1998;178:1035-1040.
53. Hassan SS, Romero R, Berry SM: Patients with an ultrasonographic cervical length ≤15 mm have nearly a 50% risk of early spontaneous preterm delivery. Am J Obstet Gynecol 2000;182:1458-1467.
54. Heath VC, Daskalakis G, Zagaliki A, et al: Cervicovaginal fibronectin and cervical length at 23 weeks of gestation: Relative risk of early preterm delivery. Br J Obstet Gynaecol 2000;107:1276-1281.
55. Guzman ER, Mellon C, Vintzileos AM, et al: Longitudinal assessment of endocervical canal length between 15 and 24 weeks' gestation in women at risk for pregnancy loss or preterm birth. Obstet Gynecol 1998;92:31-37.

56. Fleischer AC, Lombardi S, Kepple DM: Guidance for cerclage using transrectal sonography. J Ultrasound Med 1989;8:589-590.

57. Rozenberg P, Goffinet F, Hessabi M: Comparison of the Bishop score, ultrasonographically measured cervical length, and fetal fibronectin assay in predicting time until delivery and type of delivery at term. Am J Obstet Gynecol 2000;182:108-113.

58. Rozenberg P, Gillet A: Endovaginal ultrasonography of the uterine cervix in asymptomatic populations at high risk and at low risk for premature birth: To do or not to do? Gynecol Obstet Fertil 2001;29:148-158.

59. Rozenberg P, Rudant J, Chevret S, et al: Repeat measurement of cervical length after successful tocolysis. Obstet Gynecol 2004;104:995-999.

60. To MS, Alfirevic Z, Heath VC, et al: Cervical cerclage for prevention of preterm delivery in women with short cervix: Randomized controlled trial. Lancet 2004;363:1849-1853.

61. Rozenberg P, Gillet A, Ville Y: Transvaginal sonographic examination of the cervix in asymptomatic pregnant women: Review of the literature. Ultrasound Obstet Gynecol 2002;19:302-311.

62. Berghella V, Talucci M, Desai A: Does transvaginal sonographic measurement of cervical length before 14 weeks predict preterm delivery in high-risk pregnancies? Ultrasound Obstet Gynecol 2003;21:140-144.

63. Conoscenti G, Meir YJ, D'Ottavio G, et al: Does cervical length at 13-15 weeks' gestation predict preterm delivery in an unselected population? Ultrasound Obstet Gynecol 2003;21:128-134.

64. Carvalho MH, Bittar RE, Brizot ML, et al: Cervical length at 11-14 weeks' and 22-24 weeks' gestation evaluated by transvaginal sonography, and gestational age at delivery. Ultrasound Obstet Gynecol 2003;21:135-139.

65. Shalev J, Mashiach R, Bar-Chava I, et al: The "virtual" cervical internal os: Diagnosis during the first trimester of pregnancy. Ultrasound Obstet Gynecol 2003;21:145-148.

66. Hoesli IM, Surbek DV, Tercanli S, Holzgreve W: Three dimensional volume measurement of the cervix during pregnancy compared to conventional 2D-sonography. Int J Gynaecol Obstet 1999;64:115-119.

67. Bega G, Lev-Toaff A, Kuhlman K, et al: Three-dimensional multiplanar transvaginal ultrasound of the cervix in pregnancy. Ultrasound Obstet Gynecol 2000;16:351-358.

68. Rozenberg P, Rafii A, Senat MV, et al: Predictive value of two-dimensional and three-dimensional multiplanar ultrasound evaluation of the cervix in preterm labor. J Matern Fetal Neonatal Med 2003;13:237-241.

69. Towner D, Boe N, Lou K, Gilbert WM: Cervical length measurements in pregnancy are longer when measured with three-dimensional transvaginal ultrasound. J Matern Fetal Neonatal Med 2004;16:167-170.

70. Severi FM, Bocchi C, Florio P, et al: Comparison of two-dimensional and three-dimensional ultrasound in the assessment of the cervix to predict preterm delivery. Ultrasound Med Biol 2003;29:1261-1265.

71. Goldstein SR, Horii SC, Snyder JR, et al: Estimation of nongravid uterine volume based on a nomogram of gravid uterine volume: Its value in gynecologic uterine abnormalities. Obstet Gynecol 1988;72:86-90.

72. Platt JF, Bree FL, Davidson D: Ultrasound of the normal nongravid uterus: Correlation with gross anatomy histopathology. J Clin Ultrasound 1990;18:19.

73. Warwick W (ed): Gray's Anatomy. Edinburgh, Churchill Livingstone, 1973.

74. Birnholz JC: Ultrasonic visualization of endometrial movements. Fertil Steril 1984;41:157-158.

75. de Vries K, Lyons EA, Ballard G, et al: Contractions of the inner third myometrium. Am J Obstet Gynecol 1990;172:679-682.

76. Lyons EA, Taylor PJ, Zheng XH, et al: Characterization of sub-endometrial myometrial contractions throughout the menstrual cycle in normal fertile women. Fertil Steril 1991;55:771-774.

77. Abramowicz JS, Archer DF: Uterine endometrial peristalsis, a transvaginal ultrasound study. Fertility 1990;54:451-454.

78. Bulletti C, De Ziegler D, Rossi S, et al: Abnormal uterine contractility in nonpregnant women. Ann N Y Acad Sci 1997;828:223-229.

79. Bulletti C, De Ziegler D, Polli V, et al: Uterine contractility during the menstrual cycle. Hum Reprod 2000;15:81-89.

80. Fanchin R, Righini C, De Ziegler D, et al: Effects of vaginal progesterone administration on uterine contractility at the time of embryo transfer. Fertil Steril 2001;75:1136-1140.

81. Ayoubi JM, Fanchin R, Kaddouz D, et al. Uterorelaxing effects of vaginal progesterone: Comparison of two methodologies for assessing uterine contraction frequency on ultrasound scans. Fertil Steril 2001;76:736-740.

82. De Ziegler D, Bulletti C, Fanchin R, et al: Contractility of the nonpregnant uterus: The follicular phase. Ann N Y Acad Sci 2001;943:172-184.

83. Bulletti C, de Ziegler D: Uterine contractility and embryo implantation. Curr Opin Obstet Gynecol 2005;17:265-276.

84. Fleischer AC, Kepple DM, Entman SS: Transvaginal sonography of uterine disorders. In Timor-Tritsch IE, Rottem S (eds): Transvaginal Sonography, 2nd ed. New York, Chapman & Hall, 1991, p 113.

85. Timor-Tritsch IE, Rottem S: Transvaginal Sonography. New York, Elsevier, 1988.

86. Fleischer AC, Kalemeris GC, Entman SS: Sonographic depiction of the endometrium during normal cycles. Ultrasound Med Biol 1988;12:271-272.

87. Detchert U, Hackketoer BJ, Duame E: The sonographic and endocrinologic evaluation of endometrium in the luteal phase. Hum Reprod 1986;1:219-222.

88. Fleischer AC, Kalemeris GC, Machin JE, et al: Sonographic depiction of normal and abnormal endometrium with histopathologic correlation. J Ultrasound Med 1986;5:445-452.

89. Mendelson EB, Bohm-Velez M, Joseph N, Neiman HL: Endometrial abnormalities: Evaluation with transvaginal sonography. AJR Am J Roentgenol 1988;150:139-142.

90. Fleischer AC, Herbert CM, Hill GA, et al: Transvaginal sonography of the endometrium during induced cycles. J Ultrasound Med 1991;10:93-95.

91. Grunfeld L, Walker B, Bergh PA, et al: High-resolution endovaginal endometrium: A noninvasive test for endometrial adequacy. Obstet Gynecol 1991;78:200.

92. Gonen Y, Casper RF, Jacobson W, et al: Endometrial thickness and growth during ovarian stimulation: A possible predictor of implantation in vitro fertilization. Fertil Steril 1989;52:446-450.

93. Gonen Y, Casper RF: Prediction of implantation by the sonographic appearance of the endometrium during controlled ovarian stimulation for IVF. J Vitro Fert Embryo Transf 1990;7:146-152.

94. Pierson RA: Imaging the endometrium: Are there predictors of uterine receptivity? J Obstet Gynaecol Can 2003;25:360-368.

95. Fleischer AC, Herbert CM, Sacks GA, et al: Sonography of the endometrium during conception and nonconception cycles of in vitro fertilization and embryo transfer. Fertil Steril 1986;46:442-447.

96. Santolaya-Forgas I: Physiology of the menstrual cycle by ultrasonography. J Ultrasound Med 1992;11:139-142.

97. Scholtes MCW, Wladimiroff JW, Van Rijen HJM, Hop WCI: Uterine and ovarian blood flow waveforms in the normal menstrual cycle: A transvaginal Doppler study. Fertil Steril 1989;52:981-985.

98. Bourne TH: Transvaginal color Doppler in gynecology. Ultrasound Obstet Gynecol 1991;1:359-373.

99. Sladkevicius P, Valentin L, Marsal K: Blood flow velocity in the uterine and ovarian arteries during the normal menstrual cycle. Ultrasound Obstet Gynecol 1993;3:199-208.

100. Steer CV, Campbell S, Pampiglionel I, et al: Transvaginal colour flow imaging of the uterine arteries during the ovarian and menstrual cycles. Hum Reprod 1990;5:391-395.

101. Steer CV, Tan SL, Dillon D, et al: Vaginal color Doppler assessment of uterine artery impedance correlates with immunohistochemical markers of endometrial receptivity required for the implantation of an embryo. Fertil Steril 1995;63:101-108.

102. Zaidi J, Campbell S, Pittrof R, Tan SL: Endometrial thickness, morphology, vascular penetration and velocimetry in predicting implantation in an in vitro fertilization program. Ultrasound Obstet Gynecol 1995;6:191-198.

103. Contart P, Baruffi RL, Coelho J, et al: Power Doppler endometrial evaluation as a method for the prognosis of embryo implantation in an ICSI program. J Assist Reprod Genet 2000;17:329-334.

104. Jinno M, Ozaki T, Iwashita M, et al: Measurement of endometrial tissue blood flow: A novel way to assess uterine receptivity for implantation. Fertil Steril 2001;76:1168-1174.

105. Baruffi RL, Contart P, Mauri AL, et al: A uterine ultrasonographic scoring system as a method for the prognosis of embryo implantation. J Assist Reprod Genet 2002;19:99-102.

106. Chien LW, Au HK, Chen PL, et al: Assessment of uterine receptivity by the endometrial-subendometrial blood flow distribution pattern in women undergoing in vitro fertilization-embryo transfer. Fertil Steril 2002;78:245-251.

107. Chien LW, Lee WS, Au HK, Tzeng CR: Assessment of changes in utero-ovarian arterial impedance during the peri-implantation period by Doppler sonography in women undergoing assisted reproduction. Ultrasound Obstet Gynecol 2004;23:496-500.

108. Puerto B, Creus M, Carmona F, et al: Ultrasonography as a predictor of embryo implantation after in vitro fertilization: A controlled study. Fertil Steril 2003;79:1015-1022.

109. Granberg S, Wikland M, Karlsson B, et al: Endometrial thickness as measured by endovaginal ultrasonography for identifying endometrial abnormality. Am J Obstet Gynecol 1991;164:47-52.

110. Varner RE, Sparks IM, Cameron CD, et al: Transvaginal sonography of the endometrium in postmenopausal women. Obstet Gynecol 1991;78:195-199.

111. Goldstein SR, Nachtigall M, Snyder JR, Nachtigall L: Endometrial assessment by vaginal ultrasonography before endometrial sampling in patients with postmenopausal bleeding. Am J Obstet Gynecol 1990;163:119-123.

112. Malpani A, Singer J, Wolverson MK, Merenda G: Endometrial hyperplasia: Value of endometrial thickness in ultrasonographic diagnosis and clinical significance. J Clin Ultrasound 1990;18:173-177.

113. Requard CK, Wicks JD, Mettler FA: Ultrasonography in the staging of endometrial adenocarcinoma. Radiology 1981;140:781-785.

114. Fleischer AC, Dudley BS, Entman SS, et al: Myometrial invasion by endometrial carcinoma: sonographic assessment. Radiology 1987;162:307-310.

115. Smith-Bindman R, Weiss E, Feldstein V: How thick is too thick? When endometrial thickness should prompt biopsy in postmenopausal women without vaginal bleeding. Ultrasound Obstet Gynecol 2004;24:558-565.

116. van Doorn LC, Dijkhuizen FP, Kruitwagen RF, et al: Accuracy of transvaginal ultrasonography in diabetic or obese women with postmenopausal bleeding. DUPOMEB (Dutch Study in Postmenopausal Bleeding). Obstet Gynecol 2004;104:571-578.

117. Milojkovic M, Sijanovic S: Assessment of reliability of endometrial brush cytology in detection etiology of late postmenopausal bleedings. Arch Gynecol Obstet 2004;269:259-262. Erratum in Arch Gynecol Obstet 2005;271:94.

118. Tanriverdi HA, Barut A, Gun BD, Kaya E: Is Pipelle biopsy really adequate for diagnosing endometrial disease? Med Sci Monit 2004;10:CR271-CR274.

119. Guven MA, Pata O, Bakaris S, et al: Postmenopausal endometrial cancer screening: Is there a correlation between transvaginal sonographic measurement of endometrial thickness and body mass index? Eur J Gynaecol Oncol 2004;25:373-375.

120. Bruchim I, Biron-Shental T, Altaras MM, et al: Combination of endometrial thickness and time since menopause in predicting endometrial cancer in women with postmenopausal bleeding. J Clin Ultrasound 2004;32:219-224.

121. Epstein E, Valentin L: Managing women with post-menopausal bleeding. Best Pract Res Clin Obstet Gynaecol 2004;18:125-143.

122. Erkkola R, Kumento U, Lehmuskoski S, et al: No increased risk of endometrial hyperplasia with fixed long-cycle oestrogen-progestogen therapy after five years. J Br Menopause Soc 2004;10:9-13.

123. Alcazar JL, Castillo G, Minguez JA, Galan MJ: Endometrial blood flow mapping using transvaginal power Doppler sonography in women with postmenopausal bleeding and thickened endometrium. Ultrasound Obstet Gynecol 2003;21:583-588.

124. Develioglu OH, Omak M, Bilgin T, et al: The endometrium in asymptomatic breast cancer patients on tamoxifen: Value of transvaginal ultrasonography with saline infusion and Doppler flow. Gynecol Oncol 2004;93:328-335.

125. Bourne TH, Campbell S, Steer CV, et al: Detection of endometrial cancer by transvaginal ultrasonography with color flow imaging and blood flow analysis: A preliminary report. Gynecol Oncol 1991;40:253-259.

126. Kurjak A, Zalud I: The characterization of uterine tumors by transvaginal color Doppler. Ultrasound Obstet Gynecol 1991;1:50-52.

127. Lang PC, Filly RA, Marks W, et al: Ultrasonic demonstration of endometrial fluid collections unassociated with pregnancy. Radiology 1980;137:471-474.

128. Scott WW Jr, Rosenshein NB, Siegelman SS, Sanders RC: The obstructed uterus. Radiology 1981;141:767-770.

129. Breckenridge JW, Kurtz AB, Ritchie WGM, Macht EL Jr: Postmenopausal uterine fluid collection: indicator of carcinoma. AJR Am J Roentgenol 1982;139:529-534.

130. Johnson MA, Graham MF, Cooperberg PL: Abnormal endometrial echoes: Sonographic spectrum of endometrial pathology. J Ultrasound Med 1982;1:161-166.

131. Rubin D, Graham MF, Cronheim C, Cooperberg PL: Echogenic hematometra mimicking endometrial carcinoma. J Ultrasound Med 1985;4:47-48.

132. McCarthy KA, Hall DA, Kopans DB, Swann CA: Postmenopausal endometrial fluid collections: Always an indicator of malignancy? J Ultrasound Med 1986;5:647-649.

133. Chambers CB, Unis JS: Ultrasonographic evidence of uterine malignancy in the postmenopausal uterus. Am J Obstet Gynecol 1986;154:1194-1199.

134. Carlson JA, Arger P, Thompson S, Carlson EJ: Clinical and pathologic correlation of endometrial cavity fluid detected by ultrasound in the postmenopausal patient. Obstet Gynecol 1991;77:119-123.

135. Goldstein SR: Postmenopausal fluid collections revisited: Look at the doughnut rather than the hole. Obstet Gynecol 1993;83:738-740.

136. Fleischer AC, Dudley BS, Entman SS, et al: Myometrial invasion by endometrial carcinoma: Sonographic assessment. Radiology 1987;162:307-310.

137. Conte M, Guarglia L, Panici PB, et al: Transvaginal ultrasound evaluation of myometrial invasion in endometrial carcinoma. Gynecol Oncol 1990;29:224-226.

138. Karlsson B, Norstrom A, Granberg S, Wikland M: The use of endovaginal ultrasound to diagnose invasion of endometrial carcinoma. Ultrasound Obstet Gynecol 1992;2:35-39.

139. Lehtovirta P, Cacciatore B, Wahlstrom T, Ylostalo P: Ultrasonic assessment of endometrial cancer invasion. J Clin Ultrasound 1987;15:519-524.

140. Gordon AN, Fleischer AC, Reed GW: Depth of myometrial invasion in endometrial cancer: Preoperative assessment by transvaginal ultrasonography. Gynecol Oncol 1990;39:321-327.

141. Cacciatore B, Lehtovirta P, Wahlstrom T, Ylostalo P: Preoperative sonographic evaluation of endometrial cancer. Am J Obstet Gynecol 1989;160:133-137.

142. Obata A, Akamatsu N, Sekiba K: Ultrasound estimation of myometrial invasion of endometrial cancer by intrauterine radial scanning. J Clin Ultrasound 1985;13:397-404.

143. Timor-Tritsch IE, Rottem S, Boldes R: Scanning the uterus. In Timor-Tritsch IE, Rottem S (eds): Transvaginal Sonography. New York, Elsevier, 1988, pp 27-43.

144. Van Roessel J, Wamsteker K, Exalto N: Sonographic investigation of the uterus during artificial uterine cavity distention. J Clin Ultrasound 1987;15:439-450.

145. Parsons AK, Leuse JJ: Sonohysterography for endometrial abnormalities: Preliminary results. J Clin Ultrasound 1993;21:87-95.

146. Goldstein SR: Use of ultrasonohysterography for triage of perimenopausal patients with unexplained uterine bleeding. Am J Obstet Gynecol 1994;170:565-570.

147. Goldstein SR, Monteagudo A, Popiolek D, et al: Evaluation of endometrial polyps. Am J Obstet Gynecol 2002;186:669-674.

148. Markovitch O, Tepper R, Aviram R, et al: The value of sonohysterography in the prediction of endometrial pathologies in asymptomatic postmenopausal breast cancer tamoxifen-treated patients. Gynecol Oncol 2004;94:754-759.

149. Fedele L, Bianchi S, Dorta M, et al: Transvaginal sonography versus hysteroscopy in the diagnosis of uterine submucous myomas. Obstet Gynecol 1991;77:745-748.

150. Aaron J: Ultrasound localization of intra-uterine contraceptive devices and associated pathology. Br J Radiol 1984;57:795-797.

151. Najarian KE, Kurtz AB: New observations in the sonographic evaluation of intrauterine contraceptive devices. J Ultrasound Med 1986;5:205-210.

152. Schiesser M, Lapaire O, Tercanli S, Holzgreve W: Lost intrauterine devices during pregnancy: Maternal and fetal outcome after ultrasound-guided extraction. An analysis of 82 cases. Ultrasound Obstet Gynecol 2004;23:486-489.

153. Carroll R, Gombergh R: Empty bladder (hysterographic) view on US for evaluation of intrauterine devices. Radiology 198;163:822-823.

154. Fleischer AC, Kepple DM: Transvaginal Sonography. Philadelphia, JB Lippincott, 1992.

155. American Fertility Society: The American Fertility Society classification of adnexal adhesions, distal tubal occlusion, tubal occlusion secondary to tubal ligation, adhesions. Fertil Steril 1988;49:944-955.

156. Worthern NJ, Gonzales F: Septate uterus: Sonographic diagnosis and obstetric complications. Obstet Gynecol 1984;64:345-385.

157. Fedele L, Dorta M, Vercellini P, et al: Ultrasound in diagnosis of subclasses of unicornuate uterus. Obstet Gynecol 1988;71:274-277.

158. Nicolini U, Bellotti M, Bonazzi B, et al: Can ultrasound be used to screen uterine malformations? Fertil Steril 1987;47:89-93.

159. Randolph JF, Ying YK, Majer DB, et al: Comparison of real time ultrasonography, hysterosalpingography and laparoscopy/hysteroscopy in the evaluation of uterine abnormalities and tubal patency. Fertil Steril 1986;46:828-832.

160. Funk A, Fendel H: Sonography diagnosis of congenital uterine abnormalities. Z Geburtshilfe Perinatol 1988;192:77-88.

161. Lev-Toaff AS, Toaff ME, Friedman AC: Endovaginal sonographic appearance of a DES uterus. J Ultrasound Med 1990;9:661-664.
162. Bohlman ME, Ensor RE, Sanders RC: Sonographic findings in adenomyosis of the uterus. AJR Am J Roentgenol 1987;148:765-766.
163. Siedler D, Laing FC, Jeffrey RB Jr, Wing VW: Uterine adenomyosis: A difficult sonographic diagnosis. J Ultrasound Med 1987;6:345-349.
164. Togashi K, Ozasa H, Konishi I, et al: Enlarged uterus: Differentiation between adenomyosis and leiomyoma with MR imaging. Radiology 1989;171:531-534.
165. Montgomery BE, Daum GS, Dunton CJ: Endometrial hyperplasia: A review. Obstet Gynecol Surv 2004;59:368-378.
166. Popp LW, Schwiedessen JP, Gaetje R: Myometrial biopsy in the diagnosis of adenomyosis uteri. Am J Obstet Gynecol 1993;169:546-549.
167. Timor-Tritsch IE, Rottem S, Lewitt N: The fallopian tubes. In Timor-Tritsch IE, Rottem S (eds): Transvaginal Sonography, 2nd ed. New York, Chapman & Hall, 1991, pp 131-144.
168. Timor-Tritsch IE, Rottem S: Transvaginal ultrasound study of the fallopian tube. Obstet Gynecol 1987;70:424-428.
169. Mitri FF, Andronikou AD, Peripinyal S, et al: A clinical comparison of sonographic hydrotubation and hysterosalpingography. Br J Obstet Gynaecol 1991;98:1031-1036.
170. Volpi E, De-Grandis T, Sismondi P, et al: Transvaginal salpingosonography (TSSG) in the evaluation of tubal patency. Acta Eur Fertil 1991;22:325-328.
171. Tufekci EC, Girit S, Bayirli E, et al: Evaluation of tubal patency by transvaginal sonosalpingography. Fertil Steril 1992;57:336-340.
172. Hotel J, Rassmunsen C, Morris H: First clinical experience with sonicated albumin (Albunex) as an intrafallopian ultrasound contrast medium. Ultrasound Obstet Gynecol 1993;3:106(A).
173. Deichert U, Schlief R, Sandt H, Juhnke I: Transvaginal hysterosalpingo-contrast sonography (HyCoSy) compared with conventional tubal diagnostics. Hum Reprod 1989;4:418-424.
174. Deichert U, Schlief R, van de Sandt M, et al: Transvaginal contrast hysterosalpingo-sonography with the B-image procedure and color-coded duplex sonography for the assessment of fallopian tube patency [in German]. Geburtshilfe Frauenheilkd 1990;50:717-721.
175. Fobbe F, Becker R, Koch HC, et al: The demonstration of the patency of the uterine tubes with color-coded duplex sonography in combination with ultrasonic contrast media [in German]. ROFO 1991;154:349-353.
176. Schlief R, Deichert U: Hysterosalpingo-contrast sonography of the uterus and fallopian tubes: Results of a clinical trial of a new contrast medium in 120 patients. Radiology 1991;178:213-215.
177. Venezia R, Zangara C: Echohysterosalpingography: New diagnostic possibilities with SHU 450 (Echovist). Acta Eur Fertil 1991;22:279-282.
178. Deichert U, Schlief R, van de Sandt M, Daume E: Transvaginal hysterosalpingo-contrast sonography for the assessment of tubal patency with gray scale imaging and additional use of pulsed wave Doppler. Fertil Steril 1992;57:62-67.
179. Stern J, Peters AJ, Coulam CB: Color Doppler ultrasonography assessment of tubal patency: A comparison study with traditional techniques. Fertil Steril 1992;58:897-900.
180. Peters AJ, Coulam CB: Hysterosalpingography with color Doppler ultrasonography. Am J Obstet Gynecol 1991;164:1530-1534.
181. Allahbadia GN: Fallopian tube patency using color Doppler. Int J Gynaecol Obstet 1993;40:241-244.
182. Friberg B, Joergensen C: Tubal patency studied by ultrasonography: A pilot study. Acta Obstet Gynecol Scand 1994;73:53-55.
183. Goswamy RK, Campbell S, Royston IP, et al: Ovarian size in postmenopausal women. Br J Obstet Gynaecol 1988;95:795-801.
184. Rodriguez MH, Platt LD, Medearis AL, et al: The use of transvaginal sonography for evaluation of postmenopausal ovarian size and morphology. Am J Obstet Gynecol 1988;159:810-814.
185. Sassone AM, Timor-Tritsch IE, Artner A, et al: Transvaginal sonographic characterization of ovarian disease: Evaluation of a new scoring system to predict ovarian malignancy. Obstet Gynecol 1991;78:70-76.
186. Gollub E, Westhoff C, Timor-Tritsch IE: Transvaginal sonography in 230 healthy menopausal women. Ultrasound Obstet Gynecol 1993;3:422-425.
187. Holbert TR: Screening transvaginal ultrasonography of postmenopausal women in a private office setting. Am J Obstet Gynecol 1994;170:1699-1703.
188. Granberg S, Wikland M: Comparison between endovaginal and transabdominal transducers for measuring ovarian volume. J Ultrasound Med 1987;6:649-653.
189. Timor-Tritsch IE, Goldstein SR: The complexity of a complex mass and the simplicity of a simple cyst [editorial]. J Ultrasound Med 2005;24:255-258.
190. Reynolds T, Hill MC, Glassmann LM, et al: Sonography of hemorrhagic ovarian cysts. J Clin Ultrasound 1986;14:449-453.
191. Yoffe N, Bronshtein M, Brandes J, Blumenfeld Z: Hemorrhagic ovarian cyst detection by transvaginal sonography: The great imitator. Gynecol Endocrinol 1991;5:123-129.
192. Baltarowich OH, Kurtz AB, Pasto ME, et al: The spectrum of sonographic findings in hemorrhagic ovarian cysts. AJR Am J Roentgenol 1987;148:901-905.
193. Davis JA, Gosink BB: Fluid in the female pelvis: Cyclic patterns. J Ultrasound Med 1986;5:75-79.
194. Pavlik EJ, DePriest PD, Gallion HH, et al: Ovarian volume related to age. Gynecol Oncol 2000;77:410-412.

Chapter 6

Adenomyosis

Dirk Timmerman

Uterine adenomyosis is characterized by the presence of heterotopic endometrial glands and stroma in the myometrium with adjacent smooth muscle hyperplasia. Rokitansky described its histopathologic characteristics in 1860,[1] but the etiology of the condition remains unclear even today. Adenomyosis is relatively common, estimated to affect approximately 1% of women, and the diagnosis is most common in multiparous women in their fourth and fifth decades of life. Adenomyosis is often underdiagnosed because many clinicians are not familiar with its typical features on ultrasound examination. This chapter focuses on criteria and difficulties in diagnosing uterine adenomyosis. Less common conditions, such as rectovaginal and bladder wall adenomyosis, are also discussed.

Histopathology

Histopathologic findings include a poorly circumscribed area of smooth muscle cells, stroma, and endometrial glands invading the uterine smooth muscle layers of the myometrium. The degree of invasion is variable and can involve the whole uterine wall up to the serosa. In the diffuse form of adenomyosis, the lesions are distributed within the myometrium, whereas in the focal form, nodules of adenomyosis (or "adenomyoma") are observed. Most pathologists limit the diagnosis of adenomyosis to glandular extension beneath the endometrial–myometrial interface of greater than 2.5 mm,[2] whereas adenomyosis sub-basalis can be defined as minimally invasive adenomyosis extending less than 2 mm below the basal endometrium.[3] Hyperplasia of the smooth uterine musculature is often seen, typically resulting in a globally enlarged uterus.

The wide range of reported prevalence of adenomyosis in uterine specimens is partly explained by the different diagnostic criteria and classifications based on the depth of infiltration that have been used in different studies.[4] Other reasons include the method of patient selection (e.g., proportion of pain or bleeding as indications for hysterectomy) and the motivation of the pathologist to find endometriosis. The latter is illustrated by the finding in one study that adenomyosis was found in 31% of uteri if three sections were made, whereas it was found in 61% if six sections were made through the same uteri.[3] Bazot and colleagues prospectively studied a total of 129 women scheduled for hysterectomy.[5] Group 1 ($N = 23$) consisted of patients with menometrorrhagia who were free of myoma and endometrial disorders on transabdominal ultra-

sound. Group 2 consisted of all other patients ($N = 106$). The prevalence of adenomyosis in groups 1 and 2 was 91.3% and 24.5%, respectively.[5] In general, the posterior wall of the uterus is affected more often than the anterior wall. Overall, histologic features of adenomyosis are present in 20% to 35% of women undergoing hysterectomy for benign gynecologic disorders.[5-7]

Other localizations of adenomyosis have been described, such as rectovaginal and bladder wall involvement.[8,9] Originally these lesions were considered to be deeply infiltrating endometriosis, but histologically the lesions are characterized by scarce glands with active endometrial-type endometrium and scanty stroma; secretory changes are absent, and 90% of the nodule consists of smooth muscle hyperplasia. Therefore, Donnez et al. proposed that bladder wall and rectovaginal endometriosis are adenomyosis and the consequence of metaplasia of müllerian remnants.[9]

Clinical Presentation

Among the clinical signs, a soft, tender, and diffusely enlarged uterus is most common, whereas the presenting symptoms include menorrhagia (40% to 50%), dysmenorrhea (10% to 30%), metrorrhagia (10% to 12%), dyspareunia, and dyschezia.[6] However, these symptoms and signs are nonspecific and can occur as part of many other gynecologic disorders, such as fibroids, endometriosis, and dysfunctional uterine bleeding.[6] Typically, the symptoms start 1 week before the menstrual flow. Infertility is a less frequent complaint because uterine adenomyosis is usually diagnosed in the fourth or fifth decade of life. However, because more women delay their first pregnancy until later in their thirties or forties, adenomyosis is now more frequently encountered in the fertility clinic during diagnostic work-up. In a series including 26 patients with infertility and dysmenorrhea or menorrhagia, adenomyosis was found in 14 (53.8%).[10] The impact of adenomyosis on fertility has been thoroughly reviewed.[11]

Rectovaginal adenomyosis is typically associated with deep dyspareunia and pain at rectovaginal examination, especially when this examination is performed during the menstrual period.[12] Adenomyosis in the bladder wall (i.e., full-thickness detrusor lesion) is exceedingly rare and found only in 0.2% of patients treated for endometriosis.[9] It is usually not palpable at bimanual examination but is often associated with urinary symptoms, such as micturition frequency, mictalgia, and sometimes hematuria, that characteristically flare up during menstruation.[9,13,14] Bladder wall adenomyosis is associated with rectovaginal adenomyosis in up to 35% of cases.[9]

Imaging Features

Historically, the diagnosis of adenomyosis could be established only at pathologic examination of a hysterectomy specimen. During the 1990s, however, development of several noninvasive techniques enabled the clinician to at least suspect the diagnosis before undertaking any treatment. These techniques have reduced reliance on the more invasive diagnostic methods such as percutaneous or laparoscopic uterine biopsy.[15] The noninvasive imaging modalities for diagnosis of adenomyosis have previously been reviewed in depth.[16]

Several authors have compared the accuracy of different ultrasound criteria for the diagnosis of adenomyosis. Although numbers are relatively small and inclusion criteria vary widely, overall good performance is obtained when diagnostic criteria are combined.[17-21] These data are summarized in Table 6–1.[5,19,20,22-31] Results of other studies are more difficult to interpret because of incomplete description of the study population[23] or histologic criteria used.[24]

X-ray Hysterosalpingography

Hysterosalpingography was the first imaging modality used for the diagnosis of adenomyosis. The characteristic findings on hysterosalpingography are multiple small (1- to 4-mm) spicules extending from the endometrium into the myometrium with saccular endings. Alternatively, a local accumulation of contrast material in the myometrium can sometimes provide a honeycomb appearance. Because of its low sensitivity and specificity and associated patient discomfort, hysterosalpingography is no longer used in the evaluation of patients with suspected adenomyosis. However, hysterosalpingography remains part of the routine diagnostic work-up in many fertility clinics.

Transabdominal Sonography

Because of its limited spatial resolution, transabdominal ultrasonography does not reliably permit differential diagnosis between adenomyosis and fibroids. Older studies using only abdominal access for the diagnosis of adenomyosis reported relatively poor sensitivity.[17,18] Although spatial resolution obtained with more modern transabdominal probes has improved since then, transvaginal sonography (TVS) is usually required to demonstrate the more subtle ultrasound features of adenomyosis.[11] However, in patients presenting with an enlarged uterus, transabdominal sonography should still be used in combination with TVS to obtain optimal diagnostic results.[5]

Transvaginal Sonography

Technical progress with TVS in the mid-1980s led to renewed [interest in the] diagnosis of adenomyosis. The higher frequencies [(to Hz)] reduce artifacts while improving the spatial resolution. Leading authors support the routine use of real-time TVS for a detailed depiction of the myometrium in patients with suspected adenomyosis.[16]

The ultrasound features of adenomyosis are often subtle and extremely variable. Diagnostic criteria for adenomyosis include the following (Figs. 6–1 and 6–2):

- Asymmetric uterine enlargement[17-19] (i.e., asymmetry between the anterior and posterior myometrial walls; Figs. 6–3 and 6–4)
- Uterine enlargement in the absence of fibroids (globular uterus)[18]
- Ill-defined hyperechogenic areas (i.e., heterotopic endometrial glands) and hypoechogenic areas[17-20] (i.e., smooth muscle hyperplasia; Figs. 6–5 and 6–6)
- Small, anechoic cysts measuring between 1 and 6 mm scattered throughout the myometrium (present in approximately 50% of patients with adenomyosis)[19,21,32]
- Indistinct endometrial–myometrial border (measurement of endometrial thickness is often very difficult)
- Minimal mass effect on the endometrium or the serosa relative to the size of the lesion[18]
- Increased echotexture of the myometrium[17,19]
- Elliptic rather than globular shape of the lesion
- Lack of edge shadowing; "shaggy" or whorled appearance of the endometrium
- Echogenic nodules or linear striations radiating out from the endometrium into the myometrium[30]
- Color Doppler imaging: absence of circular vascularization at the border of the lesion (see Figs. 6–4 and 6–6), contrary to what is seen in fibroids (Fig. 6–7)

Table 6–1	Sensitivity and Specificity of Transvaginal Sonography in Diagnosing Adenomyosis		
Study	**Prevalence**	**Sensitivity (%)**	**Specificity (%)**
Fedele et al., 1992[22]	23/405	87	99
Fedele et al., 1992[23]	22/43	80	74
Ascher et al., 1994[19]	17/20	53	75
Reinhold et al., 1995[24]	29/100	86	86
Brosens et al., 1995[20]	28/56	86	50
Atzori et al., 1996[25]	13/58	87	96
Reinhold et al., 1996[26]	29/119	89	89
Koçak et al., 1998[27]	18/95	89	88
Vercellini et al., 1998[28]	29/102	83	67
Bromley et al., 2000[29]	51/?	84	84
Atri et al., 2000[30]	30/102	81	71
Bazot et al., 2001[31]	40/120	65	97
Bazot et al., 2002[5]	21/23	81	100
Bazot et al., 2002[5]	26/106	38	97

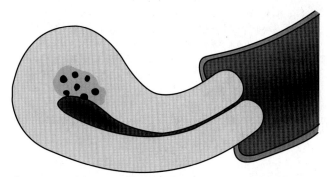

Figure 6–1. Schematic drawing summarizing the most common ultrasound findings in adenomyosis: poorly marginated hyperechogenic and hypoechogenic areas, small myometrial cysts, indistinct endometrial–myometrial border, and absence of circular vascularization at the border of the lesion.

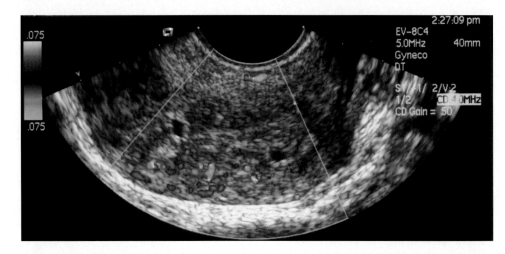

Figure 6–2. Transvaginal sonography image of small subendometrial cysts in a uterus with adenomyosis.

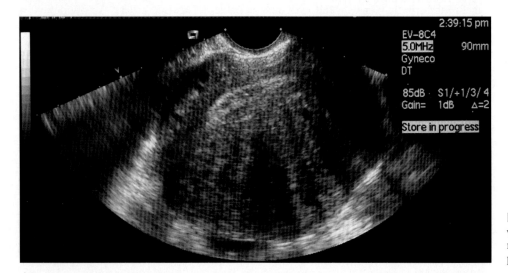

Figure 6–3. Globular enlarged uterus with strong asymmetry between anterior and posterior uterine wall and presence of diffuse adenomyosis.

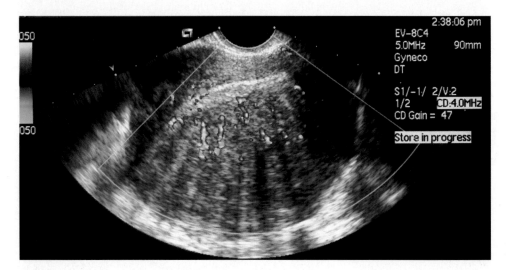

Figure 6–4. Same uterus as Figure 6–3 at color Doppler imaging; note the absence of circular vascularization.

The most common findings on TVS in the patient with adenomyosis are poorly marginated hyperechogenic and hypoechogenic areas. Atri and colleagues[30] compared ultrasound and histologic findings and demonstrated that the decreased echogenicity of the myometrium is caused by smooth muscle hypertrophy accompanying the heterotopic endometrial tissue. Small (1- to 6-mm) myometrial cysts are present (see Fig. 6–2) in approximately 50% of cases.[21] With the use of color Doppler imaging, these cysts are easily distinguished from dilated uterine veins, which are usually located in the outer third of the myometrium (see Figs. 6–4 and 6–6). The timing of the ultrasound scan in the cycle is important because the

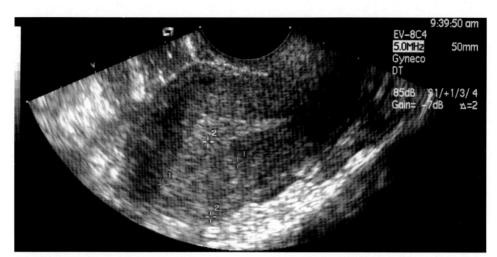

Figure 6–5. Focal adenomyosis in posterior uterine wall.

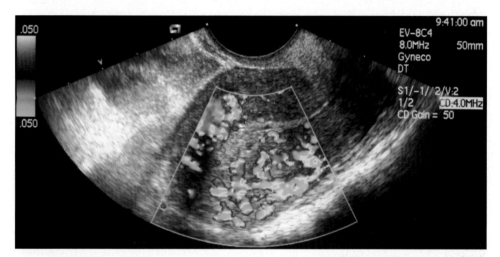

Figure 6–6. Same uterus as in Figure 6–5 at color Doppler imaging, showing radial arteries running straight through the adenomyotic lesion to the endomyometrial junction.

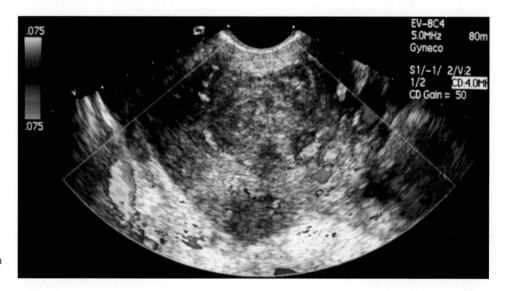

Figure 6–7. Uterine fibroid with typical circular vascularization.

uterine size has been shown to increase substantially during the menstrual period in patients with adenomyosis.

The ultrasound features of adenomyosis can overlap with those of uterine fibroids, especially in cases of focal adenomyosis. In such cases, additional imaging using magnetic resonance imaging (MRI) may be necessary. Table 6–2 summarizes helpful criteria to make the differential diagnosis between adenomyosis and fibroids.

The TVS appearance of adenomyosis can mimic the features of endometrial carcinoma, and the coexistence of

Table 6–2	Differential Diagnosis of Adenomyosis and Fibroids	
	Adenomyosis	**Fibroids**
Shape	Elliptic	Concentric, round
Borders	Poorly defined	Sharply defined
Mass effect	Absent	Present
Calcifications	Absent	Often present
Cysts	Multiple, small and regular	Single irregular cyst may be present after cystic degeneration
Color Doppler or power Doppler	Straight radial arteries running through the lesion	Circular vascularization (more prominent than internal vessels)

adenomyosis and endometrial carcinoma may lead to overstaging of endometrial or cervical cancer; conversely, these malignancies are sometimes understaged because the myometrial lesions are considered to be adenomyotic. Pulsed and color Doppler may be helpful to distinguish between adenomyosis and endometrial carcinoma.[19] Furthermore, it sometimes is difficult to differentiate between adenomyosis and myometrial contractions, hypertrophy, and vascular calcifications.

Although TVS is inexpensive, readily available, and well tolerated, the accuracy of diagnosis of adenomyosis is highly dependent on the experience and motivation of the sonographer. This limitation can hamper the acquisition of standardized images for sequential follow-up. Therefore, some authors recommend the use of MRI in the follow-up of conservatively treated patients with adenomyosis. However, both the overall image quality and clinical familiarity with ultrasound continue to improve, and thus it is not surprising that older studies report lower accuracies.

Magnetic Resonance Imaging

Magnetic resonance imaging has become an important imaging modality for uterine disease because of its excellent soft tissue differentiation. It is less operator dependent than TVS, and the images are standardized and reproducible. Several studies have demonstrated MRI—especially with T2-weighted images—to be highly accurate in the diagnosis of uterine adenomyosis, with a sensitivity and specificity ranging from 86% to 100% in a symptomatic patient population.[33] Diagnostic criteria used in these studies include the following:

- Low-signal-intensity uterine mass with ill-defined borders (T2-weighted)[34]
- Localized high signal foci within an area of low signal intensity (T2-weighted)[26,34]
- Linear striations of increased signal radiating out from the endometrium into the myometrium (T2-weighted)[34]
- Focal or diffuse thickening of the junctional zone (JZ; T2-weighted)[34]
- JZ thickness greater than 5 mm (T2-weighted)[19,35]
- JZ thickness greater than 12 mm (T2-weighted)[26,36]
- Poorly defined JZ borders (T2-weighted)[37]
- Bright foci in endometrium isointense with myometrium (T1-weighted)[37]

Adenomyotic lesions usually appear as a low-intensity area on T2-weighed images, which often gives the appearance of diffuse or focal widening of the JZ (i.e., the band of lower signal intensity representing the inner layer of the myometrium). The differential diagnosis with leiomyomas, uterine contractions, or uterine muscular hypertrophy may be difficult.[16] In infertile patients with symptoms indicative of a uterine pathologic process, MRI can be useful in differentiating the nature of the condition[10] or in evaluating conservative management.[38]

Several studies have compared the accuracy of TVS and MRI in the diagnosis of adenomyosis in the same patient population. Ascher and colleagues found MRI to be superior in a small series with a high prevalence of adenomyosis (17/20),[19] whereas Reinhold and coworkers found no differences between the sensitivities and specificities for both modalities in 119 patients undergoing hysterectomy.[26] More recently, Bazot et al. concluded that TVS is as efficient as MRI for the diagnosis of adenomyosis in women without myoma, although MRI could be recommended for women with associated leiomyoma.[31] The limited availability and high cost of MRI make it an impractical tool for the initial evaluation of patients with nonspecific gynecologic complaints suggestive of adenomyosis. However, it has its place as an adjunctive tool in the assessment of patients with clinically significant adenomyosis, especially in the presence of fibroids, and in the follow-up of patients with adenomyosis treated with hormonal therapy.

Rectovaginal Adenomyosis

Although deep nodes of endometriosis or adenomyosis of the rectovaginal wall are often clinically suspected and may be palpated by rectovaginal examination, TVS may be useful to confirm their presence and to offer precise measurements of the lesion's size. This can be clinically relevant if surgery is planned.

At TVS, rectovaginal adenomyosis is visualized as an oval solid nodule measuring 0.5 to 4 cm and without clear cystic contents.[39] The node is hypoechogenic and seems to make an impression in the rectum, which is usually seen as a thick white line partly surrounding the lesion (Figs. 6–8 and 6–9). The node can be separated from the uterus, but not from the rectum or the vagina, by gentle pressure with the transvaginal probe. Color Doppler imaging most often reveals very limited

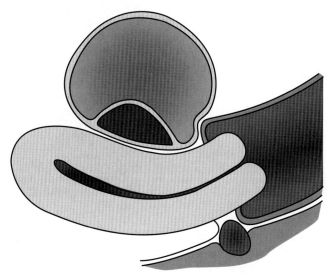

Figure 6–8. Schematic drawing of rectovaginal and bladder wall adenomyosis.

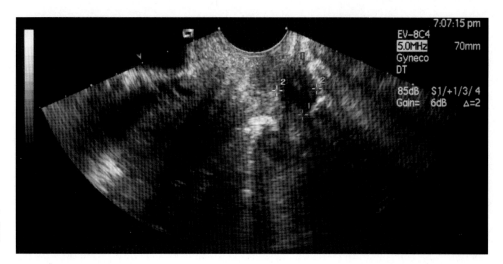

Figure 6–9. With transvaginal sonography, rectovaginal adenomyosis is visualized as an oval-shaped solid nodule.

internal vascularization.[39] Rectal endoscopic sonography has been used to evaluate the thickness of the uterosacral ligaments and degree of rectal infiltration in patients with deep endometriosis.[14,40]

Sonovaginography is a novel technique for assessing rectovaginal adenomyosis.[41] Sonovaginography is based on TVS combined with the introduction of saline solution into the vagina, which creates an acoustic window between the probe and the surrounding structures of the vagina. This technique resulted in higher sensitivity and specificity for diagnosing rectovaginal endometriosis.[41] The diagnostic role of MRI in this condition has also been described in detail.[42]

Bladder Wall Adenomyosis

Bladder wall adenomyosis is easier to detect at ultrasound than rectovaginal adenomyosis. TVS may reveal a solid nodule in the posterior bladder wall if the bladder is slightly filled[14] (see Fig. 6–8). Again, in contrast to subserous fibroids, bladder adenomyosis may easily be separated from the uterus by gentle pressure with the transvaginal probe. Furthermore, this maneuver often elicits focal pain. Color Doppler studies may detect low to moderate internal vascularization.[14,39] Fedele et al. concluded that TVS was more accurate than MRI for making the diagnosis of bladder adenomyosis.[43] However, in a more recent study using improved MRI techniques in a series of 12 women with histologically proven bladder adenomyosis that varied between 10 and 31 mm, TVS was negative in 4 patients with small lesions.[44] In contrast, MRI using a body coil enabled visualization of the lesions in all 12 patients. At cystoscopy, bladder wall adenomyosis is visualized as a protruding mass of the posterior bladder wall at the level of the fundus or the trigone. It consists of a typical bluish or brownish nodule.[9]

Conclusion

Uterine adenomyosis remains a common and clinically important disease that is still underdiagnosed. Moreover, it will be encountered with increasing incidence in the infertile female population. If proper diagnostic criteria are used, noninvasive ultrasound may lead to a correct diagnosis and proper management in many patients with adenomyosis. However, neither ultrasound nor MRI can replace histologic study.

REFERENCES

1. Rokitansky K: Ueber uterusdruesen-neubildung. Z Gesellschaft Aerzte Wien 1860;16:577.
2. Uduwela AS, Perera MAD, Aiqing L, Fraser IS: Endometrial-myometrial interface: Relationship to adenomyosis and changes in pregnancy. Obstet Gynecol Surv 2000;55:390-400.
3. Bird CC, McElin TW, Manola-Estrella P: The elusive adenomyosis of the uterus—revisited. Am J Obstet Gynecol 1972;112:583-593.
4. Bergholt T, Eriksen L, Berendt N, et al: Prevalence and risk factors of adenomyosis at hysterectomy. Hum Reprod 2001;16:2418-2421.
5. Bazot M, Daraï E, Rouger J, et al: Limitations of transvaginal sonography for the diagnosis of adenomyosis, with histopathological correlation. Ultrasound Obstet Gynecol 2002;20:605-611.
6. Azziz R: Adenomyosis: Current perspectives. Obstet Gynecol Clin North Am 1989;16:221-235.
7. Kim J, Strawn EY Jr: Adenomyosis: A frequent cause of abnormal uterine bleeding. Obstet Gynecol 2000;95[4 Suppl 1]:S23.
8. Donnez J, Nisolle M, Casanas-Roux F, et al: Rectovaginal septum, endometriosis or adenomyosis: Laparoscopic management in a series of 231 patients. Hum Reprod 1995;10:630-635.
9. Donnez J, Spada F, Squifflet J, Nisolle M: Bladder endometriosis must be considered as bladder adenomyosis. Fertil Steril 2000;74: 1175-1181.
10. de Souza NM, Brosens JJ, Schwieso JE, et al: The potential value of magnetic resonance imaging in infertility. Clin Radiol 1995;50:75-79.
11. Devlieger R, D'Hooghe T, Timmerman D: Uterine adenomyosis in the infertility clinic. Hum Reprod Update 2003;9:139-147.
12. Koninckx PR, Meuleman C, Oosterlynck D, Cornillie FJ: Diagnosis of deep endometriosis by clinical examination during menstruation and plasma CA-125 concentration. Fertil Steril 1996;65:280-287.
13. Sircus SI, Sant GR, Ucci AA Jr: Bladder detrusor endometriosis mimicking interstitial cystitis. Urology 1988;32:339-342.
14. Brosens J, Timmerman D, Starzinski-Powitz A, Brosens I: Noninvasive diagnosis of endometriosis: The role of imaging and markers. Obstet Gynecol Clin North Am 2003;30:95-114.
15. Vercellini P, Trespidi L, Panazza S, et al: Laparoscopic uterine biopsy for diagnosing diffuse adenomyosis. J Reprod Med 1996;41:220-224.
16. Reinhold C, Tafazoli F, Wang L: Imaging features of adenomyosis. Hum Reprod Update 1998;4:337-349.
17. Siedler D, Laing FC, Jeffrey RB Jr, Wing VW: Uterine adenomyosis: A difficult sonographic diagnosis. J Ultrasound Med 1987;6:345-349.
18. Bohlman ME, Ensor RE, Sanders RC: Sonographic findings in adenomyosis of the uterus. AJR Am J Roentgenol 1987;148:765-766.
19. Ascher SM, Arnold LL, Patt RH, et al: Adenomyosis: prospective comparison of MR imaging and transvaginal sonography. Radiology 1994; 190:803-806.

20. Brosens JJ, de Souza NM, Barker FG, et al: Endovaginal ultrasonography in the diagnosis of adenomyosis uteri: Identifying the predictive characteristics. Br J Obstet Gynaecol 1995;102:471-474.

21. Hirai M, Shibata K, Sagai H, et al: Transvaginal pulsed and color Doppler sonography for the evaluation of adenomyosis. J Ultrasound Med 1995; 14:529-532.

22. Fedele L, Bianchi S, Dorta M, et al: Transvaginal ultrasonography in the differential diagnosis of adenomyoma versus leiomyoma. Am J Obstet Gynecol 1992;167:603-606.

23. Fedele L, Bianchi S, Dorta M, et al: Transvaginal ultrasonography in the diagnosis of diffuse adenomyosis. Fertil Steril 1992;58:94-97.

24. Reinhold C, Atri M, Mehio A, et al: Diffuse uterine adenomyosis: Morphologic criteria and diagnostic accuracy of endovaginal sonography. Radiology 1995;197:609-614.

25. Atzori E, Tronci C, Sionis L: Transvaginal ultrasound in the diagnosis of diffuse adenomyosis. Gynecol Obstet Invest 1996;42:39-41.

26. Reinhold C, McCarthy S, Bret PM, et al: Diffuse adenomyosis: comparison of endovaginal US and MR imaging with histopathologic correlation. Radiology 1996;199:151-158.

27. Koçak I, Yanik F, Üstün C: Transvaginal ultrasound in the diagnosis of diffuse adenomyosis. Int J Gynecol Obstet 1998;62:293-296.

28. Vercellini P, Cortesi I, De Giorgi O, et al: Transvaginal ultrasonography versus uterine needle biopsy in the diagnosis of diffuse adenomyosis. Hum Reprod 1998;13:2884-2887.

29. Bromley B, Shipp TD, Benacerraf B: Adenomyosis: Sonographic findings and diagnostic accuracy. J Ultrasound Med 2000;19:529-534.

30. Atri M, Reinhold C, Mehio AR, et al: Adenomyosis: US features with histologic correlation in an in-vitro study. Radiology 2000;215:783-790.

31. Bazot M, Cortez A, Darai E, et al: Ultrasonography compared with magnetic resonance imaging for the diagnosis of adenomyosis: Correlation with histopathology. Hum Reprod 2001;16:2427-2433.

32. Fedele L, Bianchi S, Raffaelli R, et al: Treatment of adenomyosis-associated menorrhagia with a levonorgestrel-releasing intrauterine device. Fertil Steril 1997;68:426-429.

33. Reinhold C, Tafazoli F, Mehio A, et al: Uterine adenomyosis: Endovaginal US and MR imaging features with histopathologic correlation. Radiographics 1999;19[Special No.]:S147-S160.

34. Togashi K, Ozasa H, Konishi I, et al: Enlarged uterus: Differentiation between adenomyosis and leiomyoma with MR Imaging. Radiology 1989;171:531-534.

35. Mark AS, Hricak H, Heinrichs LW, et al: Adenomyosis and leiomyoma: Differential diagnosis with MR imaging. Radiology 1987;163:527-529.

36. Kang S, Turner DA, Foster GS, et al: Adenomyosis: Specificity of 5 mm as the maximum normal uterine junctional zone thickness in MR images. AJR Am J Roentgenol 1996;166:1145-1150.

37. Reinhold C, Gallix BP, Ascher SM: Uterus and cervix. In Ascher SM, Reinhold C, Semelka RC (eds): MRI of the Abdomen and Pelvis. New York, Wiley-Liss, 1997, pp 617-620.

38. Siskin GP, Tublin ME, Stainken BF, et al: Uterine artery embolization for the treatment of adenomyosis: clinical response and evaluation with MR imaging. AJR Am J Roentgenol 2001;177:297-302.

39. Timmerman D, Deprest J, Okaro E, Bourne T: Ultrasound characteristics of endometriosis. In: Timmerman D, Deprest J, Bourne TH (eds): Ultrasound and Endoscopic Surgery in Obstetrics and Gynecology. Berlin, Springer-Verlag, 2002, p 189.

40. Koga K, Osuga Y, Yano T, et al: Characteristic images of deeply infiltrating rectosigmoid endometriosis on transvaginal and transrectal ultrasonography. Hum Reprod 2003;18:1328-1333.

41. Dessole S, Farina M, Rubattu, G, et al: Sonovaginography is a new technique for assessing rectovaginal endometriosis. Fertil Steril 2003;79:1023-1027.

42. Chapron C, Liaras E, Fayet P, et al: Magnetic resonance imaging and endometriosis: Deeply infiltrating endometriosis does not originate from the rectovaginal septum. Gynecol Obstet Invest 2002;53:204-208.

43. Fedele L, Bianchi S, Raffaelli R, Portuese A: Pre-operative assessment of bladder endometriosis. Hum Reprod 1997;12:2519-2522.

44. Balleyguier C, Chapron C, Dubuisson JB, et al: Comparison of magnetic resonance imaging and transvaginal ultrasonography in diagnosing bladder endometriosis. J Am Assoc Gynecol Laparosc 2002;9:15-23.

Chapter 7

Congenital Uterine Anomalies

Rehan Salim and Davor Jurkovic

The diagnosis and management of a range of gynecologic conditions have been greatly facilitated by the advent of high-resolution B-mode transvaginal sonography (TVS). However, the impact of TVS on the diagnosis and management of congenital uterine anomalies (CUAs) has been limited, mainly because of the inability to obtain accurate information about the type and extent of fundal distortion in cases of CUAs. Without this information, it is not possible to differentiate between various types of uterine anomalies. Other diagnostic techniques, such as hysterosalpingography or hysteroscopy, suffer from similar limitations, and they are often combined with laparoscopy to perform a complete examination of the uterus.

The recent introduction of three-dimensional (3D) ultrasound has significantly improved our ability to assess uterine morphology. This new technology overcomes many problems of conventional two-dimensional (2D) B-mode scanning and has enabled for the first time an outpatient, noninvasive diagnosis of CUAs. This chapter reviews the current clinical concepts of CUAs, with particular emphasis on recent studies using 3D sonography. Further information on the sonographic evaluation of uterine malformations can be found in Chapters 5, 17, and 19.

Diagnosis of Congenital Uterine Anomalies Using Imaging Techniques

The use of the imaging techniques available for the diagnosis of CUAs is limited by the subjectivity of the operator's impressions. Until recently, no attempt was made to establish the accuracy of these methods for the diagnosis of CUAs. Also, no method for diagnosis of CUAs, including 3D ultrasound, has been evaluated for reproducibility. In addition, there is no agreement on the diagnostic criteria used to diagnose various CUAs, as reflected in the results of studies that have screened for CUAs. For instance, in women with a history of recurrent first-trimester miscarriage, the prevalence of CUAs diagnosed by hysterosalpingography has been reported as 1.8% to 37.6%, a very wide range.[1-3] 3D ultrasound has also revealed CUAs; in infertile women, Raga et al.[4] found anomalies in 6.3% overall, and 2% of the women had a subseptate uterus. In con-

trast, in a study by Kupesic and Kurjak,[5] subseptate uterus was diagnosed in 66.2% of infertile women. Such differences cannot be explained by variations in study populations and are almost certainly the result of differing criteria for diagnosing CUAs.

Hysterosalpingography and conventional 2D ultrasound are used most commonly for the diagnosis of a CUA, whereas hysteroscopy and laparoscopy are used to determine the exact nature of an anomaly. Other techniques are magnetic resonance imaging and 3D ultrasound.

Hysterosalpingography

Hysterosalpingography has been the mainstay for diagnosis and is based on the principle that filling defects in the uterine cavity are easily identifiable.[6,7] Anomalies of agenesis, such as the unicornuate uterus, and duplication anomalies, such as the arcuate, subseptate, and bicornuate uterus, in which there is an obvious deviation from the normal uterine cavity, are readily identified (Figs. 7–1 and 7–2). A significant limitation of this technique is that it provides an image only of the uterine cavity; no information on the external serosal uterine contour is available. Thus, the difficulty in differentiating between the various duplication anomalies and identifying noncommunicating rudimentary cornua, and the possibility of inadvertent insertion of the catheter into one half of a septate or bicornuate uterus, giving a false impression of a unicornuate uterus, are all causes of significant diagnostic problems that have implications for further management. Instillation of a large amount of contrast medium into the uterine cavity can also obscure the presence of small uterine septa.[8] Several studies have shown that the use of hysterosalpingography for the diagnosis of any intrauterine lesion may provide false-positive rates as high as 54% and false-negative rates of 28%, as verified with hysteroscopy.[8-10] In the context of CUAs, hysterosalpingography is unable to distinguish between subseptate and bicornuate uteri in up to 45% of cases, and it often misses a small uterine septum.[11,12] Several methods have been devised in an attempt to overcome this problem, involving complex descriptions of the angle and attitude of the medial walls of the uterine cavity. None of these, however, has been shown to be reproducible or accurate.[13]

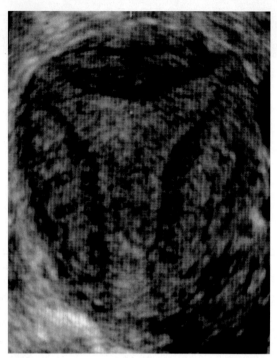

Figure 7–1. Coronal view of an arcuate uterus demonstrating both interstitial portions of the fallopian tubes. The fundal indent is concave with a central point that is obtuse, differentiating it from a subseptate uterus.

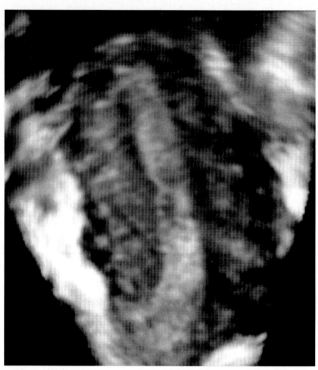

Figure 7–3. 3D ultrasound coronal view of a unicornuate uterus with a single uterine body and cavity.

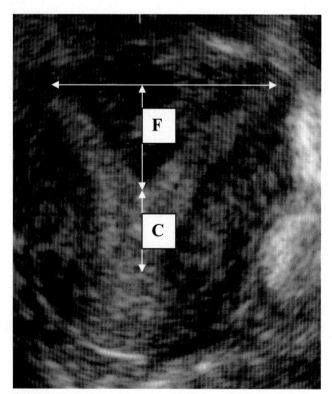

Figure 7–2. Coronal view of a subseptate uterus with intrauterine dimensions. The distortion ratio is calculated using the following formula: length of the septum (F)/[length of cavity (C) + length of septum (F)].

Two-Dimensional Ultrasound

Conventional 2D ultrasound is also a popular method for the diagnosis of CUAs. Uterine anomalies are suspected when the uterine cavity is seen to split from a fundus by myometrial tissue (a duplication anomaly) or when one of the interstitial portions of the fallopian tubes is absent (a unicornuate uterus; Fig. 7–3). Conventional ultrasound also enables the identification of both communicating and noncommunicating rudimentary cornua and the presence of endometrial tissue within them. This differentiation is important because noncommunicating rudimentary cornua may support a pregnancy, which usually ruptures at approximately 16 weeks' gestation, causing catastrophic hemorrhage.[14] Furthermore, the presence of endometrial tissue in noncommunicating cornua is likely to be associated with significant dysmenorrhea.

Conventional TVS has been reported to have high sensitivity but low specificity in the diagnosis of CUAs.[5,15,16] Jurkovic et al.[17] examined the accuracy of conventional ultrasound in the diagnosis of CUAs compared with hysterosalpingography. They reported that 2D sonography had a positive predictive sensitivity and specificity of 88% and 94%, respectively, for the diagnosis of a normal uterus; of 67% and 94% for the diagnosis of an arcuate uterus; and of 100% and 95% for the diagnosis of a major CUA. The authors concluded that conventional ultrasound should be used as a screening test rather than a definitive diagnostic test, and cases of suspected anomaly should be investigated further.

Conventional B-mode TVS has a sensitivity of 86% and a specificity of 100% in the detection of more severe anomalies, such as unicornuate uterus with a rudimentary horn.[18] However, as with hysterosalpingography, it is not possible to examine the external serosal contour of the uterus with conventional B-mode TVS, and thus it is not possible to differentiate among the various duplication anomalies. Differentiation is possible only if the uterus can be visualized in the coronal plane, which is perpendicular to the ultrasound beam.

The instillation of saline into the uterine cavity (i.e., saline infusion sonohysterography) may help to improve the specificity of B-mode scanning. In one study, saline infusion sonohysterography agreed with hysteroscopic and laparoscopic findings of uterine anomalies in 78% of cases, compared with 44% for hysterosalpingography and unenhanced B-mode TVS.[19] Although the accuracy of saline infusion sonohysterography for differentiation of duplication anomalies is reported to be as high as 100%, all studies have used hysteroscopy as the gold standard, which shares the same limitation of being unable accurately to visualize the external uterine fundal contour.[20] In addition, this procedure is associated with pain and the risk of retrograde spread of infection.[21,22]

Hysteroscopy and Laparoscopy

Whereas hysterosalpingography and 2D ultrasound have served as the first-line imaging techniques for the diagnosis of CUAs, diagnostic laparoscopy and hysteroscopy are required to confirm and accurately classify the anomalies thus identified. The use of diagnostic hysteroscopy alone is subject to the same limitations as both hysterosalpingography and conventional ultrasound in that the external serosal surface of the uterus cannot be examined. The addition of diagnostic laparoscopy overcomes this limitation, and this combination of invasive tests has been regarded as the gold standard for the diagnosis of CUAs.[23] However, laparoscopic examination of the uterine fundus remains a subjective exercise: some operators consider the presence of small indentations to be characteristic of a bicornuate uterus as opposed to some other duplication anomaly, whereas others would disagree. Furthermore, the presence of other lesions, such as uterine fibroids, may lead to further diagnostic inaccuracies. Any operative technique also carries the concomitant risks of anesthesia and complications associated with the technique itself. Given the current uncertainties regarding the true impact of CUAs in any population, as well as the lack of consensus over the management of these conditions, it remains debatable whether such invasive tests are warranted.

Magnetic Resonance Imaging

Magnetic resonance imaging (MRI) is being used increasingly to assess uterine morphology. Its multiplanar capability, good soft tissue contrast, use of nonionizing radiation, and relatively noninvasive nature make it an attractive imaging technique. It allows reconstruction of images and evaluation of both the internal and external fundal contours, thereby permitting differentiation among the various duplication anomalies and detection of the presence of rudimentary cornua. Several studies have found MRI to have excellent diagnostic accuracy, consistent with intraoperative findings.[24] MRI is also able to identify septal tissue because it contains a higher amount of fibrous tissue than the more muscular normal myometrium.[15] However, MRI is expensive and not readily accessible in all centers. Furthermore, there are some studies that question the widely held belief that MRI is highly accurate in the diagnosis of CUAs. Letterie et al.[25] compared the findings of MRI and ultrasound, in the diagnosis of 16 cases of CUA, to diagnostic laparoscopy and hysteroscopy. MRI and ultrasound correctly diagnosed subseptate uterus in 33% and 50% of cases, respectively, and MRI had an overall sensitivity of only 77% and a specificity of 33%.

Three-Dimensional Ultrasound

3D ultrasound is a major advance in the noninvasive, office-based diagnosis of CUAs. The technique enables visualization of the uterus in the coronal plane, depicting both the internal and external contours of the uterus. It is based on the principle of acquiring a large number of sequential tomograms of ultrasound data and arranging them digitally into a 3D ultrasound volume. This ultrasound image volume can then be manipulated in a number of ways, which enables examination of the organ of interest.

The optimal time to examine patients for the presence of uterine anomalies is in the luteal phase of the cycle, when the endometrium appears thick and echogenic and the uterine cavity can be clearly differentiated from the surrounding myometrium. To obtain a 3D ultrasound image of the uterus, the probe is positioned to display the uterus in longitudinal section from the outer fundal surface and the cervix in one plane. 3D volumes are then obtained by either a mechanical transducer or a manual sweep of the area of interest, depending on the mode of acquisition of the available equipment. Both methods, however, are based on the principle of obtaining a large number of consecutive tomograms in composite and storing them on a computer.

3D data may be examined by one of three methods: section reconstruction, surface rendering, or volume rendering. Section reconstruction, the most relevant for examining uterine morphology, involves generating an arbitrary sectional image through a volume by rotating and manipulating the orientation of a 3D ultrasound data set in relation to three orthogonal planes. The uterus is examined in the coronal plane, with both interstitial portions of the fallopian tubes and the internal cervical os, identified at the point of reflection of the urinary bladder, visible on the same plane.[26]

Two studies have examined the diagnostic accuracy of 2- and 3D sonography for the diagnosis of CUAs, using hysterosalpingography as the gold standard.[17,27] The first study included 61 women with a history of recurrent first-trimester miscarriage or infertility. There was complete agreement between 3D ultrasound and hysterosalpingography in classifying the uterus as abnormal or normal. This result was superior to that of 2D ultrasound, which also identified all cases of abnormal uterus but gave a number of false-positive results as well.[17] Raga and colleagues[27] reported similar results when comparing 3D ultrasound to hysterosalpingography and laparoscopy. There was complete agreement between 3D ultrasound and hysterosalpingography in all 44 cases. In one of the 12 cases of CUA, the description of the uterine fundus differed between 3D ultrasound and laparoscopy. The value of 3D ultrasound in the diagnosis of CUA was also confirmed by Merz,[28] who found it helpful in 20 cases of suspected anomaly.

3D ultrasound also enables measurement of the dimensions and volume of an organ. Thus, it is possible to measure not only endometrial volume but also the magnitude of uterine defects, such as the length of a uterine septum. This method has been shown to be accurate in both in vivo and in vitro studies.[29,30]

Two new 3D rendering modalities that recently became available can readily be used to enhance 3D ultrasound's ability to diagnose or rule out uterine anomalies. The first modality is the *inversion mode*. If saline infusion sonohysterography is used (usually in the follicular phase of the cycle), a software algorithm inverts the black, anechoic fluid contained in the distended cavity appearing in the rendering box (box D) as a "cast" of the cavity itself[31] (see Fig. 19–7). The second rendering mode is the *tomographic display*. Much like the sequential images contained on an MRI or CT film, this display enables the viewer to examine the sequential "slices" obtained in any desired plane. Such a quasi-tomographic display helps in localizing the possible uterine anomaly for a better understanding and applying of the correct treatment if necessary.

Classification of Congenital Uterine Anomalies

Classification by Anomaly

The classification of CUAs has been arbitrary and highly subjective. The most basic classification divides the müllerian anomalies into three groups[32,33]:

1. Agenesis
2. Vertical fusion defects, obstructive and nonobstructive
3. Lateral fusion defects, obstructive and nonobstructive

This classification gave rise to much confusion and debate over exactly what the terminology used in various studies was actually referring to. Many studies used the term *hemi-uterus* for cases of unicornuate uterus and *double uterus* for cases of septate and bicornuate uterus.[34,35]

Classification by Degree of Failure of Normal Development and by Clinical Manifestations, Treatment, and Prognosis

In 1979[36] (revised in 1983[37]), Buttram and Gibbons proposed a new classification for CUAs, based on the degree of failure of normal development of the female genital tract, that separated CUAs into groups based on clinical manifestations, treatment, and prognosis. The classification bases anomalies in six groups:

1. Agenesis (vagina, cervix, uterine fundus, fallopian tube)
2. Unicornuate uterus (communicating and noncommunicating)

3. Uterus didelphys
4. Bicornuate uterus (complete, partial arcuate)
5. Septate uterus (complete, partial)
6. Diethylstilbestrol use–related T-shaped uterus

Classification by Degree of Failure of Normal Development and by Presumed Clinical Significance, Treatment, and Prognosis

The 1983 classification and its current (1988) version, the American Fertility Society (AFS) classification of CUAs,[37] together constitute the most widely accepted working classification of CUAs. The AFS system also groups anomalies based on their presumed clinical significance, treatment, and prognosis.

A major limitation of the AFS classification is that it is based on a retrospective analysis of a small group of women with a previous diagnosis of CUA. It does not specify the diagnostic methods or criteria that should be used to analyze uterine morphology. It also includes only one case of bicornuate uterus and excludes all arcuate uteri. Therefore, since its introduction, the AFS classification has not been universally accepted, although it does in principle form the basis for practice for most clinicians. Furthermore, this classification, although used repeatedly in studies and clinical work, has never been assessed for interobserver and intraobserver reproducibility.

Three-Dimensional Classification

A revised 3D ultrasound classification based on the 1988 AFS classification of CUAs has been proposed (Table 7–1). This system is a descriptive classification only; neither prognosis nor treatment is a factor. The classification has been investigated for reproducibility by examination of 83 3D ultrasound volumes by two blinded experienced operators.[38] They found excellent agreement in the classification of uterine morphology, with complete agreement in all cases of normal and unicornuate uteri. There was disagreement in one case of uterine anomaly, where one operator classified it as an arcuate uterus and the other a subseptate uterus. The study also investigated the accuracy of intrauterine dimension measurements in CUAs and found no statistically significant differences when repeat measurements were made by the same operator and no statistically significant differences in measurements by the two operators.[39] 3D ultrasound and the revised AFS classification are at present the only imaging technique and criteria examined for diagnostic reproducibility in CUAs.

Table 7–1	Three-Dimensional Ultrasound Classification of Congenital Uterine Anomalies	
Uterine Morphology	**Fundal Contour**	**External Contour**
Normal	Straight or convex	Uniformly convex or with indentation <10 mm
Arcuate	Concave fundal indentation with central point of indentation at obtuse angle (>90 degrees)	Uniformly convex or with indentation <10 mm
Subseptate	Presence of septum, which does not extend to cervix, with central point of septum at an acute angle (<90 degrees)	Uniformly convex or with indentation <10 mm
Bicornuate	Two well-formed uterine cornua, fundal contour convex in each	Fundal indentation >10 mm dividing the two cornua
Unicornuate	Single well-formed uterine cavity with a single interstitial portion of fallopian tube and concave fundal contour	Fundal indentation >10 mm dividing the two cornua if rudimentary horn present

Table 7–2	Prevalence of Congenital Uterine Anomalies	
Study and Populations	**Diagnostic Method**	**Prevalence (%)**
General Population		
Jarcho,[39] 1946	Clinical examination	0.005
Moore,[40] 1941	Clinical examination	0.002
Cooper et al.,[41] 1983	Hysteroscopy	6.2
Ashton et al.,[42] 1988	HSG	1.9
Simon et al.,[43] 1991	HSG	3.2
Raga et al.,[4] 1997	HSG	3.8
Jurkovic et al.,[44] 1997	Three-dimensional ultrasound	5.4
Recurrent Miscarriage		
Clifford et al.,[2] 1994	HSG/TAS	1.8
Makino et al.,[3] 1992	HSG	15.7
Raziel et al.,[8] 1994	HSG/hysteroscopy	18
Acien,[1] 1996	HSG	37.6
Infertility		
Tulandi et al.,[47] 1980	HSG	1
Raga et al.,[4] 1997	HSG/hysteroscopy	2.4

HSG, hysterosalpingography; TAS, transabdominal sonography.

Clinical Significance of Congenital Uterine Anomalies

The principal fact confounding progress in the management of CUAs is that although they are usually found in women with poor reproductive histories, they are sometimes found in women with normal reproductive histories who undergo pelvic imaging for indications unrelated to reproductive performance. The prevalence of CUAs in high-risk populations is well documented, but their prevalence in the general gynecologic population has been more difficult to ascertain because it is not possible to subject women with normal reproductive histories to the invasive diagnostic techniques that are commonly required to diagnose CUAs (Table 7–2). In the absence of these data in low-risk women, it has been difficult to assess the true significance of CUAs in the high-risk population.

Women with an Incidental Diagnosis of Congenital Uterine Anomaly

Several studies have attempted to define the prevalence of uterine anomalies as an incidental diagnosis. In one of the initial studies of this type, Jarcho[39] reported anomalies in 1 in 15,000 deliveries and 1 in 200 nonpregnant gynecologic patients. In contrast, however, a subsequent study by Moore[40] reported an incidence of CUAs of 1 in 500 to 700 deliveries. In both studies, the previous reproductive histories are unknown and the classification of anomalies is subjective and arbitrary, varying between the studies. Furthermore, the diagnosis of CUA in both studies is based on the subjective impression of the clinician on clinical examination or exploration of the uterine cavity.

In 1983, Cooper et al.,[41] using hysteroscopy in patients undergoing elective hysteroscopic sterilization, noted the incidence of CUAs. This was one of the first studies to use an imaging technique to diagnose CUAs. They reported a prevalence of 6.2%, although no attempt was made to differentiate between anomalies, and the criteria for diagnosis were not specified.

Hysterosalpingography is often used to assess the completeness of tubal sterilization procedures, and several investigators have retrospectively analyzed these images to determine the prevalence of CUAs. These studies reported a lower prevalence in such women, ranging from 1.9% to 3.8%.[4,42,43] Each of these studies used its own diagnostic criteria and classification, thus making valid comparison impossible.

3D ultrasound has also been used to investigate the prevalence of CUAs in women with apparently normal reproductive histories. Jurkovic and coworkers[44] used the modified 3D ultrasound–based AFS classification of CUAs and 3D ultrasound as the sole diagnostic modality in a screening study of 1046 women. They found CUAs in 5.4% of women. Arcuate uterus was the most common anomaly, found in 3.1% of women, and subseptate uterus was the most frequent major anomaly, present in 1.6% of women, followed by bicornuate uterus, with a prevalence of 0.4%.

A more recent study used 3D sonography to screen for CUAs in 1089 women who presented for pelvic imaging for indications unrelated to reproductive performance.[45] In this study, the most common CUA was the arcuate uterus, which was associated with a significantly higher risk of preterm delivery and second-trimester miscarriages than was a normal uterus. Similarly, women with a subseptate uterus, the most common major anomaly, were significantly more likely to have had a first-trimester miscarriage. This was the first study to differentiate accurately between the duplication anomalies and to analyze past reproductive performance in the low-risk group.

The impact of arcuate, subseptate, and bicornuate uterus on reproductive performance has remained unresolved. Ashton et al.[42] reported that all of the 16 women in their study with an incidental finding of uterine anomaly had had multiple successful pregnancies and concluded that CUAs in low-risk women have limited impact on reproductive performance. However, this study did not differentiate between bicornuate and subseptate uteri, the latter being more commonly found and associated with a much poorer prognosis for pregnancy. Furthermore, the study focused only on live births and did not elaborate on previous miscarriages or gestation of delivery, preterm delivery being considered to be more common in women with a bicornuate uterus.

Women with Poor Reproductive Histories

The most common indication for screening for CUAs is a history of recurrent first-trimester miscarriage. In this group of women, the subseptate uterus is specifically implicated as a cause, with treatment being resection of the uterus.[23]

Most studies have used hysterosalpingography as a screening tool. The limitations of this technique are evident in the wide range of prevalences of CUAs found in this population of women by different operators, ranging from 1.8% to 37.6%.[1-3] A more recent study, using 3D ultrasound and its classification of CUAs (see Table 7–1), has reported on the incidence of CUAs in women with recurrent first-trimester miscarriages.[46] In this study, CUAs were found in 23.8% of women with recurrent miscarriage. The most common anomaly was the arcuate uterus, considered to be a minor anomaly. Major anomalies were present in 6.9% of women, the most common major anomaly being the subseptate uterus. The study further compared the severity of CUAs found in women with recurrent first-trimester miscarriage and low-risk women by calculating a distortion ratio (see Fig. 7–2). Women with a history of recurrent first-trimester miscarriage had significantly shorter unaffected uterine cavities and significantly higher distortion ratios, suggesting that CUAs found in this group of women are indeed more severe.[46]

The prevalence of CUAs in women with a history of infertility is also highly variable, ranging from 1% to 26%.[4,27,47] A recent meta-analysis of the prevalence of CUAs in women with infertility reported a median prevalence of 3.4%, which is comparable to that in low-risk women.[48] A workshop sponsored by the European Society of Human Reproduction and Embryology (ESHRE) came to the indirect conclusion that CUAs have no impact on women's fertility.[49]

Conclusion

Ultrasound offers a noninvasive and accurate method for diagnosing CUAs. Conventional 2D ultrasound should be used as the first-line investigative tool and has a high sensitivity but a low specificity. In those women in whom CUAs are suspected, 3D ultrasound should be used as a primary diagnostic tool to accurately define the exact nature of the anomaly. Whereas other methods for diagnosing CUAs are limited by their invasive and subjective nature and by their inability to assess uterine morphology completely, 3D ultrasound is the only diagnostic modality that has been assessed and found to be highly accurate for this purpose.

Ultrasound screening for CUAs has shown that they are more common and more severe in women with recurrent miscarriages than when found incidentally. The differences in morphologic severity of anomalies in these two groups of women suggest a threshold of severity above which the chances of reproductive failure are higher. Further research should be directed toward collecting data on large numbers of women with these anomalies and defining a cut-off level for severity. These data may potentially then be used to triage those women who are most likely to benefit from resection of uterine septa.

REFERENCES

1. Acien P: Uterine anomalies and recurrent miscarriage. Infertil Reprod Med Clin North Am 1996;7:698-719.
2. Clifford K, Rai R, Watson H, Regan L: An informative protocol for the investigation of recurrent miscarriage: Preliminary experience of 500 consecutive cases. Hum Reprod 1994;9:1328-1332.
3. Makino T, Hara T, Oka C, et al: Survey of 1120 Japanese women with a history of recurrent spontaneous abortions. Eur J Obstet Gynecol Reprod Biol 1992;44:123-130.
4. Raga F, Bauset C, Remohi J, et al: Reproductive impact of congenital uterine anomalies. Hum Reprod 1997;12:2277-2281.
5. Kupesic S, Kurjak A: Septate uterus: Detection and prediction of obstetrical complications by different forms of ultrasonography. J Ultrasound Med 1998;17:631-636.
6. Cary WH: Note on determination of patency of fallopian tubes by the use of Collargol and x-ray shadow. Am J Obstet Dis Women Child 1914;69:462.
7. Rindfleisch W: Darstellung des cavum uteri. Klin Wochenschr 1910; 47:780.
8. Raziel A, Arieli S, Bukovsky I, et al: Investigation of the uterine cavity in recurrent aborters. Fertil Steril 1994;62:1080-1082.
9. Mencaglia L, Tantini C: Hysteroscopic treatment of septate and arcuate uterus. Gynecol Endosc 1996;5:151-154.
10. Taylor PJ, Goswamy RK: Hysteroscopy in infertility and habitual abortion. Hum Reprod 1989;4:13-16.
11. Golan A, Ron-El R, Herman A, et al: Diagnostic hysteroscopy: Its value in an in vitro fertilisation/embryo transfer unit. Hum Reprod 1992;7:1433-1434.
12. Reuter KL, Daly DC, Cohen SM: Septate versus bicornuate uteri: Errors in imaging diagnosis. Radiology 1989:172:749-752.
13. Barbot J: Hysteroscopy and hysterography. Obstet Gynecol Clin North Am 1995;22:591-603.
14. Daskalakis G, Pilalis A, Lykeridou K, Antsaklis A: Rupture of noncommunicating rudimentary uterine horn pregnancy. Obstet Gynecol 2002;100:1108-1110.
15. Pellerito JS, McCarthy SM, Doyle MB, et al: Diagnosis of uterine anomalies: Relative accuracy of MR imaging, endovaginal sonography and hysterosalpingography. Radiology 1992;183:795-800.
16. Storment JM, Kaiser JR, Sites CK: Transvaginal ultrasonographic diagnosis of uterine septa. J Reprod Med 1998;43:823-826.
17. Jurkovic D, Geipel A, Gruboeck K, et al: Three-dimensional ultrasound for the assessment of uterine anatomy and detection of congenital anomalies: A comparison with hysterosalpingography and two-dimensional sonography. Ultrasound Obstet Gynecol 1995;5:233-237.
18. Fedele L, Ferrazzi E, Dorta M, et al: Ultrasonography in the differential diagnosis of "double" uteri. Fertil Steril 1988;50:361-364.
19. Soares SR, Barbosa dos Reis MM, Camargos AF: Diagnostic accuracy of sonohysterography, transvaginal sonography and hysterosalpingography in patients with uterine contour diseases. Fertil Steril 2000;73:406-411.
20. Keltz MD, Olive DL, Kim AH, Arici A: Sonohysterography for screening in recurrent pregnancy loss. Fertil Steril 1997;67:670-674.
21. Ayida G, Kennedy S, Barlow D, Chamberlain P: A comparison of patient tolerance of hysterosalpingo-contrast sonography (HyCoSy) with Echovist-200 and x-ray hysterosalpingography for outpatient investigation of infertile women. Ultrasound Obstet Gynecol 1996;7:201-204.
22. Forsey JP, Caul EO, Paul ID, Hull MG: Chlamydia trachomatis, tubal disease and the incidence of asymptomatic infection following hysterosalpingography. Hum Reprod 1990;5:444-447.
23. Homer HA, Li TC, Cooke ID: The septate uterus: A review of management and reproductive outcome. Fertil Steril 2000;73:1-4.
24. Fischetti SG, Politi G, Lomeo F, Garozzo G: Magnetic resonance in evaluation of mullerian duct anomalies. Radiol Med (Torino) 1995;89:105-111.
25. Letterie GS, Haggerty M, Lindee G: A comparison of pelvic ultrasound and magnetic resonance imaging as diagnostic studies for mullerian tract abnormalities. Int J Fertil Menopausal Stud 1995;40:34-38.
26. Jurkovic D, Aslam N: Three-dimensional ultrasound for diagnosis of congenital uterine anomalies. In Merz E (ed): 3-D Ultrasound in Obstetrics and Gynaecology. Philadelphia, Lippincott Williams & Wilkins, 1998, pp 27-29.
27. Raga F, Bonilla-Muscoles F, Blanes J, Osbourne NG: Congenital mullerian anomalies: Diagnostic accuracy of three-dimensional ultrasound. Fertil Steril 1996;65:523-528.
28. Merz E: Three-dimensional transvaginal ultrasound in gynecological diagnosis. Ultrasound Obstet Gynecol 1999;14:81-86.
29. Gilja OH, Thune N, Matre K, et al: In vitro evaluation of three-dimensional ultrasonography in volume estimation of abdominal organs. Ultrasound Med Biol 1994;20:157-165.
30. Kyei-Mensah A, Zaidi J, Pitroff R, et al: Transvaginal three-dimensional ultrasound: Accuracy of follicular measurements. Fertil Steril 1996; 65:371-376.
31. Timor-Tritsch IE, Monteagudo A, Tsymbal T, Strok I: Three-dimensional inversion rendering: A new sonographic technique and its use in gynecology. J Ultrasound Med 2005;24:681-688.
32. Jones WS: Obstetric significance of female genital anomalies. Obstet Gynecol 1957;10:113-127.
33. Rock JA, Schlaff WD: The obstetric consequences of uterovaginal anomalies. Fertil Steril 1985;43:681-692.
34. Buttram VC Jr: Mullerian anomalies and their management. Fertil Steril 1983;40:159-163.
35. Heinonen PK, Pystynen PP: Primary infertility and uterine anomalies. Fertil Steril 1983;40:311-316.
36. Buttram VC, Gibbons WE: Mullerian anomalies: A proposed classification (an analysis of 144 cases). Fertil Steril 1979;32:40-46.
37. The American Fertility Society: The American Fertility Society classifications of adnexal adhesions, distal tubal occlusion, tubal occlusion secondary to tubal ligation, tubal pregnancies, mullerian anomalies and intrauterine adhesions. Fertil Steril 1988;49:944-955.
38. Salim R, Woelfer B, Backos M, et al: Reproducibility of three-dimensional ultrasound diagnosis of congenital uterine anomalies. Ultrasound Obstet Gynecol 2003;21:578-582.

39. Jarcho J: Malformations of the uterus: Review of the subject, including embryology, comparative anatomy, diagnosis and report of cases. Am J Surg 1946;71:106-166.
40. Moore O: Congenital abnormalities of female genitalia. South Med J 1941;34:610.
41. Cooper JM, Jouch RM, Rigberg HS: The incidence of intrauterine abnormalities found at hysteroscopy in patients undergoing elective hysteroscopic sterilization. J Reprod Med 1983;28:659-661.
42. Ashton D, Amin HK, Richart RM, Neuwirth RS: The incidence of asymptomatic uterine anomalies in women undergoing transcervical tubal sterilization. Obstet Gynecol 1988;72:28-30.
43. Simon C, Martinez L, Pardo F, et al: Mullerian defects in women with normal reproductive outcome. Fertil Steril 1991;56:1192-1193.
44. Jurkovic D, Gruboeck K, Tailor A, Nicolaides KH: Ultrasound screening for congenital uterine anomalies. Br J Obstet Gynaecol 1997;104:1320-1321.
45. Woelfer B, Salim R, Banerjee S, et al: Reproductive outcomes in women with congenital uterine anomalies detected by three-dimensional ultrasound screening. Obstet Gynecol 2001;98:1099-1103.
46. Salim R, Regan L, Woelfer B, et al: A comparative study of the morphology of congenital uterine anomalies in women with and without a history of recurrent first trimester miscarriage. Hum Reprod 2003;1:162-166.
47. Tulandi T, Arronet GH, McInnes RA: Arcuate and bicornuate uterine anomalies and infertility. Fertil Steril 1980;34:362-364.
48. Grimbizis GF, Camus M, Tarlatzis BC, et al: Clinical implications of uterine malformations and hysteroscopic treatment results. Hum Reprod Update 2001;7:161-174.
49. ESHRE Capri Workshop: Infertility revisited: The state of the art today and tomorrow. Hum Reprod 1996;11:1779-1807.

Chapter 8

Adnexal Masses

Ilan E. Timor-Tritsch

Transvaginal sonography (TVS) is the imaging tool of choice for scanning the adnexa. The high-resolution pictures generated by the 5- to 7.5-MHz probes greatly enhance diagnostic accuracy and have led to a major advance in our understanding of adnexal inflammatory processes, especially of ovarian lesions. This chapter provides a detailed discussion of the ultrasound appearance and evaluation of fallopian tube and ovarian pathologic processes. The interested reader is directed to the pertinent textbooks for a complete reference base.[1-6]

Ultrasound Appearance of the Pathologic Fallopian Tube

Sonography can explore the fallopian tube's wall structure, luminal contents, and adherence to surrounding structures. The great majority of tubal disease is related to inflammatory processes (see Chapter 21 for a complete discussion of the inflammatory pathology of the tube), which produce changes in wall thickness as well as some fluid collection in the lumen of the tube. This intraluminal fluid helps the examiner locate the tube and diagnose the disease.[7] A distinct advantage of TVS in the setting of pelvic inflammatory disease (PID) is that the vaginal probe is much better tolerated by patients than the transabdominal probe, which is typically operated through a full bladder. For some patients, the abdominal pressure in this case can be intolerable.[8-10]

Sonography in the form of ultrasound-guided puncture also has a role in treating the most feared complications of PID, such as ectopic pregnancy. These puncture procedures, discussed in detail in Chapter 16, are used in conjunction with antibiotic therapy.

The contents of the tube may be anechoic or uniformly echogenic, with low-level echoes (mucus or purulent fluid). Ruptured or bleeding tubal ectopic pregnancies may fill the tubal cavity with blood clots. An unruptured gestational sac with or without embryonic heartbeats also is occasionally identified in the tube. Any heterogeneous structure that is not normally present in the general area of the adnexal area should raise the suspicion of ectopic pregnancy, with necessary measures taken to rule it out. The ultrasound features of tubal pregnancy are discussed fully in Chapter 13.

Tubal malignancy is very rare, although an increasing number of reports have appeared regarding its ultrasound recognition.[11-18] The ultrasound picture of tubal carcinoma is not pathognomonic. Tubal malignancy can show a mixture of echogenicities, similar to the appearance of a pyosalpinx, or it can be imaged as a fluid-filled tube with a significant solid component adjacent to the tube that is evidently not part of the ovary, cervix, or uterus (Fig. 8–1). Sometimes a typical component or ultrasound marker, such as a mural nodule or an incomplete septum, can lead to the correct diagnosis (Fig. 8–2). Color Doppler has been used to evaluate tubal carcinoma,[19] and a leiomyoma of the fallopian tube scanned sonographically was also reported.[20] It is extremely difficult to determine whether the malignancy is a primary carcinoma of the tube or secondary to an ovarian primary cancer.

Torsion of the adnexa, with or without involvement of the fallopian tube, can be diagnosed using ultrasonography[21] (see Chapter 17, Fig. 17–22). Color Doppler flow detection in a twisted adnexa enhances the accuracy of this diagnosis.[22,23] Ultrasound diagnosis of adnexal torsion may obviate the need to resect the tube and ovary, thus preserving reproductive function with conservative follow-up.[24] Torsion of the fallopian tube is discussed in greater detail in Chapters 17 and 21 (see Fig. 21–26).

Ultrasound Appearance of Ovarian Lesions

The normal ovary and corpus luteum are described in Chapter 5. Some benign and malignant ovarian lesions and their ultrasound appearance are discussed in the following.

Benign Ovarian Masses

Functional Ovarian Cyst

The most common ovarian lesion in the reproductive years is the functional cyst. To understand the pathophysiologic process behind this and other benign functional structures in the ovary, it is important to remember that the ovary is an extremely dynamic organ: it changes its size, shape, and structural anatomy over the menstrual cycle. Best diagnosed on TVS, functional simple cysts are usually unilocular and anechoic follicular cysts with thin, smooth outer and inner walls, measuring 6 cm or less in diameter (usually 2 to 3 cm). However, if no ovulation occurs, the cysts can increase in size to approximately 6 cm. They usually shrink spontaneously and are best scanned if the patient is on day 5 to 10 of the

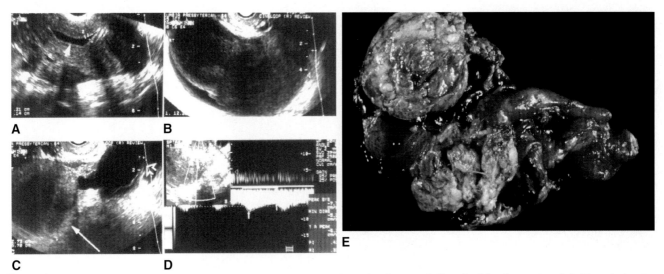

Figure 8–1. Fallopian tube cancer. **A,** Fluid in the endometrial cavity *(arrow),* a frequent hallmark of the disease. **B** and **C,** The tubular character of the lesion. The *arrow* points to the thick wall of the tube. **D,** Determination of low resistance to flow can help establish the malignant nature of the disease. **E,** Macroscopic specimen.

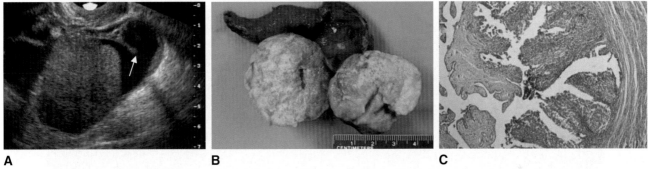

Figure 8–2. Fallopian tube cancer. **A,** The *arrow* points to the incomplete septum, a highly suggestive feature in identifying the target organ of the cancer. **B,** The macroscopic specimen. **C,** Microscopic histology on a cross section of the affected tube. (Courtesy of Dr. Natan Haratz-Rubinstein, Long Island College Hospital, Brooklyn Heights, New York. Reprinted by permission.)

subsequent cycle. If they do not shrink spontaneously, hormonal suppression therapy can be tried and the progress monitored by TVS.

Polycystic Ovary Syndrome

Polycystic ovary syndrome was first described by Stein and Leventhal.[25] This type of ovary has a typical ultrasound appearance. It is recognized as an enlarged, almost spheric ovary with multiple small (<10 mm), immature follicles crowded along its surface[10-12] (Fig. 8–3). These follicles, lined up side by side, give the ovary a "beads-on-a-string" appearance.[26-33] If the patient is hormonally stimulated, the polycystic ovary gives an even more distinctive image, sometimes described as the "stained glass window" appearance. The most common ultrasound finding in polycystic ovaries, however, is enlargement, usually to greater than 12 cm³. Color Doppler evaluation demonstrates a rich central blood supply within the echogenic hilus of the polycystic ovary (Fig. 8–4). TVS is the best modality for diagnosis of polycystic ovaries and subsequent follow-up in these patients, such as monitoring the effects of gonadotropin-releasing hormone therapy.

Hyperstimulated Ovary

An increasing number of centers and obstetrician-gynecologists offer reproductive technologies and fertility enhancement procedures. Thus, physicians now treat patients who have been administered menotropins, resulting in ovarian hyperstimulation. These patients have enlarged ovaries with many follicles or corpora lutea of variable appearance. Hyperstimulated ovaries are sometimes surrounded by ascites (Fig. 8–5A).

It may be more advantageous initially to scan patients with ovarian hyperstimulation syndrome by the transabdominal (see Fig. 8–5A) rather than transvaginal (Fig. 8–5B and C) route because the transvaginal scan may not be able to include the entire enlarged ovary in the focal range. Chapter 14 is devoted to the imaging of patients with fertility problems.

Ovarian Torsion

Ovarian torsion usually involves both the ovary and the fallopian tube; however, a severely dilated fallopian tube may twist separately. Chapter 17 describes the ultrasound features of ovarian torsion. The typical ultrasound picture of a twisted

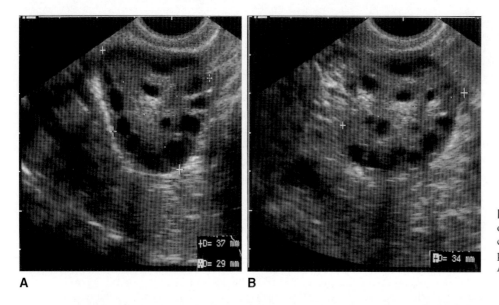

A   **B**

Figure 8–3. This typical polycystic ovary has a volume of 15.5 mL and contains many subcapsular follicles approximately 0.6 to 0.8 cm in diameter. **A,** Longitudinal section. **B,** Cross section.

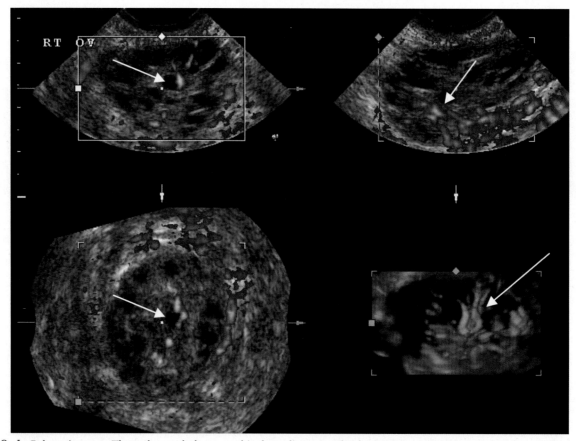

Figure 8–4. Polycystic ovary. The orthogonal planes on this three-dimensional color Doppler acquisition of the ovary show an enlarged ovary containing small follicles at its periphery. The *arrows* point to the high vascularity of the central hilar area of the ovary. Box D is a rendered three-dimensional power Doppler angiogram of the vessels.

ovary includes enlargement, a hyperechoic hilus, follicles pushed to the surface, and no visible blood flow. The ovary is also tender to the touch of the transvaginal probe. The diagnosis of ovarian (as well as fallopian tube) torsion relies primarily on clinical signs and symptoms.[34-38] While an ultrasound image of the typical features (see Chapter 17, Figs. 17–20 through 17–22) greatly aids in the diagnosis, the clinical picture should take the leading role in making the diagnosis if the imaging results are inconclusive.

Cystadenoma

Cystadenoma is one of the most common ovarian cystic structures in postmenopausal women. Two variations are known: serous and mucinous. Cystadenomas can reach sizes

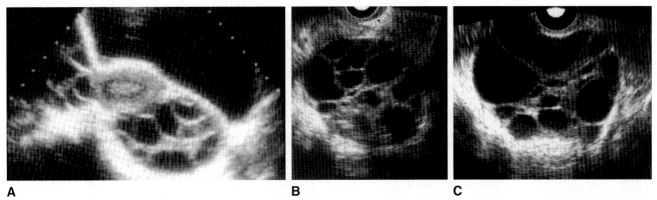

Figure 8–5. Hormonally hyperstimulated ovaries. **A,** Panoramic transabdominal view of the enlarged ovaries with multiple follicles. Note the hyperechoic endometrium. **B** and **C,** Transvaginal ultrasound view of the ovaries.

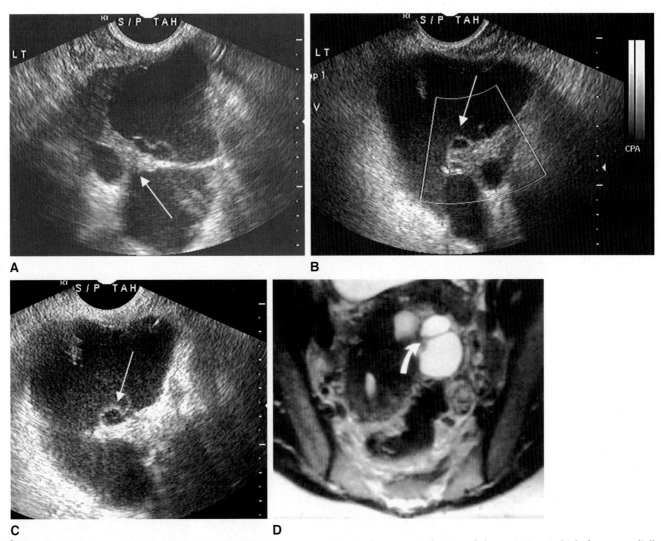

Figure 8–6. Benign ovarian cystadenoma. **A** to **C,** The *arrows* point to the common origin of the septations, which fan out radially. **B,** Only a small number of blood vessels are highlighted by power Doppler. **D,** The magnetic resonance imaging scan is similar to the ultrasound picture. The *arrow* points to the origin of the radiating septa.

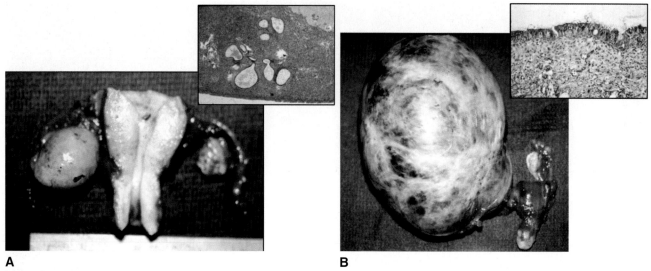

Figure 8–7. Two pathologic specimens of adnexal masses. **A,** Benign right serous cystadenoma; *inset* shows its histologic appearance. **B,** Benign right mucinous cystadenoma; *inset* shows its histologic appearance. (Courtesy of Dr. Robert Wallach, New York University, New York.)

of 4 to 5 cm or more and usually show a simple multilocular architecture; however, they also may have minimal solid components from which septations emanate, usually radially. A septate cystic structure 5 cm or larger persisting over two or three menstrual cycles may be a cystadenoma (Figs. 8–6 and 8–7).

It is difficult to distinguish cystadenomas with a serous content from those with a mucinous content (see Fig. 8–7). The fluid in the mucinous cystadenoma often shows low-level echogenicity (see Fig. 8–6), whereas its serous counterpart usually contains anechoic fluid-filled compartments, and its septa fan out from a common point within an area of ovarian stroma (see Fig. 8–6). Color or power Doppler evaluation of either type may show minimal flow in the septa, and the resistance-to-flow values will be in the benign range (pulsatility index [PI] > 0.46, resistance index [RI] > 0.62). They usually do not have shadowing.

Ovarian Endometrioma

Endometriosis is a common disease, estimated to occur in 5% to 20% of women in their reproductive years.[39,40] It is characterized by the presence of functional endometrial tissue in an ectopic location and can occur almost anywhere in the abdominal cavity; however, it is predominantly seen in the lesser pelvis, and commonly in the ovaries. Like normally located endometrial tissue, the ectopic endometrial tissue responds to hormonal changes throughout the menstrual cycle and at times during pregnancy and bleeds into the cyst during the period of normal menstrual flow, which slowly enlarges the cyst.

Sonography cannot detect small endometrial implants; however, the larger, more localized, more cystlike structures, such as endometriomas or so-called chocolate cysts, can be detected easily by TVS. Their ultrasound appearance is typical: they have thick walls, and some have septations. They may contain solid components or can be of mixed echogenicity.[41-45] In my experience, however, the most prevalent ultrasound appearance of an endometrioma is that of a spheric cyst with a diffuse, low-level echogenicity produced by the thickened blood (Fig. 8–8). It is sometimes difficult to differentiate a small endometrioma from a hemorrhagic corpus luteum (see Fig. 8–8). However, the endometrioma typically lacks significant blood vessels on color or power Doppler (Fig. 8–9). In this case, a follow-up scan in 2 to 3 months on days 5 to 9 of

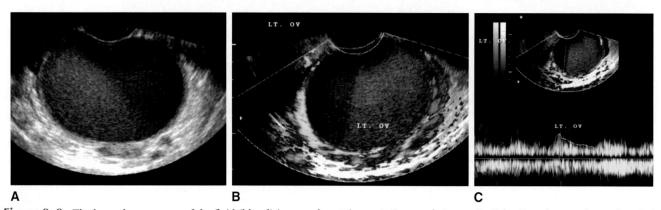

Figure 8–8. The layered appearance of the fluid (blood) in an endometrioma. **A,** Gray-scale image. **B,** Color Doppler reveals vessels only in the wall. **C,** Flow velocity waveforms show normal diastolic flow.

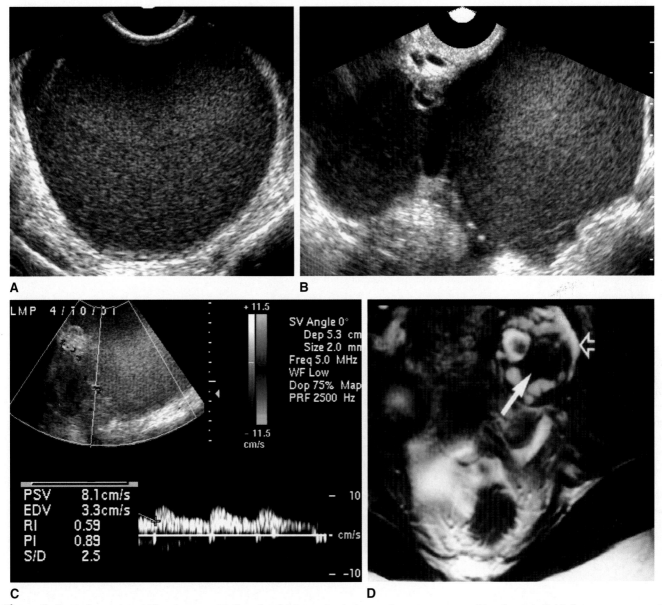

Figure 8–9. Endometrioma. The ultrasound hallmarks of this ovarian lesion are homogeneous, weakly echogenic fluid, few or no septa, and a paucity of blood vessels. **A,** Unilateral typical endometrioma. **B,** Bilateral endometriomas. **C,** Doppler interrogation. Resistance indices are in the normal range. **D,** Magnetic resonance imaging is redundant in these cases, although it confirms the blood content.

the cycle may help in the differential diagnosis, as can the patient's history. The hemorrhagic corpus luteum disappears or shrinks over 1 or 2 months.

Rarely, malignancy is found in an endometrioma. This usually is defined as endometrioid carcinoma or clear cell carcinoma. The pathognomonic feature of this lesion is the presence of vascularized papillary projections on its internal walls (Fig. 8–10).

Ovarian Fibroma

Four types of ovarian fibroma have been identified: granulosa cell tumors, theca cell tumors, Sertoli and Leydig cell tumors, and pure fibromas. Ovarian fibromas are also regarded as variants of serous cystadenoma, termed *cystadenofibroma* or *adenofibroma* depending on the amount of fibrous stroma in the tumor. They account for 5% to 10% of all ovarian neoplasms

and are formed from undifferentiated mesenchymal cells and their endocrine derivatives.

Fibromas consist of spindle cells and abundant collagen. They may grow to large sizes and demonstrate cystic degeneration. Their malignant potential is reported to be under 1%. In the predominantly solid variety, sonography shows a solid hypoechoic mass with marked sound attenuation (Fig. 8–11). They may be bilateral in up to 10% of the cases.

Approximately 20% of fibromas are predominantly cystic, with several small (<5 mm), extremely hyperechoic internal mural nodules that have no vascularity. This ultrasound picture does not change significantly over time (Fig. 8–12). Careful evaluation is suggested to identify avascular mural nodules, because whereas cystic fibromas can be managed conservatively, a tumor with true vessels containing mural papillae is usually malignant.

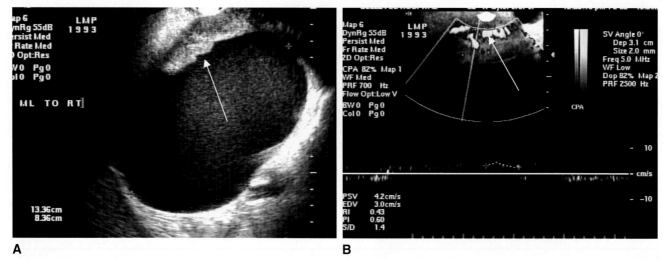

Figure 8–10. Endometrioid (clear cell) carcinoma of the ovary. **A,** Note the weakly echogenic fluid and the papilla *(arrow)*. **B,** Power Doppler shows flow in the papilla *(arrow)* with low resistance and pulsatility indices.

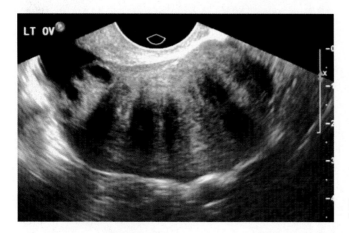

Figure 8–11. Solid ovarian fibroma. Note the dense solid tissue "texture" with areas of shadowing due to excess density.

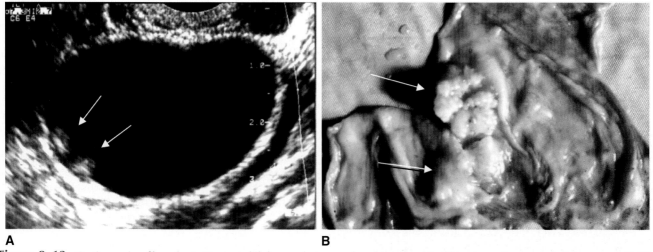

Figure 8–12. Cystic ovarian fibroma. **A,** Dense, solid, hyperechoic mural nodules devoid of blood vessels are marked by *arrows*. **B,** The pathologic specimen. The mural excrescences are marked by *arrows*.

Parovarian Cysts and Cysts of Morgagni

Parovarian cysts and cysts of Morgagni can reach large sizes and have a simple cystic architecture. These cysts originate in the wolffian or müllerian duct or are of mesothelial origin.[46] Internal ultrasound echoes are seen very rarely; the cysts' typical feature is a degree of mobility in the pelvis. Occasionally, they are found serendipitously during an imaging study or even at pelvic surgery. The diagnosis can be based on a single important feature—namely, the demonstration of an ovary separate from the cyst in question[47-49] (Fig. 8–13). Very rarely, they can become malignant.[46] The clinical value of aspirating these cysts is debatable.[50]

Cystic Teratoma

Benign cystic teratoma of the ovary, or dermoid cyst, originates from all three germ layers and is typically found in young women. The ultrasound appearance of dermoid cysts is extremely variable. They can be cystic and filled with a weakly echogenic content (i.e., sebaceous material) (Fig. 8–14). They are bilateral in 20% of cases (Fig. 8–15) and can also be multiloculated or solid-appearing (Fig. 8–16). The "tip of the iceberg" sign on transabdominal sonography indicates the echogenic core of this lesion.[51] On TVS, dermoid cysts may show the typical "fried egg" sign, that of a central, highly echogenic core amid a weakly echogenic rind[52] (see Fig. 8–16B). These ovarian lesions have a variable appearance (see Fig. 8–16) on computed tomography as well as sonography.[53] In the appropriate age group, cystic teratoma almost always must be included in the differential diagnosis of an ovarian lesion, especially those lesions that share the typical characteristics of cystic teratomas: low-level echoes; a central, more echogenic core; near-total absence of blood vessels on Doppler interrogation; or bilateral occurrence.

The variable appearance of ovarian teratomas creates problems in the construction and use of scoring systems[54] and complicates distinguishing between benign and malignant tumors by TVS. Because more than 80% of dermoid cysts demonstrate distal shadowing behind denser tissues,

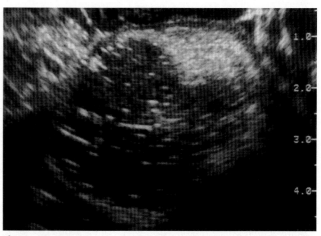

Figure 8–14. Cystic teratoma of the ovary. Note the hyperechoic solid portion and the speckled appearance of the sebaceous contents.

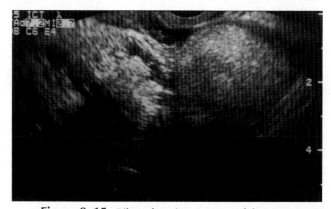

Figure 8–15. Bilateral cystic teratomas of the ovary.

one of the newer scoring systems tries to correct for the presence or absence of shadowing in ovarian lesions.[55] This has improved the ability to differentiate between a malignant lesion and a cystic teratoma. Cohen and Sabbagha[56] describe the various ultrasound appearances of cystic teratomas on TVS.

Since the introduction of TVS, the detection of small teratomas in near–normal-sized ovaries has become common. Clinicians are now faced with the problem of how to react to these tiny ovarian teratomas, which sometimes even are detected bilaterally. I recommend a conservative approach to management, with yearly follow-up.

Pelvic Kidney

Although a pelvic kidney (Fig. 8–17) is not strictly an adnexal mass, it is sometimes encountered serendipitously during a pelvic scan. The diagnosis is made based on the typical oval structure with a branching, hyperechoic central area (the fat-containing, hyperechoic renal pelvis and the calices). The correct diagnosis is important mainly to prevent additional unnecessary tests and surgery.

Myomas as an Adnexal Mass

Occasionally, a subserous or pedunculated fibroid (myoma) arising from the lateral aspect of the uterus appears as an

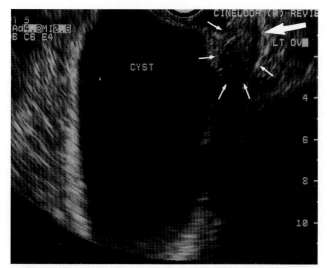

Figure 8–13. Typical parovarian cyst with simple cystic architecture. The ovary (*large arrow*) is seen (highlighted by the *small arrows*) alongside the cyst.

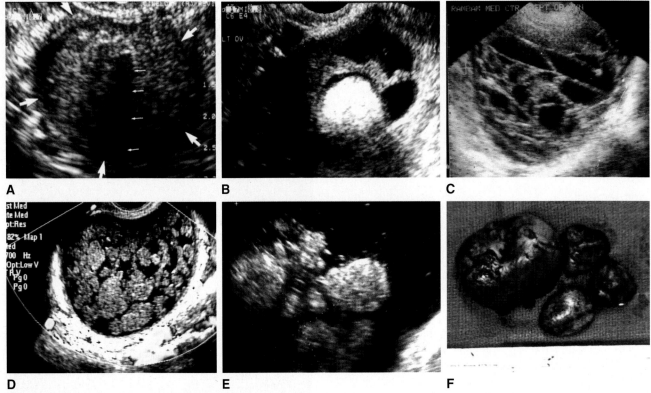

A   B   C

D   E   F

Figure 8–16. A few of the possible ultrasound appearances of the benign cystic teratoma of the ovary. **A,** Dense, hyperechoic tissue creates shadows *(small arrows).* **B,** The shadow behind the hyperechoic, solid structure is termed the *Rokitansky nodule* or the sonographic "fried egg" sign. **C,** Thin septations in an unusual presentation of a benign cystic teratoma. **D** and **E,** Hyperechoic sebaceous and hair tissue creates globular echoes as it floats in the fluid. **F,** Macroscopic appearance of the "globules" seen in **E.**

adnexal mass. Intraligamentary fibroid growths generally are the most difficult to diagnose (Fig. 8–18), and the main task of sonography is to differentiate such a growth from an ovarian mass. The simplest and least costly way to achieve this is to use color or power Doppler sonography. The vascular connection between the uterus and a lateral myoma (pedunculated, serous, or intraligamentary) will be seen in almost all instances (see Fig. 8–18), enabling the correct assessment of the "adnexal mass."

Malignant Ovarian Tumors

One of the most important reasons for scanning the female pelvis is to evaluate the ovaries and detect neoplastic processes as early as possible. Ovarian carcinoma is the most feared and the leading cause of death for gynecologic malignancy in the world. Because it usually is detected late, in stage III or IV, the overall 5-year survival rate is between 30% and 35%. Although the accurate characterization of an ovarian mass will determine its nature, the main task of sonography is to detect ovarian malignancy in its early stages. If it is detected early enough (i.e., in stage I), the patient has a 5-year survival rate of 80% to 85%.[57]

Chapter 18 deals with the subject of screening for ovarian cancer, and Chapter 9 discusses the postmenopausal ovaries; this chapter is restricted to discussion of the ultrasound appearance of ovarian cancer. Only references pertaining to the ultrasound attributes of these lesions are cited.

It is important also to mention the pathologic appearance of the most prevalent ovarian cancers because the ultrasound characterization of ovarian masses takes into consideration some of the key structural features of these neoplasms.

Usually, the malignant ovarian lesions tend to contain centrally located blood vessels. As a rule, pathologic ovarian lesions with significant central blood flow are extremely suspicious for malignancy.

Serous Cystadenocarcinoma

As opposed to serous cystadenomas, serous cystadenocarcinomas are usually multilocular, containing papillary prominences and solid, vascularized papillary nodules. The fluid content is usually bloody, making it weakly echogenic. Thirty

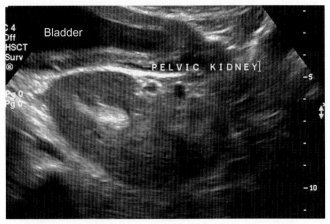

Figure 8–17. Transabdominal image of a pelvic kidney.

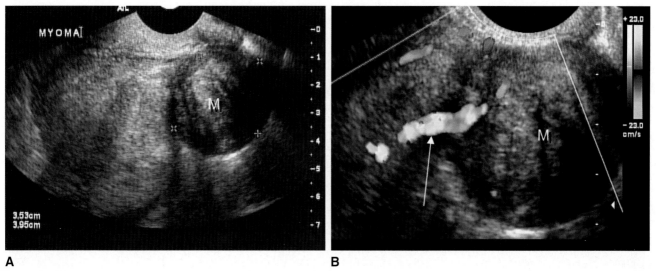

A   **B**

Figure 8–18. Intraligamentary myoma. **A,** Left lateral location of the mass (M). **B,** Color Doppler clearly shows the blood vessel *(arrow)* with flow from the uterus to the mass (M).

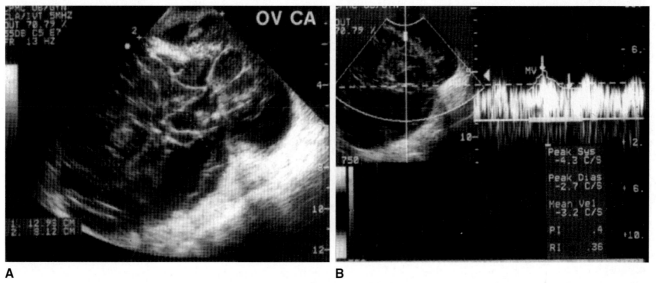

A   **B**

Figure 8–19. Cystadenocarcinoma of the ovary. Note the large number of septations in bizarre orientations (**A**), as well as the high diastolic flow *(small vertical arrows)* resulting in low resistance indices (**B**).

percent to 50% of these neoplasms are bilateral. Doppler studies (Fig. 8–19) usually show a low resistance to flow (low PI and RI).

Mucinous Cystadenocarcinoma

Mucinous tumors are usually benign; only approximately 10% are borderline malignant, and another 10% show explicit malignancy. Mucinous cystadenocarcinoma is a less frequent finding than serous cystadenocarcinoma. It should be suspected if the fluid it contains appears to be of low-level echogenicity. The ultrasound appearance of malignant mucinous cystadenocarcinoma resembles that of the malignant serous cystadenocarcinoma. Both are multilocular cystic masses; some have a centrally located solid component from which septa radiate. Their inner walls may be smooth or may have papillary nodules containing blood vessels (Fig. 8–20). The mucinous fluid filling the tumor is weakly echogenic on sonography. Approximately 10% are bilateral.

This tumor can spread into the entire peritoneal cavity (myxoma peritonei). In such cases, the characteristic ultrasound picture is a meshlike multilocular content filling and extending above the true pelvis.

Endometrioid Carcinoma

Endometrioid carcinoma is probably the third most prevalent ovarian cancer. It is a cystic mass that contains hemorrhagic, serous, or mucinous components, with an ultrasound picture very similar to that of an endometrioma (i.e., a low-level echo–filled, thick-walled cystic structure).[45] In addition, it is common to see vascularized mural papillae of variable sizes (see Fig. 8–10).

Metastatic Carcinoma

Metastatic carcinoma comprises approximately 10% of ovarian cancers. It is almost impossible to determine the exact diagnosis sonographically. The ultrasound picture may be consistent with an echo-dense, hyperchoic component.

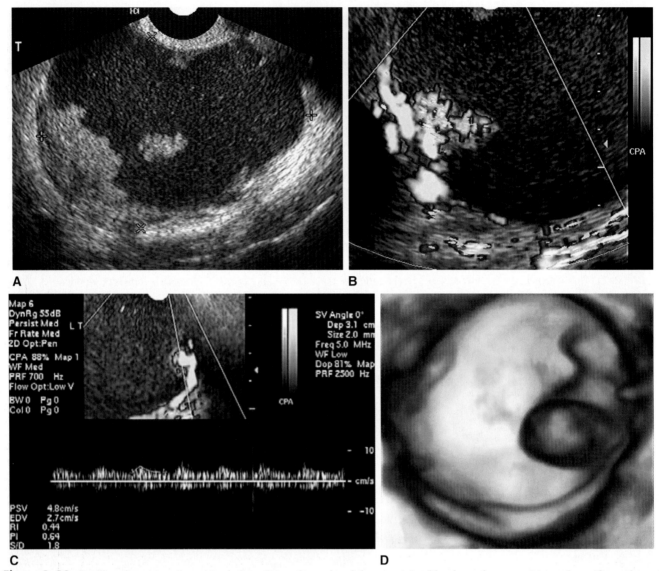

Figure 8–20. Papillary formations in ovarian lesions. Internal mural nodules containing blood vessels are sensitive and specific markers of malignancy. **A,** Gray-scale image of papillae. **B** and **C,** Power Doppler image of the papillary vessels, showing their low resistance to flow. **D,** Three-dimensional surface rendering of ovarian papillae from a different case.

However, the picture may also be totally different, as demonstrated in Figure 8–21. In this case, the lesion was a metastatic right ovarian cancer from a primary colon cancer.

Ovarian Tumors of Low Malignant Potential

Borderline ovarian tumors or ovarian tumors of low malignant potential (LMP) are histologically distinct from invasive cancer of the ovary. They account for approximately 15% of epithelial ovarian tumors. Clinically, patients with tumors of LMP are 10 to 15 years younger than those with the invasive form of the disease. Histologically, the tumors show no invasion of the underlying stroma. The survival rate for this tumor is significantly better stage by stage than for invasive ovarian cancer.

Unfortunately, no preoperative tumor marker or pathognomonic ultrasound features have been described to aid in diagnosing ovarian tumors of LMP. They may be serous or mucinous tumors, so on ultrasound their loculations may be anechoic or of low-level echogenicity. Ovarian tumors of LMP can be suspected based only on their relatively large size, uncharacteristic ultrasound picture, and occasionally bizarre vascular pattern (Fig. 8–22).

Ovarian Steroid Cell Tumors (Leydig Cell Tumors)

Although these usually small ovarian tumors are rare and comprise only 0.1% of all ovarian tumors, their recognition by TVS is relatively straightforward. They are also called *lipid cell tumors* for their high fatty content (when cut for pathology, their surface appears yellow). Leydig cell tumors contain Reinke crystals, visible on histologic sections. Their ultrasound appearance is typical,[58] consisting of a relatively discrete, small, round (spheric) structure in the ovary, which is usually small or normal-sized (Fig. 8–23A and B). Because these tumors have a high rate of hormonal secretion, they usually have a distinct vascular ring ("ring of fire") marking their size and location. This vascularity, highlighted by power

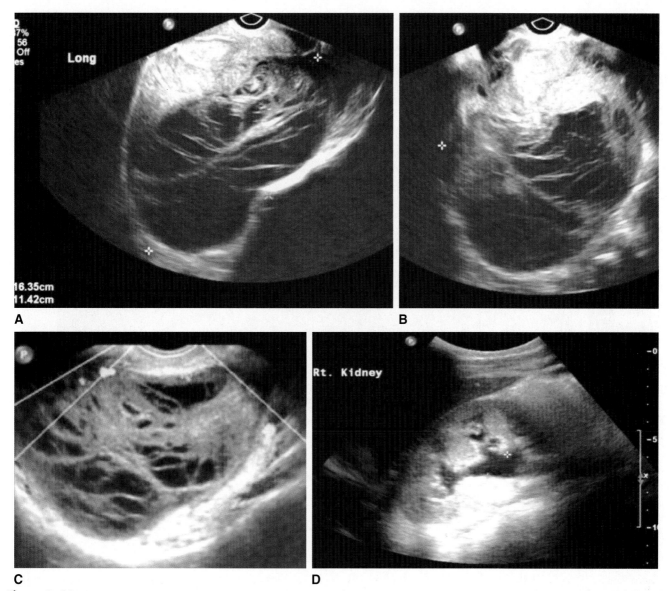

Figure 8–21. Metastatic carcinoma of the ovary originating from a primary colon cancer. **A** and **B,** Note the common origin of the septations arising from a predominantly solid area of the tumor. **C,** There is a clear lack of vessels, a somewhat atypical finding for cancerous tissue. **D,** This large right-sided ovarian mass caused pressure on the urethra, resulting in a mild right renal pyelectasis.

Doppler interrogation (Fig. 8–23C and D), resembles the circular vessel arrangement seen in the corpus luteum; in both the corpus luteum and steroid cell tumors, the dense vascularization serves to remove hormonal products from the ovary. In steroid cell tumors, however, the Doppler velocity and resistance indices are not always helpful diagnostically because the vessels are small compared with those of the corpus luteum. No studies are available to prove or disprove the value of such blood velocity measurements in steroid cell tumors.

Ultrasound Techniques for Characterization of Adnexal Tumors

Several attempts have been made to characterize adnexal masses using transabdominal sonography and TVS, with or without color flow Doppler–derived information on vascularization.[54,58-68]

In 1991, Sassone et al.[54] used TVS to characterize adnexal masses. The parameters scored were (1) the presence of irregularities or papillary projections on the inner wall, (2) the wall thickness, (3) the presence of thin or thick septations, and (4) the echogenic pattern of the mass. The possible score ranged from 1 to 14, with a score of 9 or greater deemed significant in predicting malignancy. In scanning 143 patients with a 10% prevalence of adnexal masses, the specificity was 83%, the sensitivity 100%, the positive predictive value 37%, and the negative predictive value 100%. Complex statistical analysis established the scientific validity of this scoring system.[54] The difficulty with the system, however, was that cystic teratomas could not be distinguished from frank malignancies.

One year later, a trial to correct the shortcomings of this scoring system resulted in the construction of a weighted scoring system that took into consideration the importance of

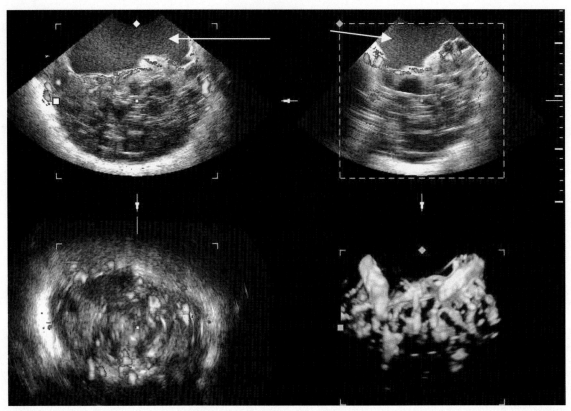

Figure 8–22. Mucinous cystadenoma of low malignant potential. This three-dimensional (3D) image depicts the structure of the tumor in orthogonal planes. The *arrows* point to the cystic area filled with weakly echogenic mucinous fluid. Numerous septa and small solid areas are evident. Box D contains the 3D power Doppler–generated "angiogram" of the tumor, showing bizarre vessels with variable calibers and multiple anastomoses.

the individual variables in the system.[55] Logistic regression analysis demonstrated that wall thickness of the adnexal masses was statistically nondiscriminatory. The scores were simplified and several categories were merged, which made the scoring system more logical (Fig. 8–24). Elimination of wall thickness made it possible to introduce a new variable, "shadowing." The presence of shadowing receives a score of 0, and its absence results in the addition of 1 point. The new scoring system enables better discrimination between malignant and benign tumors because most cystic teratomas contain tissue components that show distal shadowing, and this feature permits a more confident diagnosis of these usually benign tumors.

Clearly, TVS characterization of adnexal masses by gray scale alone is feasible, but the user should not expect to determine the exact histologic diagnosis or even the stage of the disease. The different scoring systems bring us a step closer to a more accurate identification of ovarian malignancies.[69] After initial attempts to apply more or less strict ultrasound guidelines to the definition of adnexal masses, several other scoring systems were published.[70-72] Most of the proposed scoring systems are based on the same building blocks: the data obtained by high-frequency TVS examination. Computer-enhanced models were suggested by Timmerman,[73] and these

seem to be reasonably accurate in predicting ovarian malignancy.

Gray-scale examination of adnexal masses using TVS, however, represents only one dimension of the diagnostic capabilities of ultrasound (i.e., study of the lesion's morphology). Color Doppler examination of flow velocity and resistance to flow introduces a new dimension, the study of the blood supply or physiology of these lesions. The addition of color-coded flow studies to transvaginal gray-scale characterization of adnexal masses may add to the sensitivity, specificity, and positive predictive value of ultrasound in the diagnosis of ovarian malignancy.[66-68,74-81]

Tumor cells multiply and grow quickly; they need a constant and increasing blood supply. Folkman and colleagues[82-84] hypothesized and proved that an abundance of newly formed vessels supply the tumor. This neovascularization or angiogenesis consists of a rapid growth of capillaries. Because the newly generated blood vessels lack a muscular layer, having only an inner and an outer layer, they do not pose significant resistance to flow. The downstream resistance can be determined sonographically using Doppler flow methods, and analysis of the systolic and diastolic wave frequencies gives some indication as to whether there is a low or high resistance to flow in the system. The PI and RI of vessels supplying blood

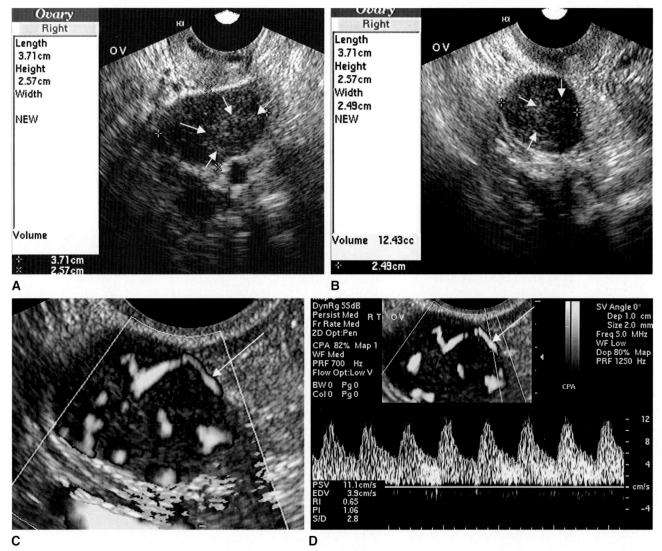

Figure 8–23. Steroid cell tumor of the ovary. In this postmenopausal patient, the ovaries are devoid of follicles. **A** and **B,** The round area marked by *arrows* has a slightly different, somewhat higher echogenicity. **C,** The *arrow* indicates the circularity of the blood flow. **D,** Power Doppler interrogation of the vessel around the lesion gives an unusually high (11 cm/s) peak systolic velocity in this postmenopausal ovary. The resistance indices are not indicative of an increased diastolic flow.

to pathologic adnexal structures and to normal ovaries were studied by Fleischer and coworkers,[77,81] Kurjak et al.,[66,75,78,80] Bourne and colleagues,[85] and others.[55,67,76,79,86,87] This topic is discussed in greater detail in Chapters 17 and 18.

More recently, serious doubts have been voiced in the literature regarding the diagnostic power of flow velocity and resistance indices in predicting ovarian malignancy or reassuring the patient that the ovarian lesion is benign.[88-91] The focus has shifted back to a thorough gray-scale characterization of lesions as well as the detection of centrally located blood vessels to increase the detection rate of malignancy.[92-95]

Controversy notwithstanding, however, it is clear that our constantly improving and updated knowledge of the ultrasound characteristics of adnexal masses, together with ongoing innovation and refinement in ultrasound equipment, are of the utmost importance in the correct classification of these lesions.

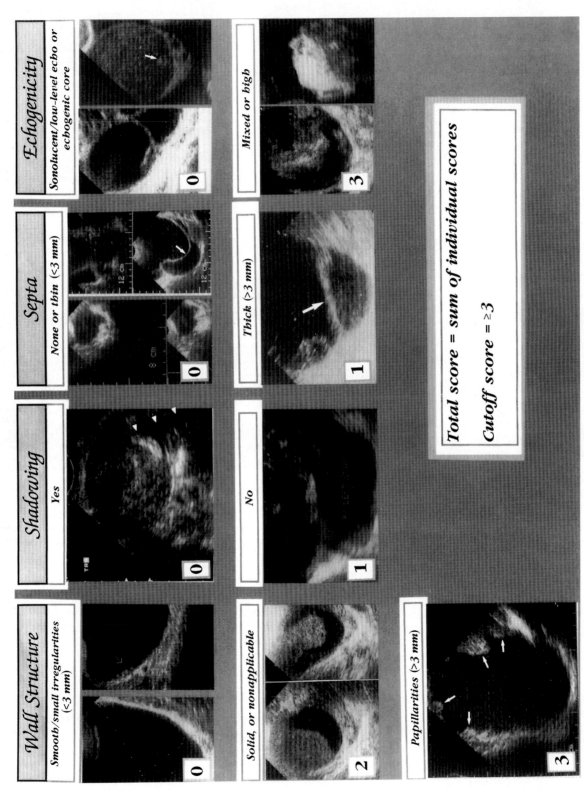

Figure 8–24. The Sassone scoring system designed to differentiate between benign and malignant ovarian tumors. A score of 3 or more is associated with a high risk of malignancy.

REFERENCES

1. Fleischer AC, Romero R, Manning FA: The Principle and the Practice of Ultrasonography in Obstetrics and Gynecology, 4th ed. East Norwalk, Conn, Appleton & Lange, 1991.
2. Timor-Tritsch IE, Rottem S: Transvaginal Sonography, 2nd ed. New York, Chapman & Hall, 1991.
3. Goldstein SR: Endovaginal Sonography, 2nd ed. New York, Wiley-Liss, 1991.
4. Sabbagha RE: Diagnostic Ultrasound Applied to Obstetrics and Gynecology, 3rd ed. Philadelphia, JB Lippincott, 1994.
5. Chervenak FA, Isaacson GC, Campbell S: Ultrasound in Obstetrics and Gynecology. Boston, Little, Brown, 1993.
6. Nyberg DA, Hill LM, Bohm-Velez M, Mendelson EB: Transvaginal Ultrasound. St. Louis, Mosby-Yearbook, 1992.
7. Tessler FN, Perrella RR, Fleischer AC, Grant EG: Endovaginal sonographic diagnosis of dilated fallopian tubes. AJR Am J Roentgenol 1989; 153:523-525.
8. Timor-Tritsch IE, Rottem S, Lewitt N: The fallopian tubes. In Timor-Tritsch IE, Rottem S (eds): Transvaginal Sonography, 2nd ed. New York, Chapman & Hall, 1991, pp 131-144.
9. Timor-Tritsch IE, Rottem S: Transvaginal ultrasound study of the fallopian tube. Obstet Gynecol 1987;70:424-428.
10. Patten RM, Vincent LM, Wolner-Hanseen P, Thorpe E Jr: Pelvic inflammatory disease: Endovaginal sonography with laparoscopic correlation. J Ultrasound Med 1990;9:681-689.
11. Subramanyam BR, Raghavendra BN, Whaler CA, Yee J: Ultrasonic features of fallopian tube carcinoma. J Ultrasound Med 1984;3:391-393.
12. Ajjimakorn S, Bhamarapravati Y, Israngura N: Ultrasound appearance of fallopian tube carcinoma (case report). J Clin Ultrasound 1988;16:516-518.
13. Hinton A, Bea C, Winfield AC, Entman SS: Carcinoma of the fallopian tube. Urol Radiol 1988;10:113-115.
14. Granberg S, Jansson I: Early detection of primary carcinoma of the fallopian tube by endovaginal ultrasound. Acta Obstet Gynecol Scand 1990;69:667-668.
15. Ajjimakorn S, Bhamarapravati Y: Transvaginal ultrasound and the diagnosis of fallopian tubal carcinoma. J Clin Ultrasound 1991;19:116-119.
16. Chang HC, Hwueh S, Soong YK: Malignant mixed mullerian tumor of the fallopian tube. Case report and review of the literature. Chang Keng I Hsueh 1991;14:259-263.
17. Kol S, Gal D, Friedman M, Paldi E: Preoperative diagnosis of fallopian tube carcinoma by transvaginal sonography and CA-125. Gynecol Oncol 1990;37:129-131.
18. Podobnik M, Singer Z, Ciglar S, Bulic M: Preoperative diagnosis of primary fallopian tube carcinoma by transvaginal ultrasound, cytological finding and CA-125. Ultrasound Med Biol 1993;19:587-591.
19. Shalan H, Sosic A, Kurjak A: Fallopian tube carcinoma: recent diagnostic approach by color Doppler imaging. Ultrasound Obstet Gynecol 1992;2:297-299.
20. Schust D, Stovall DW: Leiomyomas of the fallopian tube: A case report. J Reprod Med 1993;38:741-742.
21. Sherer DM, Liberto L, Abramowicz JS, et al: Endovaginal sonographic features associated with isolated torsion of the fallopian tube. J Ultrasound Med 1991;10:107-109.
22. Rosado WM, Trambert MA, Gosink BB, Pretorius DH: Adnexal torsion: Diagnosis by using Doppler sonography. AJR Am J Roentgenol 1992;159:1251-1253.
23. Gordon JD, Hopkins KL, Jeffrey RB, Giudice LC: Adnexal torsion: Color Doppler diagnosis and laparoscopic treatment. Fertil Steril 1994;61:383-385.
24. Oelsner G, Bider D, Goldenberg M, et al: Long-term follow-up of the twisted ischemic adnexa managed by detorsion. Fertil Steril 1993;60:976-979.
25. Stein IF, Leventhal ML: Amenorrhea associated with bilateral polycystic ovaries. Am J Obstet Gynecol 1935;29:181-186.
26. Swanson M, Sauerbrei EE, Cooperberg PL: Medical implication of ultrasonically detected polycystic ovaries. J Clin Ultrasound 1981;9:219-222.
27. Parisi L, Tramonti M, Casciano S, et al: The role of ultrasound in the study of polycystic ovarian disease. J Clin Ultrasound 1982;10:167-172.
28. Hall DA: Sonographic appearance of the normal ovary of polycystic ovary and of functional ovarian cysts. Semin Ultrasound 1983;4:149.
29. Hann LE, Hall DA, McArdle CR, Siebel M: Polycystic ovarian disease: Sonographic spectrum. Radiology 1984;150:531-534.
30. Nicolini U, Ferrazzi E, Bellotti M, et al: The contribution of sonographic evaluation of ovarian size in patients with polycystic ovarian disease. J Ultrasound Med 1985;4:347-351.
31. Yeh H-C, Futterwert W, Thornton JC: Polycystic ovarian disease: US features in 104 patients. Radiology 1987;163:111-116.
32. Takahashi K, Nishigaki A, Eda Y, et al: Transvaginal ultrasound is an effective method for screening in polycystic ovarian disease: Preliminary study. Gynecol Obstet Invest 1990;30:34-36.
33. Orsini LF, Venturoli S, Lorusso R, et al: Ultrasonic findings in polycystic ovarian disease. Fertil Steril 1985;43:709-714.
34. Graif M, Shalev J, Strauss S, et al: Torsion of the ovary: Sonographic features. AJR Am J Roentgenol 1984;143:1331-1334.
35. Warner MA, Fleischer AC, Edell SL, et al: Uterine adnexal torsion: Sonographic findings. Radiology 1985;154:773-775.
36. Graif M, Itzchak Y: Sonographic evaluation of ovarian torsion in childhood and adolescence. AJR Am J Roentgenol 1988;150:647-649.
37. Halvie MA, Silver TM: Ovarian torsion: Sonographic evaluation. J Clin Ultrasound 1989;17:327-332.
38. Sommerville M, Grimes DA, Koonings PP, Campbell K: Ovarian neoplasms and the risk of ovarian torsion. Am J Obstet Gynecol 1991;164:577-578.
39. Dawood MY: Endometriosis. In Gold JF, Josimovich JB (eds): Gynecologic Endocrinology, 4th ed. New York, Plenum Press, 1987, p 387.
40. Cramer DW: Epidemiology of endometriosis. In Wilson EA (ed): Endometriosis. New York, Alan R. Liss, 1987, pp 5-22.
41. Sandler MA, Karo JJ: The spectrum of ultrasonic findings in endometriosis. Radiology 1978;127:229-231.
42. Coleman BG, Arger PH, Mulhern CB Jr: Endometriosis: Clinical and ultrasonic correlation. AJR Am J Roentgenol 1979;132:747-749.
43. Friedman H, Vogelzang RL, Mendelson EB, et al: Endometriosis detection by US with laparoscopic correlation. Radiology 1985;157:217-220.
44. Athey PA, Diment DD: The spectrum of sonographic findings in endometriomas. J Ultrasound Med 1989;8:487-491.
45. Kupfer MC, Schwimer SR, Lebovic J: Transvaginal sonographic appearance of endometriomata: Spectrum of findings. J Ultrasound Med 1992; 11:129.
46. Stenback F, Kauppila A: Development and classification of parovarian cysts: An ultrastructural study. Gynecol Obstet Invest 1981;12:1-10.
47. Alpern MB, Sandler MA, Madrazo BL: Sonographic features of parovarian cysts and their complications. AJR Am J Roentgenol 1984;143:157-160.
48. Athey P, Cooper NB: Sonographic features of parovarian cysts. AJR Am J Roentgenol 1985;144:83-86.
49. Reuter KL, Meyer RN: Unusual features of parovarian cyst: A report of two cases. J Reprod Med 1987;32:371-374.
50. Stein AL, Koonings PP, Schlaerth JB, et al: Relative frequency of malignant parovarian tumors: Should parovarian tumors be aspirated? Obstet Gynecol 1990;75:1029-1031.
51. Guttman PH: In search of the elusive benign cystic ovarian teratoma: Application of the ultrasound "tip of the iceberg" sign. J Clin Ultrasound 1977;5:403-406.
52. Quinn SF, Erickson S, Blach WC: Cystic ovarian teratomas: The sonographic appearance of the dermoid plug. Radiology 1985;155:477-478.
53. Sheth S, Fishman EK, Buck JL, et al: The variable sonographic appearances of ovarian teratomas: Correlation with CT. AJR Am J Roentgenol 1988;151:331-334.
54. Sassone AM, Timor-Tritsch IE, Artner A, et al: Transvaginal sonographic characterization of ovarian disease: Evaluation of a new scoring system to predict ovarian malignancy. Obstet Gynecol 1991;78:70-76.
55. Lerner JP, Timor-Tritsch IE, Federman A, Abramovich G: Transvaginal sonographic characterization of ovarian masses using an improved, weighted scoring system. Am J Obstet Gynecol 1994;170:81-85.
56. Cohen LS, Sabbagha RE: Echopatterns of benign cystic teratomas by transvaginal ultrasound. Ultrasound Obstet Gynecol 1993;3:120-123.
57. Swenerton KD, Hislop TG, Spinelli J, et al: Ovarian carcinoma: A multivariate analysis of prognostic factors. Obstet Gynecol 1985;65:264-270.
58. Monteagudo A, Heller D, Husami N, et al: Ovarian steroid cell tumors: Sonographic characteristics. Ultrasound Obstet Gynecol 1997;10:282-288.
59. Finkler NJ, Benacerraf B, Lavin PT, et al: Comparison of serum CA 125, clinical impression and ultrasound in the postoperative evaluation of ovarian masses. Obstet Gynecol 1988;72:659-664.
60. Herrmann UJ, Locher GW, Goldhirsch A: Sonographic patterns of ovarian tumors: Prediction of malignancy. Obstet Gynecol 1987;69:777-781.

61. Granberg S, Norstrom A, Wikland M: Tumors in the lower pelvis as imaged by vaginal sonography. Gynecol Oncol 1990;37:224-229.

62. Benacerraf BR, Finkler NJ, Wojciechowski C, Knapp RC: Sonographic accuracy in the diagnosis of ovarian masses. J Reprod Med 1990;35:491-495.

63. Luxman D, Bergman A, Sagi J, David MP: The postmenopausal adnexal mass: Correlation between ultrasonic and pathologic findings. Obstet Gynecol 1991;77:726-728.

64. Granberg S, Wikland M, Jansson I: Macroscopic characterization of ovarian tumors and the relation to histologic diagnosis: Criteria to be used for ultrasound evaluation. Gynecol Oncol 1989;35:139-144.

65. Benacerraf B, Finkler NJ, Wojciechowski C, Knapp RC: Sonographic accuracy in the diagnosis of ovarian masses. J Reprod Med 1990;35:491-495.

66. Kurjak A, Predanic M: New scoring system for prediction of ovarian malignancy based on transvaginal color Doppler sonography. J Ultrasound Med 1992;11:631-638.

67. Timor-Tritsch IE, Lerner JP, Monteagudo A, Santos R: Transvaginal sonographic characterization of ovarian masses using color flow directed Doppler measurements and a morphologic scoring system. Am J Obstet Gynecol 1993;168:909-913.

68. Bromley B, Goodman H, Benacerraf BR: Comparison between sonographic morphology and Doppler waveform for the diagnosis of ovarian malignancy. Obstet Gynecol 1994;83:434-437.

69. Deligdisch L, Altchek A, Cohen CJ: Atlas of Ovarian Tumors. New York, Igaku-Shoin, 1994.

70. Ferrazzi E, Zanetta G, Dordoni D, et al: Transvaginal ultrasonographic characterization of ovarian masses: Comparison of five scoring systems in a multicenter study. Ultrasound Obstet Gynecol 1997;10:192-197.

71. Merz E, Weber G, Bahlmann F, Kiesslich R: A new sonomorphologic scoring system (Mainz Score) for the assessment of ovarian tumors using transvaginal ultrasonography: Part I. A comparison between the scoring-system and the assessment by an experienced sonographer. Ultraschall Med 1998;19:99-107.

72. Valentin L: Use of morphology to characterize and manage common adnexal masses. Best Pract Res Clin Obstet Gynecol 2004;18:71-89.

73. Timmerman D: The use of mathematical models to evaluate pelvic masses: Can they beat an expert operator [review]? Best Pract Res Clin Obstet Gynaecol 2004;18:91-104.

74. van Nagell JR, Higgins RV, Donaldson ES: Transvaginal sonography as a screening method for ovarian cancer. Cancer 1990;65:573-577.

75. Kurjak A, Zalud I, Jurkovic D, et al: Transvaginal colour Doppler for the assessment of pelvic circulation. Acta Obstet Gynecol Scand 1989;68:131-135.

76. Kawai M, Kano T, Kikkawa F, et al: Transvaginal Doppler ultrasound with color flow imaging in the diagnosis of ovarian cancer. Obstet Gynecol 1992;79:163-167.

77. Fleischer AC, Rodgers WH, Rao BK, et al: Assessment of ovarian tumor vascularity with transvaginal color Doppler sonography. J Ultrasound Med 1991;10:563-568.

78. Kurjak A, Zalud I, Alfievic Z: Evaluation of adnexal masses with transvaginal color ultrasound. J Ultrasound Med 1991;10:295-297.

79. Weiner Z, Thaler I, Beck D, et al: Differentiating malignant from benign ovarian tumors with transvaginal color flow imaging. Obstet Gynecol 1992;79:159-162.

80. Kurjak A, Schulman H, Sosic A, et al: Transvaginal ultrasound, color flow and Doppler waveform of the postmenopausal adnexal mass. Obstet Gynecol 1992;80:917-921.

81. Fleischer AC, Rodgers WH, Kepple DM, et al: Color Doppler sonography of ovarian masses: A multiparameter analysis. J Ultrasound Med 1993;12:41-48.

82. Folkman J, Shing Y: Angiogenesis [minireview]. J Biol Chem 1992;267:10931-10934.

83. Folkman J, Meirel E, Abernethy C, Williams G: Isolation of a tumor factor responsible for angiogenesis. J Exp Med 1971;133:275-278.

84. Folkman J: Tumor angiogenesis. Adv Cancer Res 1985;43:175-180.

85. Bourne T, Campbell S, Steer C, et al: Transvaginal colour flow imaging: A possible new screening technique for ovarian carcinoma. BMJ 1989;299:1367-1370.

86. Tekay A, Jouppila P: Validity of pulsatility and resistance indices in classification of adnexal tumors with transvaginal color Doppler ultrasound. Ultrasound Obstet Gynecol 1992;2:338-344.

87. Tekay A, Jarvela I, Jouppila P: Reproducibility of transvaginal Doppler velocimetry measurements in the uterine arteries of postmenopausal women. Ultrasound Obstet Gynecol 1997;10:198-204.

88. Tekay A, Jouppila P: Controversies in assessment of ovarian tumors with transvaginal color Doppler ultrasound. Acta Obstet Gynecol Scand 1996;75:316-329.

89. Tekay A, Jouppila P: Intraobserver reproducibility of transvaginal Doppler measurements in uterine and intraovarian arteries in regularly menstruating women. Ultrasound Obstet Gynecol 1996;7:129-134.

90. Hata K, Hata T, Manabe A, et al: A critical evaluation of transvaginal Doppler studies, transvaginal sonography and magnetic resonance imaging and CA 125 in detecting ovarian cancer. Obstet Gynecol 1992;80:922-926.

91. van Nagell JR Jr, DePriest PD, Reedy MB, et al: The efficacy of transvaginal sonographic screening in asymptomatic women at risk for ovarian cancer. Gynecol Oncol 2000;77:350-356.

92. Ueland FR, DePriest PD, Pavlik EJ, et al: Preoperative differentiation of malignant from benign ovarian tumors: The efficacy of morphology indexing and Doppler flow sonography. Gynecol Oncol 2003;91:46-50.

93. DePriest PD, DeSimone CP: Ultrasound screening for the early detection of ovarian cancer. J Clin Oncol 2003;21:194-199.

94. Modesitt SC, Pavlik EJ, Ueland FR, et al: Risk of malignancy in unilocular ovarian cystic tumors less than 10 centimeters in diameter. Obstet Gynecol 2003;102:594-599.

95. Bailey CL, Ueland FR, Land GL, et al: The malignant potential of small cystic ovarian tumors in women over 50 years of age. Gynecol Oncol 1998;69:3-7.

Chapter 9

Menopausal Dilemmas: How Ultrasound Has Changed Clinical Management

Steven R. Goldstein

Initially, sonography was a tool of the obstetrician. Early equipment had barely enough resolution to localize the placenta, find the fetal lie, and measure biparietal diameter. As equipment and resolution improved, sonography began to be used in gynecology, including examination of menopausal patients. Introduction of the vaginal probe, and the "sonomicroscopy" it allows, has opened new doors in the application of ultrasound to postmenopausal patients. Transvaginal sonography (TVS) allows magnification and resolution of images such that, for example, if one were viewing a 3-mm embryo attached to its yolk sac at 45 days since last menstrual period, one could visualize distinct cardiac pulsations *within* the embryo. In comparison, if one were holding a structure of this size grossly in one's hand at arm's length, squinting at it, it would not be possible to appreciate cardiac pulsations in it. Such resolution is possible only with the image magnification available with the vaginal probe—hence "sonomicroscopy."

Menopause

A patient is considered menopausal after cessation of menstruation for at least 12 months because of depletion of ovarian follicles. The climacteric is the phase in the aging process that marks the transition from the reproductive stage of life to the nonreproductive stage.

In 1850, when the average age of menopause was 46 years, life expectancy was 50 years. Today, the average age of menopause in the United States is 51.4 years, and it is thought that a 50-year-old woman who does not already have cancer or heart disease has a life expectancy of 91 years. Thus, modern women live an abundant portion of their lives in a postmenopausal state. Diseases and pathologic abnormalities that are more common in menopause are becoming increasingly clinically relevant and will become more so as the baby boomer population continues to age.

The Postmenopausal Ovary

Increasingly, clinicians are ordering imaging studies to assess gynecologic complaints in the postmenopausal woman; for example, the internist treating a postmenopausal woman with vague lower abdominal complaints may order a pelvic-abdominal computed tomography scan. Often, the only positive finding is a small cystic structure thought to be adnexal in origin. Such patients often then present to the gynecologist, for whom ultrasound now plays a primary role.

Historical Perspective

In 1971, Barber and Graber described the palpable postmenopausal ovary syndrome. In a now classic editorial[1] based on three cases, two of which were malignancies, they stated:

> The palpation of what is interpreted as a normal sized ovary in the premenopausal woman represents an ovarian tumor in the postmenopausal woman. There is no such thing as physiologic enlargement of the postmenopausal ovary. Physiologic cysts can only arise from the nonrupture of a follicle (follicular cysts) or cystic degeneration of the corpus luteum (hemorrhagic corpus luteum cysts). There are no such cysts in a postmenopausal ovary, simply because there are no follicles or corpora lutea.

Barber and Graber further stated that "the contrast between the premenopausal and postmenopausal ovary is striking." They concluded that "when such an ovary is palpable it is not a normal ovary for this stage of life."

Based on this, an entire generation of gynecologists was taught that the ability to palpate a postmenopausal ovary was grounds for exploratory laparotomy and total abdominal hysterectomy with bilateral salpingo-oophorectomy. As late as 1984, Barber[2] was still stating that

> patients with Palpable Postmenopausal Ovary Syndrome should not be followed or re-evaluated but must be

investigated promptly for the presence or absence of an ovarian tumor. . . . The only method of diminishing the mortality from ovarian cancer is the acceptance of more liberal indications of surgery.

In 1989, Goldstein et al.[3] published an article on postmenopausal cystic adnexal masses and the potential role of ultrasound in conservative management. The study consisted of 48 postmenopausal patients who ranged in age from 46 to 86 years. None had had any menses for at least 12 months before the study. They all had unilateral, simple-appearing cysts detected with transabdominal sonography. The maximal diameter of the cysts was 5 cm. None of the cysts had septations or solid components, and none of the patients had ascites.

Of the 48 patients, 26 had prompt surgical evaluation. Sixteen had serial ultrasound evaluation every 3 to 6 months. Six patients were lost to follow-up. Of the 26 surgical cases, 16 had serous cysts, 1 had a mucinous cyst, 4 had hydrosalpinges, 2 had endometriotic cysts, and 3 had parovarian cysts.

Two of the 16 patients evaluated sonographically were operated on subsequently. One was operated on at 6 months of observation for increasing size and development of a septation. Pathologic study revealed a cystadenofibroma. One patient was operated on at 9 months of observation for increased pain; the lesion in this case proved to be a degenerating myoma. The other 14 patients were followed from 10 to 73 months (average, 29 months), with no change in size or character of the cyst.

Goldstein et al. concluded that "small (5 cm or less) unilocular, unilateral postmenopausal adnexal cystic masses, without septations or ascites, will have a very low incidence of malignant disease and therefore serial ultrasound follow-up without surgical intervention may play a role in clinical management of such patients."[3]

Goldstein et al. reviewed the two papers that had preceded theirs. Hall and McCarthy[4] reported on 13 postmenopausal cysts (only 10 were unilocular). There was one borderline malignancy in a 3.5-cm simple cyst. Thus, their incidence of malignancy was 8% of the total cases, or 10% of the cases with unilocular cysts. They concluded that the "simple postmenopausal adnexal cyst may not necessarily be an ominous finding." I do not agree with their conclusions. Surgical removal is the proper management for even borderline malignancies, and in clinical medicine, 10% is a relatively large pick-up rate.

Rulin and Preston[5] reported on a 4-year experience with adnexal masses (not simple cysts). They divided their findings into three groups of lesions based on size: (1) 5 cm or less, (2) between 5 and 10 cm, and (3) greater than 10 cm. Of the 33 masses measuring 5 cm or less, there was one 3-cm endometrioid carcinoma. Apparently, this was a complex cystic and solid-appearing ovary. They stated, "Our findings cast doubt on the concept that all postmenopausal women with minimally enlarged ovaries should undergo laparotomy."[5]

Ultrasound and Postmenopausal Ovarian Anatomy

To understand the application of ultrasound to the evaluation of the postmenopausal reproductive system, the anatomy of the postmenopausal ovary should be appreciated. A thorough knowledge of in vivo appearance and anatomy equips the clinician to understand and correctly interpret ultrasound images.

In postmenopause, folliculogenesis ceases. The tunica albuginea becomes very dense, causing the surface of the ovary to become scarred and shrunken. Eventually, the ovary becomes inert, consisting mainly of connective tissue, and clings to the posterior leaf of the broad ligament. Thus, it can no longer be palpated on standard palpatory bimanual examination. This was the basis for Barber and Graber's original thesis in 1971.

It is useful to contrast the ultrasound images of premenopausal and postmenopausal ovaries. In premenopausal patients, the sonolucencies of follicles make visualization relatively simple. Furthermore, when a woman assumes the lithotomy position, a freely mobile premenopausal ovary will be located lateral to the uterus and is easily seen with a vaginal probe immediately adjacent to the pelvic side wall, overlying the iliac artery and iliac vein (Fig. 9–1). These iliac vessels are retroperitoneal. If the patient then assumes a knee–chest position, the freely mobile ovaries move somewhat toward the anterior abdominal wall, whereas the iliac vessels do not because of their retroperitoneal location.

The postmenopausal ovary lacks folliculogenesis and thus should have no small sonolucencies that allow easy ultrasound identification (Fig. 9–2). It does not reach the pelvic side wall; therefore, the iliac vessels are not as helpful in identification (Figs. 9–3 and 9–4). In addition, the vaginal probe shows loops of bowel throughout the pelvis; these contain bizarre and confusing echo patterns produced by gas and fecal material.

Evaluation of the ovary requires seeing an ovary in two planes at right angles to each other to assess the three-dimensional nature of the structure. The ability to visualize one or both ovaries in postmenopausal women varies depending on the experience, equipment, and patience of the observer.[6]

The lingering question is whether a normal image in a postmenopausal patient not showing the ovary owing to its nonlucence will be as reassuring as an image that definitively

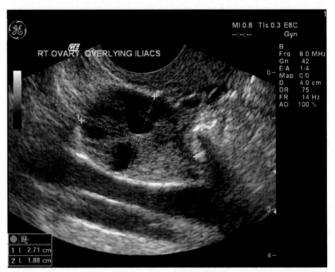

Figure 9–1. Right ovary in a premenopausal patient showing folliculogenesis is seen immediately adjacent to the iliac artery and iliac vein. The iliac vessels are retroperitoneal, whereas the ovaries are intraperitoneal structures. A premenopausal patient without any adhesive disease who assumes the lithotomy position can expect to have her ovaries visualized immediately adjacent to these iliac vessels. The ovary is outlined by the *calipers* and measures 2.7 × 1.9 cm.

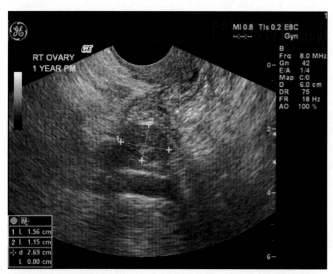

Figure 9–2. Right ovary measuring 1.6 × 1.2 cm *(calipers)* is still seen in its normal anatomic relationship relative to the iliac vessel in this patient who is 1 year since her final menstrual period.

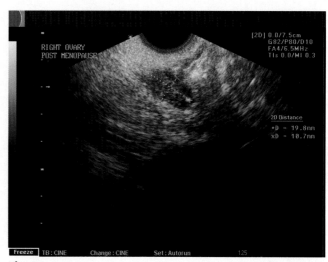

Figure 9–4. The right ovary, seen here in a patient distantly menopausal, can often be challenging to locate because of lack of folliculogenesis and absence of the iliac vessels as anatomic landmarks. Often, the echogenicity of surrounding bowel helps delineate the less echogenic ovarian stroma, as shown here.

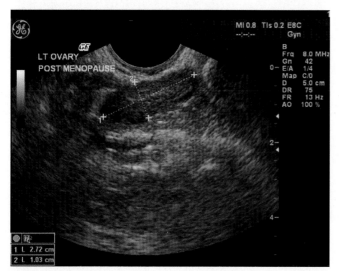

Figure 9–3. This patient was 3 years postmenopausal. The left ovary, outlined by *calipers* (2.7 × 1 cm), contains no folliculogenesis and is not immediately adjacent to the iliac vessels.

locates it and verifies it as atrophic. Rodriguez et al.[6] were able to image the ovaries in 82% of the postmenopausal women they studied. All women were also explored surgically for definitive diagnosis. All abnormal ovaries were visualized. The mean surgical diameter of nonvisualized ovaries was 7.3 mm (range, 5 to 12 mm). No ovaries that appeared normal on sonography were abnormal at surgery. One ovary that appeared grossly normal on TVS and to the surgeon's eye had a microscopic Brenner's tumor at pathologic study.

Ultrasound and Adnexal Cysts

Sonographers have long been interested in cystic structures in the adnexa because cystic structures are so easily visualized on ultrasound and because 85% of ovarian tumors are epithelial, and virtually all epithelial ovarian tumors have some cystic component.

The incidence of adnexal cysts in postmenopausal women using TVS appears to be much greater than that indicated by transabdominal sonography (Fig. 9–5). In the first 100 patients seen at the Women's Wellness Center at New York University Medical Center, 10 had simple ovarian cysts when examined with TVS. Wolf and colleagues[7] reported on 184 women with 358 ovaries and 137 uteri. At initial examination, 17.3% had simple adnexal cysts, ranging in size from 4 to 47 mm. Of these, 58% were 1 cm or less and 90% were 3 cm or less. There was no statistically significant difference in incidence associated with hormone replacement therapy. The article did not discuss what percentage of patients with cysts had previous surgery, although from the demographic data it was obvious that 47 women had had hysterectomies. Certainly, some of these structures may have represented peritoneal inclusion cysts. Six of the patients came to surgical exploration: two with hydrosalpinges, one with papillary serous cystadenoma, one with parovarian cyst, one with a cystic teratoma, and one with stage IC ovarian cancer in a 4-cm "complex" mass.

A more recent analysis of cystic structures in asymptomatic postmenopausal women older than 50 years of age was reported by Bailey et al.[8] Of 7705 women scanned, unilocular cysts were present in 3.3% (n = 256). Of these, 49% resolved in 60 days, and 51% persisted. Forty-five women who were operated on displayed no malignancies, although cystadenomas were found in 32 of them (71%). This is the same ratio seen at surgery in simple cysts from one of the original reports of the 1980s.[3] In the series by Bailey and colleagues, 86 women were followed every 3 to 6 months, with no development of malignancy.

There continues to be tremendous interest in postmenopausal cystic adnexal masses. Another study[9] screened 1769 postmenopausal women who were asymptomatic with no previous gynecologic disease; 6.6% (n = 116) of them displayed simple ovarian cysts measuring less than 5 cm. Among those, 23% of cysts resolved spontaneously, 60% of cysts persisted, and 17% of patients were lost to follow-up. Eighteen

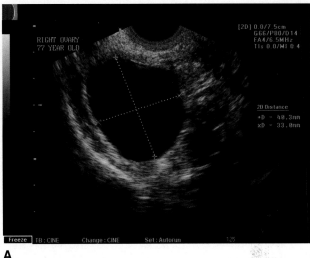

Figure 9–5. A, A unilocular, smooth-walled cystic structure measuring 4 × 3.3 cm is seen on this scan from a 77-year-old postmenopausal patient. The CA-125 level was within normal limits. This scan remained unchanged over 36 months. **B,** Transvaginal sonogram of a 71-year-old patient sent for computed tomography (CT) scan by gastrointestinal physician as part of work-up for vague lower abdominal complaints. The only positive finding on CT was this 5 × 3.8 cm cystic structure in the adnexa. It is smooth-walled and unilocular, without evidence of septation, solid components, or pelvic ascites. The CA-125 was within normal limits. The patient was followed for several years without any change. **C,** Transvaginal pelvic sonogram of the left ovary in this postmenopausal patient displays a cystic structure with a mural nodule projecting into the wall of the cyst. This solid portion had identifiable blood flow. Pathology revealed stage I papillary serous cystadenocarcinoma.

women with persistent cysts underwent surgery, and no malignancies were identified.

Modesitt et al.[10] at the University of Kentucky Ovarian Cancer Screening program identified 2763 women with unilocular ovarian cysts measuring less than 10 cm, from a population of 156,106 women older than 50 years of age who were screened. This represents an 18% incidence, similar to that reported in our series from the 1980s.[3] Of these cysts, 70% resolved, a septum developed in 17%, a solid area developed in 6%, and 7% persisted as a unilocular lesion. No woman with an isolated unilocular cystic ovarian lesion developed ovarian cancer in that study.

Finally, to improve understanding of the management of persistent unilocular ovarian cysts less than 5 cm in diameter in women with normal CA-125 levels, Nardo and coworkers[11] identified a group of postmenopausal women with such cysts and followed them for a 5-year period. This was not a screening program; the women were initially evaluated for "postmenopausal symptoms, abdominal discomfort or postmenopausal bleeding." There were 226 women with unilocular cysts of 5 cm or less and normal CA-125 levels. Of these, 76% showed no change, whereas 24% (54 women) had an increase in cyst size. Elevated levels of CA-125 also developed in 6 of these 54 women. All 54 women underwent surgical management, and 2 of them had stage 1B cystadenocarcinomas. Both were among the six women whose CA-125 levels had become elevated.

Thus, in reference to adnexal cysts in postmenopausal patients, we can conclude that (1) not all cystic adnexal structures are ovarian in origin, (2) none of the cysts we see (at least of those with surgical confirmation) are "functional" or "physiologic" cysts, and (3) the vaginal probe will identify a great many small sonolucencies (in up to 18% of women in some series). However, the evidence suggests that the majority of unilocular cysts measuring 5 cm or less are benign and remain unchanged or resolve. These lesions can be managed expectantly as long as there is no increase in size, change in morphology, or increase in CA-125 level.

Postmenopausal Ovarian Cancer

Although ovarian cancer is important enough to warrant its own chapter (see Chapter 18), an abbreviated discussion is necessary in the context of the postmenopausal woman. The statistics for ovarian cancer and its relation to the postmenopause are familiar and sobering[12-15]:

- Ovarian cancer is the leading cause of death from gynecologic cancer in the United States.
- Ovarian cancer is the fifth leading cause of all cancer deaths in women.
- Eighty percent of such cases involve women older than 50 years of age, usually during menopause.

- Approximately 1 in 70 women (1.4%) will have ovarian cancer in her lifetime. This increases to 4% to 6% if there is a history of ovarian cancer in a first-degree relative.
- Annually, there are approximately 20,700 new cases of ovarian cancer diagnosed in the United States and 12,500 deaths (more than those from endometrial and cervical cancers combined).
- More than two thirds of the cases of ovarian cancer are diagnosed as stage III or IV.
- The 5-year survival rate in advanced cases is 9% to 28%, whereas stage I disease has a 73% 5-year survival rate.

Ovarian Cancer Screening

There is more pressure on physicians to provide ovarian cancer screening regardless of whether such screening has proved to be efficacious.

Anatomic Imaging: Transvaginal Sonography

The first and largest ovarian cancer screening project was reported by Campbell et al.,[16] who screened 5479 patients over an 8-year period. The patients were older than 44 years of age and were scanned each year for 3 years. Five patients were found to have primary cancer, for a rate of 1 primary cancer per 1100 women screened. The false-positive rate was 3.5%.

Van Nagell and colleagues[17] reported on 1300 postmenopausal women screened with a 5-MHz vaginal probe. Each ovary was measured in three planes. An "abnormal" ovary was one with a volume greater than 8 cm^3, or with any complex cystic areas. They identified an abnormal ovary in 33 women (2.5%), of whom 27 had laparotomies. They identified two primary ovarian cancers that measured 4.4 × 4.0 cm and 6.7 × 6.1 cm. The benign findings on surgery included 14 serous cystadenomas, 3 leiomyomas, 3 epithelial cysts, 2 hydrosalpinges, 1 endometrioma, and 1 thecoma. The similarity of the various benign lesions to those found in the transabdominal ultrasound study by Goldstein et al.[3] mentioned previously should be noted.

Van Nagell's group updated their data in 2000.[18] From 1987 to 1999, 14,469 women were studied annually. To be included, women had to be older than 50 years of age or, if there was a positive family history, older than 25 years of age. An abnormal ovary was defined as one with an ultrasound volume greater than 10 cm^3 for postmenopausal women and greater than 20 cm^3 for premenopausal women, or with any papillary or complex projection into the cystic structure. Abnormal ultrasound results were followed up in 4 to 6 weeks. Patients with persistent ultrasound abnormality were advised to have surgical removal. There were 180 surgeries (1.2%). Seventeen cancers were detected, of which only three were palpable. This equates to 1 cancer per 10 surgeries as well as 1 cancer per 850 patients screened. Of the cancers, 11 were stage I (65%), 3 were stage II (17%), and 3 were stage III (17%). All patients with stages I and II disease were alive in 2000 (median, 4.5 years after diagnosis; range, 1.8 to 9.9 years). Two of the three patients with stage III disease died at 4.3 and 7.7 years after detection. In four patients, ovarian cancer developed within 12 months of a negative screen. Thus, these data appear to indicate that annual TVS screening is associated with detection at an earlier stage (65% stage I, 17% stage II) and a decrease in the case-specific mortality rate. TVS screening was not effective in detecting ovarian cancer when ovarian volume was normal.

It has been said that ovarian cancer screening with ultrasound would be too expensive and not "cost-effective."[19] Such analyses presuppose a separate charge per scan. We already do screen for ovarian cancer: it is the annual gynecologic visit, and it fails miserably at early detection. If we incorporated TVS into the overall gynecologic examination (see Chapter 4), the annual gynecologic visit would have a higher detection rate.

Physiologic Imaging: Color-Flow Doppler

Image magnification in ultrasound today is great enough to warrant the term *sonomicroscopy*. Paradoxically, the greater structural detail provided by TVS may actually be problematic.

It was hoped that physiologic imaging—that is, Doppler blood flow studies—might represent the next horizon. In principle, tumors are rich in neovascularization. These new vessels are often morphologically bizarre and rich in arteriovenous anastomoses. Hence, there is diminished resistance to blood flow across these vessels. Doppler assessment of resistance to flow is greatly aided by the addition of color-flow mapping, which allows easy, rapid assessment of where to place the Doppler gate to perform spectral analysis (i.e., obtain resistive indices). Researchers in Croatia[20] (formerly Yugoslavia) reported an experience with color-flow Doppler that makes one almost believe that some day we will simply point a probe at a morphologically normal ovary, obtain a resistive index, and distinguish benignity from malignancy with great accuracy. Unfortunately, this has not uniformly been the experience of all investigators.[21,22]

Many parameters may affect the ability of Doppler to detect flow within a mass, not the least of which are that not all scanning instruments have the same sensitivity to slow flow, and the equipment as well as the methods of obtaining measurements are not standardized. When no flow is detected in the periphery of a cyst or in a prominent postmenopausal ovary, is it because there truly is no flow, or is the sensitivity of the equipment inadequate? Thus, the significance of an inability to detect flow in an ovarian structure by color or pulsed Doppler has not been satisfactorily determined. It is tempting to conclude that a negative finding means absence of neovascularity, but the accuracy of the negative finding has not been established.

The location from which the pulsed Doppler waveform is obtained is another area of concern. Doppler analysis from vessels clearly within a mass should be indicative of vascular resistance at least within that part of the mass, but in some studies, the description of methods either does not mention or is ambiguous about the location of the vessels from which the Doppler waveforms are obtained. Another problem occurs with Doppler analysis of simple cysts or masses that, although not meeting all criteria for simple cysts, have little or no solid component from which the Doppler analysis can be obtained. As the probe is moved more laterally, it can be difficult to ascertain if the vessel being interrogated is within the mass in question or just outside of it, and hence whether the results reflect blood flow in the area of concern. Furthermore, diminished resistance can be seen in some benign processes, especially inflammatory disease and ovarian torsion.[22]

Observations made in the late 1980s indicated that color Doppler TVS might be useful in the detection of ovarian cancer. This led to a number of clinical trials. Tekay and Jouppila[23] analyzed 32 studies using TVS color Doppler that displayed considerable homogeneity. The sensitivity for detecting malignancy was 25% to 100%, the specificity was 46% to 100%, the positive predictive value was 29% to 100%, and the negative predictive value was 63% to 100%. The accuracy varied between 57% and 100%. They stated, however, that "an indisputable overlap was found between the ranges of pulsatility index (PI) and resistance index (RI) values from the benign and malignant adnexal tumors." The RI was less than 0.40 in 43% of benign tumors and in 25% of normal vascular ovaries. This led them to conclude that "current cut-off levels for PI or RI values should not be used in clinical decision making due to their poor specificity."

The real question is whether color Doppler is effective in detecting malignancy before anatomically recognizable change has taken place. Will physiologic assessment complement or eventually replace anatomic assessment in distinguishing benign from malignant lesions? In other words, will color-flow Doppler allow us to diagnose stage IA cancer in an ovary that appears morphologically normal? This is a very exciting possibility, but it remains unresolved.

CA-125

At least 75 antigens defined by monoclonal antibodies are associated with human epithelial ovarian carcinoma. Of these, the most widely accepted and tested is CA-125, the antigenic determinant of a high–molecular-weight glycoprotein recognized by a monoclonal antibody raised to an ovarian cancer cell line as an immunogen. Whereas CA-125 has been used effectively for the detection of cancer relapse and for monitoring patients during primary therapy for epithelial ovarian cancer,[24] its usefulness as a screening test is not as well understood. However, mainly through the efforts of Gene Wilder, people are very much aware of CA-125 and often demand that the clinician assess it. The CA-125 determinant is expressed not only by epithelial ovarian tumors but by various other pathologic and normal tissues of müllerian origin,[25] including endometrial tissue, leiomyoma uteri, embryonic tissues, and infected pelvic tissue.[26] These nonmalignant conditions significantly reduce the usefulness of CA-125 measurement in premenopausal women, but less so in the postmenopausal group. The antigen is detectable in 80% of serous tumors and in a lower proportion of mucinous tumors. It is positive in only 50% of patients with disease confined to the ovary (stage I).

One problem with the use of the CA-125 blood test by itself for screening is its low positive predictive value. In the general population, ovarian cancer has a prevalence of approximately 30 cases per 100,000 women. Because approximately 80% of women with ovarian cancer have an elevated CA-125 and 99% of healthy control subjects have a normal CA-125, the calculated positive predictive value is 2.4%—that is, 2.4% of women in the general population with elevated CA-125 levels will have ovarian cancer. Thus, nearly 98% of women with a CA-125 elevation would be shown *not* to have ovarian cancer.

More recently, Fung et al.[27] assessed the positive predictive value of elevated CA-125 from a meta-analysis of 20 studies (17 prospective cohort studies and 3 randomized, controlled trials). They concluded that of every 10,000 women participating in an annual CA-125 screening program for 3 years,

800 would have an ultrasound scan because of an elevated CA-125, 30 would undergo surgery because of an abnormal ultrasound result, and 6 would have ovarian cancer detected at surgery, of whom 3 would be diagnosed at an early stage and have a chance of cure.

The physician's response to an elevated CA-125 should depend on the degree of elevation, the change in level with time, the age and menopausal status of the patient, concurrent medical conditions, family history, and, most important, findings on pelvic examination and sonography. Premenopausal patients are far more likely to have elevated levels than are older women and in the absence of a pelvic pathologic process are best followed prospectively. Postmenopausal women with CA-125 elevations in the absence of pelvic disease must be screened for tumors that also are associated with an elevated CA-125, particularly breast and colorectal carcinomas. Thus, for our purposes, CA-125 testing is best reserved for patients who have an identified adnexal lesion in the postmenopausal state, and not used simply as a random screening test. Additional data on ovarian cancer screening are presented in Chapter 18.

Proteomics

Petricoin and associates[28] used proteomic patterns in serum and mass spectroscopy to develop a cluster of patterns that segregate malignant from nonmalignant ovarian disease. Proteomics are believed to measure specific proteins that indicate a host response to tumor cells. In their original publication, they correctly identified 50 out of 50 cases of ovarian cancer (including 18 stage I). Three of 66 nonmalignant cases (4.5%) were inappropriately deemed malignant (false positive).

Operative Endoscopy

The use of endoscopic surgery has mushroomed since the mid-1990s. There is increasing interest by some clinicians and patients in performing endoscopically procedures that previously routinely required open laparotomy. It is tempting to view operative endoscopy as a wonderful compromise for postmenopausal patients in the treatment of small adnexal masses with an unknown histology. Indeed, widespread use of operative endoscopy has already resulted in a collection of 42 patients in one series who had laparoscopic excision of ovarian neoplasms subsequently found to be malignant.[29] Certainly, laparotomy with total abdominal hysterectomy and bilateral salpingo-oophorectomy cannot be appropriate if up to 18% of postmenopausal asymptomatic patients examined by TVS have a simple cystic adnexal mass.

Clinical Management of Cystic Adnexal Masses

An increasing number of imaging studies of the female abdomen and pelvis are being ordered by internists, and routine ultrasound studies are being ordered or performed in the office as a part of the overall pelvic examination. Thus, clinicians are constantly confronted with the finding of small cystic structures in the adnexa of postmenopausal patients.

First, the physician should establish a plan with which the physician and patient are comfortable, while avoiding injection of the physician's personal bias. It is certainly appropriate to obtain a CA-125 level in postmenopausal patients. If the CA-125 level is elevated (although a standard definition of "elevated" has not been established) in association with an adnexal mass, the mass should be removed. In this particular clinical setting (postmenopause, abnormal adnexa, and elevated CA-125), exploratory laparotomy and total abdominal hysterectomy and bilateral salpingo-oophorectomy are appropriate. However, operative endoscopy should be acceptable if the physician's skills are sufficient to *remove* the mass in its entirety. In my opinion, aspiration, whether at the time of endoscopy (regardless of how benign the structure looks) or under TVS guidance, is not adequate.

Based on the data presented thus far, if the cystic structure is unilateral and unilocular, has no septation or ascites, and measures less than 5 cm, the patient should be followed conservatively. The interval of follow-up is negotiable. I see patients initially at 6 weeks and then again at 10 to 12 weeks. This algorithm still allows for early detection of any lesion (unilateral and no evidence of ascites). If there is any progression on ultrasound over time (increased size, change in internal echoes, development of bilaterality, ascites) or a subsequent elevation of CA-125, prompt surgical exploration is mandatory. If no change is seen over time, the patient may continue to be followed conservatively, and ultimately the interval between examinations may be lengthened.

Summary

Ovarian cancer is the most frustrating of gynecologic tumors. Normal postmenopausal ovaries are difficult and sometimes impossible to visualize sonographically. CA-125 is not considered an appropriate screening tool even in the postmenopausal population. Color-flow Doppler is most useful in terms of "color as morphology," that is, indicating the presence or absence of blood flow. Whether there is benefit to the strict use of quantitatively measured resistance to flow remains unresolved. Operative endoscopy, if used, must be capable of removing the cystic mass in its entirety so that prompt pathologic evaluation can be performed. Simple cysts (especially those <3 cm) are more common in postmenopausal patients than was previously thought, are very unlikely to be malignant, and are certainly capable of being followed conservatively.

The Postmenopausal Uterus

In the past, the first clue to possible endometrial cancer was bleeding. Endometrial carcinoma has a peak prevalence at 55 years of age. Thus, 75% of cases occur in postmenopausal women. The role of unopposed estrogen in the development of this disease has been known for some time. Classic risk factors include obesity, diabetes, hypertension, and low parity.

The introduction of vaginal probes has permitted visualization of endometrial detail never previously imagined. The premenopausal endometrium has been characterized extensively. After menopause there is no epithelial stimulation by estrogen, and the thin and atrophic endometrium is prone to superficial punctate ulceration. Such so-called senile endometritis is the most common cause of postmenopausal bleeding. It must, however, be distinguished from hyperplasia or adenocarcinoma.

Appearance of Endometrial Echo

Atrophic endometrium, as expected in a postmenopausal patient who is not on hormone replacement therapy, will appear on ultrasound as a thin "pencil-line" echogenicity. This is surrounded by an intact, hypoechoic halo (Fig. 9–6). The

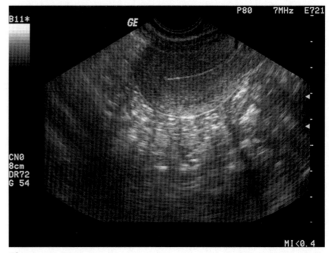

Figure 9–6. Long-axis view of the uterus revealing a thin "pencil-line" endometrium. This is the typical appearance of an inactive atrophic postmenopausal endometrium. Note how the endometrial echo can be traced from its beginning at the end of the cervical canal and then toward the uterine fundus.

thin echogenic line represents the interface between two sides of atrophic basal endometrium. The basalis of the endometrium itself is one cell layer thick in this stage. It is unclear exactly what causes the echogenicity that we routinely image as this interface.

The various appearances of the endometrium in premenopausal patients during different phases of the menstrual cycle are well described. Patients receiving therapy for endometriosis, originally danazol and more recently gonadotropin-releasing hormone agonists, show a thin pencil-line endometrial echo on TVS, similar to that in normal postmenopausal patients. This result prompted a pilot study on 30 postmenopausal women with bleeding who ranged in age from 39 to 81 years.[30] Twelve were not on hormone replacement therapy; thus, any bleeding was considered abnormal. Eighteen were on hormone replacement therapy sequentially but were bleeding at an inappropriate time. TVS was performed before endometrial sampling. The endometrial thickness was measured as a maximum anteroposterior distance on the long-axis view. Eleven of the patients had an endometrial thickness of 5 mm or less (range, 1 to 5 mm). All 11 had endometrial sampling that revealed "scant cellular material" or inactive endometrium. Seventeen patients had an endometrial thickness of 6 mm or greater (range, 6 to 25 mm). Of these, two patients also had inactive endometrium, which measured 6 mm. Also, there were six patients with proliferative endometrium, three patients with secretory endometrium, three patients with hyperplasia, two patients with polyps, and one patient with well-differentiated endometrial carcinoma. In two of the patients, the proliferative endometrium measured 6 mm. The patient with endometrial cancer had an 8-mm endometrium. Two patients with multiple myomas had an endometrium that could not be visualized. On biopsy, one of these patients had inactive endometrium, and the other had proliferative endometrium and focal glandular hyperplasia.

The pilot study concluded that an endometrial echo of 5 mm or less was uniformly associated with inactive endometrium or tissue insufficient for diagnosis. Furthermore, an endometrial echo of 6 mm or greater was associated with virtually every pathologic type known. The study concluded that when the sonographic endometrial thickness in such patients with abnormal bleeding was 6 mm or greater, histologic diagnosis should be made in the pathology laboratory. However, the potential existed for some patients with endometrial echoes of 5 mm or less (37%) in this series to be spared endometrial sampling and its risks, discomfort, and expense.

Other authors have examined this issue. Nasri and Coast[31] studied 93 women with postmenopausal bleeding and correlated the ultrasound and histologic studies. One hundred percent of patients with endometrial measurements of 1 to 5 mm (51 of 51) had inactive endometria. There were six patients with endometrial cancer; their endometrial measurements ranged from 8 to 38 mm. When endometrial fluid was present (see later), the authors incorporated the fluid and the anterior and posterior endometrial measurements in a combined total measurement.

Osmers et al.[32] studied 103 women with postmenopausal bleeding and 283 postmenopausal women without bleeding. Interestingly, 3.5% (11 of 283) of the asymptomatic group had carcinoma. Of the group with bleeding, 12.6% (8 of 103) had carcinoma. They recommended curettage for asymptomatic women with endometrial thickness greater than 4 mm. However, they measured only half the thickness, or only one side of the endometrium. Thus, this thickness would equal 8 mm using the technique from other studies. None of their patients was on hormone replacement therapy. They had no patients with cancer with a half-thickness of less than 4 mm (<8 mm full thickness). They did not mention their *thickest* measurement that was associated with atrophy on histology. They did not give the *thinnest* measurement that was associated with cancer.

Varner and colleagues[33] studied 80 women, of whom 65 were asymptomatic and 15 had postmenopausal bleeding. They used either Pipelle aspiration or a Novak curette for endometrial biopsy. All 60 women (100%) with an endometrial measurement of 4 mm or less had inactive endometrium on biopsy. Five women had an endometrial measurement of 5 mm. Of these endometria, two were inactive, one was proliferative, one was hyperplastic, and one had carcinoma (although pictures were shown for none of them). Their largest measurement associated with inactive endometrium was 5 mm. One of the cancerous endometria measured 5 mm, and the other measured 9 mm.

Granberg et al.[34] studied 205 women, all with postmenopausal bleeding. There were no cases of cancer with an endometrial thickness less than 9 mm. The mean thickness for endometrial cancer was 15.2 mm (range, 9 to 25 mm). The mean thickness for atrophic changes was 3.4 mm (range, 1 to 15 mm), although 150 of 157 were 5 mm or less. They concluded that curettage could be avoided in postmenopausal women with bleeding and an endometrial echo of 5 mm or less; no endometrial cancer would be missed, and the rate of dilation and curettage would be reduced by 70%.

Conclusions Regarding Ultrasound Measurement

There seems to be considerable confusion surrounding the use of TVS measurement of endometrial thickness in various types of postmenopausal patients. Several issues exist and should be clearly differentiated from each other. Patients who are bleeding (whether they are patients on hormone replacement therapy bleeding at an unscheduled time, or patients not on hormone replacement therapy bleeding at any time) in the past required mandatory endometrial tissue sampling. The studies reviewed here indicate that in such patients, a thin endometrial echo on TVS (e.g., ≤5 mm, ≤4 mm, "pencil line") is uniformly associated with inactive endometrium, indicating that such bleeding results from atrophic changes, and that biopsy, whether in the office or by formal curettage, can be avoided. However, acknowledging that an endometrial echo of less than 4 to 5 mm in patients with bleeding (Fig. 9–7) seems uniformly associated with inactive, atrophic endometrial tissue on pathologic study (high negative predictive value) is not at all the same as saying that endometrial measurements greater than 4 to 5 mm are pathologic, especially if they are found incidentally in a nonbleeding patient.

Because ultrasound will not yield a tissue diagnosis, it is important that it be appropriately performed and documented. By angling the transducer sufficiently, one could always locate a linear white structure, freeze the frame, place calipers, and call this the "endometrial echo." A well-defined endometrial echo should be seen taking off from the endocervical canal. It should be distinct. Often, fibroids, previous surgery, marked obesity, or an axial uterus makes visualization suboptimal. If so, it is acceptable and appropriate to conclude "endometrial echo not well visualized." In these cases, ultrasound cannot be relied on to exclude a pathologic process. Saline infusion sonohysterography or hysteroscopy is an appropriate next step in the endometrial evaluation of such patients if they have a history of bleeding. If the scan is being done for other reasons, inadequate visualization should be noted and recorded, but further evaluation is not mandatory.

Another important consideration, in addition to measured endometrial thickness, is the texture of the endometrium. If it is heterogeneous and irregular, this may be a more important determinant than simply absolute thickness.

Historical Perspective

Patients with postmenopausal bleeding are considered to have cancer until proven otherwise. Such patients routinely were subjected to dilation and curettage, first described in 1841. In the past, this was the most common operation in women. As early as the 1950s, however, a review of 6907 curettage procedures[35] found that the technique missed endometrial lesions in 10% of cases. Of these, 80% were polyps. A study of curettage before hysterectomy[36] found that in 16% of specimens less than one fourth of the cavity was curetted, in 60% less than one half of the cavity was curetted, and in 84% less than three fourths of the endometrial cavity was effectively curetted.

Ultimately, dilation and curettage was largely replaced by procedures using equipment such as the Vabra aspirator (Berkeley Medevices, Berkeley, Calif), which used a resterilizable metal cannula attached to suction and permitted performance of "mini dilation and curettage" in the office setting. This procedure was found to be 86% accurate in diagnosing cancer.[37] Subsequently, less expensive, smaller, less painful plastic catheters with their own internal pistons to generate

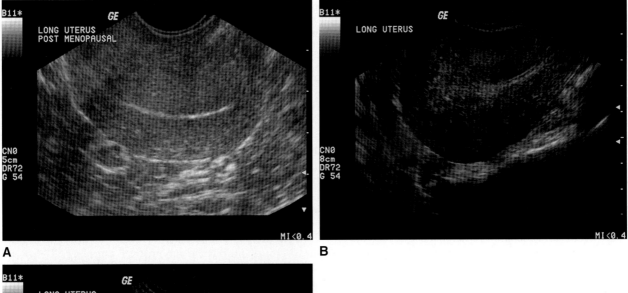

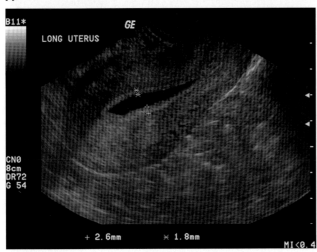

Figure 9–7. A, Postmenopausal patient with episode of vaginal staining. Long-axis view reveals an endometrial echo measuring 1.3 mm in thickness. Such a picture in a patient with bleeding has a 99% negative predictive value for exclusion of a significant pathologic process. **B,** Transvaginal pelvic sonogram of a postmenopausal patient who presented with an episode of bleeding. An endometrial echo is poorly visualized beyond the lower uterine segment. Such a picture does not reliably exclude a significant pathologic process. **C,** Same patient as in **B** after instillation of saline through a catheter for saline infusion sonohysterography (SIS). There was prompt expansion of the endometrial cavity, and the endometrium surrounding the fluid was seen to be thin (2.6 mm anteriorly and 1.8 mm posteriorly). There were no endoluminal masses. Such a picture on SIS excludes a significant pathologic process.

suction became popular. One of these, the Pipelle* device (Unimar, Wilton, Conn), was found to have similar efficacy to the Vabra and better patient acceptance.[38] Rodriguez and associates[39] did a pathologic study of 25 hysterectomy specimens. The percentage of endometrial surface sampled by the Pipelle device was 4%, versus 41% for the Vabra aspirator.

In one widely publicized study,[40] the Pipelle had a 97.5% sensitivity in detecting endometrial cancer in 40 patients undergoing hysterectomy. The shortcoming of this study was that the diagnosis of malignancy was known before performance of the specimen collection.

In another study,[41] Pipelle aspiration biopsy was performed in 135 premenopausal patients before curettage. Thirteen patients (10%) had different histologic results on Pipelle biopsy than on curettage. It is interesting that only five of these patients had polyps, of which Pipelle sampling missed three. In total, 18 patients had hyperplasia, of which Pipelle sampling missed the diagnosis in 7 (39%), thus underscoring the often focal nature of that pathologic process.

*Although many brands of this device are now available, clinicians often refer to them generically as a "Pipelle," in much the same way that we ask for a "Kleenex" when we want a tissue, or refer to the "Xerox" machine even if it is a different brand of copier.

Finally, in yet another study, Guido et al.[42] analyzed the Pipelle biopsy in 65 patients with known carcinoma undergoing hysterectomy. Pipelle biopsy provided tissue adequate for analysis in 63 of the 65 patients (97%). Malignancy was detected in only 54 samples (83%). Of the 11 with false-negative results, 5 (8%) had disease confined to endometrial polyps and 3 (5%) had tumor localized to less than 5% of the surface area. The surface area of endometrial involvement in this study was 5% or less of the cavity in 3 of 65 patients (5%); 5% to 25% of the cavity in 12 of 65 patients (18%), of which the Pipelle missed 4; 26% to 50% of the cavity in 20 of 65 patients (31%), of which the Pipelle missed 4; and greater than 50% of the cavity in 30 of 65 patients (46%), of which the Pipelle missed none. These results provide great insight into the way endometrial carcinoma can be distributed over the endometrial surface or confined to a polyp. Because tumors localized in a polyp or a small area of endometrium may go undetected, the authors concluded that the "Pipelle is excellent for detecting global processes in the endometrium."[42]

The Postmenopausal Estrogen/Progestin Interventions (PEPI) study[43] had an endometrial surveillance arm. In a multicenter trial of 448 women, the authors found that at a threshold of 5 mm for endometrial thickness, TVS had a negative predictive value of 99%. This led the authors to conclude that "when the endometrial echo measures 5 mm or less there is little need for tissue sampling for histologic evaluation." However, in this study the positive predictive value of an endometrial echo greater than 5 mm was only 9%, and for a serious pathologic process (i.e., carcinoma or hyperplasia), it was only 4%. Thus, the conclusion is that TVS is not a good screening tool in nonbleeding women.

From these data, it seems that undirected sampling, whether through curettage or various types of suction aspiration, will often be fraught with error, especially in cases in which the abnormality is not global but focal (i.e., polyps, focal hyperplasia, or carcinoma involving small areas of the uterine cavity). In this regard, it also should be stressed that endometrial measurements need to be made on a long-axis view, perpendicular to the endometrial echo. The coronal view is prone to error because it may be tangential and not perpendicular to the echo. Because carcinomas, hyperplasias, and polyps are often focal, it is not sufficient simply to produce and measure a single long-axis view. Multiple two-dimensional views in the long axis from cornua to cornua are mandatory in an attempt to recreate three-dimensional anatomy and avoid missing potentially focal changes. Saline infusion sonohysterography can also be helpful (see Chapter 15), and proof that a pathologic process is symmetric (i.e., "global" and not focal) should precede any type of blind office sampling (Fig. 9–8).

Endometrial Fluid Collections

The presence of an endometrial fluid collection was previously thought to be an ominous sign often associated with malignancy. In 1982, Breckenridge et al.[44] found that 16 of 17 patients with intrauterine fluid collections on ultrasound had carcinoma in the uterine corpus or cervix. With the development of improved transabdominal resolution, McCarthy and colleagues[45] reported in 1986 that six of eight patients with postmenopausal endometrial fluid collections had benign processes. With the image magnification afforded by the

vaginal probe, fluid is easily seen in ovarian follicular changes, in the cul-de-sac after ovulation, and increasingly within the endometrial cavity of postmenopausal women.

In 1991, Goldstein[46] postulated that fluid collections seen in the endometrium of many postmenopausal women actually represent transudate associated with cervical stenosis. More recently, a paper describing 30 cases of postmenopausal endometrial fluid collection emphasized the need to measure the endometrial tissue *peripheral* to the fluid.[47] This is the significant tissue, not the mere presence of fluid itself. Initially, during routine ultrasound-enhanced bimanual examination, nine postmenopausal women with unremarkable palpatory examinations were found to have endometrial fluid collections. None had any history of bleeding, and none was on hormone replacement therapy. The patients were 9 to 24 years postmenopause. Because of concern that the endometrial fluid signaled an abnormality,[44,45] each of the women in the study group underwent endometrial sampling. There was some degree of cervical stenosis in each case. Scant tissue was obtained and was reported by the pathologist as "inactive endometrium." Subsequently, the sonograms on each patient were re-reviewed, and it was found that the endometrium surrounding the fluid was uniformly 3 mm thick or less (Fig. 9–9).

After the original 9 patients, 21 additional patients with endometrial fluid collections were identified. None had any history of bleeding, and none was taking any hormone replacement therapy. These patients were 3 to 26 years postmenopause. Eighteen of the 21 additional patients had tissue surrounding the fluid measuring 3 mm thick or less. These patients were followed conservatively for 6 to 26 months, with scans at 3- to 6-month intervals. Six showed resolution of the fluid, and 12 cases remained unchanged. Three of the 21 had thickened, heterogeneous endometrium (≥3 mm) peripheral to the fluid. In one, two attempts at dilation and curettage were unsuccessful because of cervical stenosis, and total abdominal hysterectomy and bilateral salpingo-oophorectomy was performed; a 15-mm endometrial polyp

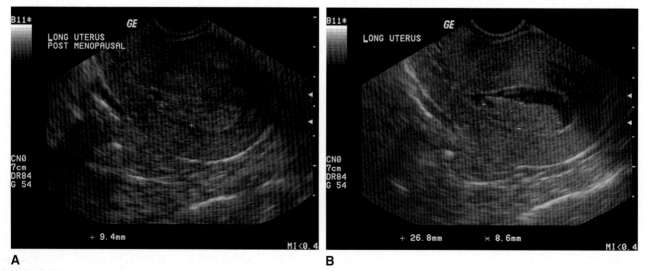

A   **B**

Figure 9–8. **A,** In a postmenopausal patient with an episode of bleeding, the unenhanced endometrial echo is thick, measuring 9.4 mm. This is incompatible with atrophic endometrium. **B,** In the same patient, after instillation of saline through a catheter for saline infusion sonohysterography, the actual endometrium is seen to be thin, compatible with atrophy. There is a large posterior wall sessile polyp *(calipers)* measuring 2.7 × 0.9 mm. The pathologic specimen obtained at dilation and curettage hysteroscopy revealed inactive endometrial polyp.

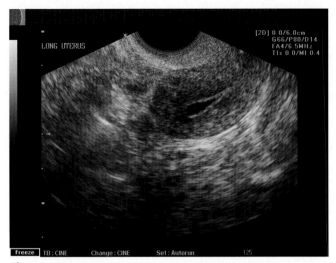

Figure 9–9. Long-axis view of the endometrium in a 65-year-old asymptomatic patient. Endometrial fluid is identified. The endometrial tissue surrounding the fluid is thin and typical of inactive atrophic endometrium. Such a picture is seen with clinical cervical stenosis. Histopathologic study revealed inactive atrophic endometrium at the time of hysterectomy performed for uterine prolapse.

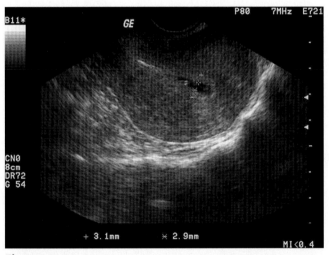

Figure 9–10. Long-axis view of the endometrium in a postmenopausal patient with a history of cervical conization 35 years previously. The patient was diabetic and obese. The naturally occurring endometrial fluid collection shows the anterior and posterior endometrium to measure 2.9 mm and 3.1 mm, respectively. At dilation and curettage hysteroscopy, the fluid was found to be blood tinged, and the diagnosis of atypical adenomatous hyperplasia was made.

was found. The other two patients had thickened endometrium surrounding the fluid (Fig. 9–10). Dilation and curettage and hysteroscopy in both revealed simple hyperplasia without atypia. It appears that normal atrophic postmenopausal endometrium, when associated with cervical stenosis, can be accompanied by endometrial fluid collections, easily seen on TVS. When the endometrial layer peripheral to the fluid collection is no thicker than 3 mm, the endometrial pathology result is invariably inactive endometrium, and sampling is not indicated. If the peripheral endometrium is thicker than 3 mm, the endometrium cannot be expected to be inactive, and sampling is necessary. Thus, the important

issue is not the fluid itself, but the thickness and character of the tissue surrounding it.

Conclusions Regarding Indications for Ultrasound

In summary, in postmenopausal women with bleeding, TVS (and sonohysterography when necessary) is a simple, inexpensive, well-tolerated office procedure to triage patients to

1. No anatomic endometrial pathologic process (treated expectantly or hormonally);
2. Globally thickened endometrial tissue (candidates for blind sampling); or
3. Abnormally thickened but focal tissue (including polyps and nonglobal pathologic processes) in need of visually directed sampling.

In women without bleeding, incidental abnormal findings on various imaging studies have not been scientifically evaluated. Benign quiescent anatomic structures may be common, hitherto undetected, and now easily seen with the improved resolution of all imaging modalities. Additional testing and evaluation have not been shown to be necessary or clinically relevant and in some cases may result in more harm than good to patients. Decisions about how to proceed with incidental unexpected findings should be made on a case-by-case basis and depend on a multitude of factors, but certainly a thin, distinct endometrial echo in a woman with bleeding has a very high negative predictive value, whereas a thick endometrial echo in a woman without bleeding is unvalidated and does not require automatic tissue sampling.

Conclusion

Sonographic assessment of adnexal structures and endometrial detail has provided new insights into the physiologic and pathologic changes of menopausal patients. These insights have in turn guided modifications in the clinical approach to many of these patients.

REFERENCES

1. Barber H, Graber E: The PMPO syndrome (postmenopausal palpable ovary syndrome). Obstet Gynecol 1971;38:921-923.
2. Barber H: Ovarian cancer: Diagnosis and management. Am J Obstet Gynecol 1984;150:910-916.
3. Goldstein SR, Subramanyam B, Snyder JR, et al: The postmenopausal cystic adnexal mass: The potential role of ultrasound in conservative management. Obstet Gynecol 1989;73:8-10.
4. Hall DA, McCarthy KA: The significance of the postmenopausal simple adnexal cyst. J Ultrasound Med 1986;5:503-505.
5. Rulin MC, Preston AL: Adnexal masses in postmenopausal women. Obstet Gynecol 1987;70:578-581.
6. Rodriguez MH, Platt LD, Medearis AL, et al: The use of transvaginal sonography for evaluation of postmenopausal ovarian size and morphology. Am J Obstet Gynecol 1988;159:810-814.
7. Wolf SI, Gosink BB, Feldesman MR, et al: Prevalence of simple adnexal cysts in postmenopausal women. Radiology 1991;180:65-71.
8. Bailey CL, Ueland FR, Land GL, et al: The malignant potential of small cystic ovarian tumors in women over 50 years of age. Gynecol Oncol 1998;69:3-7.
9. Conway C, Zalud I, Dilena M, et al: Simple cyst in the postmenopausal patient: Detection and management. J Ultrasound Med 1998;17:369-372; quiz 373-374.
10. Modesitt SC, Pavlik EJ, Ueland FR, et al: Risk of malignancy in unilocular ovarian cystic tumors less than 10 centimeters in diameter. Obstet Gynecol 2003;102:594-599.

11. Nardo LG, Kroon ND, Reginald PW: Persistent unilocular ovarian cysts in a general population of postmenopausal women: Is there a place for expectant management? Obstet Gynecol 2003;102:589-593.

12. Whittemore AS: Characteristics relating to ovarian cancer risk: Implications for prevention and detection. Gynecol Oncol 1994;55:S15-S19.

13. Schildkraut JM, Thompson WD: Familial ovarian cancer: A population-based case-control study. Am J Epidemiol 1988;128:456-466.

14. NIH Consensus Development Panel on Ovarian Cancer: NIH consensus conference: Ovarian cancer: Screening, treatment, and follow-up. JAMA 1995;273:491-497.

15. Cannistra SA: Medical progress: Cancer of the ovary. N Engl J Med 2004;351:2519-2529.

16. Campbell S, Royston P, Bhan V, et al: Novel screening strategies for early ovarian cancer by transabdominal ultrasonography. Br J Obstet Gynaecol 1990;797:304-311.

17. Van Nagell JR Jr, Higgins RV, Donaldson ES, et al: Transvaginal sonography as a screening method for ovarian cancer. Cancer 1990;65:573-577.

18. Van Nagell JR Jr, DePriest PD, Reedy MB, et al: The efficacy of transvaginal sonographic screening in asymptomatic women at risk for ovarian cancer. Gynecol Oncol 2000;77:350-356.

19. Crane JP, Gray DL, Mulch DG: Routine ultrasound screening for ovarian cancer: Can we afford it? [Editorial] J Ultrasound Med 1991;00:543.

20. Kurjak A, Zalud I, Alfirevic Z: Evaluation of adnexal masses with transvaginal color ultrasound. J Ultrasound Med 1991;10:295-297.

21. Bourne T, Campbell S, Steer C, et al: Transvaginal color flow imaging: A possible new screening test for ovarian cancer. BMJ 1989;289:1367-1370.

22. Fleischer AC, Rodgers WH, Rao B, et al: Assessment of ovarian tumor vascularity with transvaginal color Doppler sonography. J Ultrasound Med 1991;10:563-568.

23. Tekay A, Jouppila P: Controversies in assessment of ovarian tumors with transvaginal color Doppler ultrasound. Acta Obstet Gynecol Scand 1996;75:316-329.

24. Niloff JM, Bast RC, Schoetzl EM, et al: Predictive value of CA 125 antigen levels in second look procedures for ovarian cancer. Am J Obstet Gynecol 1985;151:981-986.

25. Kabowat S, Bast R, Knapp RC, et al: Immunopathologic characterization of a monoclonal antibody that recognizes common surface antigens of human ovarian tumors of serous, endometrioid and clear cell types. Am J Clin Pathol 1983;79:98-104.

26. Niloff JM, Knapp RC, Schoetzl EM: CA 125 antigen levels in obstetrics and gynecologic patients. Obstet Gynecol 1984;64:703-707.

27. Fung MF, Bryson P, Johnston M, Chambers A, Cancer Care Ontario Practice Guidelines Initiative Gynecology Cancer Disease Site Group: Screening postmenopausal women for ovarian cancer: A systematic review. J Obstet Gynaecol Can 2004;26:717-728.

28. Petricoin EF, Ardekani AM, Hitt BA, et al: Use of proteomic patterns in serum to identify ovarian cancer. Lancet 2002;359:572-577.

29. Maiman M, Seltzer V, Boyce J: Laparoscopic excision of ovarian neoplasms subsequently found to be malignant. Obstet Gynecol 1991;77:563-565.

30. Goldstein SR, Nachtigall M, Snyder JR, Nachtigall L: Endometrial assessment by vaginal ultrasonography before endometrial sampling in patients with postmenopausal bleeding. Am J Obstet Gynecol 1990;163:119-123.

31. Nasri MN, Coast GJ: Correlation of ultrasound findings and endometrial histopathology in postmenopausal women. Br J Obstet Gynaecol 1989;96:1333-1338.

32. Osmers R, Volksen M, Schauer A: Vaginosonography for early detection of endometrial carcinoma? Lancet 1990;335:1569-1571.

33. Varner RE, Sparks JM, Cameron CD, et al: Transvaginal sonography of the endometrium in postmenopausal women. Obstet Gynecol 1991;78:195-199.

34. Granberg S, Wikland M, Karlsson B, et al: Endometrial thickness as measured by endovaginal ultrasonography for identifying endometrial abnormality. Am J Obstet Gynecol 1991;164:47-52.

35. Word B, Gravlee LC, Widemon GL: The fallacy of simple uterine curettage. Obstet Gynecol 1958;12:642-645.

36. Stock RJ, Kanbour A: Prehysterectomy curettage. Obstet Gynecol 1975;45:537-541.

37. Vuopala S: Diagnostic accuracy and clinical applicability of cytological and histological methods for investigating endometrial carcinoma. Acta Obstet Gynecol Scand Suppl 1977;70:1-72.

38. Kaunitz AM, Masciello AS, Ostrowsky M, Rovvira EZ: Comparison of endometrial Pipelle and Vabra aspirator. J Reprod Med 1988;33:427-431.

39. Rodriguez MJ, Platt LD, Medearis AL, et al: The use of transvaginal sonography for evaluation of postmenopausal size and morphology. Am J Obstet Gynecol 1988;159:810-814.

40. Stovall TG, Photopulos GJ, Poston WM, et al: Pipelle endometrial sampling in patients with known endometrial cancer. Obstet Gynecol 1991;77:954-956.

41. Goldchmit R, Katz A, Blickstein I, et al: The accuracy of endometrial Pipelle sampling with and without sonographic measurement of endometrial thickness. Obstet Gynecol 1993;82:727-730.

42. Guido RS, Kanbour A, Ruhn M, Christopherson WA: Pipelle endometrial sampling sensitivity in the detection of endometrial cancer. J Reprod Med 1995;40:553-555.

43. Langer RD, Pierce JJ, O'Hanlan KA, et al: Transvaginal ultrasonography compared with endometrial biopsy for the detection of endometrial disease. Postmenopausal Estrogen/Progestin Interventions Trial. N Engl J Med 1997;337:1792-1798.

44. Breckenridge JW, Kurta A, Ritchie W, Macht E: Postmenopausal uterine fluid collection: Indicator of carcinoma. AJR Am J Roentgenol 1982;139:529-534.

45. McCarthy KA, Hall DA, Swann CA: Postmenopausal endometrial fluid collections: Always an indicator of malignancy? J Ultrasound Med 1986;5:647-649.

46. Goldstein SR: Endovaginal Ultrasound, 2nd ed. New York, John Wiley & Sons, 1991.

47. Goldstein SR: Postmenopausal endometrial fluid collections revisited: Look at the doughnut rather than the hole. Obstet Gynecol 1994;83:738-740.

Chapter 10

Lower Urinary Tract

Ilan E. Timor-Tritsch

Urinary incontinence is a common complaint in women of all ages, but it becomes more frequent and severe with advancing age. The most common underlying cause is genuine stress incontinence, with or without instability of the detrusor mechanism.[1] Complete urodynamic tests are required to differentiate detrusor instability from genuine stress incontinence. Classically, these tests and investigations have included lateral (chain) cystourethrography,[2] pelvic viscerography,[3] pad testing,[4] urethral pressure profilometry,[5] videocystourethrography,[6] and electrical conductance measurements.[7,8] All or almost all these tests are invasive to some degree and require a special environment (urodynamic laboratory equipment, special examination table, etc.) to be performed.[9] Another consideration is that most of the tests use x-rays, with consequent radiation exposure to the pelvis.

External and internal ultrasound examination of the lower urinary tract circumvents the invasiveness of the aforementioned techniques. The external transabdominal and perineal approaches preceded the internal approach.[10,11] Internal ultrasound evaluation is conducted using the transvaginal and the transrectal routes. Transvaginal sonography (TVS), a minimally invasive and easily applied imaging technique, opened new horizons and possibilities for the study of urinary incontinence and several other diseases of the bladder wall.[1,12,13] TVS can image target structures such as the bladder neck and wall more easily than transabdominal sonography because the transducer's tip can be positioned nearer these structures. The transvaginal route seems to be better tolerated by patients than the transrectal route.[1,14] An increasing number of TVS studies are being published in the urologic, surgical, gynecologic, and sonographic literature. Lately, three-dimensional (3D) transperineal ultrasound has been tested in obtaining volume scans of the perineal and lower pelvic structures.[15-17]

Transducers and Techniques

Ultrasound techniques used to image the lower urinary tract depend on availability of probes and personal preference of the examiner. Urologists primarily use perineal and introital techniques, whereas gynecologists use the transvaginal and transrectal routes.

Relatively high frequency (6.5 to 7.5 MHz) transrectal or transvaginal transducers with a scanning field of view of at least 110 degrees, producing clear pictures, must be used in urogynecologic ultrasound examinations. The mechanical or electronic sector scan heads need to be set off-axis by 20 to 30 degrees to be able to capture the region of interest. Patients are examined in the dorsal recumbent position and sometimes in the sitting position, using a specially adapted chair that enables easy introduction of the vaginal probe.

Preparation of the probe is similar to that of the customary TVS examination. The examination is started with a relatively full urinary bladder. At or near the end of the examination, the bladder is emptied, after which the residual urine volume is estimated. Excessive distention of the bladder should be avoided so as not to distort the anatomy (or the pathologic findings) by pressure from the probe.

The image is usually generated in the sagittal and coronal planes. After proper probe angling, a clear picture should be displayed on the monitor. Several transvaginal probes (mechanical as well as electronic) are provided with scanning field steering capabilities, a clear advantage if such scanning is required. Various's patient maneuvers, such as coughing and straining (i.e., Valsalva's maneuver), can be used to enhance the diagnostic yield of the examination.

The more recent introduction of three-dimensional ultrasound provides an additional technique to evaluate the lower urinary tract.[15-17] The interested reader is referred to relevant chapters in several textbooks on ultrasonography.[18-20]

Ultrasound Evaluation of the Bladder and Urethra

Normal Ultrasound Anatomy of the Lower Urinary Tract

In the sagittal plane, as the urethra enters the bladder, the bladder neck is at the junction of the urethra and the urinary bladder (Fig. 10–1). If the probe is placed on the introitus or inserted into the lower fourth to fifth of the vagina, three parallel structures can be imaged in the sagittal plane: the urethra anteriorly, the rectum posteriorly, and the vagina between the two (Fig. 10–2). Normally, the angle between the urethra and the posterior bladder neck measures 100 to 110 degrees (Fig. 10–3; see Figs. 10–1 and 10–2). The thickness of the bladder will vary depending on the amount of urine in the bladder. A technique for measuring bladder wall thickness using TVS was described in patients with

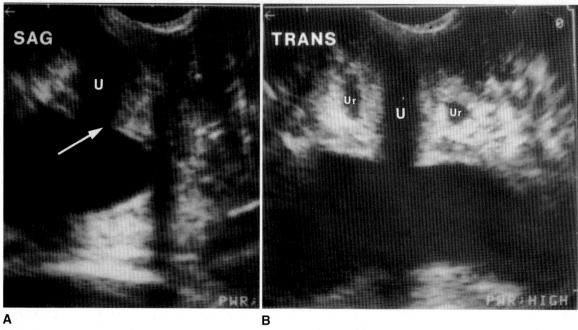

A   **B**

Figure 10–1. Sagittal **(A)** and transverse (coronal) **(B)** views of the bladder imaged by the transvaginal probe. The sagittal view shows the urethra (U) and the posterior angle of the bladder neck *(arrow)*. On the transverse view, the ureters (Ur) are seen on both sides of the urethra. In cases of stress incontinence, the urethra is hypermobile.

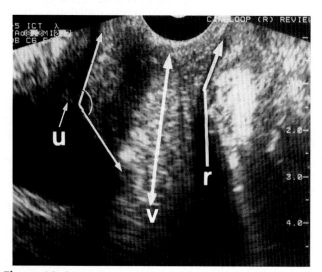

Figure 10–2. Sagittal view of the urethra (u), the vagina (v), and the rectum (r) as imaged by the transvaginal probe placed over the vaginal introitus. The angle of the posterior bladder neck is highlighted by the *arrows*.

urodynamically diagnosed detrusor instability.[21] These patients were found to have significantly thicker bladder walls than women with urodynamically diagnosed genuine stress incontinence.

In the coronal plane the bladder resembles an inverted capital T; the horizontal component is always thicker than the vertical component, which is the urethra (see Figs. 10–1 and 10–3A). This scanning section enables a thorough investigation of the bladder wall. Discrete "jets" of urine can be seen pulsing into the urinary bladder from the two laterally located ureters.[22-26] Color-coded flow scanning detects these jets somewhat better than gray scale (see Fig. 10–3B). The urethra, which is approximately 4 cm long in the woman, can be detected by its sonolucency, which is attributed to its fixed, immobile muscle layers. In cases of stress incontinence, the urethra is hypermobile. It is important to observe any changes in the anatomic location of the bladder neck during straining or coughing; whereas the normal bladder neck should always remain in a retropubic location (Fig. 10–4), with a pathologic process this relationship may be altered.

Ultrasound Evaluation of Pathologic Processes of the Bladder and Urethra

Urinary Incontinence

Transvaginal sonography is the modality of choice for convenient evaluation of the lower urinary tract. Descent of the bladder neck greater than 1 cm during straining is considered diagnostic for bladder neck hypermobility.[27,28] Some authors note the position of the bladder neck in relation to the pubic bone at rest as well as when intra-abdominal pressure is rising[18] (Figs. 10–4 and 10–5). Several publications show results with ultrasound studies that correlate well with those obtained by the gold standard examination, cystourethrography. One of the advantages of ultrasound-based tests is that they can be repeated many times during the session and can also assess the results of surgical procedures used to correct the pathologic process.[27-29]

The feasibility of TVS evaluation of urinary stress incontinence was tested by Leroy and Jeny.[30] They scanned 25 patients with urinary stress incontinence and showed a sensitivity of 94% and a specificity of 100% for establishing the diagnosis. They also reported good correlation between urodynamic test results and TVS.[30] Descent or distortion of the bladder neck below the level of the symphysis pubis was used as an end point to define urinary stress incontinence.

The determination of postvoid residual (PVR) urine volume by sonography is noninvasive, easy, and informative. Whereas measurements in the three basic planes obtained by transab-

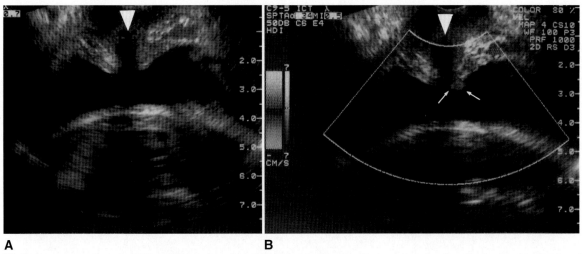

Figure 10–3. **A,** Transverse (coronal) views of a normal bladder partially filled with urine. **B,** Color flow detected a urine jet *(small arrows)* arising from the left ureter. The urethra is indicated by *arrowheads.*

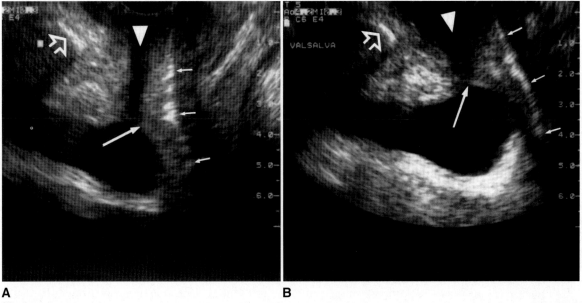

Figure 10–4. Sagittal bladder views in a healthy woman. The urethra *(arrowheads)*, the symphysis *(open arrows)*, the posterior bladder angle *(long arrows)*, and the anterior vaginal wall *(small arrows)* are indicated. **A,** Normal anatomy in the sagittal plane. **B,** Valsalva's maneuver in a patient causes a small bulge of the posterior bladder wall, but the bladder neck stays above the level of the symphysis. (Caudal is toward the top of the picture.)

dominal sonography have been disappointing in assessing bladder volume,[31] TVS allows for easy assessment of the bladder PVR volume. The normal amount left behind after voiding is about 30 to 50 mL. Haylen[32,33] used TVS to assess bladder residual volumes. The best approximation occurred if the bladder contained 50 to 200 mL of urine; the mean error was 46%. Haylen suggested the following formula:

$$\text{Bladder volume (mL)} = 5.9 \times (\text{height} \times \text{depth in cm}) - 14.6$$

Mouritsen and Strandberg,[34] in 44 women with incontinence, and Yalcin and colleagues,[35] in 96 women before surgery for incontinence, compared ultrasound with colpocystourethrography in the evaluation of female incontinence. In both studies, the investigators concluded that ultrasound measurements were more accurate than those obtained by colpocystourethrography and recommended ultrasound as

the most practical and economic modality for the evaluation of bladder neck anatomy. In another article, Mouritsen[36] reiterated that dynamic ultrasonography is the first-line imaging method for studying bladder support.

Badder et al.[37] evaluated the ultrasound parameters for the assessment of female urinary stress incontinence. They found that stress incontinence was associated with the occurrence of cystoceles, bladder neck funneling, increased retrovesical β angle, and descent of the bladder neck. Bladder neck position was strongly related to parity. Later studies by this group reinforce the importance of sonography in the diagnosis of urinary stress incontinence.[38,39]

Khullar and associates[21,41] correlated bladder wall thickness with detrusor instability. They concluded that a bladder wall thickness greater than 5 mm correlated positively with detrusor instability. Meyer et al.[42] used perineal ultrasound to assess

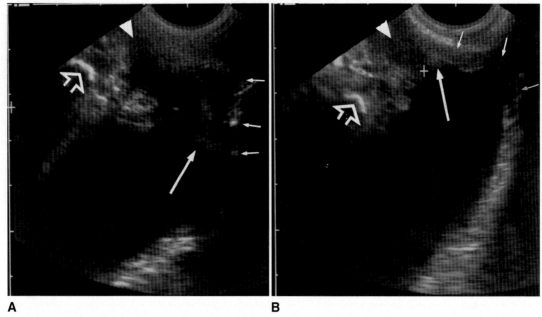

A   **B**

Figure 10–5. Sagittal view of the bladder in a patient complaining of slight stress incontinence. The urethra *(arrowheads),* the symphysis *(open arrows),* the bladder neck (posterior angle; *long arrows*), and the anterior vaginal wall *(small arrows)* are indicated. **A,** Anatomy in the sagittal plane. **B,** Valsalva's maneuver causes the bladder neck to sink below the level of the symphysis while the posterior bladder wall bulges significantly into the vagina. (Caudal is toward the top of the picture.)

the position and mobility of the bladder neck in (1) continent nulliparous and multiparous women and (2) continent and incontinent women whose infants were delivered by forceps. The investigators measured bladder neck position using the two-coordinate system. In continent women with normal vaginal deliveries and in those delivered by forceps, a lower bladder neck position was measured during Valsalva's maneuver than in continent nulliparous women. Women with stress incontinence had a more mobile bladder neck than continent women. They concluded that ultrasound is useful for the evaluation of bladder neck anatomy in symptomatic patients.

Howard and colleagues[43] studied the effect of stress (cough and Valsalva's maneuver) on vesical neck movement and its relationship to continence status. They concluded that in normal nulliparous woman, activation of the muscles of the pelvic floor during coughing stabilizes the urethra, preventing its descent. With damage to the muscles or nerve supply, activation of this system is impaired, and stabilization of the urethra is impossible.

Virtanen and Kiilholma[44] used ultrasound to observe descent of the urethrovesical angle in women with urinary stress incontinence. They found that urogynecologic perineal ultrasound examination strongly supported the anamnestic diagnosis of genuine stress incontinence, proving to be a safe and effective ambulatory procedure.

Other Lesions of the Bladder

Calculi are often seen in the bladder; they are echogenic and usually cast shadows. They move freely if the probe is pushed toward their location in the bladder. Sometimes, stones situated in the lower fifth of the ureter can also be seen by TVS, causing a slight but detectable dilation above the calculus.

Malignancies of the bladder are also detectable by TVS. Granberg et al.[45] identified 5 bladder tumors in a prospective

TVS study of 100 women with postmenopausal bleeding. They emphasized the importance of scanning all women with postmenopausal bleeding with TVS.[46] Leiomyomata of the bladder also have been detected by TVS.[46,47]

An endometrioma in the bladder arising from the bladder wall is shown in Figure 10–6. Occasionally, a thorough vaginal scan may reveal an ectopic kidney. With all the differential diagnostic problems involved, the correct identification of such a case is obviously important (Fig. 10–7).

Urethral diverticula occur in approximately 2% to 5% of women. This lesion has been detected by transabdominal sonography[48] as well as TVS.[49] TVS detection of bladder invasion by cervical cancer also has been reported.[50]

If it is necessary to remove urine from the urinary bladder, some clinicians prefer to perform a suprapubic puncture. Such a procedure can be carried out with greater ease and precision with ultrasound guidance.[51]

Standardization of Techniques for Evaluating the Lower Urinary Tract

In reading the pertinent literature, it is clear that there is a lack of standardization in the techniques for evaluating the lower urinary tract. A commendable effort to establish some common ground for the sonographic evaluation of the bladder and the urethra was made by the German Association of Urologists (GAU).[52] Their recommendations are as follows:

1. The image should be oriented with the urethra pointing to the bottom of the picture (in the United States, the urethra is directed toward the top of the image).
2. The imaged structures should include the urethra, pubic bone, bladder, vagina, and rectum.
3. The measurements should be related to an x-y coordinate system (Fig. 10–8), and the retrovesical β angle must be measured.

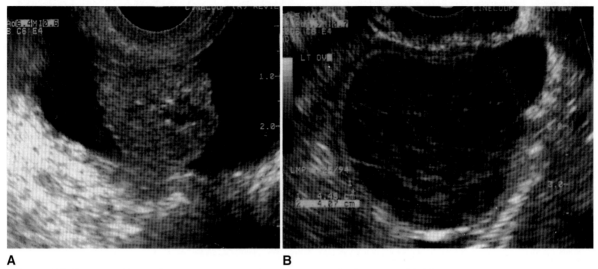

A   **B**

Figure 10–6. Sagittal (**A**) and coronal (**B**) views of endometrioma in the urinary bladder. It measures 4.4 × 4.0 × 4.5 cm.

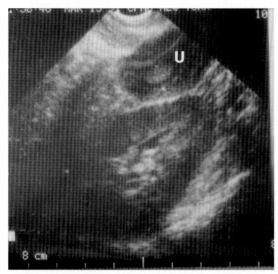

Figure 10–7. Slightly above the uterus (U), a right pelvic kidney is imaged by transvaginal sonography.

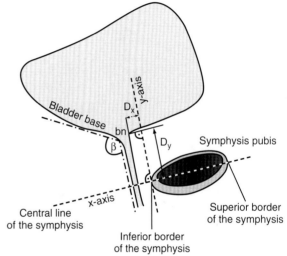

Figure 10–8. Measurement method for perineal ultrasound and lateral-chain urethrocystography. D_x = distance between y-axis and bladder neck; D_y = distance between x-axis and bladder neck; bn = bladder neck; β = posterior urethrovesical angle. (From Schaer GN: Ultrasonography of the lower urinary tract. Curr Opin Obstet Gynecol 1997;9:313-316, with permission.)

4. The patient should be examined in the supine or standing position.
5. The bladder should be filled to 300 mL.
6. Stress tests, such as Valsalva's maneuver, coughing, and straining, can be used.
7. The examiner must minimize the pressure effect of the transducer probe.

Schaer's suggested coordinate system has not been adopted in the daily practice of most urologists. The multiple measurements tend to be cumbersome, necessitating many on-screen measurements to determine the x-y coordinates for each position of the bladder neck at rest or peak effort. The system also does not lend itself to describing the angle at which the vesical neck moves relative to the pubic axis.

Reddy et al.[53] suggested an on-screen, vector-based ultrasound assessment of vesical neck movement. A mid–pubic axis line serves as the zero-degree baseline for measurements

of direction (Fig. 10–9A and B). After compensating for transducer movement, the difference between the baseline vector and the vesical neck vector represents the final real motion of the neck (Fig. 10–9C). They evaluated the corrected and the uncorrected vectors of 10 nulliparous continent, 10 primiparous continent, and 10 primiparous incontinent women during Valsalva's maneuvers. The distance and the angle were greatest in women with stress incontinence (Fig. 10–9D).

Three-Dimensional Imaging

The versatility of 3D acquisition in displaying various planes of the pelvic floor has increased the diagnostic ability of ultrasonography. Figures 10–10 and 10–11 demonstrate how the rendering (thick-slice mode) of the pelvic floor is performed.

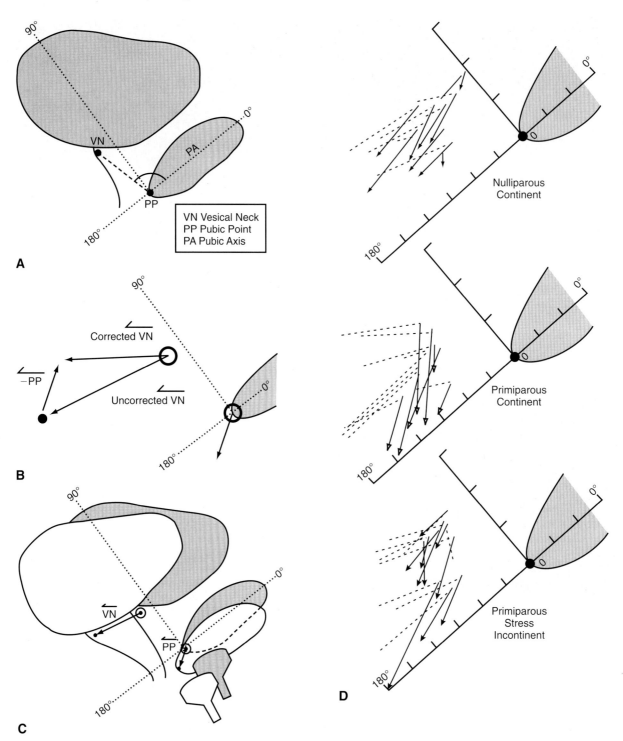

Figure 10–9. The "Reddy coordinate." **A,** The inferior border of the pubic point (PP) acts as a reference point for vesical neck position (VN). **B,** Transducer motion relative to pubic axis movement is measured by determining the distance and direction of apparent pubic point movement. **C,** Subtracting the pubic point vector from the uncorrected vesical neck movement vector yields the vesical neck vector corrected for movement of pubic point. **D,** A comparison of the distances and the angles obtained in continent nulliparous and primiparous women and primiparous women with stress incontinence shows that these were greatest in the incontinent group. (From Reddy AP, DeLancey JO, Zwica LM, Ashton-Miller JA: On-screen vector-based ultrasound assessment of vesical neck movement. Am J Obstet Gynecol 2001;185:65-70, with permission.)

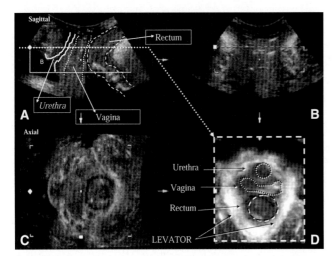

Figure 10–10. 3D evaluation of the pelvic floor and its structures. Box A is the sagittal plane demonstrating the bladder, urethra, vagina, and rectum. Boxes B and C are the coronal and the axial planes, respectively. Box D is the rendering box of the 3D images. If a horizontal plane (*dotted line* in box A) is selected, the rendering box displays the cross sections of the urethra, vagina, rectum, and levators.

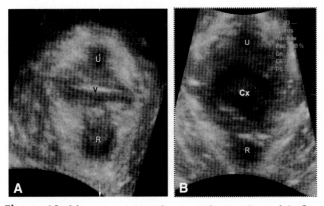

Figure 10–11. Comparison of a normal-appearing pelvic floor (**A**) and a prolapsed cervix (**B**). Cx, cervix; R, rectum; U, urethra; V, vagina.

With experience, this technique may significantly contribute to the diagnosis of pelvic floor pathology.

Conclusion

Ultrasound evaluation of the lower urinary tract remains the simplest, fastest, and most cost-effective way to diagnose urinary stress incontinence and cystocele in the obstetrician-gynecologist's office. Dynamic magnetic resonance imaging (MRI) using ultrafast spin technology has recently shown great promise in demonstrating pathologic processes of the female pelvic floor.[54-57] Also, with the maturation of three-dimensional ultrasound techniques, recent interest has been shown in assessing their usefulness for imaging the female lower urinary tract.[16,17,58-65] However, notwithstanding the aforementioned research and achievements in the field of ultrasound urogynecology, very few obstetrician-gynecolo-

gists and specialists in urogynecology use ultrasound to assess urinary incontinence and bladder descent.

Sonography has several practical advantages over more traditional diagnostic techniques. Its use in the evaluation of detrusor instability needs further study. Transvaginal or introital sonography probably cannot yet replace all the tests used in urodynamic evaluation; however, it may permit elimination of some of these tests and enhance the diagnostic predictability of others.

REFERENCES

1. Hilton P: Urinary incontinence in women. BMJ 1987;299:455-460.
2. Green TH: Urinary stress incontinence: Differential diagnosis, pathophysiology and management. Am J Obstet Gynecol 1967;29:324-327.
3. Richter K, Hausegger K, Lissner J, et al: Die Dochtmethode, eine Vervollkommende Ansatz an der Kolpozystourethrographie. Geburtshilfe Frauenheil 1974;34:711-719.
4. Sutherst J, Brown M, Shawer M: Assessing the severity of urinary incontinence in women by weighing perineal pads. Lancet 1981;1:1128-1129.
5. Hilton P, Stanton SL: Urethral pressure measurement by microtransducer: I. An analysis of variance; II. An analysis of rotation variation. In Sundin T, Mattiasson A (eds): Proceedings of the 11th Annual Meeting of the International Continence Society, Lund, Sweden. 1981, p 69.
6. Bates CP, Whiteside CG, Turner-Warwick R: Synchronous cine/pressure/flow cystourethrography with special reference to stress and urge incontinence. Br J Urol 1970;42:714-723.
7. Plavnik S: Urethral electric conductance. In Drife JO, Hilton P, Stanton SL (eds): Micturition. New York, Springer Verlag, 1990, p 111.
8. Kirby RS, Eardley R: Role of electrophysiological studies. In Drife JO, Hilton P, Stanton SL (eds): Micturition. New York, Springer Verlag, 1990, p 143.
9. Stanton SL: What is the place of urodynamic investigations in a district general hospital [editorial]? Br J Obstet Gynaecol 1983;90:97-99.
10. Bhatia NN, Ostergard NN, Ostergard DR, McQuown D: Ultrasonography in urinary incontinence. Urology 1987;29:90-94.
11. White RD, McQuown D, McCarthy TA, Ostergard DR: Real-time ultrasonography in the evaluation of urinary stress incontinence. Am J Obstet Gynecol 1980;138:235-237.
12. Koelbl H, Bernscheck G, Deutinger J: Assessment of female urinary incontinence by introital sonography. J Clin Ultrasound 1990;18:370-374.
13. Quinn MJ, Beynon J, Mortensen NJ, Smith PJ: Transvaginal endosonography: A new method to study the anatomy of the lower urinary tract in urinary stress incontinence. Br J Urol 1988;62:414-418.
14. Richmond D, Sutherst JR, Brown MC: Screening of the bladder base and urethra using array transrectal ultrasound scanning. Am J Obstet Gynecol 1983;90:97-99.
15. Defreitas GA, Wilson TS, Zimmern PE, Forte TB: Three-dimensional ultrasonography: An objective outcome tool to assess collagen distribution in women with stress urinary incontinence. Urology 2003;62:232-236.
16. Robinson D, Toozs-Hobson P, Cardozo L, Digesu A: Correlating structure and function: Three-dimensional ultrasound of the urethral sphincter. Ultrasound Obstet Gynecol 2004;23:272-276.
17. Dietz HP, Wilson PD: The "iris effect": How two-dimensional and three-dimensional ultrasound can help us understand anti-incontinence procedures. Ultrasound Obstet Gynecol 2004;23:267-271.
18. Quinn M: Transvaginal ultrasound of the lower urinary tract. In Timor-Tritsch IE, Rottem S (eds): Transvaginal Sonography, 2nd ed. New York, Chapman & Hall, 1991, p 175.
19. Cardozo L, Tapp AJS, Wise B: Ultrasonography of the lower urinary tract. In Chervenak FA, Isaacson GC, Campbell S (eds): Ultrasound in Obstetrics and Gynecology. Boston, Little, Brown, 1993, p 1675.
20. Debus-Thiede G: Ultrasound in urinary incontinence. In Sabbagha RE (ed): Diagnostic Ultrasound Applied to Obstetrics and Gynecology, 3rd ed. Philadelphia, JB Lippincott, 1994, p 691.
21. Khullar V, Salvatore S, Cardozo L, et al: A novel technique for measuring bladder wall thickness in women using transvaginal ultrasound. Ultrasound Obstet Gynecol 1994;4:220-223.
22. Dubbins PA, Kurty AB, Darby J, Goldberg BB: Ureteric jet effect: The echogenic appearance of urine entering the bladder. Radiology 1981;140:573-575.

23. Haratz-Rubinstein N, Murphy KE, Monteagudo A, Timor-Tritsch IE: Transvaginal gray-scale imaging of ureteral jets in the evaluation of ureteral patency. Ultrasound Obstet Gynecol 1997;10:342-345.

24. Timor-Tritsch IE, Haratz-Rubinstein N, Monteagudo A, et al: Transvaginal color Doppler sonography of the ureteral jets: A method to detect ureteral patency. Obstet Gynecol 1997;89:113-117.

25. Abulafia O, Sherer DM, Lee PS: Postoperative color Doppler flow ultrasonographic assessment of ureteral patency in gynecologic oncology patients. J Ultrasound Med 1997;16:125-129.

26. Matsuda T, Saitoh M: Detection of the urine jet phenomenon using Doppler color flow mapping. Int J Urol 1995;2:232-234.

27. Johnson JD, Lamensdorf H, Hollander IN, Thurman AE: Use of transvaginal endosonography in the evaluation of patients with stress urinary incontinence. J Urol 1992;147:421-425.

28. Bergman A, Koonings P, Ballard CA, Platt LD: Ultrasonic prediction of stress urinary incontinence development in surgery for severe pelvic relaxation. Gynecol Obstet Invest 1988;26:66-72.

29. Quinn MJ, Beynon J, Mortensen NN, Smith PJ: Vaginal endosonography in the postoperative assessment of colposuspension. Br J Urol 1989; 63:295-300.

30. Leroy B, Jeny B: Contribution of vaginal echography in urinary incontinence. Arch Gynecol Obstet 1988;244:530-537.

31. Holm H, Dristensen J, Rasmussen S, et al: Abdominal Ultrasound. Baltimore, University Park Press, 1976.

32. Haylen B: Verification of the accuracy and range of transvaginal ultrasound in measuring bladder volumes in women. Br J Urol 1981;64:350-352.

33. Haylen B: Residual urine volumes in a normal female population: Application of transvaginal ultrasound. Br J Urol 1989;64:347-349.

34. Mouritsen L, Strandberg C: Vaginal ultrasonography versus colpo-cysto-urethrography in the evaluation of female urinary incontinence. Acta Obstet Gynecol Scand 1994;73:338-342.

35. Yalcin OT, Hassa H, Ozalp S: Effectiveness of ultrasonographic parameters for documenting the severity of anatomic stress incontinence. Acta Obstet Gynecol Scand 2000;79:421-426.

36. Mouritsen L: Techniques for imaging bladder support. Acta Obstet Gynecol Scand Suppl 1997;166:48-49.

37. Bader W, Degenhardt F, Kauffels W, et al: Ultrasound morphologic parameters of female stress incontinence. Ultraschall Med 1995;16:180-185.

38. Bader W, Tunn R, Viereck V, Merz E: Introital and perineal sonography in diagnosing stress urinary incontinence: Possible clinical applications. Ultraschall Med 2004;25:181-190.

39. Viereck V, Bader W, Skala C, et al: Determination of bladder neck position by intraoperative introital ultrasound in colposuspension: Outcome at 6-month follow-up. Ultrasound Obstet Gynecol 2004;24:186-191.

40. Robinson D, Anders K, Cardozo L, et al: Can ultrasound replace ambulatory urodynamics when investigating women irritative urinary symptoms? Br J Obstet Gynaecol 2002;109:145-148.

41. Khullar V, Cardozo LD, Salvatore S, Hill S: Ultrasound: A noninvasive screening test for detrusor instability. Br J Obstet Gynaecol 1996;103:904-908.

42. Meyer S, De Grandi P, Schreyer A, Caccia G: The assessment of bladder neck position and mobility in continent nullipara, multipara, forceps-delivered and incontinent women using perineal ultrasound: A future office procedure? Int Urogynecol J Pelvic Floor Dysfunct 1996;7:138-146.

43. Howard D, Miller JM, Delancey JO, Ashton-Miller JA: Differential effects of cough, Valsalva, and continence status on vesical neck movement. Obstet Gynecol 2000;95:535-540.

44. Virtanen HS, Kiilholma P: Urogynecologic ultrasound is a useful aid in the assessment of female stress urinary incontinence: A prospective study with TVT procedure. Int Urogynecol J Pelvic Floor Dysfunct 2002; 13:218-222.

45. Granberg S, Wikland M, Norstrom A: Endovaginal ultrasound scanning to identify bladder tumors as the source of vaginal bleeding in postmenopausal women. Ultrasound Obstet Gynecol 1991;1:63-65.

46. Caspi B, Weinberg D, Weissman A, et al: Leiomyosarcoma of the bladder: Ultrasonographic features. Ultrasound Obstet Gynecol 1992;2:432-433.

47. Fernandez-Fernandez A, Mayayo-Dehesa T: Leiomyoma of the urinary bladder floor: Diagnosis by transvaginal ultrasound. Urol Int 1992;48:99-101.

48. Lee T, Keller F: Urethral diverticulum: Diagnosis by ultrasound. AJR Am J Roentgenol 1977;128:690-691.

49. Peat B, Korda A, Boogert A, et al: Transvaginal ultrasound for the detection of urethral diverticula at urodynamic assessment. Int Urogynecol J Pelvic Floor Dysfunct 1992;3:118-120.

50. Iwamoto K, Kigawa J, Minagawa Y, et al: Transvaginal ultrasonographic diagnosis of bladder-wall invasion in patients with cervical cancer. Obstet Gynecol 1994;83:217-219.

51. Goldberg BB, Meyer H: Ultrasonically guided suprapubic urinary bladder aspiration. Pediatrics 1973;51:70-74.

52. Schaer GN: Ultrasonography of the lower urinary tract. Curr Opin Obstet Gynecol 1997;9:313-316.

53. Reddy AP, DeLancey JO, Zwica LM, Ashton-Miller JA: On-screen vector-based ultrasound assessment of vesical neck movement. Am J Obstet Gynecol 2001;185:65-70.

54. Kaufman HS, Buller JL, Thompson JR, et al: Dynamic pelvic magnetic resonance imaging and cystocolpoproctography and surgical management of pelvic floor disorders. Dis Colon Rectum 2001;44:1575-1583.

55. Dohke M, Mitchell DG, Vasavada SP: Fast magnetic resonance imaging of pelvic organ prolapse. Tech Urol 2001;7:133-138.

56. Kelvin FM, Maglinte DD: Dynamic evaluation of female pelvic organ prolapse by extended proctography. Radiol Clin North Am 2003;41:395-407.

57. Cortes E, Reid WM, Singh K, Berger L: Clinical examination and dynamic magnetic resonance imaging in vaginal vault prolapse. Obstet Gynecol 2004;103:41-46.

58. Wisser J, Schar G, Kurmanavicius J, et al: Use of 3D ultrasound as a new approach to assess obstetrical trauma to the pelvic floor. Ultraschall Med 1999;20:15-18.

59. Fiori M, Gunelli R, Bercovich E: Echo-dynamic study of female urinary incontinence: Our experience with the use of tridimensional ultrasonography. Arch Ital Urol Androl 2002;74:171-176.

60. Defreitas GA, Wilson TS, Zimmern PE, Forte TB: Three-dimensional ultrasonography: An objective outcome tool to assess collagen distribution in women with stress urinary incontinence. Urology 2003;62:232-236.

61. Jurgens J: Perineal sonography: Using time modulated 2D-ultrasound in a freehand 3D ultrasound technique. Ultraschall Med 2004;25:54-57.

62. Dietz HP, Steensma AB, Hastings R: Three-dimensional ultrasound imaging of the pelvic floor: The effect of parturition on paravaginal support structures. Ultrasound Obstet Gynecol 2003;21:589-595.

63. Dietz HP: Ultrasound imaging of the pelvic floor. Part II: Three-dimensional or volume imaging. Ultrasound Obstet Gynecol 2004;23:615-625.

64. Dietz HP, Shek G, Clarke B: Biometry of the pubovisceral muscle and levator hiatus by three-dimensional pelvic floor ultrasound. Ultrasound Obstet Gynecol 2005;25:580-585.

65. Dietz HP, Barry C, Lim YN, Rane A: Two-dimensional and three-dimensional ultrasound imaging of suburethral slings. Ultrasound Obstet Gynecol 2005;26:175-179.

SECTION IV

Ultrasound and Reproduction

One might wonder why a book dedicated to gynecologic ultrasound has chapters on early pregnancy and its failure. With minimal reflection, however, one realizes that early pregnancy forms a bridge between the fields of obstetrics and gynecology. Certainly, the specialist in maternal–fetal medicine cannot dispute the overwhelming importance of early pregnancy to the development of the fetus. Similarly, gynecologists, even if they no longer practice obstetrics, are constantly confronted with patients of reproductive age who are amenorrheic. Availability of reliable pregnancy test results on urinary samples in 2 minutes' time has changed the clinician's approach to many such patients. However, gynecologists as well as specialists in infertility must have adequate knowledge of early pregnancy—know how to diagnose it, understand if it is normal or destined to fail, and know how to judge its continued well-being to move the patients into the appropriate obstetric prenatal care (whether in the gynecologists' own hands or referred to others). Furthermore, only a firm understanding of normal early pregnancy will allow the clinician to detect abnormal intrauterine pregnancies destined to fail (see Chapter 12), and it is essential as well for diagnosing extrauterine pregnancy. Finally, patients who are pregnant but who will not be continuing the pregnancy should have accurate assessment of gestational age before the pregnancy is terminated to ensure the safety of the procedure.

Chapter 11

Early Pregnancy

Steven R. Goldstein and Ilan E. Timor-Tritsch

The process of conception, implantation, development, and birth is a difficult journey. Infertility encompasses the multitude of reasons why that process may never initiate. Naturally occurring losses at varying stages after fertilization are becoming better understood. Twenty-five percent of all pregnant women will experience bleeding in the first trimester, and of those, 50% will abort.[1] This information has been provided to patients by physicians as well as appearing in books written for the nonmedical lay public. The questions surrounding pregnancy failure—how often, when, and why it happens—have been subjects of great interest in clinical research. High-resolution ultrasound (especially the newer transvaginal probes and the "sonomicroscopy" they afford), the ability to detect minute levels of human chorionic gonadotropin (hCG) in urine and blood, the abundant data from in vitro fertilization programs, and continued interest in background loss rates for procedures such as chorionic villus sampling have all contributed to our increased level of understanding.

Nomenclature of Embryogenesis

The definition of "pregnancy" is ambiguous. Consider the patient who does a home pregnancy test (sensitivity to 50 mIU/mL hCG, International Reference Preparation [IRP]) when she is 2 days late for her menses. The result is positive, but shortly thereafter she has vaginal bleeding slightly heavier than her regular menses. She believes she has "miscarried," and when the scenario repeats itself 2 months later, she requests a work-up for "habitual abortion." The woman has experienced a *chemical pregnancy*, one in which conception takes place but loss occurs before the embryonic period. The woman can be reassured that a chemical pregnancy is a good prognostic sign in terms of her fertility and ultimately having a liveborn baby. Wilcox et al.[2] studied 221 women attempting to conceive by obtaining daily urinary hCG using radio-immunoassay. Twenty-two percent of pregnancies detected by assay were lost at or around the time of the expected menses, and hence before their clinical recognition. Of these women, however, 35% became clinically pregnant in the next cycle, 65% by the third cycle, 93% by the sixth cycle, and 95% within 2 years.

With our increasing ability to detect hCG earlier and more conveniently (over-the-counter home pregnancy tests are very sensitive monoclonal antibody tests), the concept of a chem-

ical pregnancy's preceding clinical recognition of pregnancy loses its meaning. Not all chemical pregnancies are failures to implant, because implantation takes place at the blastocyst stage and is complete before the menses are missed. Abnormal hormone production (estrogen and progesterone) from the corpus luteum may be implicated in some early pregnancy losses. An abnormal chromosome number is often also cited as a main source of early pregnancy failure. Ohno and colleagues[3] studied 144 spontaneous abortions by performing direct preparations of the chorionic villi. Of these, 69.4% had abnormal chromosomes, of which 64% were autosomal trisomies and 7% monosomy X. Nine percent were polyploidy and 6% were structural rearrangements. This does not indicate a problem with parental chromosomes or gametes, but simply demonstrates that nature's method of reducing the chromosome number for gametes from 46 to 23 (meiosis) is an imperfect process. Fortunately, the high wastage is nature's selection process. Stated another way, the small percentage of chromosomally aberrant individuals who survive to birth are the hardiest and strongest of that group.

Even the concept of the "first trimester" is an arbitrary time divider, originally applied to the point at which the pregnant uterus changes from a pelvic organ to an abdominal one. Adherence to this terminology prevents us from seeing more naturally occurring processes anatomically and developmentally, and it falsely promotes the clustering of pregnancy losses that in fact have very different contributing factors.[4] Much clinical confusion emanates from the shoehorning of events into the chronologic first trimester that would be more appropriately divided, anatomically, morphologically, and in terms of risk of spontaneous loss, into an embryonic period and a fetal period.

The *embryonic period* begins at 3 weeks postconception (5 weeks from the last menstrual period [LMP]), when the cardiovascular system and the central nervous system begin to form. It is the period of organogenesis (thus, concerns about teratogens are appropriate) and morphogenesis—the development of shape.

Before the embryo is 18 mm in length, a true "crown" and "rump" do not exist.[5] Therefore, early embryonic size (EES) is measured as the greatest length along the long axis of the embryo.[6] Initially, at the somite stage, the embryo is a linear structure 2 to 3 mm in length (Fig. 11–1). The rostral neuropore closes and develops into the forebrain prominence and then the head. The caudal neuropore elongates into a tail. As it grows, the embryo is a C-shaped, tadpole-like structure (Fig. 11–2). The primitive heart has great prominence, often allowing the sonographer to detect, early on, the pulsations of cardiac activity before visualizing an embryo distinct from the adjacent yolk sac. With further development, the tail regresses, the head unfolds from its flexed position, and limb buds develop and are replaced by hands and feet. By 18 to 22 mm, we can measure a recognizable crown–rump length (CRL; Fig. 11–3). By 10 postmenstrual weeks, with the further unfolding

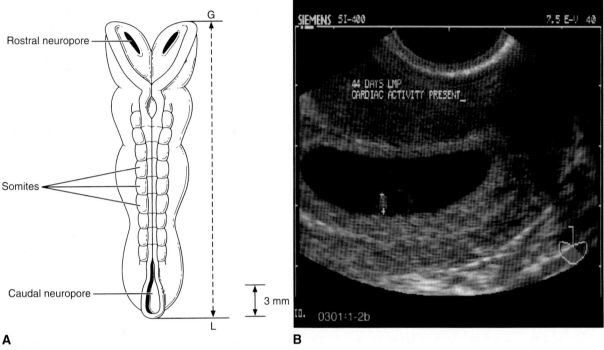

Figure 11–1. **A,** Schematic drawing of an embryo at 3 mm greatest length, at 45 days from the last menstrual period. Note that the embryo is a linear structure with rostral and caudal neuropores distally. **B,** Somite-stage embryo measuring 2.7 mm at 44 days from the last menstrual period. Cardiac activity was clearly present.

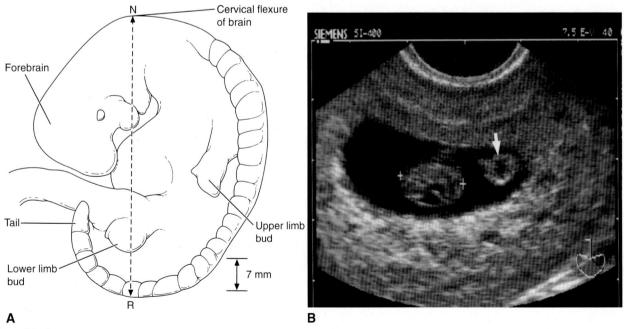

Figure 11–2. **A,** Schematic drawing of an embryo at 7 mm greatest length, at 49 days from the last menstrual period. The rostral neuropore has developed into the forebrain. The caudal neuropore has developed into a tail. The heart has great prominence. Limb buds begin to develop. **B,** A C-shaped, tadpole-like embryonic structure whose greatest length is 11 mm *(calipers)* at 53 days from the last menstrual period is clearly seen adjacent to but separate from its yolk sac *(white arrow).*

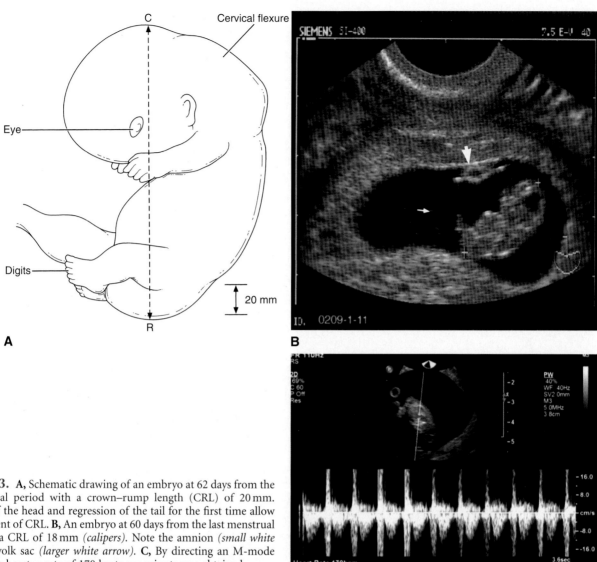

Figure 11–3. A, Schematic drawing of an embryo at 62 days from the last menstrual period with a crown–rump length (CRL) of 20 mm. Unfolding of the head and regression of the tail for the first time allow a measurement of CRL. **B,** An embryo at 60 days from the last menstrual period with a CRL of 18 mm *(calipers)*. Note the amnion *(small white arrow)* and yolk sac *(larger white arrow)*. **C,** By directing an M-mode cursor on the heart, a rate of 170 beats per minute was obtained.

of the head, final regression of the tail, regression of the heart prominence, and development of the limbs and eyes, this hitherto primitive, tadpole-like form is now recognizable as human in form—hence, *fetus* (from the Latin word for "offspring"). Thus, the *fetal period* begins at 70 days post-LMP (Fig. 11–4).

This natural demarcation seems to be borne out in newer studies of loss rates. Studies by Wilson et al.[7] indicate an overall loss rate of 2.3% in embryos between 7 and 12 weeks; the rate was 5% for embryos 7 to 9 weeks and 1% to 2% in embryos between 10 and 12 weeks. A study by Goldstein[4] chose to express anatomic landmarks instead of postmenstrual weeks because of the uncertainty of menstrual data (see Table 11–1). In this series, there were no losses between the anatomic markers of 17-mm embryonic length (8 postmenstrual weeks, 3 days) and a biparietal diameter of 3.4 cm (15.5 postmenstrual weeks). However, 2.0% of pregnancies that entered the fetal period intact were lost spontaneously after 15.5 postmenstrual weeks. In other words, an embryo that survives the embryonic period intact has very little risk of

spontaneous loss until the mid-trimester, when it may succumb to an entirely different presumed set of etiologic factors, such as abnormalities of placentation or perfusion, uterine defects, chronic or acute maternal illness, and incompetent cervix. This is in contradiction to the preponderance of early embryonic losses, in which an abnormal chromosome number is found in approximately 70% of cases.[3]

Ultrasound Approach to Early Pregnancy

Previously, only pregnancies with a suspected problem (e.g., bleeding, size–date discrepancy) came to ultrasound evaluation. Increasingly, however, pregnancies are being evaluated sonographically routinely.[5] This is especially true of patients involved in various forms of assisted reproductive technologies. The widespread use of transvaginal sonography has made routine visualization of uterine contents at the first obstetric visit more common. Thus, a firm understanding of what early

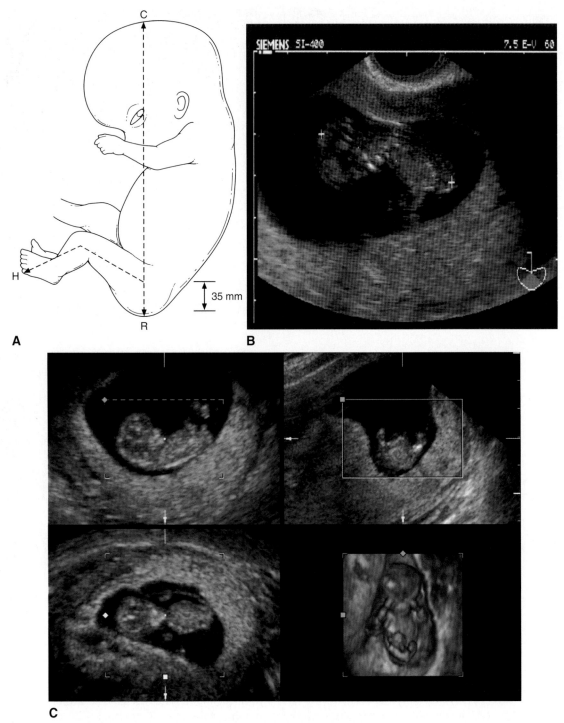

Figure 11–4. A, At 70 days from the last menstrual period, this schematic drawing shows a crown–rump length (CRL) of 35 mm. The embryonic period has ended and the fetal period now begins. **B,** A fetus at 70 days from the last menstrual period with a CRL of 35 mm *(calipers).* Even the most unsophisticated observer (the patient herself and her husband) now recognize this as the "baby." **C,** Multiplanar (orthogonal planes) display of a fetus with a CRL of 3.6 mm. Box D shows a three-dimensional display of the fetus.

pregnancy looks like on ultrasound examination, and why; what landmarks are reached, and when; and how to differentiate acceptable growth and continued well-being from a pregnancy that is definitively destined for failure is essential if the expanding use of ultrasound is indeed going to enhance our attempts to improve reproductive outcome. We have the

ability to date pregnancy with exquisite accuracy, definitively diagnose its failure before spontaneous passage, and directly diagnose ectopic pregnancy or at least suspect it so that diagnosis can precede rupture, thus allowing management to be more conservative and less destructive. However, we must use our enhanced understanding of early pregnancy and its failure

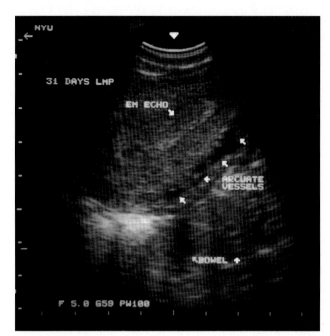

Figure 11–5. Patient at 31 days since last menstrual period with biochemical evidence of an early pregnancy event. The endometrium (EM) is thick and echogenic. The arcuate vessels *(small white arrows)* are prominent. However, these are nondiagnostic findings and can often be seen in the normal late secretory phase.

to provide better counsel to patients and alleviate their fears, anxiety, and self-doubt, not increase them.

Chorionic (Gestational) Sac

Before the gestational sac appears, the endometrium is markedly echogenic and the arcuate vessels are somewhat prominent (Fig. 11–5). This appearance, however, is nondiagnostic of pregnancy and can often be seen in the normal late secretory phase. Although the blastocyst begins to implant in the endometrium at 3 postmenstrual weeks (1 week postconception), the first definitive ultrasound sign of pregnancy is the gestational (chorionic) sac. This is a sonographic term, not an anatomic term.

In ultrasound images, the chorionic sac (Fig. 11–6) appears as a thick, echogenic rind surrounding a sonolucent center. It appears embedded deep in the thick endometrium (decidua) on one side of the cavity line, not in the middle of it (Fig. 11–7). The sonolucent center is actually the fluid within the chorionic sac. The sac already contains the amnion, a bilaminar embryonic disc, and yolk sac, but these structures are too small to be imaged even with the high magnification of our current scanners. The echogenic rind is the result of a trophoblastic decidual reaction. Early on, the entire chorionic sac is surrounded by chorionic villi (Fig. 11–8). These villi are symmetrically located. Some villi will bud and branch into secondary and tertiary villi and become chorion frondosum (the forerunner of the placenta). Other primary villi will regress and become chorion laeve. The appearance of the gestational sac predates the fusion of the decidua parietalis to decidua capsularis. In fact, one can occasionally image a sonolucent area caused by implantation bleeding that separates the sac from the contralateral decidua. Knowing the stage

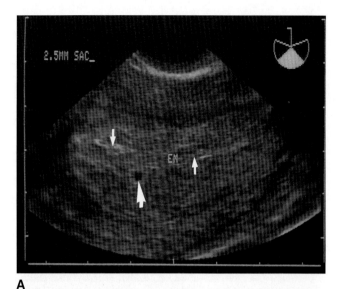

A

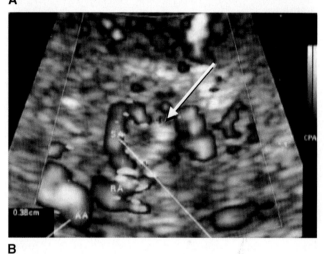

B

Figure 11–6. Early chorionic sac measuring 2.1 mm at 34 days from the last menstrual period. **A,** An echogenic rim is clearly seen around a sonolucent center *(large white arrow)*. The central endometrial echo line is labeled *(small white arrows)*. Note that the sac is embedded in the endometrium on one side of the cavity line. **B,** Color Doppler evaluation of the area of implantation at this age demonstrates an increased vascular supply to and around the tiny chorionic sac *(arrow)*.

at which the sac can first be seen (threshold level; Fig. 11–9) is not as important to us as determining at what stage all normal sacs should be imaged (discriminatory level). Expressed in days from the LMP, this is 34.8 ± 2.2 days,[8] not dismissing the occasional vagaries of menstrual data even in the seemingly most reliable historian. In terms of levels of hCG, the discriminatory level has been reported to range from 935 to 2388 mIU/mL IRP.[8-18] The presence of fibroids, coexisting intrauterine devices, or multiple gestations, however, may create exceptions.[15,19,20]

The chorionic sac grows approximately 1 mm/day in mean diameter during early pregnancy.[21] Several attempts have been made to use the mean chorionic sac growth as a yardstick to assess not only gestational age but also the normal or abnormal development of the pregnancy. Several graphs and tables are available for these purposes. However, none of them was

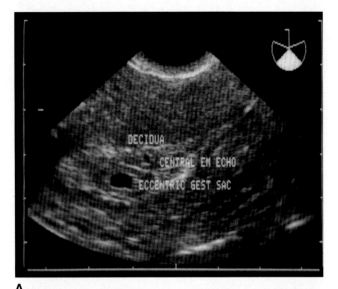

A

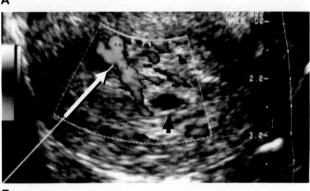

B

Figure 11–7. The chorionic sac at 5 postmenstrual weeks and 2 days (38 days). **A,** Eccentric chorionic sac showing its relationship to the central endometrial (EM) echo contained within the overall decidualized endometrium. **B,** At this age, the blood supply to the sac *(black arrow)* becomes distinct and discrete *(white arrow)*.

clinically useful because of the very wide confidence limits, so they never became known and widely used.[14,21]

With further growth, first the yolk sac and later the embryo become visible sonographically inside the chorionic cavity. The yolk sac has a very bright echogenic rim around a sonolucent center. When it first appears at approximately 5 weeks, it may be only 1 to 2 mm in diameter (Fig. 11–10). Discriminatory size of the chorionic sac for transvaginal sonographic visualization of the yolk sac is reported to range from 8 to 13 mm in mean diameter.[6,14,18] Rowling et al.[22] found that transducer frequency contributes to the smallest (earliest) chorionic sac (threshold level) as well as the largest chorionic sac in which a normal yolk sac should absolutely be seen (discriminatory level). The secondary yolk sac, the one readily detectable by ultrasound in early pregnancy, is visible using transabdominal sonography at or after 6 weeks; however, transvaginal sonography reveals it at or soon after 5 weeks in normal intrauterine pregnancies.

The practical clinical importance of sonographic imaging of the yolk sac has become increasingly evident. In abnormal pregnancies, the yolk sac may be enlarged or irregular, or sometimes described as "floating." An unusual use of the sonographic image of the yolk sac is based on its relatively stable size during the weeks that it can be seen. The section on Gestational Age Assessment, later, deals with this aspect of the yolk sac.

The embryo has been present since 9 days postconception.[9] Sonographically, it is first recognized as a thickening along the yolk sac (Fig. 11–11). As discussed, the early embryo goes through a somite stage in which it is linear, then elongates and curves into a C-shaped, tadpole-like structure, and undergoes further development of the head and regression of the tail, reduction in heart prominence, and development of limbs, a process that finally culminates in the transformation from embryo to fetus at approximately 70 days from the LMP.

Formation of the Early Placenta

With implantation, the inner cytotrophoblast and the outer syncytiotrophoblast layers proliferate rapidly. Sonographically, they are the source of the somewhat enhanced echogenicity of the chorionic sac wall. The endometrium, which is also echogenic (in the late secretory phase), is invaded by the trophoblast, giving rise to the decidua basalis and chorion frondosum on one side and the decidua capsularis and parietalis (or vera) on the other side. The echo-dense structure around the chorionic sac is thus formed. It is possible that the ringlike echogenicity of the chorionic sac is generated by the fuzzy villi surrounding the sac itself.

Later, after the fifth postmenstrual week, small, 2- to 3-mm, sonolucent "lacunar structures" appear approximately 3 to 4 mm from the chorionic sac and tend to cluster only on one side of it. Classic embryology textbooks describe the lacunar structures as the forerunners of the placental feeding vessels, but this is in slight contrast to the observation of Hill and colleagues,[23] who found that before the eighth postmenstrual week it is hard to pinpoint the exact location of the primordial placental tissue. The entire chorionic sac appears to have uniform thickness and echogenicity, without any indication of a differentiation process in a specific chorionic area to herald the shape and function of a placenta. The practical application of these observations is that whenever a slight sonolucency is observed around or beneath the chorionic echogenic rind, with or without overt vaginal bleeding, the term used to describe this should be *subchorionic bleeding*. The term "early placental separation" or "subplacental bleeding" should be reserved for pregnancies in which a discrete picture of the placenta can be seen.

Appearance and Clinical Value of Heart Activity

One of the more common clinical problems in obstetrics and gynecology is the demonstration of viability. In early pregnancy, this may be necessary to exclude ectopic pregnancy, to rule out embryonic demise in case of vaginal bleeding or abdominal pain, or to clarify uncertain dates. Cardiac activity starts at 21 to 22 days of embryonic or conceptual age, or approximately 36 days post-LMP.[6] At this time, the cardiac tube folds on itself and, after the appropriate fusion, becomes active. The embryonic pole is now approximately 1 to 3 mm.

Transabdominal sonography can detect cardiac activity by 41 to 43 days' gestation.[24] High-frequency transvaginal probes are able to demonstrate embryonic cardiac activity 3 to 4 days after it begins.[25,26] Using a 5-MHz transvaginal probe, heartbeats were detected at or after 46 days' gestation, at or above

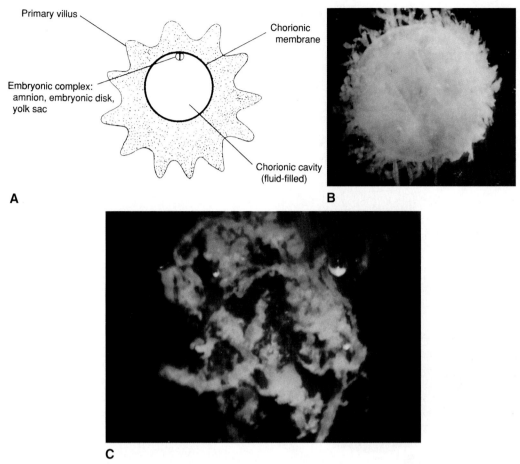

Figure 11–8. A, Schematic drawing of a conceptus at 5.5 postmenstrual weeks. The chorionic membrane surrounds the fluid-filled chorionic cavity. This already contains the embryonic complex, consisting of amnion, embryonic disc, and yolk sac (although these are too small to be imaged at this stage). Projecting from the chorionic membrane are primary trophoblastic villi. As they invade maternal decidua, they cause an echogenic trophoblastic decidual reaction that surrounds the fluid-filled cavity and constitutes the gestational sac. **B,** Pathology specimen of a conceptus at 5.5 postmenstrual weeks. The chorionic membrane has the consistency of a soft contact lens. The primary trophoblastic villi are shown projecting from the surface of the chorionic membrane. **C,** High-power view of chorionic villi. When they are examined grossly, it is sometimes said that the villi float. It is our experience that they do not float, but sink very slowly.

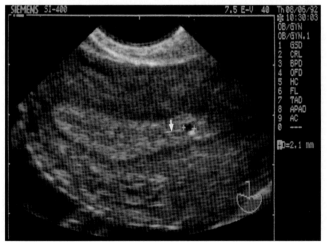

Figure 11–9. The 2.1-mm chorionic sac *(calipers)* is clearly eccentric relative to the central endometrial echo *(white arrow).* This patient had a human chorionic gonadotropin (hCG) level of 645 mIU/mL (International Reference Preparation). The concept of a "threshold" hCG level—the lowest level at which one may image a sac—must be contrasted with a "discriminatory" level—the level at which all gestational sacs, if normal, should be imaged regardless of variations in maternal anatomy or equipment used.

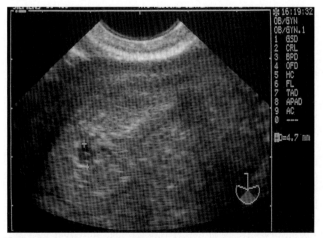

Figure 11–10. A 2-mm yolk sac appears as an echogenic circular structure around a fluid-filled center. It is seen here contained within a gestational sac with a mean diameter of 4.7 mm *(calipers).*

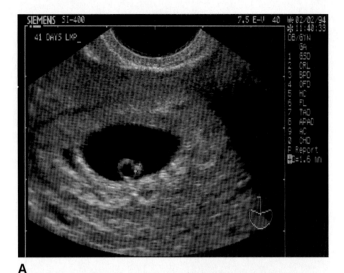

A

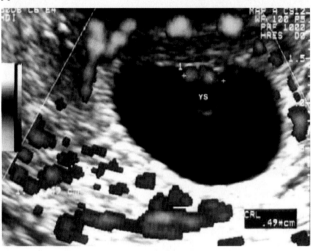

B

Figure 11–11. Early pregnancy at 41 to 46 days from the last menstrual period (LMP). **A,** First visualized, the embryo appears as a thickening along the edge of the yolk sac. This embryo at 41 days post-LMP measured 1.3 mm. Cardiac pulsations were not appreciated on real-time ultrasound. Although present from 21 days postconception, cardiac activity is often not discernible with standard ultrasound equipment before an embryonic size of 3 mm is achieved. **B,** At 46 days post-LMP, the embryo measures 4.9 mm, and on color Doppler interrogation clear cardiac activity is seen.

a β-hCG level of 47,171 mIU/mL, at a mean chorionic cavity diameter of 18.3 mm or larger.[27] Heartbeats quickly increase from approximately 100 beats per minute at 5 postmenstrual weeks to 170 beats per minute at 9 postmenstrual weeks, and then stabilize at approximately 160 beats per minute[27-32] (see Fig. 11–3C).

The clinically pertinent questions are, first, whether there is any embryonic size at which, if no cardiac activity is seen, one can diagnose early pregnancy failure beyond any doubt, and second, what the clinical implications are of a very slow embryonic heartbeat.

The answer to the first question can be found in articles by Levi et al.,[21,33] Brown and associates,[34] Howe et al.,[35] and Goldstein.[36] The consensus is that the absence of cardiac activity on real-time transvaginal sonography in embryos measuring more than 4 mm is always associated with embryonic demise. Most authors suggest rescanning patients with absent embryonic cardiac activity when the embryonic size is no larger than 3 to 4 mm. Given that the embryonic growth rate is 1 mm/day,[37] it is easy to project the expected size after a certain number of days have elapsed, and to schedule the rescan at a time when cardiac activity should definitely be seen.

With regard to the predictive value of a very slow embryonic heart beat, several reports are available. A rate of 80 to 85 beats per minute or less for a sustained period is considered ominous.[37-43] Long-term observations of pregnancies complicated by slow embryonic heart rates in the early first trimester are also available.[43] Rapid embryonic heart rate in early pregnancy was also studied.[44] Vaccaro et al.[45] considered arrhythmia in early pregnancy as a predictor of pregnancy loss. As a rule, and based on personal experience, patients with an embryo with bradycardia, tachycardia, or arrhythmia should be scheduled for a follow-up scan. The chance of a poor outcome is higher if other pathologic ultrasound signs, such as growth discrepancy, subchorionic hemorrhages, or an abnormal yolk sac, are associated with the aforementioned heart rate changes.

Early Detection of Multifetal Pregnancy

Assessment of the amnionicity and chorionicity of a multifetal gestation is important because multifetal pregnancies have an increased incidence of complications. Among the problems are preterm labor and delivery, placental complications, intrauterine growth restriction, and malformations. Complications specific to monoamniotic pregnancies are twin-to-twin transfusion, cord entanglement (leading to complete cut-off of the fetal circulation), and various degrees of conjoined twins. It is therefore imperative to determine the risk level in multifetal pregnancies.[46] Transvaginal sonography is the easiest method to perform this diagnostic task.[47-49]

The number of chorionic sacs in the uterus can be accurately assessed by 5 postmenstrual weeks (Fig. 11–12). Unfortunately, the chorionic sac count is only the beginning of the diagnostic process and will predict only the chorionicity of the multifetal pregnancy. The determination of the exact number of fetuses must wait until the sixth postmenstrual week, after the onset of cardiac activity, when the number of embryos can be determined by the number of embryonic heartbeats. We advise against using the number of yolk sacs as a marker of embryonic number because if the cleavage of the yolk sac occurs later than day 12 after conception, a set of twins may have only one yolk sac. At or after 8 weeks, it is possible and also mandatory to detect the amnion in the chorionic cavity (Fig. 11–13). Usually the content of the amniotic sac is sonolucent, as opposed to that of the extraembryonic coelom of the chorion, which is filled with low-level echoes (and also contains the yolk sac). The detection of the individual amniotic sacs in the case of monochorionic–diamniotic twins becomes possible at 7.5 postmenstrual weeks or immediately thereafter because the amnion separates from the embryo and is easily imaged.[15,47-51]

It is extremely helpful to scrutinize the way the partitioning membrane originates or separates from the uterine wall. If this area contains a triangular projection reaching deeply into the dividing membrane and has the ultrasound properties of the early placenta, it represents the joining of two chorionic membranes. The placental tissue "escorts" the chorions

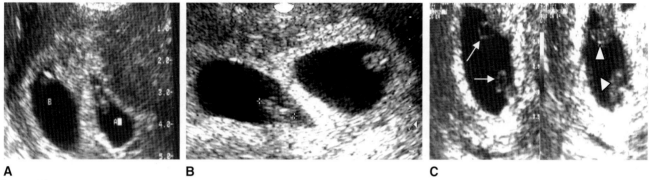

A   B   C

Figure 11–12. Early detection of chorionicity in multifetal pregnancies. **A,** At 5 postmenstrual weeks, two chorionic sacs (A and B) can be detected. This is a dichorionic twin pregnancy. The number of embryos cannot yet be determined. **B,** In the same pregnancy at 6 postmenstrual weeks, in addition to the chorionic sacs, the two embryonic poles with heartbeats can be seen. **C,** In this pregnancy at 6 postmenstrual weeks, only one chorionic sac is present; however, in it two yolk sacs *(arrows)* and two embryos *(arrowheads)* are seen. This is a monochorionic twin pregnancy.

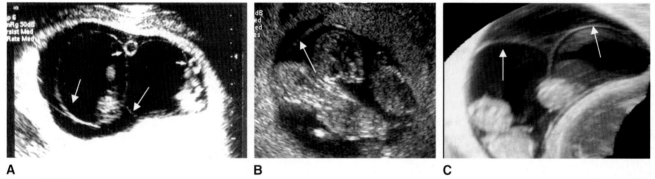

A   B   C

Figure 11–13. Early detection of amnionicity in multifetal pregnancies. **A,** At 8 postmenstrual weeks, the single chorionic sac contains two amnions *(arrows)* and two embryos. This is a monochorionic diamniotic twin pregnancy. **B,** At 8 postmenstrual weeks and 5 days, the single chorionic sac contains only one amnion *(arrow)* but two embryos. This is a monochorionic monoamniotic twin pregnancy. **C,** Using three-dimensional ultrasound, the amnions *(arrows)* in this monochorionic diamniotic twin pregnancy are distinctly seen.

as they join to form the dividing membrane. In the literature describing more advanced pregnancies, this triangular pattern is referred to as the lambda sign,[51] delta sign,[52] or twin peak sign,[53] among other terms. If the membrane take-off is abrupt or T-shaped, one can assume that it is generated by the fusion of amnions. Because there is no ingrowing (placental) tissue to generate the wedge-shaped fusion, this membrane has a clean, T-shaped take-off (Fig. 11–14).

In conclusion, early pregnancy is the preferred time to ascertain chorionicity (starting at 5 completed menstrual weeks), amnionicity (from 8 to 12 postmenstrual weeks), and number of fetuses (after 6.5 postmenstrual weeks).[54,55] Technically, the transvaginal probe should be used. Ultrasound evaluation of chorionicity in the second or third trimester is cumbersome, time-consuming, and less accurate than in the first trimester.[52,56]

Gestational Age Assessment

Previously, embryonic CRL was considered the most accurate method of sonographically dating a pregnancy. With current methods, chorionic sac size, expressed as mean sac diameter, can be correlated with postmenstrual age before visualization of an embryo (Fig. 11–15). Measurements of the sac are taken

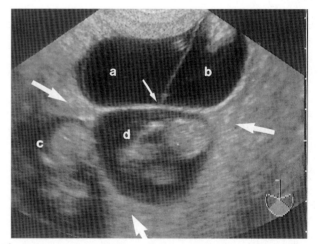

Figure 11–14. A trichorionic quadamniotic quadruplet pregnancy: Embryos a and b are sharing one chorion and therefore are monochorionic-diamniotic. The three *large arrows* point to the delta- or lambda-shaped partition between the chorions. The *small arrow* points to the T-shaped take-off of the two amnions.

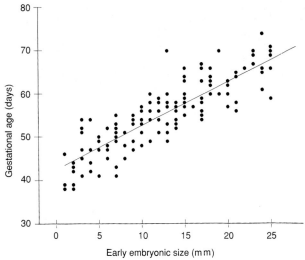

Figure 11–15. Scatter of data points from patients with embryonic size measurements up to 25 mm plotted against gestational age and day since the last menstrual period.

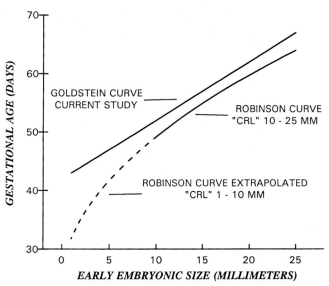

Figure 11–16. Comparison of Robinson curve to Goldstein curve: gestational age versus embryonic size.

at the interface of the trophoblastic tissue and the fluid filling the sac. Such measurements ideally come from two planes at right angles to each other. Many formulas have been described to relate chorionic sac size to menstrual age.[8,19,20] One or more such tables are usually included in the software of commercially available ultrasound machines. A quick rule of thumb, however, is expressed by the following formula[18]:

$$\text{Menstrual age (days)} = \text{mean sac diameter (mm)} + 30$$

The data for the original regression curve established by Robinson and Fleming[57] in 1973 were collected using static arm scanners. The work has been duplicated with real-time equipment by many investigators. Its extrapolation may underestimate the true menstrual age in very early pregnancy.[58,59] Robinson and Fleming's nomogram was constructed from a regression curve, with the bulk of the data derived from small fetuses (CRL >18 to 22 mm) and then extrapolated to very small embryos. Newer transvaginal probes, however, allow identification of embryonic structures as soon as they are distinct from the yolk sac (see Fig. 11–11). (Measurements of such early embryonic structures have mistakenly been referred to as CRL.) Goldstein and Wolfson[60] studied 143 women with reliable LMP dates (see Fig. 11–8) who delivered within 2 weeks of estimated date of conception, had no history of bleeding, and had EES measurements between 1 and 25 mm. The regression curve was linear (Fig. 11–16):

$$\text{Gestational age (days)} = \text{EES (mm)} + 42$$

With a correlation coefficient of 0.87, the 95% confidence limit is ±3 days.

This formula allows for easy gestational age assessment. By adding 42 to the embryonic length in millimeters, one can calculate days from the LMP ± 3 (Table 11–1). This provides very accurate dating, especially in patients with irregular menstrual cycles. Use of such dating at the first obstetric visit may reduce the number of "postdate" pregnancies, as calculated in the traditional fashion.

Table 11–1	Early Pregnancy Loss
Stage of Pregnancy	**Subsequent Loss Rate in Embryonic Period (%)**
Gestational sac present	11.5
Yolk sac present	8.8
Embryo ≤5 mm EES	7.1
Embryo 5-10 mm EES	3.3
Embryo ≥10 mm EES	0.5

EES, early embryonic size.

Practical and Simple "Gestalt Sonographic Dating" in Early Pregnancy Using Sequential Appearance of Embryonic and Extraembryonic Structures

Recognizing the ultrasound appearance of embryonic, extraembryonic, and fetal structures enables us to determine the progress of normal development. Simple and easy observations of the chorionic sac, the yolk sac, the fetal pole with heart motion, the appearance of the brain vesicles (ventricles), the appearance of the falx, and the appearance and disappearance of the physiologic midgut herniation enable the examiner to make a "gestalt" dating of the early pregnancy. It should be emphasized, however, that precise dating is not possible using these techniques.

A fairly accurate estimate of the postmenstrual age may be performed by examining the order of detection (or disappearance) of the six structures listed in Table 11–2. The percentage of these six embryonic and extraembryonic structures detected is seen as a function of the "unknown or desired" gestational age. For example, most normally developing early

Table 11–2	Percentage Detection of the Six Structures at Increasing Gestational Age								
	Weeks of Gestation								
Structure	4	5	6	7	8	9	10	11	12
Gestational sac only	100								100
Yolk sac	0	91	100						100
Fetal pole with heartbeats	0	0	86	100					100
Single-brain ventricle	0	0	6	82	70	20	0	0	0
Falx	0	0	0	0	30	75	100	100	100
Midgut herniation	0	0	0	0	100	100	100	50	0

Adapted from Warren WB, Timor-Tritsch IE, Peisner DB, et al: Dating the pregnancy by sequential appearance of embryonic structures. Am J Obstet Gynecol 1989;161:747-753, with permission.

pregnancies are at 6 weeks if they have a gestational sac, a yolk sac, and an embryonic pole with heartbeats but do not yet have a visible single-brain sonolucency. The pregnancy is probably at 9 to 10 weeks if the head contains the falx and the midgut hernia is still seen.

Summary

Early anatomic landmarks and their normal appearance on ultrasound serve as the basis for understanding normal fetal development as a function of gestational age and their pathologic conditions, which in a combined fashion will ultimately reflect on management (see Chapter 12). This is especially important in pregnant patients who present with some bleeding but a clinically closed cervical os. All such patients should also be considered as suspect for ectopic pregnancy, the approach to which is considered in detail in Chapter 13. An additional area in which early sonographic evaluation of the pregnancy is important is the multifetal pregnancy. The management of such pregnancies depends on timely definition of chorionicity and amnionicity.

REFERENCES

1. Hellman L, Pritchard J: Abortion and premature labor. In Williams Obstetrics, 14th ed. New York, Appleton-Century-Crofts, 1971, p 504.
2. Wilcox AJ, Weinberg CR, O'Connor JF, et al: Incidence of early pregnancy loss. N Engl J Med 1988;319:189-194.
3. Ohno M, Maeda T, Matsunobo A: A cytogenetic study of spontaneous abortions with direct analysis of chorionic villi. Obstet Gynecol 1991; 77:394-398.
4. Goldstein SR: Embryonic demise in early pregnancy: A new look at the first trimester. Obstet Gynecol 1994;84:294-297.
5. Goldstein SR: Embryonic ultrasonographic measurements: Crown-rump length revisited. Am J Obstet Gynecol 1991;165:497-501.
6. Moore KL: The Developing Human: Clinically Oriented Embryology, 4th ed. Philadelphia, WB Saunders, 1988.
7. Wilson RD, Kendrick V, Wittman BK, et al: Spontaneous abortion and pregnancy outcome after normal first trimester ultrasound examination. Obstet Gynecol 1986;67:352-355.
8. Bernaschek G, Rudelstorfer R, Csaicsich P: Vaginal sonography versus serum human chorionic gonadotropin in early detection of pregnancy. Am J Obstet Gynecol 1988;158:608-612.
9. Fossum GT, Davajan V, Kletzky OA: Early detection of pregnancy with transvaginal US. Fertil Steril 1988;49:788-791.
10. Cacciatore B, Titinen A, Stenman U-H, Ylostalo P: Normal early pregnancy: Serum hCG levels and vaginal ultrasonography findings. Br J Obstet Gynaecol 1990;97:889-903.
11. Bree RL, Edwards M, Bohm-Velez M, et al: Transvaginal sonography in the evaluation of normal early pregnancy: Correlation with hCG level. AJR Am J Roentgenol 1989;153:75-79.
12. Goldstein SR, Snyder JR, Watson C, et al: Very early pregnancy detection with endovaginal ultrasound. Obstet Gynecol 1988;72:200-204.

13. Nyberg DA, Mack LA, Laing FC, Jeffrey RB: Early pregnancy complications: Endovaginal sonographic findings correlated with hCG levels. Radiology 1988;167:619-622.
14. Bateman BG, Nunley WC, Kolp LA, et al: Vaginal sonography findings and hCG dynamics of early intrauterine and tubal pregnancies. Obstet Gynecol 1990;75:421-427.
15. Nyberg DA, Filly RA, Mahony BS, et al: Early gestation: Correlation of hCG levels and sonographic identification. AJR Am J Roentgenol 1985; 144:951-954.
16. Dashefsky SM, Lyons EA, Levi CS, et al: Suspected ectopic pregnancy: Endovaginal and transvesical US. Radiology 1988;169:181-184.
17. Bree RL, Marn CS: Transvaginal sonography in the first trimester: Embryology anatomy and hCG correlation. Semin Ultrasound CT MRI 1990; 11:12-21.
18. Nyberg DA, Mack LA, Laing FC, Patten RM: Distinguishing normal from abnormal gestational sac growth in early pregnancy. J Ultrasound Med 1988;6:23-27.
19. Hellman LF, Kobayashi M, Fillisti L, et al: Growth and development of the human fetus prior to the 20th week of gestation. Am J Obstet Gynecol 1969;103:784-800.
20. Daya S, Woods S, Ward S, et al: Early pregnancy assessment with transvaginal ultrasound scanning. CMAJ 1991;144:441-446.
21. Levi CS, Lyons EA, Lindsay DJ: Early diagnosis of nonviable pregnancy with endovaginal US. Radiology 1988;167:383-385.
22. Rowling SE, Langer JE, Coleman BG, et al: Sonography during early pregnancy: Dependence of threshold and discriminatory values on transvaginal transducer frequency. AJR Am J Roentgenol 1999;172:983-988.
23. Hill LM, DiNofrio D, Chenevey P: Transvaginal sonographic evaluation of first-trimester placenta previa. Ultrasound Obstet Gynecol 1995;5:301-303.
24. Cadkin AV, McAlpin J: Detection of fetal cardiac activity between 41 and 43 days of gestation. J Ultrasound Med 1984;3:499-503.
25. Rempen A: Vaginal sonography of viable gestation in the first trimester [in German]. Geburtshilfe Frauenheilkd 1987;47:477-482.
26. Timor-Tritsch IE, Farine D, Rosen MG: A close look at early embryonic development with the high frequency transvaginal transducer. Am J Obstet Gynecol 1988;159:676-681.
27. Rempen A: Diagnosis of early pregnancy with vaginal sonography. J Ultrasound Med 1990;9:711-716.
28. Jouppila P: Ultrasound in the diagnosis of early pregnancy and its complications: A comparative study of the A-, B- and Doppler methods. Acta Obstet Gynecol Scand Suppl 1971;15:3-56.
29. Robinson HP, Shaw-Dunn J: Fetal heart rates as determined by sonar in early pregnancy. J Obstet Gynaecol Br Commonw 1973;80:805-809.
30. Piiroinen O: Studies in diagnostic ultrasound: Size of the non-pregnant uterus in women of child-bearing age and uterine growth and foetal development in the first half of normal pregnancy. Acta Obstet Gynecol Scand Suppl 1975;46:1-60.
31. Hertzberg BS, Mahony BS, Bowie JD: First trimester fetal cardiac activity. J Ultrasound Med 1988;7:573-575.
32. VanHeeswijk M, Nijhuis JG, Hollanders HMG: Fetal heart rate in early pregnancy. Early Fetal Dev 1990;20:151-156.
33. Levi CS, Lyons EA, Zheng XH, et al: Endovaginal US: Demonstration of cardiac activity in embryos of less than 5.0 mm in crown-rump length. Radiology 1990;176:71-74.
34. Brown DL, Emerson DS, Felker RE, et al: Diagnosis of early embryonic demise by endovaginal sonography. J Ultrasound Med 1990;9:631-636.

35. Howe RS, Issacson K, Albert JL, Coutifaras CD: Embryonic heart rate in human pregnancy. J Ultrasound Med 1991;10:367-371.

36. Goldstein SR: Significance of cardiac activity on endovaginal ultrasound in very early embryos. Obstet Gynecol 1992;80:670-672.

37. Schatz R, Jansen CAM, Wladimiroff JW: Embryonic heart activity: Appearance and development in early human pregnancy. Br J Obstet Gynaecol 1990;97:989-994.

38. Timor-Tritsch IE: Pathology of the early intrauterine pregnancy. In Timor-Tritsch IE, Rottem S (eds): Transvaginal Sonography, 2nd ed. New York, Elsevier, 1991, p 299.

39. Laboda LA, Estroff JA, Benacerraf BR: First trimester bradycardia: A sign of impending fetal loss. J Ultrasound Med 1989;8:561-563.

40. Tejuka N, Sato S, Kanasugi H, Hiroi M: Embryonic heart rates: Development in early first trimester and clinical evaluation. Gynecol Obstet Invest 1991;32:210-212.

41. Benson CB, Doubilet PM: Slow embryonic heart rate in early first trimester: Indicator of poor pregnancy outcome. Radiology 1994;192:343-344.

42. Doubilet PM, Benson CB: Embryonic heart rate in the early first trimester: What rate is normal? J Ultrasound Med 1995;14:431-434.

43. Doubilet PM, Benson CB, Chow JS: Long-term prognosis of pregnancies complicated by slow embryonic heart rates in the early first trimester. J Ultrasound Med 1999;18:537-541.

44. Doubilet PM, Benson CB, Chow JS: Outcome of pregnancies with rapid embryonic heart rates in the early first trimester. AJR Am J Roentgenol 2000;175:67-69.

45. Vaccaro H, Amor F, Leyton M, Sepulveda W: Arrhythmia in early pregnancy: A predictor of first-trimester pregnancy loss. Ultrasound Obstet Gynecol 1998;12:248-251.

46. Machin GA: Why is it important to diagnose chorionicity and how do we do it [review]? Best Pract Res Clin Obstet Gynaecol 2004;18:515-530.

47. Warren WB, Timor-Tritsch IE, Peisner DB, et al: Dating the pregnancy by sequential appearance of embryonic structures. Am J Obstet Gynecol 1989;161:747-753.

48. Monteagudo A, Timor-Tritsch IE, Sharma S: Early and simple determination of chorionic and amniotic type in multifetal gestations in the first fourteen weeks by high-frequency transvaginal ultrasonography. Am J Obstet Gynecol 1994;170:824-829.

49. Bromley B, Benacerraf B: Using the number of yolk sacs to determine amnionicity in early first trimester monochorionic twins. J Ultrasound Med 1995;14:415-419.

50. Babinszki A, Mukherjee T, Kerenyi T, et al: Diagnosing amnionicity at 6 weeks of pregnancy with transvaginal three-dimensional ultrasonography: Case report. Fertil Steril 1999;71:1161-1164.

51. Bessis VA, Papiernik E: Echographic imagery of amniotic membranes in twin pregnancies. In Gedda L, Parisi P (eds): Twin Research. Vol. 3: Twin Biology and Multiple Pregnancy. New York, Alan R. Liss, 1981, pp 183-187.

52. Kurtz A, Mata J, Wapner R, et al: Twin pregnancies: Accuracy of first trimester abdominal US in predicting chorionicity and amnionicity. Radiology 1992;185:759-762.

53. Finberg HJ: The "twin peak" sign: Reliable evidence of dichorionic twinning. J Ultrasound Med 1992;11:571-577.

54. Monteagudo A: Sonographic assessment of chorionicity and amnionicity in twin pregnancies: How, when and why? Croat Med J 1998;39:191-196.

55. Hill LM, Chenevey P, Hecker J, Martin JG: Sonographic determination of first trimester twin chorionicity and amnionicity. J Clin Ultrasound 1996;24:305-308.

56. Monteagudo A, Timor-Tritsch IE: Second- and third-trimester ultrasound evaluation of chorionicity and amnionicity in twin pregnancy: A simple algorithm. J Reprod Med 2000;45:476-480.

57. Robinson HP, Fleming JEE: A critical evaluation of sonar crown-rump length measurement. Br J Obstet Gynaecol 1975;82:702-710.

58. MacGregor SN, Tamura RK, Sabbagha RE, et al: Underestimation of gestational age by conventional crown-rump length dating curves. Obstet Gynecol 1987;70:344-348.

59. Hadlock FP, Shah YP, Kanon DJ, Lindsey JV: Fetal crown-rump length: Reevaluation of relation to menstrual age (5 to 18 weeks) with high-resolution real-time US. Radiology 1992;1982:501-515.

60. Goldstein SR, Wolfson R: Endovaginal ultrasound measurement of early embryonic size as a means of assessing gestational age. J Ultrasound Med 1994;13:27-31.

Chapter 12

Pregnancy Failure

Steven R. Goldstein

Twenty-five percent of pregnancies bleed in the embryonic period. Of these, 50% will abort. Transvaginal sonography has become the standard approach for timely diagnosis of the failed pregnancy.

Threatened abortion is a clinical term, defined as a pregnancy of less than 20 weeks' gestation with vaginal bleeding in the presence of a closed cervical os. In the past, it was the most common indication for performing sonography in an early pregnancy. Ultrasound findings in most patients with threatened abortion show a normal-appearing intrauterine gestation (Fig. 12–1; findings depend on the age of the gestation) with no obvious reason for or source of the clinically apparent vaginal bleeding. If a definitive intrauterine gestation is identified based on the landmarks outlined in Chapter 11 or the presence of embryonic cardiac activity, then even if sonography does not indicate the cause of the vaginal bleeding, usually the bleeding will stop and the pregnancy progress.

Ectopic Pregnancy

All patients with a positive pregnancy test and vaginal bleeding must be examined to rule out an extrauterine pregnancy, which is diagnosed when a gestational sac is not evident in the uterus (Fig. 12–2). Heterotopic pregnancy (a simultaneous intrauterine and extrauterine pregnancy) is said to occur in 1 of 30,000 spontaneous pregnancies.[1] In women being treated with assisted reproductive technologies, this frequency increases to approximately 1 in 6000.[2,3] A diagnosis of ectopic pregnancy allows the clinician to proceed immediately to therapeutic intervention.

The combined sonographic–clinical approach to rule out ectopic pregnancy is complex. Intrauterine pregnancy is definitively defined clinically by the milestones outlined in Chapter 11, and a definitive intrauterine pregnancy viewed sonographically virtually excludes ectopic pregnancy. However, if no intrauterine gestation is seen on ultrasound (Fig. 12–3), the quantitative human chorionic gonadotropins (hCG) level must be determined, and the concept of a discriminatory level (described in Chapter 11) applied. If the hCG level is less than the discriminatory level, serial β-subunit determination must be made (current assays, however, actually measure the intact hCG molecule). In a normal pregnancy the hCG will rise a minimum of 66% every 48 hours, or effectively double every 2 to 3 days. Once the hCG level surpasses a discriminatory level, an intrauterine gestation should be able to be imaged. The absence of an intrauterine gestation suggests that the pregnancy is not capable of continuing (i.e., it represents either a failing intrauterine gestation or an extrauterine pregnancy). Similarly, a subnormal rate of rise of hCG also indicates a failing intrauterine gestation or extrauterine pregnancy.

When ongoing normal pregnancy has been excluded, curettage and examination of tissue for the presence or absence of chorionic villi may be useful to distinguish an intrauterine gestation from an ectopic gestation. The presence of chorionic villi (Fig. 12–4) proves an intrauterine gestation. The presence of only decidual tissue (Fig. 12–5) raises the index of suspicion for an ectopic pregnancy, although, especially when the patient has experienced bleeding, complete abortion (possibly tubal abortion, as well) can account for such findings. Follow-up quantitative hCG level, which may be rising, plateauing, or falling, may help to distinguish an ectopic gestation from completed abortion (Fig. 12–6).

A new category of "early pregnancy failure of unknown location" is emerging. This label is applied when hCG levels are low and not rising at the expected rate, but neither are they falling to levels with which the clinician is comfortable in choosing expectant observation. A single injection of methotrexate will reliably eradicate any lingering trophoblastic tissue, regardless of its location. The clinician must determine which is better for an individual patient—a single injection of methotrexate, assuming none of the contraindications,[4] or dilation and curettage (D&C). If the D&C shows no chorionic villi, such a patient would need an injection of methotrexate anyway to eradicate any lingering trophoblastic tissue. Banerjee et al.[5] prospectively studied 1625 women with pregnancy and bleeding or pain. In 135 (8%) of the patients, the location of the gestation by transvaginal sonography was unknown. Using serial hCG, observation, and follow-up ultrasound, the definitive diagnosis proved to be intrauterine gestation in 27%, pregnancy failure in 9%, definitive ectopic pregnancy in 14%, and spontaneous resolution without determination of location (i.e., completed abortion, possibly tubal) in 50%. Based on these findings, routine use of D&C in patients with a pregnancy failure of unknown location would result in 73% ultimately having a D&C. If one is willing to bypass D&C, however, then only 9% of patients would receive a single course of unnecessary methotrexate. It is important

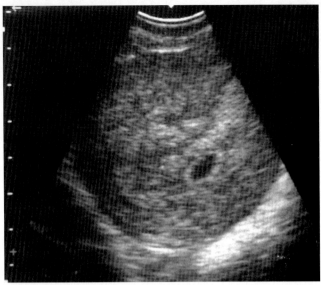

Figure 12–1. Patient with uncertain date of last menstrual period, positive home pregnancy test, vaginal spotting, and a closed cervical os. Sonogram reveals an intrauterine gestation, thereby practically excluding ectopic pregnancy.

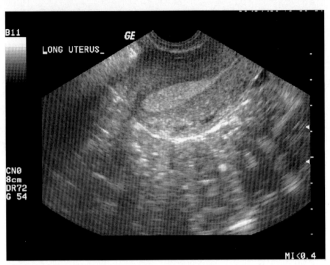

Figure 12–3. Patient with positive home pregnancy test and vaginal staining noted clinically. Long-axis view of the uterus reveals nondiagnostic echogenic endometrium without evidence of any intrauterine gestation. Quantitative human chorionic gonadotropin level was 420 mIU/mL (IRP). Subsequent follow-up revealed development of a normal gestation and ultimate delivery of a liveborn, healthy infant.

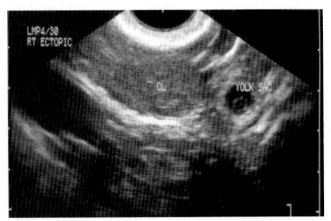

Figure 12–2. Patient at 40 days after last menstrual period with vaginal spotting. Scan reveals a normal-appearing right ovary that contains a corpus luteum (CL). Adjacent to the ovary is an extrauterine gestational sac containing a normal-appearing yolk sac. Such a definitive diagnosis of extrauterine gestation allows for immediate therapeutic intervention.

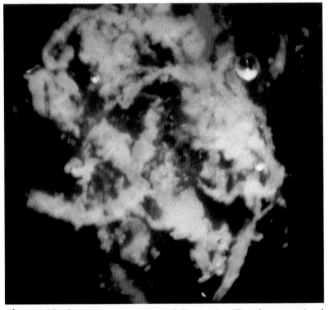

Figure 12–4. High-power view of chorionic villi. When examined grossly, it is sometimes said that the villi float. It is our experience that they do not float, but sink very slowly.

to know that inadvertent administration of methotrexate in an early ongoing intrauterine gestation that has not failed has been associated with multiple fetal abnormalities.[6] Thus, ultrasound and hCG should be used properly and consistently for diagnosis, and close follow-up is mandatory.

The ability to recognize a pregnancy sonographically depends not on the pregnancy's location but on its appearance. The more normal the gestation appears, the more likely it will be recognized as a pregnancy, regardless of whether it is located inside or outside the uterus. Similarly, the concept that extrauterine ultrasound findings reflect in vivo findings is important, because the more one appreciates the in vivo range of appearances for an entity, the better one understands why the ultrasound images appear the way they do. Figures

12–7 through 12–10 should be carefully examined. Although Figure 12–7 is an outdated static arm scan with mediocre resolution, it shows a cornual pregnancy that has developed to a 13-week size in a relatively normal anatomic manner, as cornual pregnancies often do. The scan in Figure 12–8 looks somewhat nondescript because, although it was identified as an ectopic pregnancy, the hCG was only 850 mIU/mL (International Reference Preparation [IRP]), and it is mainly hematosalpinx with some disorganized villi, blood clots, and

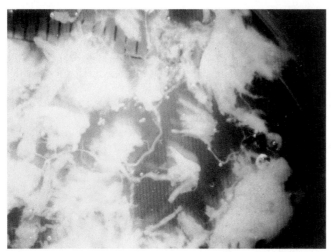

Figure 12–5. Petri dish filled with maternal decidual tissue. The ability to distinguish this tissue from villus is an essential step in ruling out ectopic pregnancy.

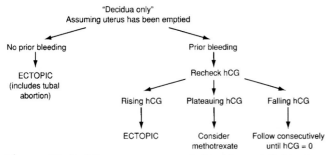

Figure 12–6. When curettage reveals "decidua only," this algorithm maps appropriate clinical management. It is assumed that the uterus has been emptied.

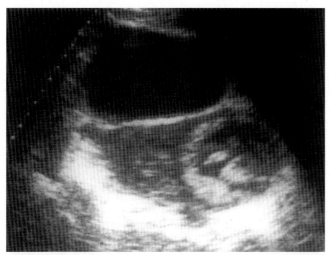

Figure 12–7. Static arm scan of a patient with a cornual pregnancy at 13 weeks since last menstrual period. Even with this level of resolution, one can appreciate the fetal structure (see Fig. 12–9).

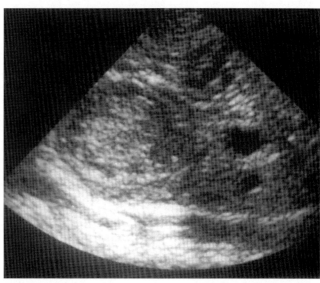

Figure 12–8. Patient with an ectopic pregnancy. The findings here are somewhat nondiagnostic (see Fig. 12–10).

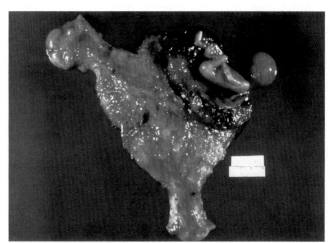

Figure 12–9. Pathology specimen from the patient in Figure 12–7. The sonogram in Figure 12–7 appears as it does exactly because of the appearance of the in vivo specimen.

fibrin. It does not look like a pregnancy (see Figs. 12–1 and 12–2) on ultrasound because it failed to recapitulate a normal gestation.

Fifteen percent to 28% of ectopic pregnancies develop to the point of yolk sac formation or cardiac activity.[7,8] Some-

times, these pregnancies follow the normal hCG doubling times. In such pregnancies, the familiar gestational sac appearance with its sonolucent center will be visible outside the uterus on ultrasound. This is especially true if there is cardiac activity present. Nevertheless, not all sonolucent or complex adnexal structures are extrauterine gestations. The ovaries should be identified on the side in question to avoid misidentifying a corpus luteum or corpus luteum cyst as an extrauterine gestation (see Fig. 12–2). Free fluid in the cul-de-sac may be helpful in diagnosing ectopic pregnancy but is not pathognomonic, being present in 41% to 83% of extrauterine pregnancies.[7,9] Finally, some intrauterine fluid collections may look like gestational sacs. The presence of the yolk sac precludes a diagnosis of such "pseudosacs." If any doubt exists about the legitimacy or normality of a gestational sac before the yolk sac or embryo is present, follow-up sonography is warranted.

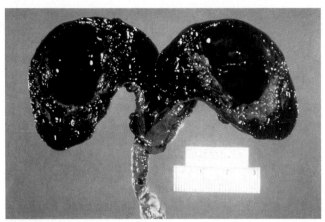

Figure 12–10. Pathology specimen on the tube removed from the patient in Figure 12–8. Note that this ectopic pregnancy is a mass of disorganized villi, blood clots, and fibrin. The appearance on ultrasound thus reflects the in vivo appearance.

Intrauterine Pregnancy Failure

Once the diagnosis of an intrauterine gestation is firmly established by ultrasound criteria, with or without serial hCG determination, further questions may arise regarding the normality of that gestation. Researchers have long attempted to identify parameters, both sonographic and biochemical, that would enhance our prognostic capacity in cases of threatened abortion.[10] Various biochemical markers have been investigated, including hCG, serum progesterone, and even serum human placental lactogen levels. On transabdominal sonography, the presence of a fetal heartbeat was found to be associated with an approximately 95% continuation rate.[11] This ultrasound finding appeared to be a better prognosticator than any of the aforementioned biochemical markers.

Appearance of Gestational Sac

Previously, a so-called blighted ovum was thought of as an anembryonic pregnancy.[12] On transabdominal sonography, this was defined by a gestational sac with a mean diameter greater than 20 mm without a yolk sac, as determined in the classic work by Nyberg and colleagues[13] on the major and minor criteria of abnormal gestational sacs. The vaginal probe has further refined these definitions. It would appear that once the mean sac diameter exceeds 8 to 13 mm (measurement including only the sonolucent portion of the chorionic cavity), a yolk sac should become visible.[14,15] However, the important issue is not how early one can see a yolk sac (threshold level), but rather at what point the lack of such a structure is absolutely pathognomonic of nonviable pregnancy, especially allowing for variability in equipment, biology, and measuring error. This also depends on transducer frequency (see Chapter 11).[16]

Embryonic Cardiac Activity

The S-shaped endothelial heart tube folds on itself and begins to beat by 21 days postconception. Thus, it is present and beating in normal pregnancy before it can be imaged with the equipment available today (at 34.8 ± 2.2 days). Occasionally, placement of an M-mode cursor can document cardiac activity on the edge of the yolk sac.[17]

The important issue is at what point the absence of cardiac activity is a definitive sign of pregnancy failure. Some investigators have attempted to relate cardiac activity to hCG levels, to determine what may be called "discriminatory" hCG levels for the first detectable heart activity. These levels show a wide range, from 6636 to 26,356 mIU/mL (IRP).[18-21] The use of "threshold" hCG levels will be fraught with error because of the different standards in units expressing hCG and conversion between them, the low reproducibility of quantitative levels from laboratory to laboratory, and differences in transducers used and scanning routes.

Because the ability to image cardiac activity depends on the type and frequency range of the equipment used, the degree of magnification available, the visual acuity of the operator, and any confounding anatomic variables (e.g., maternal obesity, coexisting myomas), it is preferable to relate the presence or absence of cardiac activity to embryonic size. By any criteria, cardiac motion is always present by embryonic size of 5-mm or more.[22-25] Thus, embryos of 4 mm or less without discernible cardiac activity should have a follow-up examination.

Embryonic Resorption

Use of the vaginal probe has led to the realization that many "blighted ova," so named because of the appearance of an empty sac when imaged by transabdominal scanning, are really cases of intrauterine pregnancy failure with subsequent embryonic resorption. The vaginal probe has often imaged a small embryonic structure of 2 to 4 mm with cardiac activity, only to demonstrate when the patient returns 2 weeks later what appears to be a large, empty sac, although sometimes a small remaining embryonic structure can still be visualized (Fig. 12–11). What we see sonographically depends on at what stage in development viability is lost and the resorption process begins, and at what stage in the resorption process we study the patient. Certainly, resorption explains the process by

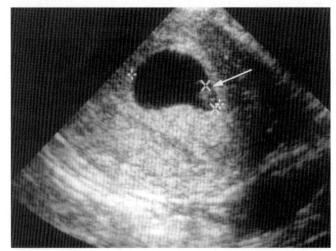

Figure 12–11. A 6-mm amorphous embryonic structure in the corner of the gestational sac (arrow). Two weeks earlier, there had been a 4-mm embryo with discernible cardiac activity. This is an example of embryonic demise with resorption. In the past, when examined transabdominally, such cases gave the appearance of a seemingly empty sac and hence were referred to as "blighted ovum" or "anembryonic pregnancy." This phenomenon actually represents embryonic demise with resorption.

which a multiple pregnancy is spontaneously reduced to a singleton (previously called the "vanishing twin"; Fig. 12–12).

The incidence of chromosomal abnormalities is generally reported to be higher in such cases of early pregnancy failure.[26-28] Ultrasound abnormalities may be seen in these cases before the embryo is visualized but after the yolk sac has become apparent. Often such a yolk sac is enlarged,[29] "floating," or poorly formed or even solid (Fig. 12–13). An abnormal yolk sac is a nonspecific sign of actual or impending embryonic demise but is seen in cases with both normal and abnormal karyotypes.

The yolk sac, embryonic disc, and amnion are present in the earliest gestational sac, but they are too small to be imaged even with the highest-frequency vaginal probes. The yolk sac portion of this complex is imaged first as the complex enlarges. This prominence is due to its sonolucent center and echogenic rim, which make it appear very bright and distinct as opposed to the early, ambiguously echogenic thickening of the embryo, which, as already discussed, is best recognized at this very early stage by its cardiac pulsations. The endothelial heart tube has folded on itself by 21 days postconception, and the cardiovascular system is the first organ system to form in the developing embryo. It, too, is present and active before it can be imaged by current techniques.[17]

The hCG levels in pathologic pregnancies, whether rising or falling, and at what rate, are a function of the condition of trophoblastic tissues, not the embryonic structures. Sonographically, the trophoblast is depicted as an echogenic rind (trophoblastic decidual reaction). Many cases of intrauterine pregnancy failure are accompanied by high levels of hCG and seemingly normal-appearing villi at curettage. Others have much lower hCG levels associated with a very weak trophoblastic decidual reaction sonographically. These findings may represent separate etiologies for failure, with mechanisms such as poor implantation, inadequate blood supply, or poor flow, as opppposed to a "fetal factor" such as abnormal chromosomal number or poor embryonic cleavage. However, the different findings may also represent the same process observed at different points along a naturally occurring continuum.

Subchorionic Hemorrhage

The finding of subchorionic bleeding has been shown to enhance our prognostic capability in cases of threatened abortion. Subchorionic hemorrhage appears as a crescent-shaped, sonolucent collection outside of the chorionic sac in a patient with threatened abortion (Fig. 12–14). In an early description of the condition,[10] patients with fetal heart activity and no evidence of subchorionic bleeding had a pregnancy continuation rate that approached 100%. In patients with fetal heart activity along with evidence of subchorionic bleeding, the continuation rate seemed to be in the range of 60% to 70%. There appeared to be no good correlation between the size and amount of subchorionic blood and the eventual outcome. Subchorionic bleeding manifests in approximately 20% of cases of threatened abortion.

Full-term pregnancy outcomes also may be less favorable in the presence of such subchorionic hematomas. The risk of preterm delivery is increased fourfold ($P = .009$) in patients with subchorionic hematomas.[30] Furthermore, in a prospective study of 187 pregnant women with intrauterine hematomas and 6488 control subjects in whom hematomas were not detected in early pregnancy, the incidence of pregnancy-induced hypertension was increased twofold, preeclampsia fourfold, and placental abruption fivefold in the group with intrauterine hematomas, suggesting that presence of an intrauterine hematoma may identify a population of patients at increased risk for adverse pregnancy outcome.[31]

Hydatidiform Mole

The classic ultrasound appearance of a hydatidiform mole is that of multiple small, sonolucent areas (Figs. 12–15 and 12–16) that correspond to the grapelike vesicles seen on gross pathologic examination. These features rarely are sonographically apparent before 10 weeks' postmenstrual age because the trophoblastic proliferation and hydropic changes seen grossly with hydatidiform mole are not yet present. However, we expect to see an increase in the number of cases diagnosed by microscopic pathology after a diagnosis of intrauterine pregnancy failure has been made sonographically. There is evidence suggesting that more widespread use of transvaginal sonography has resulted in a decrease in the incidence of molar pregnancy, presumably because products of conception are evacuated before they can undergo further hydropic change and proliferation.[32,33]

Chromosomal Pregnancy Loss

Studies have shown that in up to 70% of spontaneous abortions, the conceptus exhibits chromosomal abnormality.[26,27,34] Most of these are numeric abnormalities due to errors occurring during gonadogenesis (chromosomal nondisjunction during meiosis), fertilization (triploidy from digyny or dispermy), or the first division of the fertilized ovum (tetraploidy or mosaicism). Overall, two thirds of the abnormalities are autosomal trisomies, followed by monosomy X and structural rearrangements. Thus, except for a very small percentage of parental balanced translocations or inversions, the overwhelming majority of women whose failed pregnancies have

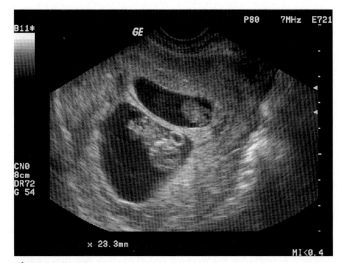

Figure 12–12. Example of a vanishing twin. One sac contains a 23-mm embryo with normal yolk sac and cardiac activity. Adjacent to it is a second sac with a 7-mm embryo that has demised and begun to resorb. In a follow-up scan 2 weeks later, there was normal progression of a singleton pregnancy without discernible evidence of the prior second sac.

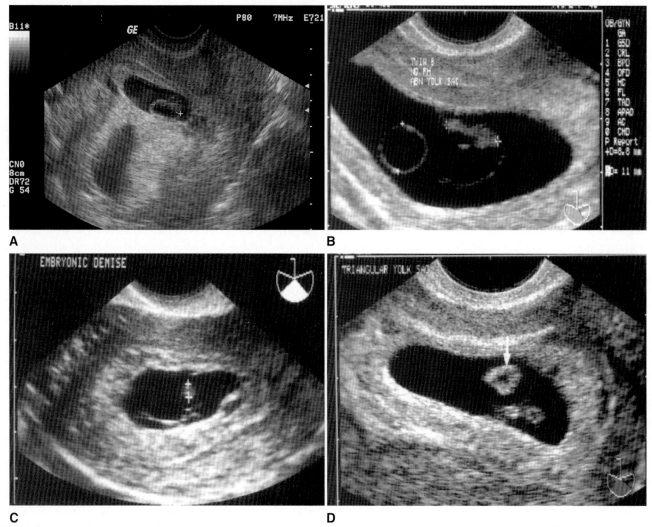

Figure 12–13. **A,** Abnormal yolk sac, ovoid in appearance and with an 11.6-mm greatest diameter, indicative of pregnancy failure. **B,** Twin pregnancy with hydropic enlarged yolk sac measuring 8.8 mm. Embryonic structure of 11 mm adjacent to it had no discernible cardiac activity. This is an intrauterine pregnancy failure. **C,** Irregular, enlarged hydropic yolk sac with 2.8-mm embryonic thickening *(calipers)*. This is another presentation of early embryonic demise. **D,** Triangular yolk sac that is abnormal in appearance *(arrow)*. Adjacent to it is an amorphous embryonic structure of 7 mm with no discernible cardiac activity, another of the many appearances of the abnormal yolk sac associated with embryonic demise and resorption.

abnormal karyotypes would not be expected to experience recurrent pregnancy failure.

Nonchromosomal Pregnancy Failure

Presumably, however, the 30% of women with early pregnancy losses in which the conceptus shows a normal karyotype are at greater risk for subsequent loss.

Some uterine abnormalities (e.g., in utero diethylstilbestrol exposure, intrauterine adhesions, and incompetent cervix) are suspected based on the clinical history. Others (e.g., congenital müllerian defects, submucous myomas, polyps), however, do not necessarily lend themselves to diagnosis by history or simple bimanual pelvic examination. Further diagnostic work-up (i.e., saline infusion sonohysterography[35] or conventional radiographic hysterosalpingography) is usually required. Some of the issues surrounding intracavitary pathologic processes and congenital uterine anomalies, and their

sonographic features, are discussed in Chapters 5 and 7. Endocrine causes, such as luteal phase deficiency, may also require further work-up in terms of invasive endometrial sampling.

Immunologic factors have been implicated in early pregnancy loss. Human leukocyte antigens (HLA) of the major histocompatibility complex may cause the maternal immune system to fail to produce blocking antibody, thus rejecting the fetus because it produces foreign antigens. Although some clinicians do HLA typing on both partners in cases of recurrent pregnancy failure, there is controversy over whether this is truly a cause of pregnancy loss.[36-38]

The presence of lupus anticoagulant as well as elevated levels of certain antiphospholipid antibodies, particularly anticardiolipin antibody, are associated with an increased risk of spontaneous abortion.[39] Ten percent of women with recurrent spontaneous abortion of undetermined etiology have

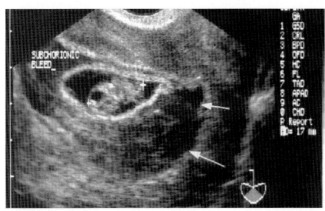

Figure 12–14. Patient with clinical history of vaginal bleeding and closed cervical os (i.e., "threatened abortion"). Note the area of blood outside the gestational sac *(arrows),* which is the classic presentation of subchorionic hemorrhage. This lowers the pregnancy continuation rate to 60% to 70%. There is no good correlation between the ultrasonically detectable amount of blood and the eventual outcome.

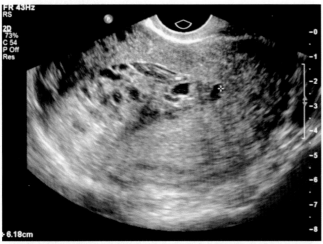

Figure 12–15. Long-axis view of hydatidiform mole 12 weeks after last menstrual period. Note that the entire uterine cavity is filled with multiple sonolucent areas. This corresponds to the typical grapelike vesicles seen on gross pathology.

lupus anticoagulant activity, whereas 13% to 40% of such individuals have anticardiolipin antibody.[40] We do not know of any sonographically detectable features of pregnancy failures caused by these factors.

Infectious agents in the cervix, uterine cavity, or seminal fluid have been implicated as etiologic factors for abortion. Although clinical endometritis due to any infectious agent can produce pregnancy loss, it is less clear whether subclinical infection can and, if so, with what organisms. The T-strain mycoplasmas, both *Ureaplasma urealyticum* and *Mycoplasma hominis,* have been suggested as causes of abortion. Endometrial colonization with *U. urealyticum* is associated with increased risk of pregnancy loss, whereas cervical colonization apparently is not.[41]

Increased pregnancy loss is also associated with maternal smoking and maternal alcohol ingestion. These risks, however, can be evaluated with historical data.

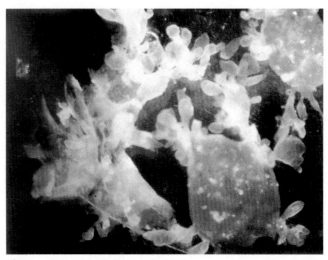

Figure 12–16. Modified gross pathologic appearance of early mole at 7 weeks after last menstrual period. Sonographically, this appeared simply as a case of intrauterine pregnancy failure. The typical sonolucent structures shown in Figure 12–15 were not yet present. However, the villi coming off the chorionic membrane are seen here to be obviously hydropic.

New Approach to the Patient with Pregnancy Failure

Cytogenetic analysis of the conceptus of a failed pregnancy will be helpful in subsequent management. If the conceptus is chromosomally normal, the couple should undergo evaluation for the various other causes discussed under Nonchromosomal Pregnancy Failure, earlier. If, however, the chromosomes of the conceptus are abnormal, then no further work-up or evaluation is necessary at that point, and the likelihood of recurrent loss is very small (unless multiple factors are at play).

Two advances have made chromosomal analysis possible. First, the use of high-resolution transvaginal ultrasound transducers has enhanced our understanding of early pregnancy and its normal milestones, making it possible to consistently diagnose pregnancy failure before spontaneous passage of the conceptus. In my private practice, I have not had a patient with spontaneous abortion in more than 15 years: The pregnancy failure rate has not changed, but virtually every case has been diagnosed before miscarriage. Ultrasound is used at the first examination after the missed menses, usually accompanied by a positive home monoclonal antibody pregnancy test. The patient returns every 2 weeks until embryonic size is greater than 10 mm and cardiac activity is present. The embryonic loss rate at that point is less than 1%.[42] If intrauterine pregnancy failure is diagnosed sonographically, elective D&C can be carried out the following day, before the patient experiences cramping, bleeding, and spontaneous passage of the conceptus (Fig. 12–17).

The second advance is our ability routinely to examine embryonic tissue at the time of curettage. Such embryonic tissue can be easily used for cytogenetic evaluation. Although initially performed to diagnose unsuspected ectopic pregnancy at the time of elective termination,[43] such tissue

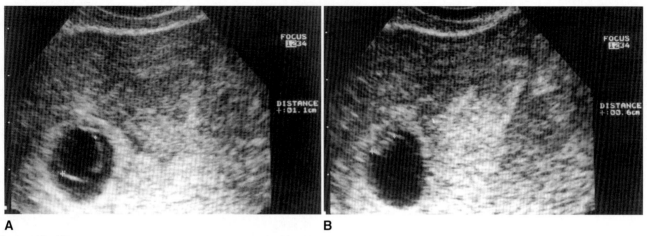

A   **B**

Figure 12–17. **A,** Patient at 54 days after last menstrual period. This intrauterine gestational sac reveals an enlarged, hydropic yolk sac measuring 11 mm *(calipers).* **B,** Adjacent to the hydropic yolk sac is a 6-mm embryonic structure *(calipers),* which showed normal cardiac activity.

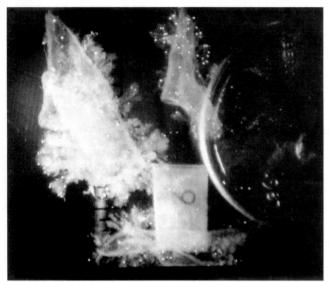

Figure 12–18. Portion of chorionic membrane with attached villi, with Lincoln penny for size reference. The ability to distinguish this tissue from maternal decidua is of utmost importance in cases of ruling out ectopic pregnancy as well as in offering patients the option of chromosomal analysis in cases of pregnancy failure.

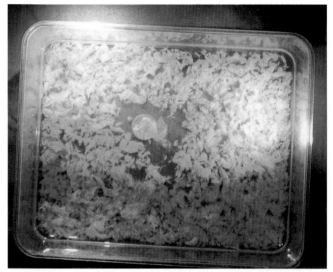

Figure 12–19. The "products of conception" displayed in a Pyrex cooking dish. The chorionic sac to the right of the Lincoln penny is a normal size for 6 to 7 weeks after last menstrual period. There is a voluminous amount of homogeneous decidua because the patient has a 12-week-sized uterus with intramural fibroid changes, resulting in an increased endometrial cavity surface area. This surface area becomes decidualized in pregnancy, and the amount of decidua present is a function of the size of the cavity, not the length of the gestation. The entire specimen is sent for chromosomal analysis. It is easy to understand how there may be contamination with maternal decidua. Furthermore, in cases where it is necessary to rule out ectopic pregnancy, if one simply sends the entire products of conception, it is understandable how the pathologist might miss the small portion of chorionic sac.

examination in cases of failed intrauterine pregnancy allows a portion of chorion and attached villi to be separated from maternal decidua and submitted for chromosomal study (Fig. 12–18). This avoids the maternal decidual contamination (46XX) that precludes simply submitting products of conception from curettage for chromosomal studies (Fig. 12–19). In addition, normal cells grow better in tissue culture. It seems plausible that some of the older studies looking at rates of abnormal karyotypes in spontaneous abortions may have underestimated the incidence of abnormal karyotypes because contamination with karyotypically normal maternal decidua (i.e., 46XX) may have raised the false-negative rate.[44]

The 70% of women with abnormal karyotypes require no further evaluation and do not need to delay conceiving again.

The 30% of failed pregnancies with normal karyotypes need not await subsequent loss but can immediately be evaluated, as clinically suspected or indicated, for a variety of other causes, such as lupus anticoagulant and anticardiolipin antibodies, luteal phase deficiencies, endometrial (and possible cervical) *U. urealyticum* infection, congenital müllerian abnormalities, and submucous myomas.

Avoiding Pitfalls

There are some practical guidelines for the clinician to keep in mind to avoid pitfalls when dealing with suspected cases of pregnancy failure. For all practical purposes, the presence of an intrauterine gestation excludes ectopic pregnancy. Once ectopic pregnancy is ruled out, embryonic well-being is proved by normal progression on serial sonograms, and not by serial hCG determinations. The gestational sac grows approximately 1 mm/day.[45] Less important than how early one can see cardiac activity is the point at which the pregnancy is definitively nonviable if cardiac activity is not seen. The ability to see cardiac activity depends on the normality of the pregnancy, the type and frequency of equipment used, the degree of image magnification, and the operator's visual acuity.

Once ectopic pregnancy is ruled out, the clinician should use the sonographic landmarks discussed in Chapter 11 and this chapter to distinguish normal pregnancies from those pregnancies destined to fail. By the time an embryo reaches 5 mm, cardiac activity must be seen sonographically if the outcome is to be normal.[22-25] Our goal should be to allow not one normal, wanted intrauterine gestation to be unnecessarily interrupted because of our zeal to diagnose pregnancy failure as early as possible. Very early gestations, as long as they are definitively intrauterine, can undergo follow-up ultrasound and are very unlikely to be associated with significant bleeding or infection if spontaneously passed. If there is even the slightest doubt about normality, the clinician should always be as conservative as possible when conducting follow-up examinations to evaluate progression.

Summary

Transvaginal sonography and a better understanding of anatomic landmarks and expected growth rates can improve clinical management and patient counseling.

REFERENCES

1. DeVoe RW, Pratt JH: Simultaneous intrauterine and extrauterine pregnancy. Am J Obstet Gynecol 1948;56:1119-1126.
2. Gamberdella FR, Marrs RP: Heterotopic pregnancy associated with assisted reproductive technology. Am J Obstet Gynecol 1989;160:1520-1524.
3. Fernandez H, Gervaise A: Ectopic pregnancies after infertility treatment: Modern diagnosis and therapeutic strategy. Hum Reprod Update 2004;10:503-513.
4. American College of Obstetricians and Gynecologists: Medical Management of Tubal Pregnancy: ACOG Practice Bulletin Number 3. Washington, DC, American College of Obstetricians and Gynecologists, 1998.
5. Banerjee S, Aslam N, Zosmer N, et al: The expectant management of women with early pregnancy of unknown location. Ultrasound Obstet Gynecol 1999;14:231-236.
6. Nguyen C, Duhl AJ, Escallon CS, et al: Multiple anomalies in a fetus exposed to low-dose methotrexate in the first trimester. Obstet Gynecol 2002;99:599-602.
7. Stiller RJ, de Regt RH, Blair E: Transvaginal ultrasonography in patients at risk for ectopic pregnancy. Am J Obstet Gynecol 1989;161:930-933.
8. Fleischer AC, Pennell RG, McKee MS, et al: Ectopic pregnancy: Features at transvaginal sonography. Radiology 1990;174:375-378.
9. de Crespigny LC: Demonstration of ectopic pregnancy by transvaginal ultrasound. Br J Obstet Gynaecol 1988;95:1253-1256.
10. Goldstein SR, Subramonyan BR, Raghavenolre BN, et al: Subchorionic bleeding in threatened abortion: Sonographic findings and significance. AJR Am J Roentgenol 1983;141:975-978.
11. Wilson RD, Kendrick V, Wittman BK, et al: Spontaneous abortion and pregnancy outcome after normal first trimester ultrasound examination. Obstet Gynecol 1986;67:352-355.
12. Nyberg DA, Laing C: Threatened abortion and abnormal first trimester intrauterine pregnancy. In Nyberg DA, Hill LM, Bohm-Velez M, Mendelson E (eds): Transvaginal Ultrasound. St. Louis, Mosby Yearbook, 1992, p 86.
13. Nyberg D, Filly R, Filho D, et al: Abnormal pregnancy: Early diagnosis by ultrasound and serum chorionic gonadotropin levels. Radiology 1986;158:393-396.
14. Elson J, Salim R, Tailor A, et al: Prediction of early pregnancy viability in the absence of an ultrasonically detectable embryo. Ultrasound Obstet Gynecol 2003;21:57-61.
15. Stampone C, Nicotra M, Muttinelli C, Cosmi EV: Transvaginal sonography of the yolk sac in normal and abnormal pregnancy. J Clin Ultrasound 1996;24:3-9.
16. Goldstein SR, Snyder JR, Watson C, et al: Very early pregnancy detection with endovaginal ultrasound. Obstet Gynecol 1988;72:200-204.
17. Fine C, Cartier M, Doubilet P: Fetal heart rates: Values throughout gestation. J Ultrasound Med 1988;7(Suppl):39-40.
18. Fossum GT, Davajan V, Kletzky OA: Early detection of pregnancy with transvaginal US. Fertil Steril 1988;49:788-791.
19. Schouwink MH, Fong BF, Mol BW, van der Veen F: Ultrasonographic criteria for non-viability of first trimester intra-uterine pregnancy. Early Pregnancy 2000;4:203-213.
20. Bree RL, Edwards M, Bohm-Velez M, et al: Transvaginal sonography in the evaluation of normal early pregnancy: Correlation with hCG level. AJR Am J Roentgenol 1989;153:75-79.
21. Bateman BG, Nunley WC, Kolp LA, et al: Vaginal sonography findings and hCG dynamics of early intrauterine and tubal pregnancies. Obstet Gynecol 1990;75:421-427.
22. Goldstein SR: Significance of cardiac activity on endovaginal ultrasound in very early embryos. Obstet Gynecol 1992;80:670-672.
23. Steinkampf MP, Guzick DS, Hammond KR, Blackwell RE: Identification of early pregnancy landmarks by transvaginal sonography: Analysis by logistic regression. Fertil Steril 1997;68:168-170.
24. Levi CS, Lyons EA, Zheng FIX, et al: Endovaginal US: Demonstration of cardiac activity in embryos of less than 5 mm in crown-rump length. Radiology 1990;176:71-74.
25. Brown DL, Emerson DS, Felker RE, et al: Diagnosis of early embryonic demise by endovaginal sonography. J Ultrasound Med 1990;9:711-716.
26. Ohno M, Maeda T, Matsunobo A: A cytogenetic study of spontaneous abortions with direct analysis of chorionic villi. Obstet Gynecol 1991;77:394-398.
27. Schmidt-Sarosi C, Schwartz LB, Lublin J, et al: Chromosomal analysis of early fetal losses in relation to transvaginal ultrasonographic detection of fetal heart motion after infertility. Fertil Steril 1998;69:274-277.
28. Coulam CB, Goodman C, Dorfmann A: Comparison of ultrasonographic findings in spontaneous abortions with normal and abnormal karyotypes. Hum Reprod 1997;12:823-826.
29. Lindsay DJ, Lovett IS, Lyons EA, et al: Early diagnosis of nonviable pregnancy with endovaginal ultrasound. Radiology 1992;183:115-118.
30. Sharma G, Kalish RB, Chasen ST: Prognostic factors associated with antenatal subchorionic echolucencies. Am J Obstet Gynecol 2003;189:994-996.
31. Nagy S, Bush M, Stone J, et al: Clinical significance of subchorionic and retroplacental hematomas detected in the first trimester of pregnancy. Obstet Gynecol 2003;102:94-100.
32. Jakob A Jr, Overi L, Ditroi P, et al: How does first trimester ultrasound influence the incidence of molar pregnancies? Ultrasound Obstet Gynecol 1994;4:50.
33. Sasaki S: Clinical presentation and management of molar pregnancy [review]. Best Pract Res Clin Obstet Gynaecol 2003;17:885-892.
34. Kajii T, Ferrier A, Niikawa N, et al: Anatomic and chromosomal anomalies in 639 spontaneous abortuses. Hum Genet 1980;55:87-98.
35. Goldstein SR: Use of ultrasonohysterography for triage of perimenopausal patients with unexplained uterine bleeding. Am J Obstet Gynecol 1994;170:565-570.
36. Backos M, Rai R, Regan L: Antiphospholipid antibodies and infertility [review]. Hum Fertil (Camb) 2002;5:30-34.
37. Smith JB, Cowchock FS: Immunological studies in recurrent spontaneous abortion: Effects of immunization of women with paternal mononuclear cells on lymphocytotoxic and mixed lymphocyte reaction blocking antibodies and correlation with sharing of HLA and pregnancy outcome. J Reprod Immunol 1988;14:99-113.
38. Krabbendam I, Dekker GA: Pregnancy outcome in patients with a history of recurrent spontaneous miscarriages and documented thrombophilias. Gynecol Obstet Invest 2004;57:127-131.

39. Deleze M, Alarcon-Segovia D, Valdes-Macho E, et al: Relationship between antiphospholipid antibodies and recurrent fetal loss in patients with systemic lupus erythematosus and apparently healthy women. J Rheumatol 1989;16:768-772.
40. Mishell DR: Recurrent abortion. J Reprod Med 1993;38:250-259.
41. Stray-Pedersen B, Eng J, Reikvan TM: Uterine T-mycoplasma colonization in reproductive failure. Am J Obstet Gynecol 1978;130:307-311.
42. Goldstein SR: Embryonic demise in early pregnancy: A new look at the first trimester. Obstet Gynecol 1994;84:294-297.
43. Goldstein SR, Snyder JR, Watson C, Danon M: Combined sonographic-pathologic surveillance in elective first-trimester termination of pregnancy. Obstet Gynecol 1988;71:747-750.
44. Goldstein SR, Kerenyi T, Scher J, Papp C: Correlation between karyotype and ultrasound findings in patients with failed early pregnancy. Ultrasound Obstet Gynecol 1996;8:314-317.
45. Nyberg DA, Mack LA, Laing FC, Patten RM: Distinguishing normal from abnormal gestational sac growth in early pregnancy. J Ultrasound Med 1988;6:23-27.

Chapter 13

Ectopic Pregnancy

Faye C. Laing

In the United States, the incidence of ectopic pregnancy (EP) continues to rise such that it has reached epidemic proportions. Statistics for the last decade are not readily available, but during the 19-year interval between 1970 and 1989, the reported number of hospitalizations almost quintupled, increasing from 17,800 to more than 88,400.[1] In 1992, EPs accounted for approximately 2% of reported pregnancies, and EP-related deaths accounted for 9% of all pregnancy-related deaths.[2]

Factors contributing to the increased incidence of EP include improved therapy for salpingitis that results in scarred, albeit patent fallopian tubes; surgical procedures such as tuboplasty with a subsequent pregnancy; pregnancy in women with a history of EP who have not undergone salpingectomy; and an increasing population of women undergoing assisted reproduction procedures. Despite the increasing incidence of EP, hospitalizations for this condition have decreased dramatically. In 1992, hospitalizations occurred in approximately 50% of cases, reflecting improved methods for earlier diagnosis and the introduction of more conservative outpatient therapies.[3]

The role of ultrasound in EP is expanding. Its primary role remains diagnosis. More recently introduced applications include screening women at high risk for development of an EP, providing information that can be used to determine therapy in women with a documented EP, providing guidance (either transabdominally or transvaginally) for injecting either methotrexate or potassium chloride (KCl) to ablate a visible EP, and serially monitoring women with EP who are treated with systemic methotrexate or who are followed expectantly. This chapter focuses on elucidating an ultrasound strategy that will optimize its application in women with suspected or proven EP.

Role of Ultrasound in Diagnosing Ectopic Pregnancy

Clinical Considerations

The clinical triad of bleeding, pain, and a palpable mass has been reported as "classic" for EP. If this classic presentation were both sensitive and specific for EP, it would be very attractive from a clinical perspective. Unfortunately, this has not proven to be the case. In one study of more than 200 patients who were clinically suspected of having EP, only 10% to 15% with the triad had one, and of those who did have an EP, the classic clinical triad was present only 45% of the time.[4] Most patients with these clinical findings are not even pregnant and have pelvic inflammatory disease, a ruptured ovarian cyst, or pain of unknown etiology. Because the clinical evaluation of patients at risk for EP is so limited, it is important for clinicians to have a low threshold for ordering reliable diagnostic tests to distinguish between the diagnostic possibilities and specifically to identify women with an EP. At the forefront for evaluating these patients is sonography, with a transvaginal approach considered the state of the art. Many of these women suspect or know they are pregnant, based on the result of either a home pregnancy test or a positive urine test performed at the time of initial clinical presentation. A specific serum β-human chorionic gonadotropin (β-hCG) level often is not available when the initial sonogram is done.

Evaluate the Uterus

The optimal approach when evaluating a woman with suspected extrauterine pregnancy is to first direct attention toward the uterus in an effort to detect an intrauterine pregnancy (IUP). Approximately 90% of women with a positive pregnancy test who are referred to "rule out EP" are ultimately shown to have an IUP. This frequency, combined with the knowledge that coexistent intrauterine and extrauterine pregnancies are rare, makes it logical to search initially for an IUP. A second and important practical reason to begin at the level of the uterus is that it is technically easier to visualize an IUP than an EP. Although some would recommend starting with a transabdominal or combined transabdominal/transvaginal pelvic ultrasound examination, our laboratory favors an initial transvaginal approach because of its better resolution. Pelvic transabdominal scanning is performed when the transvaginal approach is suboptimal with respect to complete visualization of the ovaries, adnexa, and uterus.[5] Transabdominal imaging of the upper flank areas, however, is done routinely to evaluate for the presence or absence of a large hemoperitoneum.

To evaluate the uterus and detect either a small intrauterine gestational sac or endometrial changes associated with an EP, the highest-frequency transducer that can penetrate a particular region of interest should be chosen. Broad-band technology gives greater flexibility by permitting use of a single transducer and changing its frequency assignment electronically. When beginning a study and deciding which of several frequencies to select, a good rule of thumb is to "start high, and then go low." In most patients, 7 to 8 MHz is ideal and, if available, harmonic imaging should be used.

Criteria for Diagnosing Very Early Intrauterine Pregnancy

The gestational sac can be detected sonographically when it is 2 to 3 mm in diameter, which corresponds to a gestational age between 29 days and 31 days.[6-8] The appearance of a normal early gestational sac is a small fluid collection surrounded completely by an echogenic rim of tissue. As the sac enlarges, the echogenic rim, which is due to developing chorionic villi and adjacent decidual tissue, should be at least 2 mm thick, and its echogenicity should exceed that of the myometrium.[9]

To determine whether this small, saclike structure is an IUP and not a pseudosac associated with an EP, close inspection should be made of its position relative to the central cavity stripe of the endometrium. Because a true gestational sac implants into the thick decidualized endometrium, it should be located adjacent to the linear central cavity echo complex, and it should not displace or deform this echogenic anatomic landmark (Fig. 13–1). In 1986, Yeh and colleagues used this physiologic description of sac implantation to describe the intradecidual sign.[10] In their investigation, which used a transabdominal approach, early IUP was diagnosed with a reported sensitivity of 92%, specificity of 100%, and accuracy of 93%.[10] In a more recent effort to validate the effectiveness of this sign using a transvaginal approach, Laing and associates were not nearly as successful, with a reported sensitivity of 34% to 66%, specificity of 55% to 73%, and accuracy of 38% to 65%.[11] On the basis of these relatively poor results, the authors recommend that in cases of very early pregnancy, follow-up sonography should be obtained to document conclusively the appearance of the yolk sac or embryo.

Criteria for Diagnosing Ectopic Pregnancy

Despite one report suggesting a unique "endometrial three-layer" pattern as specific for EP,[12] others have not been able to confirm this endometrial appearance as either sensitive or specific for diagnosing EP.[13] Most investigations conclude that based on the gray-scale appearance of the endometrium, there is no specific endometrial pattern or thickness that can be used to suggest an EP, or to differentiate the endometrial appearance in women subsequently shown to have an EP versus a normal or abnormal IUP.[14]

Most often when there is an EP, the endometrium is "empty." In this context, the term *empty* implies that the sonogram fails to detect any visible endometrial fluid. However, in up to 20% of women with EP, the endometrium undergoes visible decidual changes that are reflected on sonography as an intrauterine fluid collection, or pseudosac[15] (Fig. 13–2). To the uninitiated, this appearance can mimic an early intrauterine gestational sac. As noted previously, an important differentiating feature is the location of the fluid. A true gestational sac is intradecidual, whereas a pseudosac develops within the uterine cavity.[10] Unfortunately, because the central cavity echo complex is not always visible or clearly defined, it may not be possible to determine if a fluid collection is intradecidual or is located in the uterine cavity (Fig. 13–3). This significantly

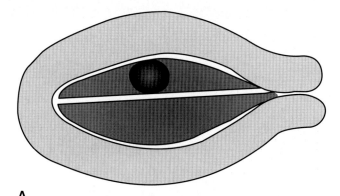

A

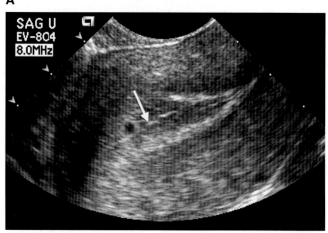

B

Figure 13–1. Normal sac at 5 weeks' gestational age. **A,** Graphic depiction of the intradecidual sac (IDS) sign shows the gestational sac *(closed black circle)* not displacing or deforming the central cavity echo complex *(straight white line)*. The gray area represents the thickened decidua. (From Laing FC, Brown DL, Price JF, et al: Intradecidual sign: Is it effective in diagnosis of an early intrauterine pregnancy? Radiology 1997;204:655-660, with permission.) **B,** A sagittal endovaginal sonogram demonstrates the IDS sign. Note the opposed walls of the central uterine cavity *(arrow)* are not displaced or deformed. The intradecidual gestational sac is implanted in the anterior endometrium.

limits the effectiveness of the intradecidual sign.[11] Imaged sonograpically, a pseudosac is relatively elliptic, is often filled with low-level echoes or debris, has relatively irregular margins, and lacks a well-defined rim of surrounding echoes.[16,17] Because the appearance of a pseudosac is often similar to that of a failed IUP, the diagnosis of EP associated with a pseudosac should be considered whenever a nonviable pregnancy is suspected.

Occasionally, well-defined "decidual cysts" are visible in the endometrium, and at least one study suggests that such cysts may be an indicator for an EP.[18] In contrast to a sac associated with an early IUP, these cysts do not abut the endometrial stripe and are not surrounded by an echogenic rim of tissue. Based on personal experience, similar-appearing cysts may also be seen in women with bona fide IUPs, as well as in nonpregnant women. They are also common with adenomyosis and tamoxifen therapy. The usefulness of this finding as an indicator of EP, therefore, remains to be confirmed.

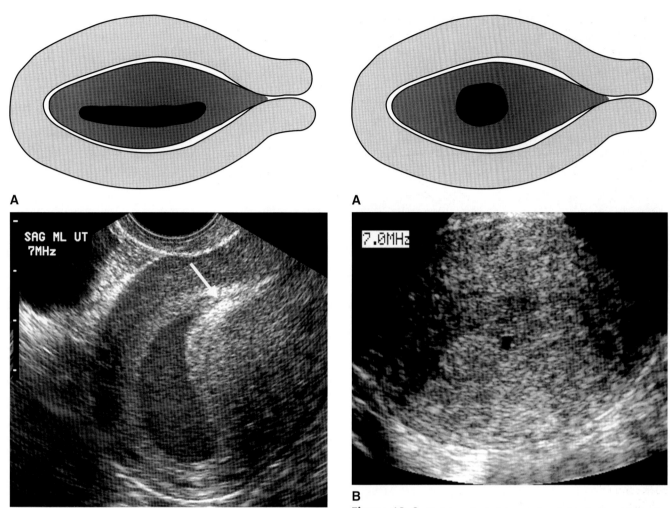

A

B

Figure 13–2. Pseudosac due to an ectopic pregnancy. **A,** Graphic depiction of a negative or absent intradecidual sac (IDS) sign shows fluid in the uterine cavity (the central black ovoid area). The gray area represents the thickened decidua. (From Laing FC, Brown DL, Price JF, et al: Intradecidual sign: Is it effective in diagnosis of an early intrauterine pregnancy? Radiology 1997;204:655-660, with permission.) **B,** Note the inferior aspect of this echogenic fluid collection tapers and is continuous with the opposed walls of the lower uterine segment *(arrow)*. This is consistent with fluid within the uterine cavity. In a patient with a positive pregnancy test, this appearance can be seen with either an abnormal intrauterine pregnancy or, as in this case, a pseudosac due to an ectopic pregnancy.

A

B

Figure 13–3. Indeterminate intrauterine fluid. **A,** Graphic depiction of an indeterminate scan. Because the central cavity echo complex line is not visible, precise location of the fluid collection *(central black circle)* is not possible. The gray area represents the thickened decidua. (From Laing FC, Brown DL, Price JF, et al: Intradecidual sign: Is it effective in diagnosis of an early intrauterine pregnancy? Radiology 1997;204:655-660, with permission.) **B,** A sagittal endovaginal sonogram demonstrates a small intrauterine fluid collection. Without visualization of the central cavity complex, it is not possible to determine whether this fluid is intradecidual or intracavitary.

Role of Endometrial Doppler in Diagnosis

Applying color and duplex Doppler to the endometrium has been recommended as a way to elicit the presence of an otherwise still-invisible IUP and to help differentiate a pseudosac from a true gestational sac[19-21] (Fig. 13–4). The rationale for using Doppler with an early IUP is to identify a high-velocity, low-resistance peritrophoblastic arterial flow pattern associated with developing chorionic villi. The resistance index for this type of flow should be less than 0.6.[21] Because pseudosacs are surrounded by decidual tissue but not chorionic villi, they should not demonstrate this flow pattern. A recent study reported that when flow consistent with a peritrophoblastic pattern is detected in the endometrium, an EP could be

excluded 97% of the time.[21] The specificity of this sign remains to be determined, because a failing or failed IUP may or may not demonstrate peritrophoblastic flow.[20,21] Increased venous flow is often detected with a nonliving IUP.[20]

Determine the Human Chorionic Gonadotropin Level and Correlate It with the Ultrasound Findings

If transvaginal sonography does not clearly identify an intrauterine gestational sac, and if the adnexa do not reveal findings consistent with an EP (see below), it is imperative to determine the quantitative serum level of β-hCG. This glycoprotein is normally elaborated by trophoblastic tissue beginning just 8 days after conception.[22] In a normal pregnancy, it doubles approximately every 2 days for 6 weeks, at which time

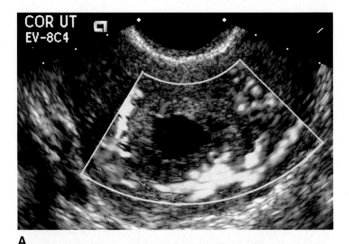

A

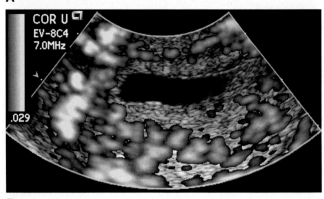

B

Figure 13–4. Comparative power Doppler studies. **A,** The presence of vascular flow suggests developing trophoblastic tissue in an early intrauterine pregnancy (IUP). **B,** Absent vascular flow in peripheral echogenic tissue is consistent with a pseudosac due to an ectopic pregnancy. This may also occur with a failed IUP.

its concentration peaks at a level of 100,000 mIU/mL.[23] Using extremely sensitive radioimmunoassays, the precise serum level of β-hCG can be determined as early as 23 days after a normal menstrual period (8 days after ovulation).[24]

If the result of this test is negative, a developing pregnancy, either intrauterine or extrauterine, is excluded. A rare exception is the presence of a chronic (nonliving) EP. When the pregnancy test is positive, the precise β-hCG level should be determined and correlated with the ultrasound findings. Depending on the study, and using the most recently introduced quantitative measuring standard (i.e., the International Reference Preparation [IRP]), state-of-the-art transvaginal sonography should identify a normal intrauterine gestational sac when the β-hCG value is 1000 to 2000 mIU/mL or greater.[25-28] Failure to identify a normal early sac when the serum β-hCG has reached this discriminatory level suggests either an abnormal IUP with a spontaneous abortion, or an EP. A history of heavy bleeding with passage of a large amount of clotlike material is often obtained when a miscarriage has occurred. In these cases, one option is to follow serially the level of the pregnancy test. If the β-hCG value is decreasing steadily, the patient is presumed to have had a miscarriage; if it is increasing, she is presumed to have an EP. If the level plateaus, an EP or retained intrauterine products of concep-

tion may be present. When this happens, repeat ultrasound may be able to solve the diagnostic dilemma.

When the β-hCG value exceeds the discriminatory level and the ultrasound examination fails to disclose a gestational sac or evidence for an EP, a second option is to perform a uterine dilation and curettage (D&C). This approach was usually implemented before the introduction of highly sensitive and specific pregnancy tests in combination with state-of-the-art transvaginal sonography. If chorionic villi are obtained, the diagnosis of a failed pregnancy is confirmed; failure to obtain villi is strong evidence for an EP. More recent, less aggressive approaches typically favor serial quantitative β-hCG determinations and, if necessary, follow-up ultrasound examinations.

With regard to the use of a discriminatory quantitative β-hCG value and an absent IUP on transvaginal sonography to diagnose or exclude EP, it is important to emphasize that controversy exists regarding the precise β-hCG level that should be used as a cut-off value. One report suggests that when 1500 mIU/mL is used as a discriminatory level in the absence of an IUP, the diagnosis of EP can be made with a sensitivity of 100% and specificity of 99%.[29] However, the accuracy depends on the equipment used and the expertise of the sonographers. In another report, Mehta et al. noted that one third of 51 pregnancies that lacked an IUP on transvaginal sonography at a discriminatory β-hCG level of greater than 2000 mIU/mL were found subsequently to have a normal IUP.[30] Accordingly, before using these criteria to establish the diagnosis of EP, each institution should establish its own realistic discriminatory β-hCG level and ensure the optimal training and expertise of its sonographers.

Not infrequently, the β-hCG value is less than the discriminatory level and the ultrasound examination fails to disclose either an intrauterine or extrauterine pregnancy. Diagnostic considerations include an early normal or abnormal IUP or an EP. Assuming that the patient is clinically stable, the β-hCG level should be repeated serially at 48-hour intervals. If it is doubling normally, a repeat ultrasound examination should be done when the pregnancy test level exceeds the discriminatory level. This approach can often be used to determine the correct diagnosis. If the serially obtained pregnancy test result is increasing but fails to double normally, the patient does not have a normal early IUP and the diagnosis is either an abnormal IUP or an EP. Depending on the clinical condition of the patient, she may be treated by D&C, receive methotrexate medical therapy, or be observed. If the serially obtained pregnancy test result is decreasing rapidly, the most likely diagnosis is a miscarriage; less likely is an EP that is no longer developing. In either of these situations, the patient most likely will be observed and will undergo frequent quantitative β-hCG monitoring until the test result becomes negative.

Be Aware of Exceptions!

With few exceptions, when the quantitative β-hCG value exceeds the discriminatory level and the uterus lacks a visible intrauterine gestational sac, the patient has an EP. One exception, as already discussed, is a patient who has recently experienced a spontaneous abortion. In this situation, the history is often pivotal for suggesting the correct diagnosis. Another exception is a patient with a multifetal pregnancy in whom the β-hCG level is greater than expected for the calculated gestational age. This occurs when multiple independent sources for

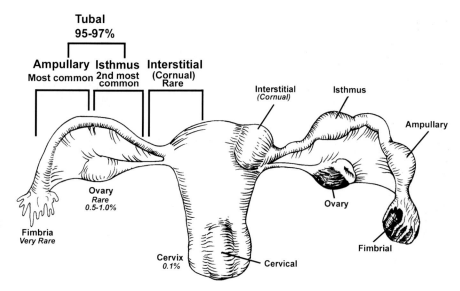

Figure 13–5. Locations for ectopic pregnancy. Note that at least 95% of the time, implantation is in the portion of the tube that is located close to the ovary. (From Schoenbaum S, Rosendorf L, Kappelman N, Rowan T: Gray-scale ultrasound in tubal pregnancy. Radiology 1978:127;757-761, with permission.)

β-hCG are summated, because the total amount of β-hCG exceeds the discriminatory level before the multiple intrauterine sacs are large enough to cross the threshold of visibility. In these women, β-hCG levels are often monitored as a result of assisted reproduction, and the suspicion for multifetal pregnancy is raised on the basis of patient history and an accelerated β-hCG doubling time.

Evaluate the Adnexa

Approach to Scanning

In women who conceive naturally, approximately 80% of extrauterine pregnancies develop in the ampullary portion and 12% develop in the isthmic portion of the fallopian tube (Fig. 13–5). In women who conceive as a result of assisted reproduction, more than 90% of EPs are ampullary.[31] The simplest way to begin searching for most EPs is to locate the ovary, which is typically positioned anterior and medial to the iliac vessels. In most women, the portions of the tube that harbor the EP are anatomically contiguous to the ovary, and because it is easier to identify the ovary than an EP, this organ serves as a useful anatomic landmark. Once the ovary is identified, the vaginal transducer should sweep carefully through all structures near the ovary. While scanning in this manner, it is useful to apply moderate pressure to the vaginal transducer, while also applying steady pressure using the nonscanning hand on the patient's low anterior abdominal wall. By compressing overlying bowel loops, these maneuvers often facilitate visualizing the EP. Asking the patient to report any area that is particularly sensitive to probe pressure also facilitates the search for an EP.

Most EPs are located between the ovary and uterus, although they may implant anywhere in the pelvis, and it may be necessary to extend the examination to include the regions adjacent to the uterine fundus, the cul-de-sac, and the lateral margins of the pelvis. In women undergoing assisted reproduction, careful attention should also be given to the cornual and cervical areas of the uterus because the reported incidence of EP in these locations is 7.3% and 1.5%, respectively.[31] If transvaginal sonography fails to identify an EP, transabdominal scanning should be considered.[5,32]

Criteria for Diagnosing Ectopic Pregnancy

Based on adnexal findings, the accuracy of transvaginal sonography for diagnosing EP varies considerably. In part, this is due to the equipment used and the experience of the examiner,[33] but it is also due to the varied criteria used to make this diagnosis.[34-37] The strictest criterion, with the highest specificity (100%) but lowest sensitivity (15% to 20%), is identifying an extrauterine gestational sac that contains a yolk sac or embryo (with or without cardiac activity)[37,38] (Fig. 13–6). A less stringent criterion in a patient with a positive pregnancy test and no IUP is a complex adnexal mass. The presence of this finding has a reported sensitivity of 21% to 84%, and a specificity of 93% to 99.5%.[37,38]

In an effort to determine the performance characteristics for these multiple criteria, one group of investigators

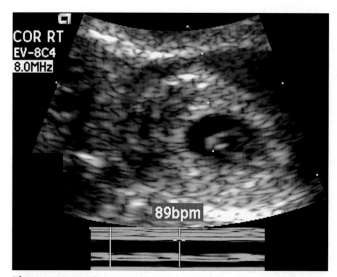

Figure 13–6. Transvaginal scan reveals a 6-week, living ectopic pregnancy in the right adnexa. Because the image is so magnified, unless labeling is accurate and precise, it would not be possible to differentiate this gestational sac from one located in the uterus. M-mode scanning reveals a heart rate of 89 beats per minute.

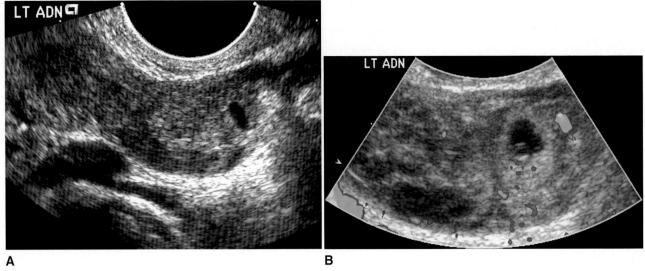

A   **B**

Figure 13–7. Scan optimization to differentiate an ectopic sac from a corpus luteum of pregnancy. **A,** On the basis of this image, the ovoid hypoechoic structure is probably a corpus luteum. Neither its peripheral echogenicity nor its location suggests it is actually an extraovarian ectopic gestational sac. **B,** After optimizing technical factors, a yolk sac becomes clearly visible. This clinches the diagnosis of ectopic pregnancy.

combined the results of 10 previously reported studies.[38] The authors concluded that with a clinical suspicion for EP, the most appropriate diagnostic criterion was the presence of any noncystic, extraovarian adnexal mass. This criterion, which included living EPs, tubal rings, and complex cystic or solid masses, had both a high specificity (98.9%) and positive predictive value (96.3%), as well as acceptable sensitivity (84.4%) and negative predictive value (94.8%). Therefore, in the absence of an IUP, the ultrasound identification of any nonsimple, nonovarian adnexal lesion can be used to diagnose EP.

Subtle Findings and Diagnostic Dilemmas

Demonstrating a living extrauterine pregnancy is usually straightforward, but diagnostic dilemmas do exist. Confusion sometimes occurs with respect to differentiating a living interstitial EP from an IUP that is eccentrically positioned owing to myomas, a focal contraction, or a duplication anomaly. Even a very advanced tubal or abdominal pregnancy can be misdiagnosed if the sonographer fails to appreciate that myometrial tissue does not surround the living fetus.[39,40] Also, an aborting sac located in the region of the cervix or upper vagina can also be misconstrued as a cervical EP (see comments later under Role of Ultrasound in Detecting Unusual and Nontubal Ectopic Pregnancies).

Every effort should be made to detect an ectopically located echogenic tubal ring because the sensitivity of this criterion for diagnosing an EP is approximately 65%. This is in contrast to the sensitivity for detecting a living EP, which is much lower, approximating 20%.[38] A tubal ring is characterized as a spheric structure with an anechoic or hypoechoic center and an echogenic periphery. If this structure is contiguous to the ovary, it may be misconstrued as the corpus luteum. There are several ways to minimize this potential error. One way is to optimize the scanning technique to determine if the tubal ring contains a yolk sac (Fig. 13–7). To visualize a yolk sac, which clinches the diagnosis of an EP, it is often beneficial to enlarge a suspect area using high-resolution computer processing, and to confirm that the transducer focal zone is optimally posi-

tioned. In addition to selecting the highest possible transducer frequency, harmonic imaging should be used, if available. A second way to differentiate a tubal ring from a corpus luteum is to compare the echogenicity of the questionable ringlike structure to the background echogenicity of the ovarian parenchyma (Fig. 13–8). In a recent report, the tubal ring of an EP was more echogenic than the ovarian parenchyma 88% of the time; in contrast, the tissue surrounding a corpus luteum was more echogenic than ovarian parenchyma only 7% of the time.[41] This observation strongly supports the thesis that the tubal ring of an EP is more echogenic than the peripheral echogenicity of the corpus luteum. A third way to determine if the ringlike structure is an ectopic tubal ring or a corpus luteum is to use transvaginal transducer pressure or anterior transabdominal wall palpation in an effort to sepa-

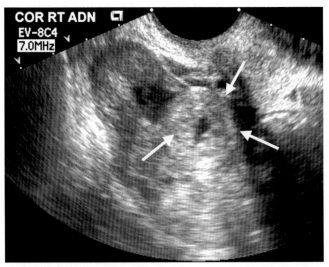

Figure 13–8. Nicely shown in this case is that the peripheral echogenicity of an ectopic sac *(arrows)* exceeds both the echogenicity of ovarian parenchymal tissue and the peripheral echogenicity of the adjacent corpus luteum.

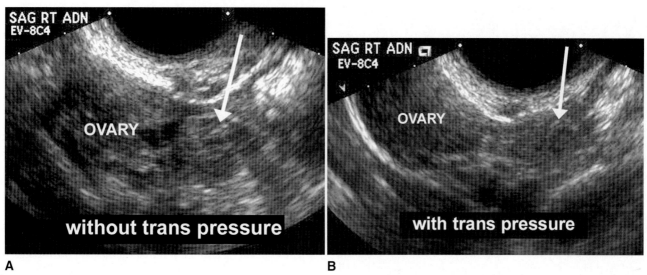

Figure 13–9. The beneficial effect of "probing" with the probe. **A,** Initially, a mass is visible contiguous with and inseparable from the medial aspect of the ovary *(arrow)*. It is not possible to state whether this structure is intraovarian or extraovarian. **B,** When the vaginal transducer was used to apply gentle but firm pressure to the mass, real-time imaging clearly showed it was separate because it was observed to move away from the ovary *(arrow)*. Based on this observation, the diagnosis of ectopic pregnancy was made with confidence.

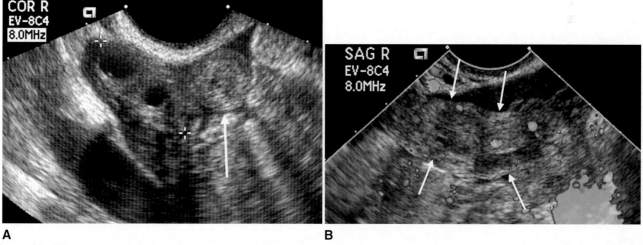

Figure 13–10. Diagnosing an ectopic pregnancy on the basis of visualizing an extraovarian solid mass. **A,** This coronal transvaginal image reveals a round, solid-appearing echogenic mass *(arrow)* just medial to the right ovary *(between calipers)*. A trace of free fluid surrounds the mass, and this helps to separate it from the more deeply located bowel loops (which on real-time observation were visibly peristalsing). **B,** After the transducer was rotated into a sagittal plane, the previously seen round mass assumed a tubular configuration *(arrows)*. This structure is a dilated fallopian tube filled with echogenic material. Because color Doppler did not document significant blood flow, most likely the tube contents are due to clotted blood, although concomitant nonliving trophoblastic tissue is not excluded.

rate the ovary from the questionable tubal ring (Fig. 13–9). Having a video clip or tape available to document that the ovary is indeed separate from the tubal ring supports the diagnosis of EP.

Not infrequently in patients with an EP, the diagnosis is determined merely on the basis of visualizing an extraovarian mass[38] (Fig. 13–10A). Most often, this mass has a complex or heterogeneous echotexture due to clotted blood or trophoblastic tissue. It may be confined to the fallopian tube (hematosalpinx; Fig. 13–10B),[42,43] but more often it is visible as a variably sized complex mass with poorly defined borders. Within this mass, meticulous ultrasound scanning sometimes confirms the diagnosis of EP by revealing an adnexal tubal ring (Fig. 13–11). Rupture of a tubal pregnancy, which results

from trophoblastic growth into and through the tubal wall, can lead to significant intraperitoneal hemorrhage and even exsanguination. A similar-appearing hemoperitoneum can occur in the absence of tubal rupture, however, if blood escapes into the peritoneal cavity from the fimbriated end of an intact tube. Unfortunately, no specific ultrasound criteria can be used to determine whether tubal rupture has occurred.[44]

Identifying a simple ovarian cyst should not raise the possibility of an EP because it is usually the corpus luteum. A complex intraovarian lesion is also unlikely to represent an EP because true ovarian pregnancies constitute fewer than 1% of all EPs[45] (Fig. 13–12). Also, the location of an ovarian cyst (right versus left) does not aid in localizing the side of the EP

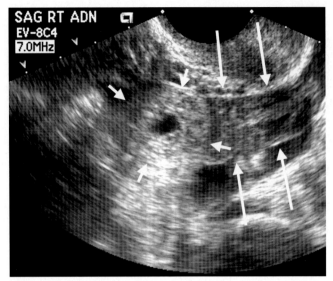

Figure 13–11. This sagittal image reveals a hematosalpinx filled with heterogeneously echogenic material *(long arrows)*. Careful examination of the anterior aspect of the tube shows the contained ectopic sac with a tubal ring *(short arrows)*.

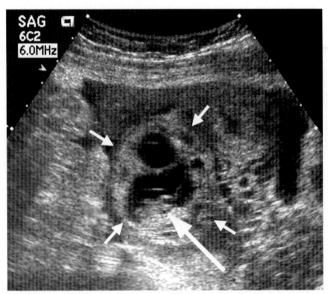

Figure 13–12. This is an unusual example of an intraovarian ectopic pregnancy (EP), reported to occur in fewer than 1% of cases. The ovary is visible *(short arrows)* and contains a few peripheral follicles. The *large arrow* indicates the EP, which was easily diagnosed because it had vigorous cardiac activity. Note also a small quantity of superficially located echogenic free fluid, due to a hemoperitoneum.

because contralateral implantation occurs in up to one third of cases.[46]

In 15% to 35% of patients with EP, no adnexal mass will be identified despite meticulous scanning technique.[37,44,47,48] In these women, free intraperitoneal fluid may be helpful for suggesting the diagnosis. In morbidly obese patients and in patients with large uterine fibroids or preexisting adnexal disease, the diagnostic accuracy of sonography can be quite limited, and negative findings at examination should be interpreted with caution.[38]

Role of Adnexal Doppler

In the experience of several investigators, the addition of color and pulsed Doppler has improved the sensitivity for making the diagnosis of EP.[49,50] The rationale for using Doppler is to detect a high-velocity, low-resistance arterial flow pattern within ectopically developing trophoblastic tissue. Once color flow identifies a possible EP, pulsed Doppler interrogation of the suspect area with calculation of the resistance index (RI) has been proposed as a method to differentiate a corpus luteum from an EP.[49] In theory this is attractive, but in a practical sense it is of limited value because the RI associated with EP frequently overlaps that of the corpus luteum.[51] Because many developing EPs have a large amount of visible flow within the surrounding trophoblastic tissue, another proposed use for Doppler is to use color to detect a prominent, peripherally located "ring of fire."[50] Unfortunately, because corpus luteal cysts can have similar peripheral flow characteristics, this appearance by itself cannot be used to differentiate an EP from a corpus luteum[52] (Fig. 13–13).

Although the presence of flow on color and pulsed Doppler is consistent with an EP, lack of flow cannot be used to exclude an EP. This is because a very small EP, or one that is nonviable, lacks flow. A tubal or peritoneal hematoma associated with an EP also lacks flow. Some investigators have taken advantage of the fact that some EPs demonstrate flow, whereas others do not, to suggest that Doppler flow indicates trophoblastic activity. In this manner, Doppler can differentiate a developing from an inactive EP. This approach, therefore, may be useful to assist in the choice of therapy and for monitoring the therapeutic response.[53-56]

In summary, Doppler may provide additional information about the vascularity of some ectopic adnexal masses, but because the actual diagnosis of EP rests on its gray-scale features, Doppler should not be considered mandatory when performing ultrasound examinations.[57]

Evaluate for Free Fluid

Free intraperitoneal fluid is the least specific criterion for diagnosing EP. Although it usually accompanies other findings that suggest the diagnosis, isolated free fluid has been reported in approximately 15% of patients with proven EP.[37,48] Causes of free intraperitoneal fluid include active bleeding from the fimbriated end of the fallopian tube, tubal rupture, and tubal abortion.[37,44,48] Occasionally, the source may be a ruptured corpus luteum. Even a small amount of free fluid in the pelvis may contribute to a superior examination by outlining the uterus, dilated tubes, ovaries, and any abnormal pelvic mass. In at-risk patients, any amount of cul-de-sac fluid greater than a trace should be considered abnormal.

Compared with transabdominal scanning of the pelvis, transvaginal sonography is superior for detecting small quantities of free intraperitoneal fluid. In part, this is because when a transabdominal scan is done with a distended bladder, the bladder tends to displace small quantities of free fluid out of the pelvis, rendering it invisible.[58] If, as has been advocated recently, a transabdominal scan is done with a decompressed bladder, small quantities of free fluid may go undetected because overlying bowel loops may preclude an optimal ultrasound acoustic window into the deep pelvis. In contrast, bladder decompression and the lithotomy position used for the transvaginal examination allow fluid to descend into the

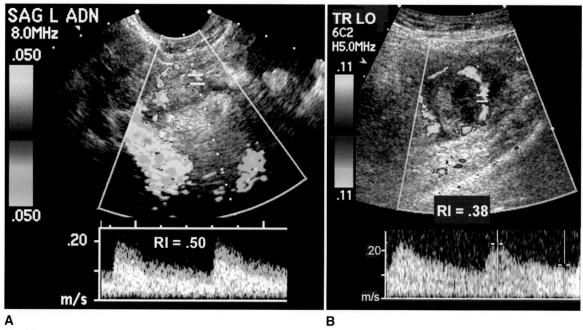

Figure 13–13. Peripheral "ring of fire." In two different patients, prominent vascular flow with a low resistance pattern is visible surrounding two similar-appearing, ringlike structures. **A,** The appearance in this patient is due to flow in trophoblastic tissue associated with an ectopic pregnancy (EP). **B,** Here, it is due to flow in the wall of a corpus luteum of pregnancy. Although this ring-of-fire appearance has been equated with an EP, most sonologists do not consider this sign to be specific for the diagnosis. RI, resistance index.

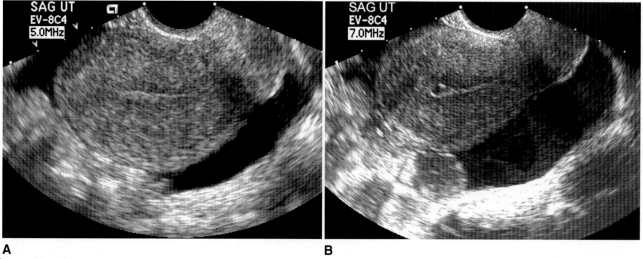

Figure 13–14. Detecting a hemoperitoneum. **A,** Using a 5-MHz transducer, free fluid is visible in the cul-de-sac. This transducer setting, however, was insufficient to resolve the low-level echoes associated with blood. **B,** On changing the transducer frequency to 7 MHz, low-level echoes become immediately visible. In the appropriate clinical setting, this appearance is highly suggestive for nonclotted blood. When the transducer is used to ballot the fluid, the echoes demonstrate a characteristic swirling pattern.

pouch of Douglas. Although the pelvis is optimally examined using a transvaginal approach, it is important also to use a transabdominal approach to examine the upper abdomen and flank areas to evaluate for fluid in Morison's pouch and the paracolic gutters.

Although free fluid of any character increases the likelihood of EP, several studies note that echogenic fluid is particularly worrisome for a hemoperitoneum.[37,59,60] To detect echogenic free fluid, which is reported in up to 56% of patients with EP, optimal equipment settings are required[37] (Fig. 13–14). One

useful adjustment is to increase the gain control to a level that is just beneath introducing artifactual echoes into urine within the bladder. Another way to confirm subtle echogenic particles within fluid is to use the vaginal probe repeatedly to apply gentle but deliberate pressure to the area of interest. As the fluid is balloted in this manner, observation during real-time scanning often reveals a continuous swirling motion to these echoes. In addition, with color Doppler turned on, particulate echoes within fluid may also begin to show slow but deliberate motion.

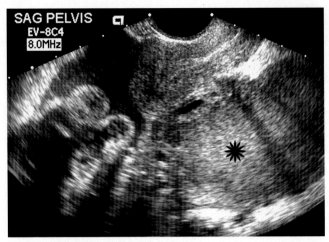

Figure 13–15. When blood clots, it becomes increasingly echogenic and difficult to detect, and it is often misconstrued as bowel. In this patient, echogenic clot is visible in the cul-de-sac (⋆), whereas nonclotted, hypoechoic blood is seen superior to the uterus. Note the appearance of undulating bowel loops located deep to the liquefied blood.

Several pitfalls have been reported with respect to detecting and diagnosing blood on the basis of its echogenic nature. One is that occasionally a hemoperitoneum may appear as a completely anechoic fluid collection.[37] Another potential problem is that with increasingly sensitive transducers, particulate echoes within nonsanguineous fluid may be observed and can be misconstrued as blood.[61] Also, because clotted blood is no longer in a fluid state, it can appear as an amorphous echogenic mass or masses[5,62] (Fig. 13–15). An inexperienced observer may fail to recognize this appearance for a significant hemoperitoneum. Indeed, because of indistinct and poorly defined margins, a large amount of clotted blood can be overlooked entirely, or it may be misconstrued as bowel gas[5,62] (Fig. 13–16A). If, under these circumstances, a culdocentesis is attempted, it will usually be unsuccessful in obtaining free fluid. In these cases, transabdominal examination of the upper abdomen usually reveals liquefied, echogenic blood (Fig. 13–16B).

In patients suspected of EP whose only abnormal ultrasound finding is free fluid, the ratio of β-hCG in the maternal serum to that in cul-de-sac fluid has been shown to provide important diagnostic information. In a study of 129 cases, this ratio was greater than unity in 42 of 44 patients subsequently shown to have an IUP, whereas it was less than unity in 82 of 85 patients with an EP.[63]

Role of Ultrasound in Detecting Unusual and Nontubal Ectopic Pregnancies

The incidence of EPs that develop in an unusual location, as well as heterotopic pregnancies, increases dramatically after use of assisted reproduction technologies. With natural conception, the incidence of interstitial pregnancy is approximately 1.9%, whereas after assisted reproduction technology it increases to 7.3%. Similarly, the rates of cervical EP increase from 0.15% to 1.5%, of ovarian or abdominal pregnancies from 1.5% to 4.6%, and of heterotopic pregnancies from approximately 0.03% to almost 12%.[31]

Interstitial Pregnancy

Interstitial pregnancies, which account for 2% to 4% of EPs, occur when the products of conception implant within the interstitial or intramural portion of the fallopian tube.[64,65] The term *cornual pregnancy,* frequently used interchangeably with *interstitial pregnancy,* should be reserved for pregnancies that develop in a rudimentary uterine horn. Compared with tubal EPs, interstitial pregnancies are associated with significantly increased morbidity and mortality. Because distensible myometrium surrounds a portion of the expanding gestational sac, rupture is usually delayed until the 9th to 12th gestational week, at which time acute symptoms develop after uterine rupture and potentially exsanguinating hemorrhage (Fig. 13–17).

The diagnosis of interstitial pregnancy should be suggested when ultrasound images demonstrate eccentric implantation of the gestational sac at the superior fundic level of the uterus. In almost all cases, there is myometrial thinning or absent myometrium around portions of the sac; rarely, however, visible myometrium has been reported to surround completely a small interstitial EP.[66] To increase the predictive value of sonography for making this diagnosis, Ackerman and associates described the *interstitial line sign.*[65] This sign consists of visualizing a thin, echogenic line that extends from the central uterine cavity echo to abut the periphery of the interstitial gestational sac (Fig. 13–18). Presumably, the line represents the endometrial canal or the interstitial portion of the fallopian tube.[65] When used in combination with the ultrasound findings of an incomplete mantle and eccentric sac location, the interstitial line sign may provide a useful clue for the early diagnosis of interstitial pregnancy.

The examiner must be aware that several conditions can mimic an interstitial EP. These include an eccentric implantation with a normal early IUP or with a congenital anomaly such as a subseptus uterus. In the latter condition, a thin line may also be observed extending from the endometrial cavity to the periphery of the sac. Close scrutiny of this line, however, reveals that it curves as it extends into the contralateral uterine horn (as opposed to the straight line described with an interstitial pregnancy). Careful evaluation of nonectopic but eccentric implantations usually reveals that they are not as superiorly located within the uterine fundus. If the diagnosis of interstitial EP is questionable, either magnetic resonance imaging (MRI) or three-dimensional ultrasound should be considered for further evaluation.[67,68]

Cervical Pregnancy

The incidence of cervical pregnancy, which results from implantation of the conceptus into the cervix, is rare in naturally conceived pregnancies (0.15% of EPs) but increases 10-fold after use of assisted reproduction technology.[31] In addition to in vitro fertilization and other therapies for infertility, risk factors that predispose to this potentially life-threatening condition include procedures that involve cervicouterine manipulation, especially prior cesarean sections and uterine D&C.[69]

The ultrasound diagnosis is based on detection of a gestational sac that contains a yolk sac, embryo, or cardiac activity within the cervix[69,70] (Fig. 13–19). The differential diagnosis includes a large nabothian cyst and a spontaneous abortion in progress. A nabothian cyst can usually be distinguished from

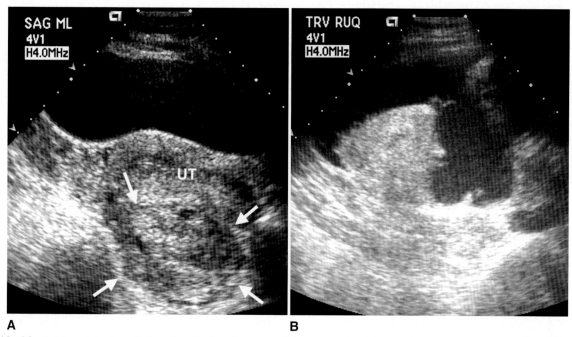

Figure 13–16. Subtle pelvic clot; obvious free fluid in the upper abdomen. **A,** On this sagittal transabdominal pelvic scan, very extensive clot *(arrows)* results in a heterogeneously echogenic mass that lacks well-defined margins. This appearance can be easily overlooked and misconstrued for bowel. UT, uterus. **B,** In the same patient, scans of the right upper quadrant reveal a large quantity of echogenic fluid, consistent with nonclotted blood.

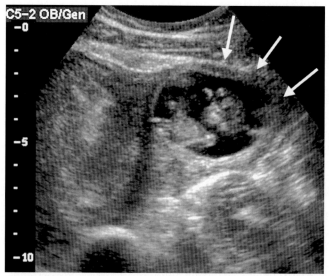

Figure 13–17. Transabdominal scan obtained at the level of the fundus reveals an interstitial ectopic pregnancy at 12.5 weeks' gestational age. Note the implantation at this level causes bulging of the lateral contour of the uterus, as well as the absence of surrounding myometrial tissue *(arrows)*.

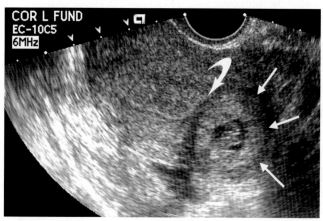

Figure 13–18. Transvaginal scan in a patient with an interstitial ectopic pregnancy at 7 weeks' gestational age. An interstitial line sign is evident as endometrial echoes extend to the periphery of the sac *(curved arrow)*. Similar to Figure 13–17, the implantation results in bulging of the lateral contour of the uterus, and there is a lack of surrounding myometrial tissue *(arrows)*.

a cervical EP by transvaginal sonography because the cyst lacks an echogenic rim, yolk sac, and embryo. Excluding a spontaneous abortion can be more problematic, and in questionable cases repeat sonography several hours later can be diagnostic by confirming sac expulsion or revealing a change in the sac shape and location. Documenting that the sac is eccentric relative to the endocervical canal suggests a cervical implantation, but this can sometimes be technically difficult to observe despite careful transvaginal or translabial scanning.

In addition, an eccentric implantation associated with a cervical EP can be mimicked by an abortion in progress if an extruded sac is in the vaginal fornix. Limited experience suggests that three-dimensional ultrasound and MRI may be useful in questionable cases.[71,72]

Abdominal Pregnancy

Abdominal pregnancies are classified as either primary or secondary, with the former considered rare and due to primary peritoneal implantation. Secondary abdominal pregnancies develop after uterine rupture, or as a result of either tubal rupture or tubal abortion with subsequent abdominal

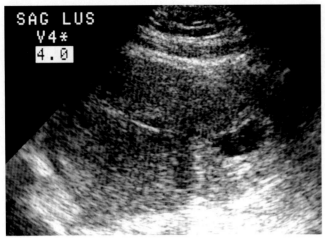

Figure 13–19. This transabdominal scan reveals a cervical implantation of a gestational sac. A yolk sac is visible and real-time imaging confirmed cardiac activity.

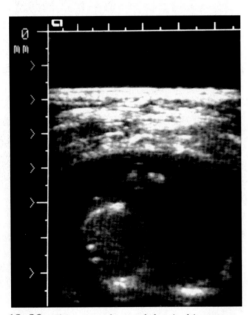

Figure 13–20. This unusual transabdominal image was obtained from a patient who, at 18 weeks' gestational age, was observed to have an abdominal pregnancy. The implantation was initially in a non-communicating rudimentary horn that ruptured several weeks before this examination. Note that despite use of a stand-off pad to eliminate near-field artifactual echoes, there is complete absence of surrounding myometrial tissue.

reimplantation. The prognosis is poor, with the maternal mortality rate reported as 7.7 times higher than for other forms of EP.[73] The ultrasound diagnosis can be difficult in both early and advanced cases and rests on demonstrating an empty uterus that is separate from the fetus.[39,74] This appearance can be mimicked by a congenital uterine duplication anomaly that consists of one empty uterus and one fetus-containing uterus. Other ultrasound features associated with an abdominal pregnancy include lack of visualization of surrounding myometrium (Fig. 13–20), extrauterine placental tissue, oligohydramnios, and an abnormal fetal lie (often above the maternal pelvis). A live fetus is born in 10% to 25% of advanced

abdominal pregnancies, but neonatal mortality is high because of the associated oligohydramnios, pulmonary hypoplasia, compression deformities of the fetal head, and other complications associated with a paucity of amniotic fluid.[75]

Significance of a Normal Ultrasound Examination

When the results of a technically satisfactory transvaginal sonographic examination are normal but an IUP is not seen and the patient is clinically stable, it is important to determine the quantitative β-hCG level. If it is above the discriminatory level and significant bleeding is absent, the possibility of an ectopic pregnancy is significant and must be excluded. If the β-hCG level is less than the discriminatory level, serial β-hCG determinations should be done and the ultrasound examination should be repeated once the discriminatory level is reached.

If significant bleeding is reported, a spontaneous abortion is likely. Under these circumstances, serial β-hCG determinations should be done to ensure that the level is decreasing rapidly, and the quantitative value should be monitored closely until the test result becomes negative. Any increase in the level of β-hCG signals the presence of trophoblastic tissue, due either to an intrauterine or an extrauterine pregnancy. Repeat sonography may be useful in these cases to document the location of this tissue.

Role of Ultrasound with Respect to Therapeutic Options

During the past decade, treatment options for EP have broadened considerably, and, not surprisingly, they favor less invasive interventions. When surgery is required, laparoscopy is the recommended approach. A variety of nonsurgical treatment options are available, with the least invasive being expectant observation. Many women respond well to systemic therapy that consists of intramuscular injection of methotrexate, or to local therapy consisting of methotrexate or KCl injection directly into the ectopic sac. The specific therapeutic approach used in an individual patient depends on a combination of factors, including the initial clinical and imaging findings, as well as the level of β-hCG. If surgery is not done initially and if the patient is stable, serial ultrasound and β-hCG determinations can often assist in deciding whether systemic or local intervention will be efficacious. Also, if a relatively noninvasive therapeutic approach is used, serial ultrasound and β-hCG determinations can subsequently monitor patient response.

An increasingly important role of interventional ultrasound is to guide therapeutic ablation of unusual ectopic pregnancies.[76] These include heterotopic pregnancies (concurrently located in an intrauterine and an extrauterine site) and implantations occurring in the cornua, cervix, or cesarean section scar. In almost all cases, treatment can be accomplished on an outpatient basis and consists of using transvaginal or transabdominal sonography to guide injection of hypertonic KCl into the ectopically located sac or embryo (Fig. 13–21). Of 27 cases recently reported from our institution, this approach was successful in 25 patients.[76] Especially gratifying is that this appears to be a safe alternative to more radical interventions such as hysterectomy or uterine artery

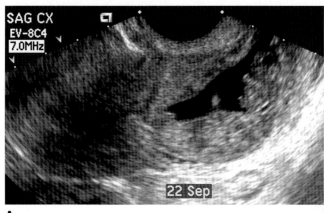

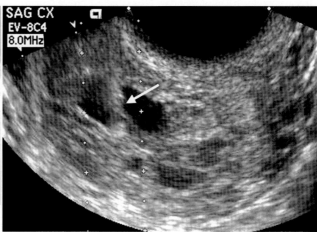

Figure 13–21. Sonographically guided ablation of cervical ectopic pregnancy. **A,** Transvaginal scan confirms the presence of a living, 8.4-week gestational age pregnancy implanted in the cervix. **B,** Using an attached needle guide, transvaginal sonography was used successfully to direct injection of 4 mL of KCl into the embryo. The *arrow* points to the needle. **C,** At 7 days postinjection, abnormal echogenic material that is nonspecific in appearance is visible in the cervix *(calipers)*. Color Doppler revealed the cervix to have increased vascularity, but compared with the initial ultrasound scan, the flow had diminished. Follow-up ultrasound imaging 5 weeks after this procedure revealed persistence of abnormal tissue in the cervix, although the β-hCG level was negative at 6 weeks. Five months later, this patient had an intrauterine pregnancy and the cervix had a normal appearance.

embolization. Not only does it ablate the ectopic pregnancy, but in cases with a concurrent, normally implanted conceptus, it permits continuation of that pregnancy, as well as preserving the uterus for subsequent reproductive potential.

Conclusion

Although EP is an increasingly common health problem, the effectiveness of quantitative β-hCG levels combined with state-of-the-art transvaginal sonography has dramatically improved our ability to detect smaller and more subtle EPs. In most cases, the standard of care remains surgical, but medical therapies using methotrexate as well as minimally invasive interventional therapies to ablate the ectopic sac directly are becoming more common. Besides being less invasive and posing less risk to the patient, these approaches have a more favorable economic and social impact and consequently greater patient acceptance. The most important task is to identify and define specific criteria that will permit successful triage of patients with EP into surgical, expectant, medical, and minimally invasive therapeutic groups. To accomplish this goal, detailed diagnostic and therapeutic protocols are required that incorporate readily available assays for determining serum β-hCG levels, high-resolution transvaginal sonography, and a support staff to monitor clinical response. The effect of this approach is to transition the con-

dition of having an EP from a surgical emergency to a medically treatable disease. These modern diagnostic advances and minimally invasive treatments permit women with EP to preserve their reproductive function and experience a normal subsequent pregnancy.

REFERENCES

1. Goldner TE, Lawson HW, Xia Z, Atrash HK: Surveillance for ectopic pregnancy—United States, 1970-1989. MMWR CDC Surveill Summ 1993;42:73-85.
2. National Center for Health Statistics: Advanced report of final mortality statistics, 1992 (Report 43, No. 6, Suppl) Hyattsville, Md, U.S. Department of Health and Human Services, Public Health Service, Centers for Disease Control and Prevention, 1994.
3. Centers for Disease Control and Prevention: Current trends: Ectopic pregnancy—United States, 1990-1992. MMWR Morb Mortal Wkly Rep 1995;44:46-48.
4. Schwartz R, Di Pietro DL: β-hCG as a diagnostic aid for suspected ectopic pregnancy. Obstet Gynecol 1980;56:197-203.
5. Hertzberg BS, Kliewer MA, Bowie JD: Sonographic evaluation for ectopic pregnancy: Transabdominal scanning of patients with nondistended urinary bladders as a complement to transvaginal sonography. AJR Am J Roentgenol 1999;73:773-775.
6. Timor-Tritsch IE, Farine D, Rosen MG: A close look at early embryonic development with the high-frequency transvaginal transducer. Am J Obstet Gynecol 1988;159:676-681.
7. Rossavik IK, Torjusen GO, Gibbons WE: Conceptual age and ultrasound measurements of gestational sac and crown-rump length in in vitro fertilization pregnancies. Fertil Steril 1988;49:1012-1017.

8. de Crespigny LC, Cooper D, McKenna M: Early detection of intrauterine pregnancy with ultrasound. J Ultrasound Med 1988;7:7-10.
9. Nyberg DA, Laing FC, Filly RA: Threatened abortion: Sonographic distinction of normal and abnormal gestation sacs. Radiology 1986;158:397-400.
10. Yeh HC, Goodman JD, Carr L, Rabinowitz JG: Intradecidual sign: A US criterion of early IUP. Radiology 1986;161:463-467.
11. Laing FC, Brown DL, Price JF, et al: Intradecidual sign: Is it effective in diagnosis of an early intrauterine pregnancy? Radiology 1997;204:655-660.
12. Lavie O, Boldes R, Neuman M, et al: Ultrasonographic "endometrial three layer" pattern: A specific finding in ectopic pregnancy. J Clin Ultrasound 1996;24:179-183.
13. Wachsberg RH, Karimi S: Sonographic endometrial three layer pattern in symptomatic first-trimester pregnancy: Not diagnostic of ectopic pregnancy. J Clin Ultrasound 1998;26:199-201.
14. Mehta TS, Levine D, McArdle CR: Lack of sensitivity of endometrial thickness in predicting presence of an ectopic pregnancy. J Ultrasound Med 1999;18:117-122.
15. Marks WM, Filly RA, Callen PW, Laing FC: The decidual cast of ectopic pregnancy: A confusing ultrasonographic appearance. Radiology 1979;133:451-454.
16. Nyberg DA, Laing FC, Filly RA, et al: Ultrasonographic differentiation of the gestational sac of early intrauterine pregnancy from the pseudogestational sac of ectopic pregnancy. Radiology 1983;146:755-759.
17. Nelson P, Bowie JD, Rosenberg ER: Early intrauterine pregnancy or decidual cast: An anatomic-sonographic approach. J Ultrasound Med 1983;2:543-547.
18. Ackerman TE, Levi CS, Lyons EA, et al: Decidual cyst: Endovaginal sonographic sign of ectopic pregnancy. Radiology 1993;189:727-731.
19. Dillon EH, Feyock AL, Taylor KJW: Pseudogestational sacs: Doppler US differentiation from normal and abnormal intrauterine pregnancies. Radiology 1990;176:359-364.
20. Emerson DS, Cartier MS, Altieri LA, et al: Diagnostic efficacy of endovaginal color Doppler flow imaging in an ectopic pregnancy screening program. Radiology 1992;183:413-420.
21. Wherry KL, Dubinsky TJ, Waitches GM, et al: Low-resistance endometrial arterial flow in the exclusion of ectopic pregnancy revisited. J Ultrasound Med 2001;20:335-342.
22. Derman R: Early diagnosis of pregnancy: A symposium. J Reprod Med 1981;26:149-178.
23. Rasor JL, Braunstein GD: A rapid modification of the beta-hCG radioimmunoassay: Use as an aid in the diagnosis of ectopic pregnancy. Obstet Gynecol 1977;50:553-558.
24. Mishell DR, Nakamura RM, Barberia JM, et al: Initial detection of human chorionic gonadotropin in serum in normal human gestation. Am J Obstet Gynecol 1974;118:990-991.
25. Cacciatore B, Stenman UH, Ylostalo P: Diagnosis of ectopic pregnancy by vaginal ultrasonography in combination with a discriminatory serum hCG level of 1000 IU/l IRP. Br J Obstet Gynaecol 1990;97:904-908.
26. Bateman MG, Nunley WC, Kolp LA, et al: Vaginal sonography findings and hCG dynamics of early intrauterine and tubal pregnancies. Obstet Gynecol 1990;75:421-427.
27. Bree RL, Edwards M, Bohm-Velez M, et al: Transvaginal sonography in the evaluation of normal early pregnancy: Correlation with hCG level. AJR Am J Roentgenol 1989;153:75-79.
28. Braffman BH, Coleman BG, Ramchandani P, et al: Emergency department screening for ectopic pregnancy: A prospective US study. Radiology 1994;190:797-802.
29. Barnhart K, Meenut MT, Benjamin I, et al: Prompt diagnosis of ectopic pregnancy in an emergency department setting. Obstet Gynecol 1994;84:1010-1015.
30. Mehta TS, Levine D, Beckwith B: Treatment of ectopic pregnancy: Is a human chorionic gonadotropin level of 2000 mIU/ml a reasonable threshold? Radiology 1997;205:569-573.
31. Pisarska MD, Carson SA: Ectopic pregnancy. In Scott JR, Saia PJ, Hammond CD, Spellacy WN (eds): Danforth's Obstetrics and Gynecology, 8th ed. Philadelphia, Lippincott Williams & Wilkins, 1999, pp 155-172.
32. Zinn HL, Cohen HL, Zinn DL: Ultrasonographic diagnosis of ectopic pregnancy: Importance of abdominal scanning. J Ultrasound Med 1997;16:603-607.
33. Wojak JC, Clayton MJ, Nolan TE: Outcomes of ultrasound diagnosis of ectopic pregnancy: Dependence on observer experience. Invest Radiol 1995;30:115-117.
34. Cacciatore B: Can the status of tubal pregnancy be predicted with transvaginal sonography? A prospective comparison of sonographic, surgical, and serum hCG findings. Radiology 1990;177:481-484.
35. Rempen A: Vaginal sonography in ectopic pregnancy. J Ultrasound Med 1988;7:381-387.
36. Fleischer AC, Pennel RG, McKee MS, et al: Ectopic pregnancy: Features at transvaginal sonography. Radiology 1990;174:375-378.
37. Nyberg DA, Hughes MP, Mack LA, Wang KY: Extrauterine findings of ectopic pregnancy at transvaginal US: Importance of echogenic fluid. Radiology 1991;178: 823-826.
38. Brown DL, Doubilet PM: Transvaginal sonography for diagnosing ectopic pregnancy: Positivity criteria and performance characteristics. J Ultrasound Med 1994;13:259-266.
39. Rice T, Bowser C: Extrauterine abdominal pregnancy: Report of a case. CRNA 1999;10:181-183.
40. Hall JM, Manning N, Moore NR, et al: Antenatal diagnosis of a late abdominal pregnancy using ultrasound and magnetic resonance imaging: A case report of successful outcome. Ultrasound Obstet Gynecol 1996;7:289-292.
41. Frates MC, Visweswaran A, Laing FC: Comparison of tubal ring and corpus luteum echogenicities: A useful differentiating characteristic. J Ultrasound Med 2001;20:27-31.
42. Atri M, deStempel J, Bret PM: Accuracy of transvaginal ultrasonography for detection of hematosalpinx in ectopic pregnancy. J Clin Ultrasound 1992;20:255-261.
43. Subramanyam BR, Goldstein SR, Balthazar EJ, et al: Hematosalpinx in tubal pregnancy: Sonographic-pathologic correlation. AJR Am J Roentgenol 1983;141:361-364.
44. Frates MC, Brown DL, Doubilet PM, Hornstein MD: Tubal rupture in patients with ectopic pregnancy: Diagnosis with transvaginal US. Radiology 1994;191:769-772.
45. Atzori E: Transvaginal ultrasonography in the diagnosis of primary ovarian pregnancy: Case report. Ultrasound Obstet Gynecol 1993;3:217-218.
46. Berry SM, Coulam CB, Hill LM, Breckle R: Evidence of contralateral ovulation in ectopic pregnancy. J Ultrasound Med 1985;4:293-295.
47. Russell SA, Filly RA, Damato N: Sonographic diagnosis of ectopic pregnancy with endovaginal probes: What really has changed? J Ultrasound Med 1993;3:145-151.
48. Rottem S, Thaler I, Timor-Tritsch IE: Classification of tubal gestations by transvaginal sonography. Ultrasound Obstet Gynecol 1991;1:197-201.
49. Kurjack A, Zalud I, Schulman H: Ectopic pregnancy: Transvaginal color Doppler of trophoblastic flow in questionable adnexa. J Ultrasound Med 1991;10:685-689.
50. Pellerito JS, Taylor KJW, Quedens-Case C, et al: Ectopic pregnancy: Evaluation with endovaginal color flow imaging. Radiology 1992;183: 407-411.
51. Taylor KJW, Ramos IM, Feyock AL, et al: Ectopic pregnancy: Duplex Doppler evaluation. Radiology 1989;173:93-97.
52. Pellerito JS, Troiano RN, Quedens-Case C, Taylor KJ: Common pitfalls of endovaginal color Doppler flow imaging. Radiographics 1995;15:37-47.
53. Cacciatore B, Korhonen J, Stenman UH, Ylostalo P: Transvaginal sonography and serum hCG in monitoring of presumed ectopic pregnancies selected for expected management. Ultrasound Obstet Gynecol 1995;5:297-300.
54. Tekay A, Jouppila P: Color Doppler flow as an indicator of trophoblastic activity in tubal pregnancies detected by transvaginal ultrasound. Obstet Gynecol 1992;80:995-999.
55. Tekay A, Martikainen H, Heikkinen H, et al: Disappearance of the trophoblastic blood flow in tubal pregnancy after methotrexate injection. J Ultrasound Med 1993;12:615-618.
56. Bonilla-Musoles FM, Ballester MJ, Tarin JJ, et al: Does transvaginal color Doppler sonography differentiate between developing and involuting ectopic pregnancies? J Ultrasound Med 1995;14:175-181.
57. Achiron R, Goldenberg M, Lipitz S, et al: Transvaginal Doppler sonography for detecting ectopic pregnancy: Is it really necessary? Isr J Med Sci 1994;30:820-825.
58. Nyberg DA, Laing FC, Jeffrey RB: Sonographic detection of subtle pelvic fluid collections. AJR Am J Roentgenol 1984;143:261-263.
59. Chen PC, Sickler GK, Dubinsky TJ, et al: Sonographic detection of echogenic fluid and correlation with culdocentesis in the evaluation of ectopic pregnancy. AJR Am J Roentgenol 1998;170:1299-1302.
60. Sickler GK, Chen PC, Dubinsky TJ, Maklad N: Free echogenic pelvic fluid: Correlation with hemoperitoneum. J Ultrasound Med 1998;17:431-435.

61. Wachsberg RH: Sonographic detection of echogenic fluid and correlation with culdocentesis in the evaluation of ectopic pregnancy [comment]. AJR Am J Roentgenol 1999;172:244-245.

62. Jeffrey RB, Laing FC: Echogenic clot: A useful sign of pelvic hemoperitoneum. Radiology 1982;145:139-141.

63. Hinney B, Bertagnoli C, Tobler-Sommer R, et al: Diagnosis of early ectopic pregnancy by measurement of the maternal serum to cul-de-sac fluid β-hCG ratio. Ultrasound Obstet Gynecol 1995;5:260-266.

64. Timor-Tritsch IE, Monteagudo A, Matera C, Veit CR: Sonographic evolution of cornual pregnancies treated without surgery. Obstet Gynecol 1992;79:1044-1049.

65. Ackerman TE, Levi CS, Dashefsky SM, et al: Interstitial line: Sonographic finding in interstitial cornual ectopic pregnancy. Radiology 1993;189:83-87.

66. Beckmann CRB, Sampson MB: Ultrasonographic diagnosis of interstitial ectopic pregnancy. J Clin Ultrasound 1984;12:304-306.

67. Takeuchi K, Yamada T, Oomori S, et al: Comparison of magnetic resonance imaging and ultrasonography in the early diagnosis of interstitial pregnancy. J Reprod Med 1999;44:265-268.

68. Lawrence A, Jurkovic D: Three-dimensional ultrasound diagnosis of interstitial pregnancy. Ultrasound Obstet Gynecol 1999;14:292-293.

69. Ushakov FB, Elchalal U, Aceman PJ, Schenker JG: Cervical pregnancy: Past and future. Obstet Gynecol Surv 1997;52:45-59.

70. Jurkovic D, Hacket E, Campbell S: Diagnosis and treatment of early cervical pregnancy: A review and a report of two cases treated conservatively. Ultrasound Obstet Gynecol 1996;8:373-380.

71. Su YN, Shih JC, Chiu WH, et al: Cervical pregnancy: Assessment with three-dimensional power Doppler imaging and successful management with selective uterine artery embolization. Ultrasound Obstet Gynecol 1999;14:284-287.

72. Jung SE, Byun JY, Lee JM, et al: Characteristic MR findings of cervical pregnancy. J Magn Reson Imaging 2001;13:918-922.

73. Atrash HK, Friede A, Hogue CJ: Abdominal pregnancy in the United States: Frequency and maternal mortality. Obstet Gynecol 1987;69:333-337.

74. Dubinsky TJ, Guerra F, Gormaz G, Maklad N: Fetal survival in abdominal pregnancy: A review of 11 cases. J Clin Ultrasound 1996;24:513-517.

75. Cartwright PS, Brown JE, Davis RJ, et al: Advanced abdominal pregnancy associated with fetal pulmonary hypoplasia: Report of a case. Am J Obstet Gynecol 1986;155:396-397.

76. Doubilet PM, Benson CB, Frates MF, Ginsburg E: Sonographically guided minimally invasive treatment of unusual ectopic pregnancies. J Ultrasound Med 2004;23:359-370.

Chapter 14

Infertility

Lawrence Grunfeld and Benjamin Sandler

Ultrasound assessment of follicle growth was introduced in the 1970s, when Hackeloer et al.[1] described a linear relationship between follicle size and estradiol levels (Fig. 14–1). The association of estrogen production with oocyte development allowed sonography to be used to detect oocyte maturity. It was not until 1978, when in vitro fertilization (IVF) was introduced, that transvaginal sonography (TVS) found a role in the treatment of infertility.[2] TVS provided a safe and effective means of retrieving oocytes in patients whose ovaries were buried under dense peritoneal adhesions. The explosion of IVF technology since the early 1990s has placed ultrasound machines in the hands of the practicing reproductive endocrinologist, making TVS an essential tool in the management of the infertile woman.

Normal Menstrual Cycle

During the normal menstrual cycle, TVS is able to discern ovarian as well as endometrial changes. Follicular growth is a continuous process that is independent of gonadotropin stimulation.

The follicle appears to develop over a period of 150 days. Three to five follicles from a cohort of approximately 1000 start developing into antral follicles beginning in the luteal phase of the previous cycle. There appear to be two or three waves of follicle development, as assessed by ultrasound observation of growth of follicles up to a diameter of 5 mm and subsequent shrinkage.[3] Gonadotropin-independent growth proceeds until the follicle reaches 5 mm.[4]

It is difficult to discern follicles that measure less than 5 mm, but ultrasound of the ovary will always demonstrate follicles at this stage of development. This is true even if ovulation is suppressed with oral contraceptives. Further growth of the follicle, however, is impossible in the absence of an appropriate gonadotropin milieu. The decline in follicle-stimulating hormone (FSH) that occurs in the late follicular phase is responsible for the selection of the single most mature follicle. Follicles with fewer FSH receptors on their surface become atretic. Once the leading follicle reaches a diameter of 14 mm, the daily growth rate is approximately 1.5 to 2 mm until ovulation, which occurs at a diameter of 20 to 24 mm.

Estradiol (E_2) is produced by the granulosa cells, and ovulation usually occurs when the serum E_2 reaches 150 to 400 pg/mL. Because the smaller atretic follicles do not contribute significantly to the pool of circulating estrogens, serum E_2 correlates with follicle diameter in the natural cycle.

Characteristic ultrasound appearance at the time of ovulation includes diminution in follicle size, blurring of the follicle borders, appearance of intrafollicular echoes, and demonstration of free fluid in the cul-de-sac. Thereafter, an irregular, mildly cystic structure representing the corpus luteum shrinks throughout the luteal phase of the cycle until luteolysis, which precedes menses. The corpus luteum can assume many forms, and there is no characteristic appearance to the ovary in the luteal phase (Fig. 14–2). Cystic corpora lutea can be sonolucent, although increasing the gain settings can usually reveal more echogenicity than in the pre-ovulatory follicle. The walls of the corpus luteum tend to be thicker and less regularly shaped than the preovulatory follicle. Many corpora lutea are echogenic and have the typical speckled appearance associated with blood. Some corpora lutea have a layered appearance owing to the presence of serum and solid clots. When there is suspicion that a luteal-phase mass is a corpus luteum, it is wise to reevaluate the patient during the follicular phase of a subsequent menstrual cycle.

The ultrasound appearance of the ovary not only evolves throughout the menstrual cycle, but also undergoes characteristic changes throughout the reproductive life of the woman. The ovary contains all the follicles it will ever have when the fetus is at 20 weeks' gestation. There is a rapid loss of follicles due to apoptosis over the woman's reproductive life. By the time menarche begins, most of the available follicles have degenerated. Only a small proportion of eggs are actually lost through ovulation. As the ovary ages, there is a noticeable diminution in ovarian volume and the number of small follicles. The number of follicles present in the ovary during menses has been called the *baseline antral follicle count* (BAFC). There is a direct correlation between age, ovarian volume, follicle count, and pregnancy rate in fertility therapy.[5] As women age, their ovaries shrink, their follicle numbers decrease, and their FSH rises.[6]

Ovarian size seems to correlate directly with oocyte reserve, as seen in women exposed to chemotherapy as children who demonstrate significantly smaller ovaries than

ACKNOWLEDGMENTS: The authors thank Dr. Martha Luna for her editorial assistance in the preparation of this chapter.

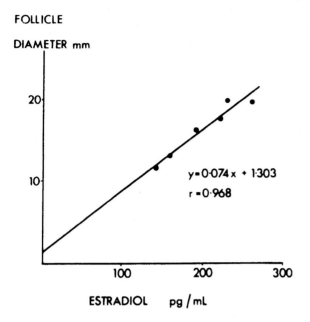

FOLLICLE

DIAMETER mm

$$y = 0.074x + 1.303$$
$$r = 0.968$$

ESTRADIOL   pg/mL

Figure 14–1. A linear relationship exists between estradiol (E_2) level and follicle size. Maturity is achieved when the follicle measures greater than 16 mm in diameter with an E_2 of 150 to 400 pg/mL.

normal women.[7] This is true even though these women preserved normal cyclicity and FSH values (Fig. 14–3).

The endometrium also demonstrates marked changes throughout the menstrual cycle (Fig. 14–4). Beginning with a thin echo during menses, the endometrium gradually thickens throughout the proliferative phase. Before ovulation, when estrogen levels peak and progesterone is not detectable, the endometrium is represented by three lines.[8] An inner luminal interface is surrounded by the functional hypoechoic endometrium and the echogenic myometrial–endometrial interface. A sonolucent halo, the origin of which is subject to debate, most likely represents the inner compact myometrium. After ovulation, the rise in progesterone causes an increase in stromal edema and the growth of spiral arterioles, which is depicted sonographically as an increase in echogenicity.[9] The luteal phase begins with an increase in peripheral echogenicity, which gradually progresses to the lumen and eventually causes its obliteration. Echogenicity in the luteal phase is maintained until menses, when there is breakdown of the endometrium.

Ovulation Induction

It is the goal of ovulation induction, in anovulatory women, to reproduce the natural menstrual cycle. Several agents are

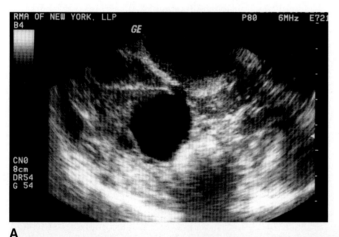

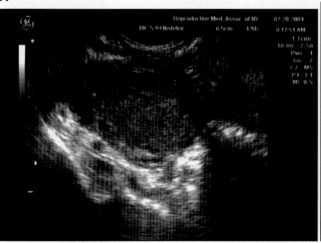

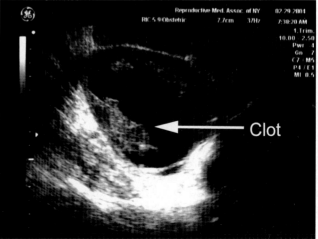

Figure 14–2. Cystic corpus luteum (**A**); hemorrhagic corpus luteum containing blood (**B**) and irregular borders and echogenic contents (**C**).

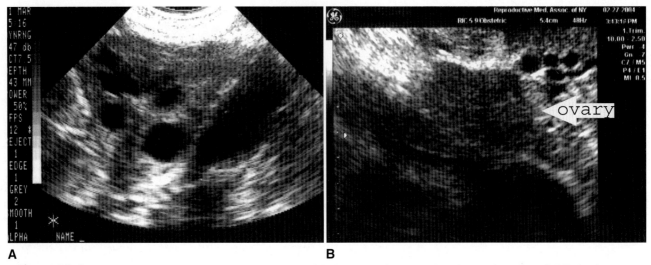

Figure 14–3. A, The normal ovary contains 4 to 10 baseline follicles. **B,** As the ovary ages, the number of small follicles decreases.

available to induce ovulation in anovulatory women. Before selecting an agent, it is important to classify the ovulation deficit. The World Health Organization[10] has devised a useful classification for this purpose:

Group I: low FSH and low estrogen (e.g., hypothalamic amenorrhea)
Group II: normal FSH and normal estrogen (e.g., polycystic ovary syndrome [PCOS])
Group III: high FSH and low estrogen (e.g., perimenopause and postmenopause)

Agents that induce endogenous FSH release through estrogen feedback (e.g., clomiphene citrate) are most productive in group II patients. Group I patients are best treated with gonadotropins (e.g., Repronex [Ferring Pharmaceuticals, Suffern, NY], Gonal-f [Serono Laboratories, Norwell, Mass], Follistim [Organon, Roseland, NJ], and Bravelle [Ferring]) to induce follicle development. Group III patients are the most challenging to treat and carry the poorest prognosis.

Induction Using Clomiphene Citrate

Clomiphene citrate induces endogenous gonadotropin release through binding of hypothalamic estrogen receptors. It is most effective in group II (normogonadotropin) anovulation. FSH and luteinizing hormone (LH) act at the ovary to stimulate follicle growth and development. It is usually initiated at a dose of 50 mg/day for 5 days, beginning on the third to fifth day of the menstrual cycle. The dosage is increased by 50 mg/day each cycle until ovulation occurs or a dose of 150 mg/day has been achieved. Exceeding this dose rarely results in pregnancy, and further diagnostic information or alternative medications should be sought.[10]

Sonography is useful in monitoring the response to clomiphene. The most important characteristic on the baseline ultrasound scan for detecting PCOS is the presence of more than five follicles measuring less than 8 mm.[11] A recent meeting of the American Society for Reproductive Medicine (ASRM) and the European Society for Human Reproduction and Embryology determined that the diagnosis of PCOS

requires either (1) 12 or more follicles measuring 2 to 9 mm in diameter or (2) increased ovarian volume (>10 cm³; Fig. 14–5). Although an ovarian volume of greater than 10 cm³ is characteristic of PCOS, approximately 30% of patients have normal ovarian volumes.[13] The definition of PCOS requires more than the above-mentioned ultrasound criteria for diagnosis. Women who are asymptomatic and have no ovulatory disturbance or elevated androgens are not considered to have PCOS[12] (Fig. 14–6).

Most patients with severe PCOS do not respond to clomiphene and may need to be treated with menotropins to induce ovulation. Insulin sensitizers such as metformin also have been extensively studied in PCOS. It appears that insulin resistance is a characteristic of polycystic ovaries.[14]

Although detection of ovulation can await luteal-phase measurements of the events that follow oocyte release, it is more practical to detect responsiveness to clomiphene before the luteal phase. Sonography performed 5 days after the last dose of clomiphene can detect enlargement of the dominant follicle. If follicular recruitment has been detected, ovulation can be expected. The luteal phase should then be evaluated for evidence of ovulation. This can be accomplished through assays of progesterone or ultrasound depiction of follicle rupture.

As an alternative to waiting for the LH surge, release of the dominant follicle can be triggered with a dose of human chorionic gonadotropin (hCG; 10,000 IU). It is imperative to use sonography to assess follicle maturity when hCG is added to stimulate follicle release. Follicle maturity is not reached with clomiphene until a diameter of 20 mm is achieved, and prematurely administering hCG will result in release of an immature oocyte.[15]

Sonography of the endometrium in clomiphene citrate therapy may demonstrate signs of premature luteal changes, even though follicle rupture has not occurred. Premature luteinization is probably one explanation for the discordance between successful induction of ovulation in more than 80% of cases and achievement of pregnancy in only 40%. The rate of multiple gestations with clomiphene treatment is 7%, with only rare cases of severe ovarian hyperstimulation.[16]

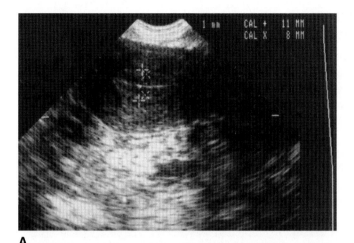

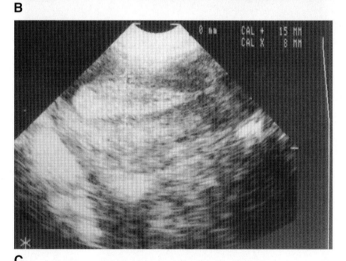

Figure 14–4. Progression of endometrial changes from a preovulatory (triple line) endometrium to the homogeneous luteal appearance. Note that echogenicity begins at the basalis and spreads into the lumen. **A,** Pattern I. **B,** Pattern II. **C,** Pattern III.

Induction Using Human Menopausal Gonadotropins

Human menopausal gonadotropins (hMGs) *(menotropins)* are available for clinical use as a combination of FSH and LH (Repronex) and a purified urinary form consisting of FSH

(Bravelle), as well as a recombinant pure FSH form (Gonal-f, Follistim). These agents achieve ovulation in group I patients who are resistant to clomiphene. They are also indicated in group II patients who fail to ovulate on clomiphene after an adequate therapeutic trial. Although they are often used in group III patients, perimenopausal women rarely become pregnant on these medications.

Menotropins are potent simulators of oocyte development and are effective only in doses that risk toxicity. These medications overcome the normal feedback mechanism that allows for only the most mature follicle to ovulate, causing maturation of a cohort of follicles at various stages of development. Spontaneous LH release occurs in approximately 20% of individuals treated with menotropins, but most need exogenous hCG to induce ovulation.[17] Because of potential toxicity when excessive drug is administered and the poor success when dosage is inadequate, sonography and serum E_2 measurement are mandatory to administer these drugs safely and effectively.

In the nonstimulated cycle, 90% of the peripheral estradiol (E_2) is secreted by the dominant follicle. In controlled ovarian hyperstimulation, the linear relationship between follicle size and E_2 is lost because peripheral E_2 reflects the sum total of all follicles. An oversupply of small follicles may significantly contribute to the circulating E_2 pool, and it is impossible to extrapolate from the E_2 level whether there are a few large follicles, several small ones, or a combination of the two. Follicle size, however, does correlate well with oocyte maturity. When the largest diameter measures between 18 and 24 mm, oocyte maturity is assumed[18] (Fig. 14–7).

A baseline ultrasound scan is recommended in the early follicular phase to ensure that the ovaries do not contain structures that may inhibit oocyte development. This is most important when the ovary was stimulated in previous cycles. Structures that may inhibit adequate stimulation include endometriomas (Fig. 14–8), corpora lutea remaining from previous stimulations, and neoplasms.

Some residual corpora lutea are normal and may permit normal responsiveness to gonadotropins. Judgment should be used regarding the initiation of gonadotropins immediately after a cycle of ovarian hyperstimulation. A single cyst as large as 5 cm was demonstrated by Penzias et al.[19] to result in normal responses. However, it is unwise to initiate gonadotropins when the ovary is completely replaced by corpora lutea after aggressive stimulation (Fig. 14–9).

The baseline scan is also useful to exclude pathologic processes such as hydrosalpinges (Fig. 14–10) (see Chapter 21). A repeat scan and E_2 measurement are performed after 5 days of stimulation. Drugs are continued until one to four mature follicles are obtained. This usually corresponds to a serum E_2 of 800 to 1500 pg/mL.

When ultrasound detects multiple small follicles and there is a high E_2 level, the dose of gonadotropin is reduced in an attempt to mature the cohort of larger follicles while smaller follicles become atretic. We have found that omitting 1 day of drug (coasting) is also helpful in obtaining this goal. In patients with a multifollicular (PCOS-like) response, follicular maturity may not be obtainable without exceeding a safety limit of 1500 pg/mL of E_2. When this occurs, it is wiser to omit hCG for fear of severe hyperstimulation and multiple gestation. Alternatively, ovulation can be induced with a gonadotropin-releasing hormone (GnRH) analog (e.g.,

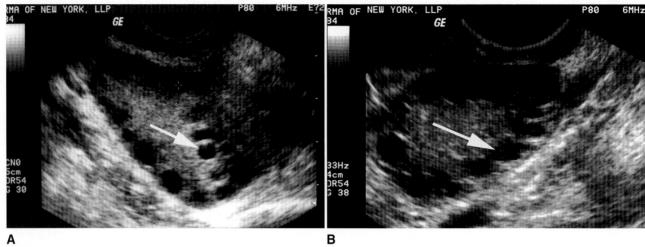

Figure 14–5. A and **B,** Ovaries with more than 10 baseline follicles *(arrow)* demonstrating the changes associated with polycystic ovary syndrome. The ovary in **B** demonstrates considerably more stromal thickening than that in **A.**

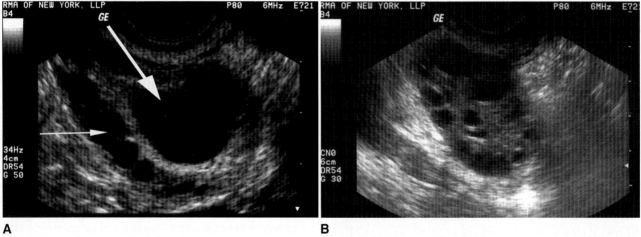

Figure 14–6. A, Ovary with multiple follicles *(small arrow)* and one mature follicle *(large arrow)*. The presence of ovulatory follicles excludes the diagnosis of polycystic ovary syndrome. **B,** An ovary with more than 10 follicles located diffusely throughout the stroma and without stromal thickening is defined as multicystic.

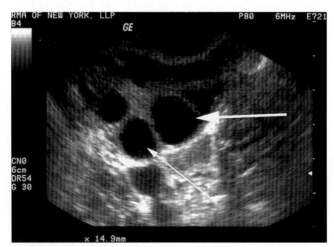

Figure 14–7. In controlled ovarian stimulation, follicles of different sizes are recruited. The mature follicle *(large arrow)* continues to grow, while the smaller follicles *(small arrow)* do not contain as many follicle-stimulating hormone receptors and become atretic.

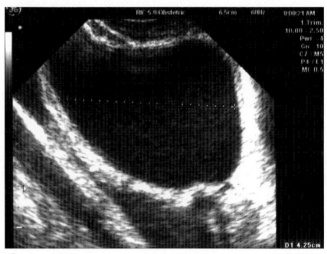

Figure 14–8. Large endometrioma (4.5 cm) found at baseline ultrasound. Note the typical speckled ultrasound appearance of endometriotic fluid.

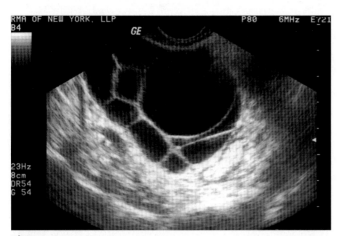

Figure 14–9. Residual corpus luteum cyst poststimulation. Note adjacent normal ovarian stroma.

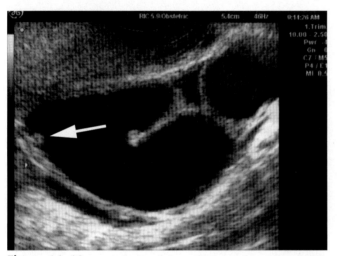

Figure 14–10. Large hydrosalpinx, which can be confused with a follicle when seen in a transverse section. Note the appearance of the fibrosed endosalpingeal folds (*arrow*) and the protruding incomplete septum.

Lupron 1 mg every 12 hours × 2 doses [TAP Pharmaceutical, Lake Forest, Ill) because significant LH will be released during the initial agonistic phase of this agent to create a "surrogate" surge.[20] The short half-life of GnRH analogs ensures LH release without prolonged luteal-phase stimulation, decreasing the risk of ovarian hyperstimulation syndrome. Luteal support, however, is mandatory.

It is safer in patients with an exaggerated response to stimulate ovulation with very low doses of pure FSH.[21] With this regimen, the dosage is increased by one half to one ampule each week until there is evidence of follicular growth. Although the mature (1.5 to 2.5 cm) follicles contain the fertilizable oocytes, the intermediate (1 to 1.5 cm) follicles also contribute to the hormonal production of the ovary. The greater number of intermediate follicles may be responsible for ovarian hyperstimulation.[22] Abdominal sonography is adequate for identification of mature follicles, but its poorer resolution can miss smaller follicles. TVS provides considerable enhancement in visualization of these smaller follicles that may be implicated in hyperstimulation. Because of the possibility of hyperstimulation, it is prudent not to trigger ovula-

tion if more than four mature or a total of nine mature and intermediate follicles appear.[23]

Ovarian Hyperstimulation Syndrome

Ovarian hyperstimulation syndrome occurs in its mild form in approximately 20% of cycles during induction therapy and in more than 50% of cycles that result in conception after hMG therapy[24] (Fig. 14–11). In its severe form, it is characterized by increased capillary permeability with consequent fluid shifts, hemoconcentration, and decreased renal perfusion. The etiology of the syndrome is not clear, but intraovarian renin production seems likely to play a role. Hyperstimulation is more common in cycles that result in multiple gestation.

Ovulation Induction and High-Order Multiple Gestation

High-order multiple gestation (HOMG; involving three or more fetuses) is a serious complication of controlled ovarian hyperstimulation. The incidence has been rapidly increasing because of the growing use of infertility treatments, especially induction of ovulation with gonadotropins and IVF. However, there is no way to reduce the risk of multiple births after induction of ovulation alone without reducing the rate of conception. As a consequence, multiple pregnancies after induction of ovulation have come to constitute the majority of all high-order multiple pregnancies related to infertility treatment. In contrast, IVF results in fewer high-order multiple pregnancies because the number of embryos replaced can be controlled.

The number and size of the follicles on the day of hCG administration are determinant factors in preventing HOMG. Gleicher and colleagues[25] reported no HOMG when less than 10 total follicles were present or E_2 levels were below 405 pg/mL on the day of ovulation. Dickey et al.[26] reported a 4% HOMG rate in women 34 years of age when fewer than six preovulatory follicles of 12 mm were present on the day of hCG administration or E_2 levels were less than 1000 pg/mL, compared with a 14% HOMG rate when there were six or more follicles of 12 mm or E_2 levels were 1000 pg/mL. However, for women 35 to 42 years of age, the HOMG rate was 5% when there were six or more follicles of 12 mm or E_2 levels were 1000 pg/mL.

It was concluded that if hCG had been withheld for women 35 years of age when six or more follicles measured 12 mm, 34% of cycles would have been canceled and the pregnancy rate in the remaining patients would have been 19%. For women 35 to 42 years of age, no cycle cancellations would be necessary.[27] Clear guidelines for cancellation to reduce HOMG can and should be established, based on the number of 10- to 12-mm preovulatory follicles and the patient's age. HOMG may be reduced by two thirds by withholding hCG when there are six or more 12-mm follicles or ten 10-mm follicles, based on the information at hand.[28]

The risk of HOMG in IVF can be considerably reduced by transferring only two embryos, with minimal effect on overall pregnancy rates. The ASRM currently recommends the transfer of a maximum of three to five embryos that have been fertilized in vitro. Furthermore, the in vitro development of embryos in the blastocyst stage now permits the transfer of fewer but more viable embryos. The transfer of only two blastocysts to the uterus can be expected to result in a clinical

Figure 14–11. Case of severe ovarian hyperstimulation syndrome. **A,** Enlarged ovary. **B,** The "floating uterus" sign due to ascites.

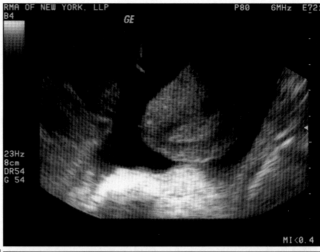

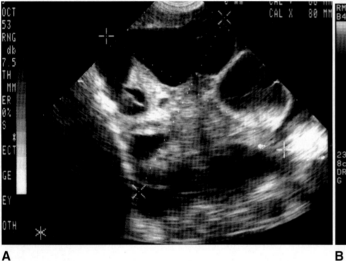

A

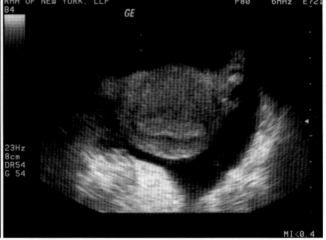

B

pregnancy in up to 60% to 70% of women, avoiding HOMG (except in case of monozygotic splitting).[28]

Initiation of Gonadotropin-Releasing Hormone and Analogs

Gonadotropin-releasing hormone is secreted by the hypothalamus, and a pulse is transported through the portal circulation to the pituitary every 90 minutes. Patients with hypothalamic amenorrhea (group I) can replace this hormone through a pulsatile delivery system that delivers a pulse of drug to the peripheral circulation at a constant interval.[29] LH surges may occur spontaneously in the cycle, stimulated by pulsatile GnRH. Sonography and E_2 measurement are helpful to time hCG administration, as in the natural cycle. After discontinuation of the pump, pituitary LH secretion is absent and luteal-phase support is mandatory.

The short-term effects of GnRH agonists are very similar to the effects of GnRH. The GnRH agonist binds to the receptors. The receptors then undergo a dimerization process and initiate a cascade of intracellular events that culminate in the synthesis and secretion of FSH and LH. Once the dimer has finished its signal transduction, it is internalized in the cell, as is the case with GnRH. However, over time, because of an overabundance of agonist with a long half-life, the dimer form of the receptor is favored and the receptors enter the cell, where they are trapped.

The lack of GnRH receptor activity results in down-regulation of GnRH activity, and the gonadotropes become desensitized to the continued presence of the GnRH agonist.[30]

During controlled ovarian hyperstimulation cycles for IVF, GnRH analogs can be initiated at different periods during the cycle to enhance stimulatory response and prevent premature LH surges. When analogs are initiated in the preceding luteal phase, desensitization is accomplished by the time gonadotropins are used (down-regulation or long protocol). This assists in synchronizing the cohort of primordial follicles as well as preventing a premature LH surge. The long protocol is not appropriate in poorly responding patients because of profound ovarian suppression. In these patients, a short protocol (flare protocol) is used to potentiate the early follicular-phase follicle recruitment. Early follicular agonist initiation induces massive release of endogenous pituitary LH and FSH during the first hours postinitiation (flare effect). It is hoped that these endogenous gonadotropins will enhance follicular response. Regardless of which protocol is used, the ultrasound assessment of follicular response is the same.

Initiation of Gonadotropin-Releasing Hormone Antagonists

The mechanism of action of the GnRH antagonist is to block the receptor directly in the pituitary gland and prevent the receptor from activating; the agonist, on the other hand, does activate the receptor and is associated with a flare effect.[31] There is no receptor dimerization with the antagonist. The GnRH antagonist outcompetes GnRH for the GnRH receptors and blocks the ability of GnRH to initiate dimer formation and signal transduction. As a result of this receptor monopolization by GnRH antagonist, there is no secretion of FSH or LH from the pituitary gonadotrope. This is true in both the short and the long term: as long as sufficient GnRH antagonist is present, suppression of FSH and LH will be sustained.[32]

One of the advantages of GnRH antagonist stimulation protocols is that they prevent premature LH surges but do not cause suppression in the early follicular phase, a crucial time for poorly responding patients.[33] GnRH antagonist treatment regimens allow for a more natural recruitment of follicles in the follicular phase in an ovary that has not been suppressed by the absence of FSH and LH due to GnRH agonist treatment.[34]

The follicular response in antagonist cycles is characterized by rapid early follicular growth, evident on ultrasound. The introduction of the antagonist too early in a cycle would be counterproductive and would lead to a shut-off of potentially helpful endogenous FSH. Conversely, if the antagonist is added too late in the cycle, it might not effectively inhibit a premature LH surge. In our program, the GnRH antagonist is administered when the largest follicle reaches 14 mm in diameter. The GnRH suppression by antagonist is profound and results in a decline in E_2 levels unless gonadotropin is added back. This is particularly important in patients who are poor responders and have fewer FSH receptors. These patients require maximal stimulation. This is why we proactively add an additional 75 IU of menotropins routinely to our antagonist/recombinant FSH stimulation protocols.

Whenever possible, it is our practice not to trigger with hCG too early (before cycle day 11, which correlates to 9 days of stimulation) in patients receiving antagonist protocols because their rapid follicular growth may not necessarily predict oocyte maturity. In the antagonist stimulation cycles at our centers, we compared pregnancy rates with administration of hCG when the lead follicle diameter was 16 to 17 mm, 18 to 19 mm, or more than 20 mm. Results of this study indicated that in GnRH antagonist cycles, as the size of the follicle increased, a concomitant increase in pregnancy rates occurred. Conversely, patients in agonist down-regulation treatment regimens did not benefit from obtaining larger follicle sizes.[35]

Clearly, the use of antagonists has advantages for patients. GnRH antagonist treatment takes less time, and there is nearly an 80% decrease in the number of injections needed compared with an agonist cycle.

Methodology of Ultrasound Assessment

It is particularly important when performing sonography in fertility therapy to avoid the use of spermicidal materials, such as lubricants, on the exterior of the probe.

Identifying the Ovaries

First, the uterus is located in the midline and is used as a reference point (Fig. 14–12). Both longitudinal and transverse

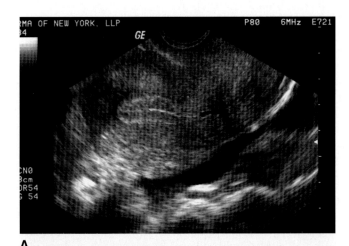

A

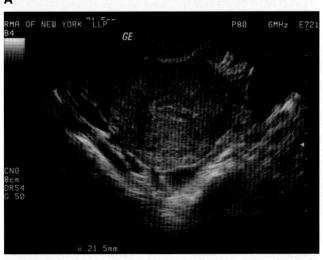

B

Figure 14–12. Longitudinal (sagittal, **A**) and transverse (coronal, **B**) views of the uterus.

sections are obtained by rotating the transducer 90 degrees. The ovaries are localized by directing the transducer lateral to the uterus. A useful landmark is the hypogastric vessels that lie lateral to the normal location of the ovaries (Fig. 14–13). The ovaries are easily identified by their echogenic stroma and sonolucent follicles. When stimulation is inadequate, however, identification of the ovary can be challenging. In patients who are obese or whose ovaries are abnormally located, the usual criteria for identifying the ovary fail. Occasionally, a full-bladder transabdominal scan can locate an ovary that is out of the focal range of the vaginal transducer.

Follicle Measurements

A follicle is an ellipsoid and has different dimensions when measured in each of its three diameters. It is easiest to use the two largest diameters when assessing follicle maturity. Research on ovarian volumes requires more complex measurements of each follicle diameter. The volume is approximated by the following formula: $(\pi/6) \times A \times B \times C$, where A, B, and C are diameters measured in three different planes. In menotropin-stimulated cycles, follicles with a mean diameter of 16 to 18 mm have fully completed the maturational process and yield fertilizable oocytes.[36] This is in contrast to

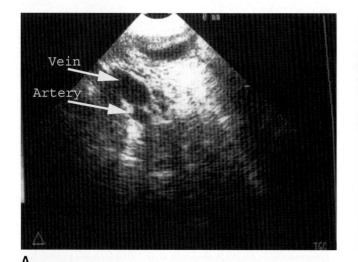

A

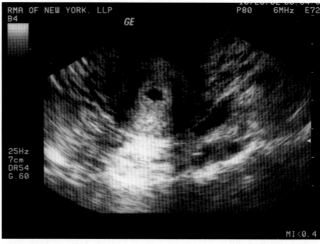

A

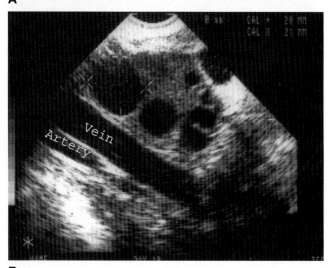

B

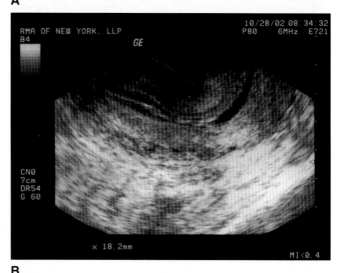

B

Figure 14–13. Coronal (**A**) and transverse (**B**) views of iliac artery and vein situated lateral to the ovary.

Figure 14–14. Transverse (**A**) and longitudinal (**B**) views of the cervical canal filled with mucus, resembling a follicle.

clomiphene-stimulated cycles, in which 20 mm is typical of mature follicles.

Follicles can be confused with other pelvic structures, mainly large-caliber blood vessels such as the hypogastric vein. They can be differentiated by rotating the transducer 90 degrees into a perpendicular plane. If the structure is a vessel, it will elongate on the screen and appear tubular. The hypogastric artery can be easily identified by its arterial pulsations. If color Doppler is available, blood vessels can be easily identified. Similarly, a hydrosalpinx can sometimes be confused with a follicle if seen in a cross-sectional plane. Bowel has a relatively greater echogenicity and continued peristaltic movements that make discrimination easy for experienced sonographers. The cervical canal can fill with mucus and may also be confused with follicles (Fig. 14–14). Other cystic structures such as loculated peritoneal cysts may also simulate the hyperstimulated ovary.

Assisted Reproductive Technology

In vitro fertilization was first successfully performed in humans in 1978.[2] Advances in ultrasound technology have decreased the invasiveness of oocyte retrieval and made IVF more acceptable for a wider range of infertility disorders. Currently, IVF is used to manage infertility due to tubal occlusion and also disorders such as unexplained infertility, immunologic infertility, male factor infertility, and endometriosis. The entire spectrum of high-technology fertility-promoting procedures that require oocyte aspiration and gamete manipulation is encompassed under the term *assisted reproductive technology.*

Superovulation

Early in the course of IVF development, it became apparent that the process of fertilizing an embryo and transferring it into the endometrial cavity is inefficient. In 1977 Steptoe and Edwards[2] transferred single embryos that were recovered in natural cycles and were able to achieve a 5% pregnancy rate. Although this was clearly a milestone in the progress of therapy for infertility, these early success rates would not be acceptable today. The major advance resulting in enhanced success was the use of superovulation (controlled ovarian hyperstimulation) for the recruitment of many oocytes[37] (Table 14–1). Today, superovulation with a combination of

Table 14–1	Controlled Ovarian Hyperstimulation versus In Vitro Fertilization	
	Ovulation Induction	**In Vitro Fertilization**
Drug dose	Low (e.g., 150 IU/day)	High (e.g., 210-450 IU/day)
Follicle number	≤4	Maximum possible
Hyperstimulation risk	High	Reduced by follicle aspiration
Multiple pregnancy risk	High	Reduced by controlling embryo transfer

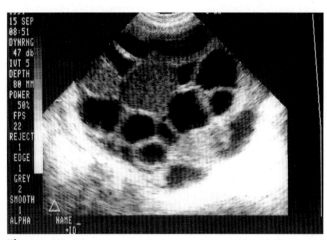

Figure 14–15. An ovary demonstrating multiple follicles and endometriomas in a patient with a known history of endometriosis undergoing in vitro fertilization.

menotropins and GnRH analogs or antagonists is standard. Controlled ovarian hyperstimulation permits the retrieval of many oocytes, whereas in natural cycles only one oocyte matures. This increase in the pool of fertilizable oocytes will increase the number of embryos transferred into the endometrial cavity, with a resultant increase in the chance of at least one embryo's implanting.

In natural cycles, ovulation occurs at follicular diameters of 1.5 to 2.5 cm. Menotropin treatment, however, is associated with more rapid increases in oocyte maturity as reflected by follicular diameters. Because only follicles that have achieved this level of stimulation contain mature oocytes, it is important that oocyte aspiration be delayed until evidence of follicular maturity exists. It is best not to trigger ovulation until most of the follicles have achieved a diameter of at least 1.5 cm.[18] GnRH analogs and antagonists offer the advantage of prolonging stimulation so that the follicle can mature without concern for premature ovulation.[38]

Hyperstimulation is less of a concern in IVF because the aspiration of follicular contents seems to protect against severe complications of overstimulation. Consequently, controlled ovarian hyperstimulation is continued until most oocytes have achieved evidence of follicular maturity. This improves fertilization rates and provides a larger pool of embryos to select from for the embryo transfer.

Once it is determined that follicular maturation has occurred, a triggering dose of hCG is administered (Fig. 14–15). This results in resumption of meiosis by the oocyte that allows the oocyte to be fertilized. With resumption of meiosis, there is a loss of the germinal vesicle and expulsion of the polar body. Only oocytes that have achieved this level of maturity are fertilizable. These events require 34 to 38 hours in humans, and oocyte aspiration is scheduled for 36 hours after injection of hCG.

Ultrasound Assessment of the Endometrium

Ultrasound assessment of the endometrium has received a great deal of attention in the analysis of factors that affect implantation. The literature has demonstrated conflicting data about the predictive value of sonography in the assessment of implantation failure. A meta-analysis of the literature demonstrates endometrial thickness to be a better negative than positive predictor of implantation.[39] Although a minimal endometrial thickness is necessary for implantation, most implantation failure is secondary to embryonic developmental arrest.

Implantation in the Late Follicular Phase

Using the classification introduced by Welker et al.,[40] Gonen et al. demonstrated improved implantation rates when a pattern associated with the late follicular phase was present on the day of hCG administration (pattern C). There is no uniformity in endometrial pattern classification, and this pattern has been described by various authors as multilayered pattern I,[6] pattern IIB,[40] or triple line. The follicular-phase pattern consists of a luminal echo surrounded by a hypoechoic endometrium and an echogenic endometrium–myometrium interface. An endometrium that is echogenic and characteristic of the luteal phase rarely results in pregnancy when present on the day of hCG administration. An advanced appearance of endometrial homogenicity on the day of hCG administration is associated with reduced pregnancy rates.[41] There is considerable overlap, however, in the endometrial patterns between those who conceived and those who did not.[42,43] Sher et al.[44] demonstrated a reduction in pregnancy rates from 29% in cycles with the multilayered pattern to 6% in more than 1300 cycles with advanced patterns. The likely explanation for this finding is that the endometrium and embryo must be synchronized, and if the endometrium is advanced or retarded in its development, implantation will not occur.

Endometrial Patterns in Patients Undergoing Drug Therapy

Investigators who have studied endometrial patterns in patients treated with GnRH analogs to suppress premature ovulation have failed to demonstrate a strong correlation between implantation and a multilayered endometrium.[45] The absence of premature luteinization diminishes the predictive value of endometrial patterns. This is probably because very few patients demonstrate advanced endometrial patterns when progesterone levels are inhibited in the late follicular phase by GnRH analogs.

Gonen and associates demonstrated that pregnancy was not associated with significantly thicker endometrium when patients were treated with a combination of clomiphene and menotropins.[46]

The endometrial thickness and pattern may provide useful information in cycles in which the endometrium is supplemented with estrogen and progesterone. Supplemented cycles are used to transfer embryos from third parties in oocyte donation. Patients who require oocyte donation do not develop eggs that can sustain pregnancy, although their endometrium is normal and can support pregnancy if healthy embryos are transferred. A minimal endometrial thickness of 6 mm is required before embryo replacement for pregnancy to be achieved.[44] Shapiro and colleagues[47] found a 60% pregnancy rate in oocyte recipients who demonstrated a favorable pattern and a 0% pregnancy rate when less than 6 mm of endometrium growth was achieved. Increasing the dosage of estrogen was shown by Sher et al.[48] to convert unfavorable to favorable endometrial patterns. In contrast, thick endometrium does not seem to affect implantation adversely.[48]

Endometrial and Uterine Contour

Although there is debate about the role of endometrial texture in implantation, endometrial contour is less disputed. Endometrial abnormalities such as fibroids and septa can cause implantation failure. Smaller cavities were also found to perform less well in IVF. On three-dimensional sonography, a cavity smaller than 2.5 mL was associated with a marked reduction in pregnancy rate[49] (Fig. 14–16). Traditionally, the uterus is evaluated by hysterosalpingography before IVF to ensure a normal-shaped cavity. The instillation of small quantities of normal saline into the uterus, a technique known as *sonohysterography,* may provide the same information. Data by Parsons and Lense[50] and Maroulis et al.[51] show good correlation between x-ray hysterosalpingography and sonohysterography (Fig. 14–17). Ultrasound has the advantages of less discomfort, less radiation, and immediate availability at the time of the preliminary evaluation.

Three-Dimensional Ultrasound Assessment of Uterine Anatomy

Three-dimensional (3D) sonography allows the computer to create a map of the uterus in a plane that is not usually visible in two-dimensional sonography (Fig. 14–18). The coronal view of the uterus is difficult to obtain because of flexion of the cavity. Conventional two-dimensional sonography with saline infusion is as effective as three-dimensional sonography at identifying filling defects due to polyps and fibroids (Fig. 14–19). 3D sonography may, however, offer an advantage in the identification of müllerian fusion abnormalities such as septa[52] (Figs. 14–20 and 14–21).

Assessment for the Presence of Endometrial Fluid

Fluid in the endometrial cavity before embryo transfer in IVF cycles is associated with implantation failure. This fluid may be cervical mucus that ascends into the endometrial cavity, but it also is associated with fluid reflux from a hydrosalpinx[53] or subclinical uterine infection[54] or could be a result of abnormal endometrial development.[55] In an IVF cycle, day 3 embryos (8 cells) or day 5 embryos (100 cells) are placed into the uterine cavity. The presence of excessive fluid inside the cavity could have adverse effects on cell proliferation or interfere with the very early stages of embryo implantation (apposition and attachment). The identification of persistent fluid accumulation may prompt the clinician to freeze all embryos and postpone the transfer. There have been reports of removal of endometrial fluid with a transfer catheter

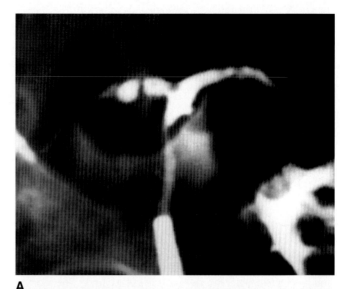

A

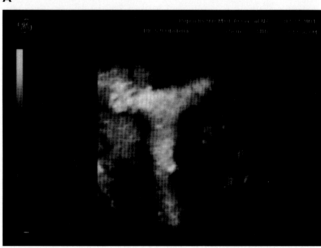

B

Figure 14–16. T-shaped uterus on hysterosalpingography (**A**) and saline infusion sonohysterography (**B**).

immediately before embryo transfer, with successful results[56] (Fig. 14–22).

Doppler Measurements of Vascular Resistance

Implantation depends on the interplay of embryonic factors and uterine receptivity. Although embryo quality is critical for successful implantation, endometrial receptivity plays a major role. Pulsed Doppler has been used to obtain flow waveforms from the uterine arteries during various phases of the menstrual cycle. Preliminary data have suggested that decreased uterine perfusion may be responsible for infertility.[57] Steer et al.[58] analyzed 82 cycles of assisted reproduction in which the flow through the uterine arteries was measured with transvaginal color-flow Doppler. The mean pulsatility index of the two uterine arteries was calculated and was used as a quantitative index of endometrial receptivity. Women whose pulsatility indices were greater than 3.0 demonstrated decreased implantation rates. It has been suggested that this new technique could lead to improved pregnancy rates in cycles of

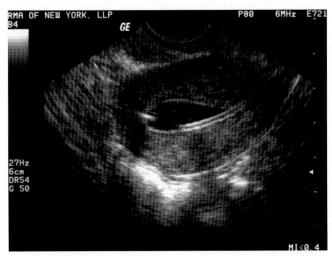

Figure 14–17. Normal endometrial cavity on saline infusion sonohysterography. Note the tip of the catheter in the posterior wall of the endometrial cavity.

assisted reproduction by demonstrating suboptimal conditions for embryo transfer. Embryo transfer can be postponed through cryopreservation to subsequent cycles in which endometrial receptivity can be manipulated through estrogen administration.

In addition to the use of 3D ultrasound as a tool for measuring uterine cavity volume, recently, subendometrial color Doppler has been used to evaluate the blood flow beneath the endometrium.[59] The vascular flow index (VFI) as calculated by a computerized nomogram has also been found to be predictive of implantation potential.[59] A VFI greater than 0.24 was associated with higher implantation potentials. The VFI was found to be more predictive of conception than was uterine artery blood flow.[60] Nevertheless, studies comparing cycles in which conception occurred with those in which conception failed have demonstrated tremendous overlap between most ultrasound criteria because, other than the requirement of an endometrial thickness of 6 mm, the overwhelming predictors of implantation are embryo quality and embryo transfer technique. In clinical practice, Doppler measurements of blood

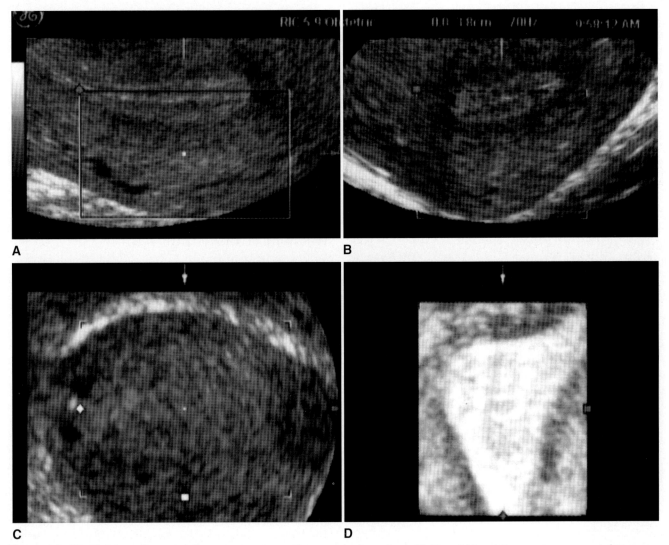

Figure 14–18. The three-dimensional sonogram captures the uterus in three planes (**A, B,** and **C**) and then creates a computed tomogram through a user-defined plane (**D**).

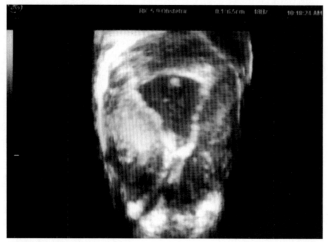

Figure 14–19. Normally shaped cavity on three-dimensional sonography.

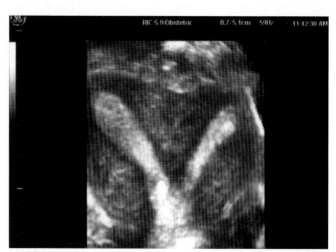

Figure 14–21. Large septum on three-dimensional sonogram without saline infusion.

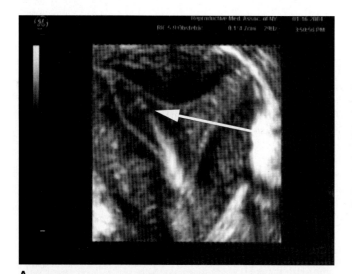

A

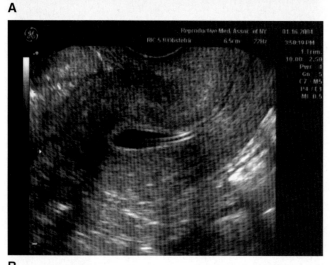

B

Figure 14–20. Septum seen on three-dimensional saline infusion hysterosonography. **A,** Three-dimensional view. The catheter is seen in one of the uterine horns *(arrow).* **B,** Sagittal view.

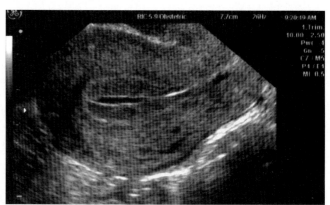

Figure 14–22. Mucus in the endometrial cavity.

flow and studies of texture are not as useful as quantifying endometrial thickness[61,62] (Fig. 14–23).

Oocyte Retrieval

The first oocyte retrieval in humans was performed in 1966 through laparotomy. With further refinements of technique, in 1977 Edwards and Steptoe successfully fertilized human oocytes recovered laparoscopically. The first ultrasound-guided aspiration of oocytes was performed by Lenz and associates[63] in Denmark. The approach used by the Danish team was transabdominal sonography with a transvesical puncture. Initially, the needle was not coupled to the transducer, but a needle guide improved the rate of oocyte recovery. The recovery rate in this series was 53%, which compares favorably with laparoscopically performed procedures. Gleicher et al.[64] were credited with the first oocyte retrieval through culdocentesis, although the technology of the time required transabdominal sonography.

A major improvement in ultrasound retrieval occurred with the development of the transvaginal transducer.[65] Ovaries that are surrounded by dense adhesions tend to be fixed to the cul-de-sac, a location that is most easily reached transvaginally. Before the development of TVS, a surgical procedure was often necessary to fix the ovaries to the fundus of

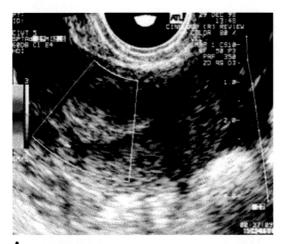

A

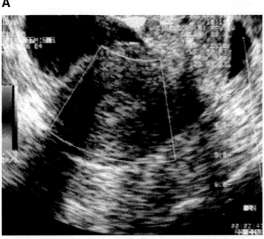

B

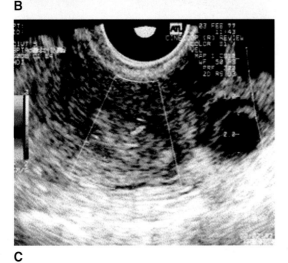

C

Figure 14–23. Doppler assessment of subendometrial flow. **A,** No detectable endometrial or subendometrial flow. **B,** Presence of subendometrial flow only. **C,** Presence of endometrial and subendometrial flow. (From Chien L-W, Au H-K, Chen P-L, et al: Assessment of uterine receptivity by the endometrial-subendometrial blood flow distribution pattern in women undergoing in vitro fertilization-embryo transfer. Fertil Steril 2002;78:245-251, with permission.)

the uterus to allow access to the ovaries by laparoscopy. Ovarian fixation in preparation for IVF is no longer recommended and should not be performed. The most appropriate place for the ovary after laparotomy undertaken for treatment of gynecologic pathology is its usual location, in the cul-de-sac. The absence of bowel gas between the vaginal fornix and the ovaries allows direct visualization of the ovaries without the need for a sonic window to enhance ultrasound transmission. In addition to easier access to the ovaries with transvaginal aspiration, the risks of bladder injury, hematuria, and infection associated with transvesical puncture are reduced when the follicle is approached transvaginally. TVS-guided follicular puncture has resulted in oocyte retrieval rates of 75%, which are comparable with those obtained by laparoscopy (Fig. 14–24).

The needle we use for aspiration has a 17-gauge outer diameter and is 11 inches long (Fig. 14–25). It is important for ultrasound visualization of the needle that the tip be echogenic to enhance reflection of the ultrasound beam. Precise placement of the needle is particularly important with regard to the major vessels of the pelvis. The stimulated ovary lies immediately adjacent to the hypogastric artery and vein. To prevent injury to these vessels, the tip of the needle must be visualized at all times. Another problem that can occur is misalignment of the needle with the ultrasound beam. It is important that the needle guide be secured to the transducer to prevent rotation from the proper axis. Misalignment of the needle guide will result in loss of visibility of the needle, with a loss of precision (Fig. 14–26).

Transvaginal approaches to the ovary are less painful than laparoscopic approaches, and this procedure can be performed on an ambulatory basis with only intravenous sedation. Patients who have a TVS-guided aspiration under local anesthesia tolerate the procedure well. Hammarberg and colleagues[66] found that 90% of patients experienced some pain or no pain, whereas none described the retrieval as very painful. Premedication with a sedative and paracervical block was sufficient anesthesia for 70% of patients, additional sedation was necessary for 20% of patients, and 10% of patients thought the procedure was painful enough to require heavier anesthesia. When only a single oocyte is retrieved, such as in the natural cycle, only local anesthetic is necessary.

Dellenbach et al.[65] reported no major complications in more than 800 transvaginal oocyte recoveries. In a series of more than 2500 retrievals, Bennett and associates[67] reported vaginal hemorrhage in 8% of cases, but most of these had insignificant blood loss. Pelvic infections occurred in 0.6% of cases. Two cases resulted in hemoperitoneum requiring laparotomy. Dicker et al.[68] reported 9 pelvic abscesses in 3600 retrievals. Most of these cases were in patients with preexisting pelvic infections. Care should be taken to avoid entering hydrosalpinges or endometriomas when performing follicle puncture because this can predispose to pelvic infection. The hypogastric vessels are easily identified by turning the transducer 90 degrees to see the long axis of the structure (Fig. 14–27).

Embryo Transfer

Embryo transfer requires the joint efforts of the reproductive biologist and the clinician. Without healthy embryos that can implant, embryo transfer is sure to fail. Likewise, the work of embryologists to maintain the viability of embryos is futile if embryo transfer is traumatic.

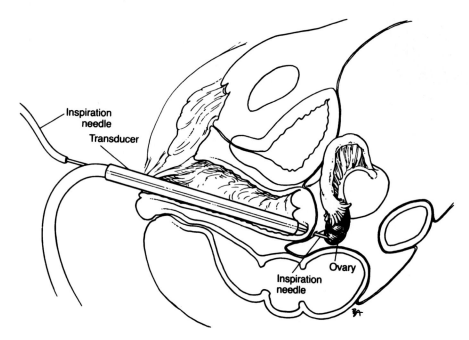

Figure 14–24. Transvaginal sonography–guided follicular aspiration. The needle punctures the lateral vaginal fornix and is introduced into the follicles. Note the position of the ovary in the cul-de-sac adjacent to the fornix. (From Grunfeld L, Fox J: Assisted reproductive technology: Surgical aspects. In Gershenson D, De Cherney A, Curry S [eds]: Operative Gynecology. Philadelphia, WB Saunders, 1993, p 551, with permission.)

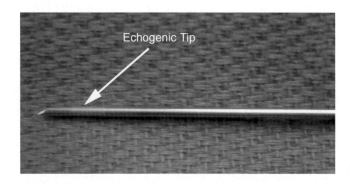

Figure 14–25. Echogenic tip *(arrow)* of the aspiration needle.

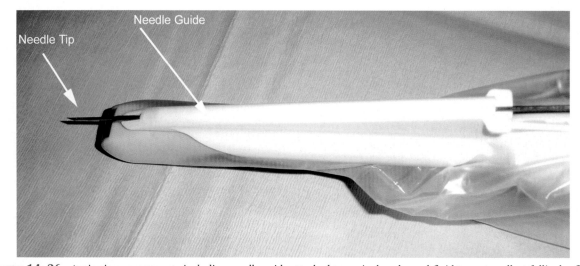

Figure 14–26. Aspiration components including needle guide attached to vaginal probe and fluid traps to collect follicular fluid.

Many factors have been proposed to explain the disparity between embryonic development and pregnancy rates. Genetic abnormalities of embryos and defects in uterine receptivity have been implicated.[69] However, much of the inefficiency of embryo implantation may stem from embryo transfer technique. Uterine contractions, expulsion of embryos, blood or mucus on the catheter tip, bacterial contamination of the catheter, and retained embryos have all been associated with problematic and unsuccessful embryo transfers.

The ultimate goal of a successful embryo transfer is to deliver the embryos precisely to the uterine fundus in a location where implantation is maximized. Because of the great variability in cervical and uterine anatomy, a trial transfer in a cycle preceding IVF allows the physician to measure the uterine cavity depth and direction in advance. The direction of the cervix and uterus can be mapped and the depth of the cavity recorded. In addition, any degree of cervical stenosis can be dealt with in advance. We therefore recommend that trial transfer be routinely performed 1 to 2 months before the IVF cycle.

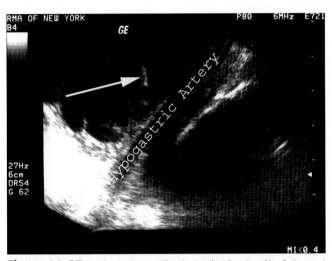

Figure 14–27. Echogenic needle tip is clearly visualized *(arrow)* entering the follicle. As follicular fluid is aspirated, the follicle will collapse. Note the proximity of the ovary to the hypogastric vessels.

Technique

In general, embryo transfer is performed by the passage of a Teflon catheter loaded with embryos through the cervical os. The column of embryos is placed between two smaller columns of media and air. The catheter is passed through the cervical os and the tip is passed to approximately 1 cm from the fundus of the uterus (without touching it), where the embryos are slowly expelled. Once the catheter is withdrawn, it is checked for the presence of residual embryos[70] (Fig. 14–28).

The use of ultrasound guidance for embryo transfer was first described by Strickler et al.[71] in 1985. Transabdominal sonography has been used to verify that the transfer catheter has passed into the endometrial cavity.[72] As the catheter is guided through the cervix, transabdominal sonography can identify the catheter tip to ensure proper fundal placement of the embryos. Ultrasound guidance has many potential advantages. It facilitates placement of soft catheters through sharp cervical uterine angles; avoids touching the fundus; confirms that the catheter is beyond the internal os in cases of an elongated cervical canal; and allows direction of the catheter along the contour of the endometrial cavity, thereby avoiding disruption of the endometrium, plugging of the catheter tip with endometrium, and initiation of bleeding (Fig. 14–29). Ancillary advantages include assessment of the ovaries and for the presence of excessive peritoneal fluid volume to confirm that the risk for ovarian hyperstimulation syndrome is not so great as to preclude embryo transfer. Fluid in the endometrial cavity can also be ruled out.

The full bladder required for transabdominal ultrasound guidance is itself helpful in pushing the uterus backward, thereby straightening the cervical–uterine angle to facilitate passage of the catheter.[73]

Potential Pitfalls

Retention of the embryos in the cervical canal is a problem sometimes encountered with embryo transfer. As the catheter passes through the cervix, cervical mucus adheres to the catheter, and embryos can get stuck to the mucus. The presence of blood on the outside of the catheter tip may indicate a traumatic embryo transfer, and Goudas et al.[74] found this to be associated with lower pregnancy rates. Visser and colleagues[75] reported that blood or mucus on the catheter tip was

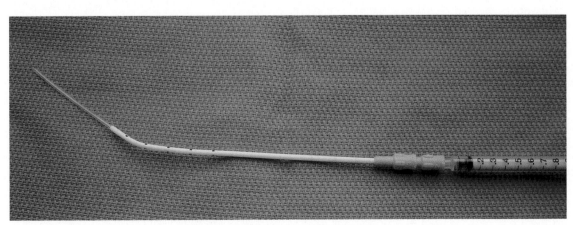

Figure 14–28. Embryo transfer catheter.

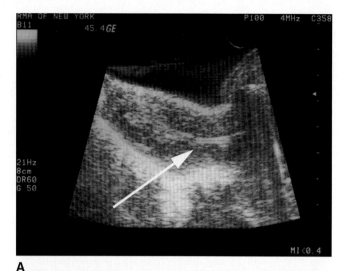

A

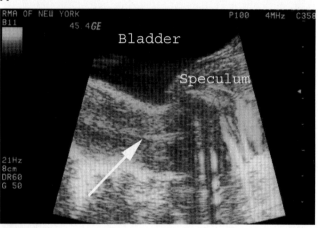

B

Figure 14–29. A, Echogenic catheter seen in the endometrial cavity *(arrow)* before advancing into the cornua **(B).** Embryo transfer is typically performed by transabdominal sonographic guidance.

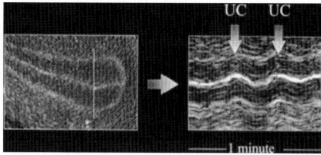

Figure 14–30. Endometrial contractility can be induced by traumatic transfers, as seen on this M-mode scan. (From Fanchin R, Ayoubi JM, Righini C, et al: Uterine contractility decreases at time of blastocyst transfers. Hum Reprod 2001;16:1115-1119. © European Society of Human Reproduction and Embryology. Reproduced by permission of Oxford University Press/Human Reproduction.)

tributing factor in the success of day 5 blastocyst–stage embryo transfer. Fewer uterine contractions are associated with improved pregnancy rates.[81]

Summary

The new reproductive technologies developed over the past 25 years are referred to collectively as *assisted reproductive technology.* They range from controlled ovarian hyperstimulation and insemination to IVF. TVS is the preferred method for monitoring endometrial and follicle development. In addition to its diagnostic capabilities, sonography plays a major role in follicle retrieval and embryo transfer. The future holds promise in the uses of embryos derived from IVF. Genetic diagnosis of embryos before implantation, oocyte preservation, and stem cell research will become prominent offshoots of IVF technology.

associated with a higher incidence of retained embryos. Mucus plugging of the catheter tip can cause embryo retention and damage (especially with assisted hatching) and improper embryo placement. Mansour et al.[76] found that cervical mucus affected the rate of embryo expulsion into the cervix. A vigorous cervical lavage with culture media performed before embryo transfer to remove all visible mucus is associated with higher pregnancy rates.[77]

Uterine contractions in the early luteal phase are usually cervicofundal in origin. This may account for some of the ectopic pregnancies seen after IVF. Alterations in the normal contraction pattern may cause expulsion of the embryos into the cervix.[78] The pregnancy and implantation rates decrease as the frequency of uterine contractions increases (Fig. 14–30). Serum progesterone levels on the day of embryo transfer, but not the day of hCG administration, correlated with the frequency of uterine contractions. As progesterone levels increase, uterine contractions decrease.[79]

It has been reported that a tenaculum applied to the cervix during mock embryo transfer increases uterine contractions.[80] Uterine junctional zone contractions progressively decrease with progression into the luteal phase, and this may be a con-

REFERENCES

1. Hackeloer B, Fleming R, Robinson H, et al: Correlation of ultrasonic and endocrinologic assessment of human follicular development. Am J Obstet Gynecol 1979;135:122-128.
2. Steptoe PC, Edwards RG: Birth after the reimplantation of a human embryo. Lancet 1978;2:366.
3. Baerwald AR, Adams GP, Pierson RA: A new model for ovarian follicular development during the human menstrual cycle. Fertil Steril 2003;80:116-122.
4. Greenwald GS, Terranova PF: Follicular selection and its control. In Knobel E, Neill JD (eds): Physiology of Reproduction. New York, Raven Press, 1988, p 387.
5. Douglas M, Addy MD, Gail F, et al: Age and resting follicle number predict response to gonadotropin stimulation in in vitro fertilization cycles. Am J Obstet Gynecol 2002;187:285-288.
6. Erdem A, Erdem M, Biberoglu K, et al: Age-related changes in ovarian volume, antral follicle counts and basal FSH in women with normal reproductive health. J Reprod Med 2002;47:835-839.
7. Larsen EC, Muller J, Rechnitzer C, et al: Diminished ovarian reserve in female childhood cancer survivors with regular menstrual cycles and basal FSH <10 IU/l. Hum Reprod 2003;18:417-422.
8. Yoshimitsu K, Nakamura G, Nakano H: Dating sonographic endometrial images in the normal ovulatory cycle. Int J Gynaecol Obstet 1989;28:33-39.
9. Grunfeld L, Walker B, Bergh PA, et al: High resolution endovaginal ultrasonography of the endometrium: A non-invasive test for endometrial adequacy. Obstet Gynecol 1991;78:200-204.
10. Gysler M, March CM, Mishell DR Jr, Bailey EJ: A decade's experience with an individualized clomiphene treatment regimen including its effect on the postcoital test. Fertil Steril 1982;37:161-167.

11. Yeh HC, Futtenweit W, Thornton JC: Polycystic ovarian disease: US features in 104 patients. Radiology 1987;163:111-116.
12. Balen AH, Laven JS, Tan SL, Dewailly D: Ultrasound assessment of the polycystic ovary: International consensus definitions. Hum Reprod Update 2003;9:505-514.
13. Takahashi K, Ucida A, Yarmasaki H, et al: Transvaginal ultrasound assessment of the response to clomiphene citrate in polycystic ovarian syndrome. Fertil Steril 1994;62:48-53.
14. Nestler JE: Should patients with polycystic ovarian syndrome be treated with metformin? An enthusiastic endorsement. Hum Reprod 2002;17:1950-1953.
15. Vargyas JM, Marrs RP, Kletzky OA, Mishell DR Jr: Correlation of ultrasonic measurement of ovarian follicle size and serum estradiol levels in ovulatory patients following clomiphene citrate for in vitro fertilization. Am J Obstet Gynecol 1982;144:569-573.
16. Garcia J, Seegar-Jones G, Wentz AC: The use of clomiphene citrate. Fertil Steril 1977;28:707-717.
17. Jones HW: Oocyte recruitment with human menopausal gonadotropin and follicle stimulating hormone. In DeCherney AH, Naftolin F (eds): The Control of Follicular Development, Ovulation and Luteal Function: Lessons from IVF. New York, Raven Press, 1987, p 211.
18. Scott RT, Hofmann GE, Muasher SJ, et al: Correlation of follicular diameter with oocyte recovery and maturity at the time of transvaginal follicular aspiration. J In Vitro Fert Embryo Transf 1989;6:73-75.
19. Penzias AS, Jones EE, Seifer DB, et al: Baseline ovarian cysts do not affect clinical response to controlled ovarian hyperstimulation for in vitro fertilization. Fertil Steril 1992;57:1017-1021.
20. Larrzone A, Fulghesu AM, Villa P, et al: Gonadotropin releasing hormone agonist versus human chronic gonadotropin as a trigger of ovulation in polycystic ovarian disease in gonadotropin hyperstimulated cycles. Fertil Steril 1994;62:35-41.
21. Kim JH, Richards CJ, Seibel MM: Proper selection of patients for intermediate dose pure follicle stimulating hormone. J Reprod Med 1994;39:1-5.
22. Navot D, Relou A, Birkenfeld A, et al: Risks factors and prognostic variables in the ovarian hyperstimulation syndrome. Am J Obstet Gynecol 1988;159:210-215.
23. Navot D, Bergh PA, Drews M, Birkenfeld A: The role of ultrasound in ovulation induction. Infertil Reprod Med Clin North Am 1991;2:741.
24. Golan A, Ron-el R, Herman H, et al: Ovarian hyperstimulation syndrome: An update review. Obstet Gynecol Surv 1989;44:430-440.
25. Gleicher N, Oleske DM, Tur-Kaspa I, et al: Reducing the risk of high-order multiple pregnancy after ovarian stimulation with gonadotropins. N Engl J Med 2000;343:2-7.
26. Dickey RP, Taylor SN, Lu PY, et al: Relationship of follicle numbers and estradiol levels to multiple implantation of 3608 intrauterine insemination cycles. Fertil Steril 2001;75:69-78.
27. Dickey RP: Prevention of high order multiple pregnancy. Hum Reprod 2002;17:1411.
28. Dickey RP, Taylor SN, Lu PY, et al: Risks of multiple pregnancy: The decision belongs to whom [letter]? Fertil Steril 2001;76:425-426.
29. Santoro N, Elzanir D: Pulsatile gonadotropin-releasing hormone therapy for ovulating disorders. Clin Obstet Gynecol 1993;36:727-736.
30. Gordon K, Hodgen GD: GnRH agonists and antagonists in assisted reproduction. Baillieres Clin Obstet Gynaecol 1992;6:247-265.
31. Diedrich K, Diedrich C, Santos E, et al: Suppression of the endogenous luteinizing hormone surge by the gonadotrophin-releasing hormone antagonist Cetrorelix during ovarian stimulation. Hum Reprod 1994;9:788-791.
32. Fluker M, Grifo J, Leader A, et al, for the North American Ganirelix Study Group: Efficacy and safety of ganirelix acetate versus leuprolide acetate in women undergoing controlled ovarian hyperstimulation. Fertil Steril 2001;75:38-45.
33. Akman MA, Erden HF, Tosun SB, et al: Comparison of agonistic flare-up-protocol and antagonistic multiple dose protocol in ovarian stimulation of poor responders: Results of a prospective randomized trial. Hum Reprod 2001;16:868-870.
34. Marci R, Caserta D, Dolo V, et al: GnRH antagonist in IVF poor-responder patients: Results of a randomized trial. Reprod Biomed Online 2005;11:189-193.
35. Copperman A: Antagonists in poor responder patients. Fertil Steril 2003;80:16-24.
36. Trounson AO, Leeton JF, Wood C: Pregnancies in humans by fertilization in vitro and embryo transfer in the controlled ovulatory cycle. Science 1981;212:681-682.
37. Sandler B, Grunfeld L: Ovulation induction and follicle surveillance. In Goldstein S (ed): Endovaginal Ultrasound. New York, Wiley-Liss, 1991, p 161.
38. Paulson RJ, Sauer MV, Francis MM, et al: In vitro fertilization in unstimulated cycles: The USC experience. Fertil Steril 1992;57:290-293.
39. Friedler S, Schenker JG, Herman A, Lewin A: The role of ultrasonography in the evaluation of endometrial receptivity following assisted reproductive treatments: A critical review. Hum Reprod Update 1996;2:323-335.
40. Welker BG, Gembruch U, Diedrich K, et al: Transvaginal sonography of the endometrium during ovum pickup in stimulated cycles for in vitro fertilization. J Ultrasound Med 1989;8:549-553.
41. Fanchin R, Righini C, Ayoubi JM, et al: New look at endometrial echogenicity: Objective computer-assisted measurements predict endometrial receptivity in in vitro fertilization-embryo transfer. Fertil Steril 2000;74:274-281.
42. Puerto B, Creus M, Carmona F, et al: Ultrasonography as a predictor of embryo implantation after in vitro fertilization: A controlled study. Fertil Steril 2003;79:1015-1022.
43. Oliveira JB, Baruffi RL, Mauri AL, et al: Endometrial ultrasonography as a predictor of pregnancy in an in-vitro fertilization programme after ovarian stimulation and gonadotrophin-releasing hormone and gonadotrophins. Hum Reprod 1997;12:2515-2518.
44. Sher G, Herbert C, Maassarani G, Jacobs MH: Assessment of the late proliferative phase endometrium by ultrasonography in patients undergoing in vitro fertilization and embryo transfer (IVF/ET). Hum Reprod 1991;6:232-237.
45. Check JH, Nowroozi K, Choe J, Dietterich C: Influence of endometrial thickness and echo patterns on pregnancy rates during in vitro fertilization. Fertil Steril 1991;56:1173-1175.
46. Gonen Y, Casper RF, Jacobson W, Blankier J: Endometrial thickness and growth during ovarian hyperstimulation: A possible predictor of implantation in in vitro fertilization. Fertil Steril 1989;52:446-450.
47. Shapiro H, Cowell Casper RF: Use of vaginal ultrasound for monitoring endometrial preparation in a donor oocyte program. Fertil Steril 1993;59:1055-1058.
48. Dietterich C, Check JH, Choe JK, et al: Increased endometrial thickness on the day of human chorionic gonadotropin injection does not adversely affect pregnancy or implantation rates following in vitro fertilization-embryo transfer. Fertil Steril 2002;77:781-786.
49. Zollner U, Zollner KP, Speckter MT, et al: Endometrial volume as assessed by three-dimensional ultrasound is a predictor of pregnancy outcome after in vitro fertilization and embryo transfer. Fertil Steril 2003;80:1515-1517.
50. Parsons AAD, Lense JJ: Sonohysterography for endometrial abnormalities: Preliminary results. J Clin Ultrasound 1993;21:87-95.
51. Maroulis GB, Parsons AK, Yeko TR: Hydrogynecography: A new technique enables vaginal sonography to visualize pelvic adhesions and other pelvic structures. Fertil Steril 1992;58:1073-1075.
52. Ayida G, Kennedy S, Barlow D, Chamberlain P: Contrast sonography for uterine cavity assessment: A comparison of conventional two-dimensional with three-dimensional transvaginal ultrasound. A pilot study. Fertil Steril 1996;66:848-850.
53. Sharara FI, McClamrock FI: Endometrial fluid collection in women with hydrosalpinx after human chorionic gonadotrophin administration: A report of two cases and implication for management. Hum Reprod 1997;12:2816-2819.
54. Drbohlav P, Halkova E, Masata J, et al: The effect of endometrial infection on embryo implantation in the IVF and ET program. Ceska Gynekol 1998;63:181-185.
55. Sharara FI, Prough SG: Endometrial fluid collection in women with PCOS undergoing ovarian stimulation for IVF: A report of four cases. J Reprod Med 1999;44:299-302.
56. Griffiths AN, Watermeyer SR, Klentzeris LD: Fluid within the endometrial cavity in an IVF cycle: A novel approach to its management. J Assist Reprod Genet 2002;19:298-301.
57. Goswamy RK, Williams G, Steptoe P, et al: Decreased uterine perfusion: A cause of infertility. Hum Reprod 1988;3:955-959.
58. Steer CV, Campbell S, Tan S, et al: The use of transvaginal color flow imaging after in vitro fertilization to identify optimum uterine conditions before embryo transfer. Fertil Steril 1992;57:372-376.
59. Wu H-M, Chiang C-H, Huang H-Y, et al: Detection of the subendometrial vascularization flow index by three-dimensional ultrasound may be useful for predicting the pregnancy rate for patients undergoing in vitro fertilization-embryo transfer. Fertil Steril 2003;79:507-511.
60. Schild RL, Holthaus S, d'Alquen J, et al: Quantitative assessment of subendometrial blood flow by three-dimensional-ultrasound is an important

predictive factor of implantation in an in-vitro fertilization programme. Hum Reprod 2000;15:89-94.

61. Schild RL, Knobloch C, Dorn C, et al: Endometrial receptivity in an in vitro fertilization program as assessed by spiral artery blood flow, endometrial thickness, endometrial volume, and uterine artery blood flow Fertil Steril 2001;75:361-366.

62. Baruffi RL, Contart P, Mauri AL, et al: A uterine ultrasonographic scoring system as a method for the prognosis of embryo implantation. J Assist Reprod Genet 2002;19:99-102.

63. Lenz S, Lauritsen J, Kjellow M: Collection of human oocytes for in vitro fertilization by ultrasonically guided follicular puncture. Lancet 1981;1:1163.

64. Gleicher N, Friberg J, Fullan N, et al: Egg retrieval for in vitro fertilization by sonographically controlled vaginal culdocentesis. Lancet 1983;1:508.

65. Dellenbach P, Nisand I, Moreau L, et al: The transvaginal method for oocyte retrieval: An update on our experience (1984-1987). Ann N Y Acad Sci 1988;541:111-124.

66. Hammarberg K, Enk L, Nilsson L, Wikland M: Oocyte retrieval under the guidance of a vaginal transducer: Evaluation of patient acceptance. Hum Reprod 1987;2:487-490.

67. Bennett SJ, Waterstone JJ, Cheng WL, Parsons J: Complications of transvaginal ultrasound directed follicle aspiration in a review of 2670 consecutive procedures. J Assist Reprod Genet 1993;10:72-77.

68. Dicker D, Ashkenaji J, Feldberg D, et al: Severe abdominal complications after transvaginal ultrasonographically guided retrieval of oocytes for in vitro fertilization and embryo transfer. Fertil Steril 1993;59:1313-1315.

69. Munne S, Alikani M, Tomkin G, et al: Embryo morphology, developmental rates, and maternal age are correlated with chromosome abnormalities. Fertil Steril 1995;64:382-391.

70. al-Shawaf T, Dave R, Harper J, et al: Transfer of embryos into the uterus: How much do technical factors affect pregnancy rates? J Assist Reprod Genet 1993;10:31-36.

71. Strickler RC, Christianson C, Crane JP, et al: Ultrasound guidance for human embryo transfer. Fertil Steril 1985;43:54-61.

72. Sundstrom P, Wramsby H, Persson PH, Liedholm P: Filled bladder simplifies human embryo transfer. Br J Obstet Gynaecol 1984;91:506-507.

73. Lewin A, Schenker JG, Avrech O, et al: The role of uterine straightening by passive bladder distention before embryo transfer in IVF cycles. J Assist Reprod Genet 1997;14:32-34.

74. Goudas VT, Hammitt DG, Damario MA, et al: Blood on the embryo transfer catheter is associated with decreased rates of embryo implantation and clinical pregnancy with the use of in vitro fertilization-embryo transfer. Fertil Steril 1998;70:878-882.

75. Visser DS, Fourie FL, Kruger HF: Multiple attempts at embryo transfer: Effects on pregnancy outcome in an in vitro fertilization and embryo transfer program. J Assist Reprod Genetics 1993;10:37-43.

76. Mansour RT, Aboulghar MA, Serour GI, Amin YM: Dummy embryo transfer using methylene blue dye. Hum Reprod 1994;9:1257-1259.

77. McNamee P, Huang T, Carwile A: Significant increase in pregnancy rates achieved by vigorous irrigation of endocervical mucus prior to embryo transfer with a Wallace catheter in an IVF-ET program [abstract]. Fertil Steril 1998;70(Suppl. 1):S228.

78. Lesny P, Killick SR, Tetlow RL, et al: Uterine junctional zone contractions during assisted reproduction cycles. Hum Reprod Update 1998;4:440-445.

79. Fanchin R, Ayoubi JM, Righini C, et al: Uterine contractility decreases at time of blastocyst transfers. Hum Reprod 2001;16:1115-1119.

80. Lesny P, Killick SR, Robinson J, et al: Junctional zone contractions and embryo transfer: Is it safe to use a tenaculum? Hum Reprod 1999;14:2367-2370.

81. Lesny P, Killick SR, Robinson J, Maguiness SD: Transcervical embryo transfer as a risk factor for ectopic pregnancy. Fertil Steril 1999;72:305-309.

SECTION V

Procedures and Applications

Chapter 15

Sonohysterography

Steven R. Goldstein

Sonohysterography consists of real-time ultrasound imaging of the uterus and uterocervical cavity during the injection of sterile saline into the uterine cavity and the use of high-resolution transvaginal probes to magnify the image. The goal is to achieve anatomic detail sufficient to detect abnormalities of the uterus and endometrium. It is an inexpensive, simple, well-tolerated office procedure that has tremendous diagnostic potential.

Initially, sonography was a tool of obstetricians. Early linear array ultrasound equipment had barely enough resolution to localize the placenta, find the fetal lie, and measure biparietal diameter. High-resolution transvaginal probes provide image magnification similar to that achieved with sonography performed through a low-power microscope (sonomicroscopy).[1] Structures that would not be appreciated with the naked eye can be discerned.

Increasingly, transvaginal ultrasound is being used in a variety of clinical situations, including in patients with abnormal uterine bleeding. If organic pathology is absent, such bleeding is either anovulatory (premenopausal) or atrophic (menopausal). Transvaginal ultrasound studies can avoid biopsy in postmenopausal patients with abnormal bleeding by revealing that the endometrial thickness and texture suggest a lack of significant tissue (4 to 5 mm or less and symmetric).[2-5]

Evolution of a Concept

Although the use of fluid enhancement was described with abdominal ultrasound for both uterine and tubal procedures,[6,7] it never gained widespread use. The introduction of the vaginal probe has changed that considerably.[8,9]

All those who perform ultrasound know that the presence of fluid is beneficial for visualization. For example, fetal structure can be clearly seen in a pregnancy with polyhydramnios; conversely, fetal anatomy is poorly visualized in a pregnancy with oligohydramnios. In a normal, unstimulated ovary at mid-cycle, the fluid of the dominant follicle allows for easy recognition. This is in contradistinction to a postmenopausal ovary or an ovary in a patient on oral contraceptives, where visualization is more difficult because of the lack of fluid-filled follicles to serve as a sonic marker. Further, a normal early pregnancy can be seen in such detail because the normal gestational sac is fluid filled.

Our understanding of naturally occurring postmenopausal endometrial fluid collections can be instructive. Previously, endometrial fluid collections were thought to be an ominous finding associated with malignancy.[10] In my early practice, I encountered nine postmenopausal women with no history of bleeding who were found to have small endometrial fluid collections on vaginal probe ultrasound performed as part of an overall bimanual examination. Attempts at endometrial sampling were unsuccessful in eight patients, owing to cervical stenosis. Prompt dilation and curettage with hysteroscopy in these patients revealed scant tissue grossly; smooth, atrophic changes on hysteroscopy; and "inactive" endometrium pathologically. In a subsequent patient with cervical stenosis, attempts at both office biopsy and operative dilation and curettage failed. Irregular, thickened tissue accompanied the endometrial fluid. This patient ultimately had a hysterectomy, and pathology revealed a benign endometrial polyp. Review of the initial nine patients revealed that the endometrium surrounding the fluid was thin (3 mm or less) and symmetric (Fig. 15–1). Subsequently, 30 patients were observed. Twenty-seven had thin tissue surrounding the fluid collection, and three had thickened tissue surrounding the endometrial fluid. Pathologic study in these three revealed a benign polyp in one and endometrial hyperplasia in the other two.

Thus, the significant factor is *not* the endometrial fluid (presumably transudate associated with cervical stenosis) but the tissue surrounding the fluid.[11] This natural occurrence is the basis for the concept of artificially creating an endometrial fluid collection to better delineate the contour and thickness of the endometrium and its cavity.

Indications and Contraindications

The indications for sonohysterography include, but are not limited to, the following:

- Abnormal bleeding in premenopausal and postmenopausal women (most common indication)
- Infertility and habitual abortion
- Congenital abnormalities or anatomic variants of the uterine cavity
- Preoperative and postoperative evaluation of the uterine cavity, especially with regard to uterine myomata, polyps, and cysts
- Suspected uterine cavity synechiae

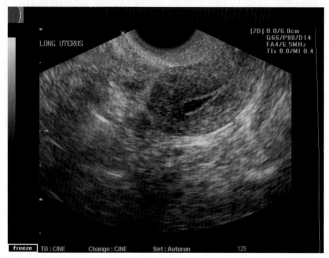

Figure 15–1. Long-axis transvaginal view in a postmenopausal patient with a naturally occurring fluid collection. The endometrium surrounding the fluid is thin. This is the typical picture of an inactive, atrophic endometrium with a degree of cervical stenosis. The resulting fluid is most likely transudate.

- Further evaluation of suspected abnormalities seen on transvaginal sonography (TVS), including focal or diffuse endometrial thickening or debris
- Inadequate imaging of the endometrium by TVS

Sonohysterography should not be performed in a woman who is pregnant or who could be pregnant. This is usually avoided by scheduling the examination in the follicular phase of the menstrual cycle, after the menstrual flow has essentially ceased but before the patient has ovulated. In a patient with regular menstrual cycles, saline infusion sonohysterography should not be performed later than the 10th day of the menstrual cycle. In addition, sonohysterography should not be performed in a patient with a pelvic infection or unexplained pelvic tenderness, which might be caused by chronic pelvic inflammatory disease.

Technique

I palpate the uterus by performing a bimanual examination, because knowing whether the uterus is anteverted or retroverted—and if so, how sharply—enhances the success and safety of any subsequent procedure. In addition, palpation can assess the presence of uterine tenderness or decreased mobility. Although TVS can identify anteversion versus retroversion, the endocervical canal is often off the midline, and identifying its direction before instrumentation makes cervical canalization easier and more successful.

Patient Preparation

If painful, dilated, or obstructed fallopian tubes are found before the saline infusion and the patient is not taking prophylactic antibiotics, the examination should be delayed until such treatment can be administered. In the presence of nontender hydrosalpinges, consideration can be given to administering antibiotics at the time of the examination. A pregnancy test is advised when clinically indicated. Patients should be asked whether they have a latex allergy before latex sheaths are used.

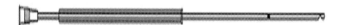

Figure 15–2. Tampa catheter for sonohysterography (Ackrad Labs, a Cooper Co., Trumbull, Conn). This single-lumen catheter is somewhat stiff and can be inserted without the use of an instrument such as a ring forceps.

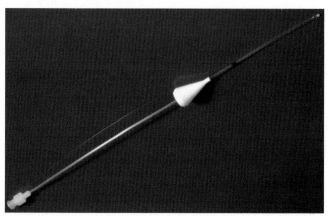

Figure 15–3. Goldstein sonohysterography catheter (Cook ObGyn, Spencer, Ind). This catheter is 25 cm long and 5.3 French (1.8 mm) in diameter. The black dot is at 7 cm. The white acorn is advanced until it is flush with the cervix and is held in place by the pressure of the vaginal probe. This catheter retards fluid run-back but does not prevent it. Thus, it does not cause the uterine cramping associated with the total occlusion of balloon catheters.

Procedure

Preliminary unenhanced endovaginal sonography should be performed to measure the endometrium and evaluate the uterus and ovaries before saline infusion sonohysterography. The speculum is inserted, and the cervix is cleansed with an antiseptic (10% iodine based) solution. A sonohysterography catheter is then inserted. Many of these are standard one-way catheters (Figs. 15–2 and 15–3), but some are bidirectional balloon catheters (Fig. 15–4). A study of six different catheters (three balloon, three standard) in 568 patients found equivalent efficacy.[12] The percentage of procedures performed correctly in that study ranged from 89.3% to 95.7%. For patient comfort, the Goldstein catheter was preferred ($P < .05$).

Before the catheter is inserted it is flushed through with sterile saline to get rid of small amounts of air, which can cause an echogenic artifact if injected (Fig. 15–5). The catheter is inserted by gently feeding it through the cervical os. The speculum is then removed carefully so as not to dislodge the catheter. The catheter may come out through the introitus despite being in the proper position relative to the uterus. The vaginal probe is then inserted. A 10-mL syringe (devoid of air bubbles) is attached to the catheter. While scanning in a long-axis projection, the clinician instills fluid while watching the video monitor. In that long-axis projection, the transducer is moved from side to side (i.e., from cornu to cornu). The amount of fluid instilled is variable and depends on the image produced on the ultrasound screen. When the uterus has been completely surveyed from cornu to cornu in a long-axis pro-

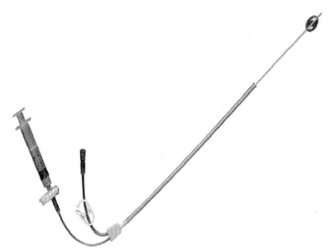

Figure 15–4. Typical bidirectional balloon catheter. One side blows up the balloon, preventing any run-back of fluid; the other lumen is for the insertion of sterile saline. These devices provide excellent pictures but increase patient discomfort and cramping.

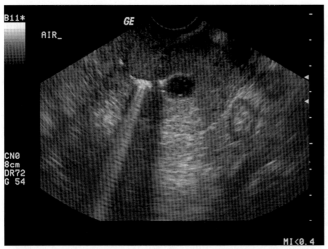

Figure 15–5. Inadvertent introduction of air during sonohysterography produces a very dense echogenic pattern with acoustic shadowing behind it. Note the loss of information in the region of the air.

jection, the transducer is rotated 90 degrees into a coronal plane, and more fluid is instilled while fanning down toward the endocervical canal and up toward the uterine fundus. This procedure allows the anatomy to be visualized in three dimensions (3D). Care must be taken not to miss any portion of the uterine cavity, because some polyps, hyperplasia, or carcinomas may be focal. It may be helpful to videotape the procedure in case a subsequent review is desired. A detailed report with representative hard-copy images is also produced.

Applications

Sonohysterography for Unscheduled Uterine Bleeding

Unscheduled uterine bleeding in perimenopausal women, as well as any bleeding in postmenopausal women not on

hormone replacement therapy, accounts for many medical interventions. Diagnostic procedures performed in the office include biopsy, suction aspiration, suction curettage, and diagnostic hysteroscopy. While occasionally invasive diagnostic procedures are therapeutic, often they are not. For instance, dysfunctional uterine bleeding in perimenopausal patients caused by a lack of ovulation is better treated hormonally, not surgically. Patients may also have curettage with or without diagnostic or operative hysteroscopy in an operating room setting. The amount of time required, the equipment needed, and the requisite skills of the operator are different for endometrial polyps, submucosal myoma, hyperplasia, and carcinoma. Some patients with submucosal myomas are inappropriate candidates for resectoscopic surgery, whereas in others it is the treatment of choice.

In a prospective pilot study, saline infusion sonohysterography was performed in 21 women with abnormal perimenopausal uterine bleeding.[13] Of the 21 patients, 8 had obvious polypoid lesions (Fig. 15–6) and were triaged for operative hysteroscopic removal. The pathology report confirmed benign polyps in all 8 patients. Three of the 21 patients had submucosal myomas. Two had wire loop resectoscopic excision (Fig. 15–7); the third, in whom the myoma extended to the serosal edge of the uterus, was managed expectantly (Fig. 15–8). Nine of the 21 patients had no obvious anatomic lesions, and the endometrial thickness of either the anterior or posterior wall was a maximum of 3.2 mm (Fig. 15–9). These studies were purposely performed on days 4 to 6 of the menstrual cycle, when early proliferative change would be expected if no anatomic abnormality existed. Biopsy in all nine of these patients revealed early proliferative endometrium. Thus, these patients had dysfunctional (anovulatory) uterine bleeding and were successfully treated with progestational agents. The final patient had an endometrial thickness along the anterior wall of 7.6 mm, although the posterior wall was thin (2.3 mm) (Fig. 15–10). Curettage with hysteroscopy revealed simple hyperplasia without atypia, and this patient was also treated with progestational agents.

Thus, we concluded that endometrial fluid instillation (sonohysterography) to enhance vaginal sonography in perimenopausal women can reliably distinguish between patients with minimal tissue (≤3 mm) whose bleeding is anovulatory and thus best treated hormonally from those with significant tissue (>3 mm) in need of formal curettage and hysteroscopy. Further, polyps can be distinguished from submucosal myomas, allowing for operative hysteroscopy in appropriate cases. Sonohysterography also eliminates the need for diagnostic hysteroscopy in patients whose bleeding is dysfunctional.

Based on the foregoing results, it seems apparent that any "blind" endometrial sampling should be preceded by fluid instillation sonohysterography. A process must be shown to be symmetrically panuterine or global to justify a blind procedure. When changes are focal (e.g., polyps, some hyperplasias, some carcinomas), they can be appreciated as such with fluid instillation sonohysterography, and directed biopsies must be carried out.

In the vast majority of patients, abnormal uterine bleeding is associated with episodes of anovulation that can be managed hormonally or expectantly with reassurance (in premenopausal patients) or endometrial atrophy (in postmenopausal patients). The value of being able to distinguish

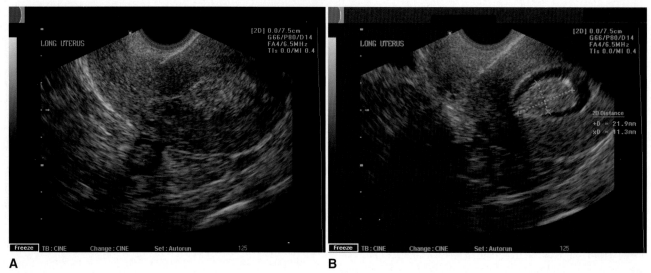

Figure 15–6. A, Long-axis view in a perimenopausal patient with abnormal bleeding. The unenhanced scan before saline infusion does not preclude the presence of abnormal tissue. **B,** The same patient after the introduction of sterile saline. Note the obvious polyp coming off the region of the lower uterine segment in this retroverted uterus. It measures 21.9 by 11.3 mm *(calipers)*. Note that the tissue surrounding the fluid is thin, typical of the early proliferative phase.

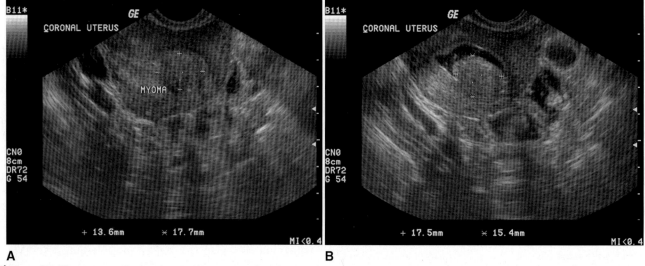

Figure 15–7. A, Coronal view in a perimenopausal patient with irregular, abnormal bleeding. The central echogenic focus (13.6 by 17.7 mm), outlined by *calipers,* is labeled myoma. **B,** The same patient after the introduction of saline. Note the myoma along the posterior wall. It measures 17.5 by 15.4 mm. Approximately 80% of the myoma extrudes into the endometrial cavity. This patient is an excellent candidate for resectoscopic surgery. The adequate amount of myometrium overlying the myoma will provide a degree of safety at the time of resection.

such patients from those with organic pathologic conditions in a safe, painless, convenient manner is obvious.

Initially, curettage was the gold standard in such patients. First described in 1843,[14] it became the most common operation performed on women in the world. As early as the 1950s, a review of 6907 curettage procedures found that the technique missed endometrial lesions in 10% of cases.[15] Of these, 80% were polyps. A study of curettage before hysterectomy found that in 16% of specimens, less than one quarter of the cavity was curetted; in 60%, less than one half of the cavity was curetted; and in 84%, less than three quarters of the endometrial cavity was effectively curetted.[16]

In the 1970s, vacuum-suction curettage devices allowed sampling without anesthesia in an office setting. The most popular was the Vabra aspirator (Berkeley Medevices, Berkeley, Calif). This was found to be 86% accurate in diagnosing cancer.[17] Subsequently, cheaper, smaller, less painful plastic catheters with their own internal pistons to generate suction became popular. One of these, the Pipelle device (Unimar, Wilton, Conn), was found to have similar efficacy but better patient acceptance compared with the Vabra.[18] Rodriguez and coworkers[19] did a pathologic study of 25 hysterectomy specimens. The Pipelle device sampled on average 4% (range, 0 to 12%) of the endometrial surface, versus 41% for the Vabra aspirator.

In one widely publicized study,[20] the Pipelle had a 97.5% sensitivity for detecting endometrial cancer in 40 patients undergoing hysterectomy. The shortcoming of that study was that malignancy had already been diagnosed before the specimen collection. In another study,[21] Pipelle aspiration biopsy was performed in 135 premenopausal patients before curettage. Thirteen patients (10%) had different histologic results on Pipelle biopsy compared with curettage. Only five of these patients had polyps, but Pipelle sampling missed the diagnosis in three. In total, 18 patients had hyperplasia, and Pipelle sampling missed the diagnosis in 7 (39%). This unreliability in the detection of hyperplasia may reflect the often focal nature of that pathologic process.

In another study, Guido et al.[22] studied the Pipelle biopsy in patients with known carcinoma undergoing hysterectomy. Among 65 patients, Pipelle biopsy provided tissue adequate for analysis in 63 (97%). Malignancy was detected in only 54 patients (83%). Of the 11 with false-negative results, 5 had

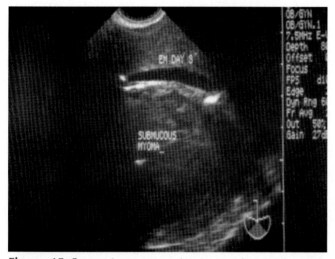

Figure 15–8. Sonohysterogram showing a submucosal myoma that extends all the way to the serosa. This patient is not a candidate for resectoscopic surgery.

disease confined to endometrial polyps, and 3 had tumor localized to less than 5% of the cavity's surface area. The surface area of endometrial involvement in that study was less than 5% of the cavity in 3 (5%); 5% to 25% of the cavity in 12 (18%), of which the Pipelle missed 4; 26% to 50% of the cavity in 20 (31%), of which the Pipelle missed 4; and greater than 50% of the cavity in 30 (46%), of which the Pipelle missed none. These results provide great insight into how endometrial carcinoma can be distributed over the endometrial surface or confined to a polyp. Because tumors localized in a polyp or a small area of endometrium may go undetected, the authors of the study concluded that the "Pipelle is excellent for detecting global processes in the endometrium."

These data show that undirected sampling, whether through curettage or various types of suction aspiration, is often fraught with error, especially when the abnormality is focal (polyps, focal hyperplasia, or carcinoma involving small areas of the uterine cavity) rather than global.

As determined by the pilot study discussed earlier,[13] the addition of saline infusion sonohysterography can reliably distinguish perimenopausal patients with dysfunctional abnormal bleeding (no anatomic abnormality) from those with globally thickened endometria or those with focal abnormalities. A clinical algorithm was proposed and studied in a large, prospective trial of perimenopausal women with abnormal bleeding.[23] Unenhanced TVS was used, followed by saline infusion sonohysterography for selected patients; this was followed by no endometrial sampling, undirected endometrial sampling, or visually directed endometrial sampling, depending on whether the sonograms revealed no anatomic abnormality, globally thickened endometrium, or focal abnormalities, respectively (Fig. 15–11). In that study, 280 of 433 patients (65%) displayed a thin, distinct, symmetric endometrial echo less than 5 mm on days 4 to 6 of the menstrual cycle, and dysfunctional uterine bleeding was diagnosed (Fig. 15–12). Among the 153 patients (35%) who had saline infusion sonohysterography, 44 procedures (29%) were

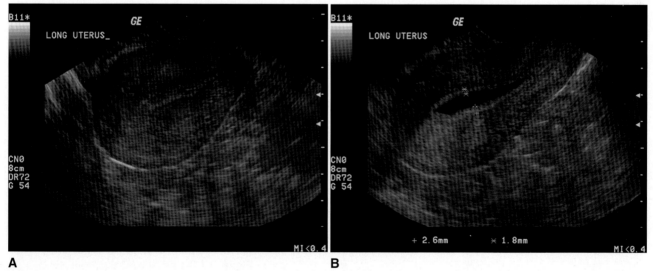

A   **B**

Figure 15–9. A, Long-axis view in a perimenopausal patient with irregular bleeding. The endometrial echo is poorly visualized. **B,** Sonohysterogram of the same patient. Fluid enhancement allows the anterior and posterior walls to be distended away from each other and measured separately. Here, the anterior wall measures 2.6 cm and the posterior wall 1.8 cm. Biopsy revealed proliferative endometrium. This is the typical picture of a patient with dysfunctional anovulatory bleeding that is best treated hormonally.

performed because of the inability to adequately characterize and measure the endometrium (Fig. 15–13), and 109 (71%) were done for endometrial measurements greater than 5 mm. Sixty-one of those patients then had both anterior and posterior endometrial thickness that was symmetric and less than 3 mm, compatible with dysfunctional uterine bleeding. Fifty-eight patients (13%) had focal polypoid masses (Fig. 15–14) that were removed hysteroscopically and confirmed patholog-

ically. Twenty-two patients (5%) had submucosal myomas, although 148 patients (34%) had clinical and ultrasound evidence of fibroids. Ten patients had single-layer endometrial measurements 3 mm or greater (range, 3 to 9 mm) on saline infusion sonohysterography. Of these, the histologic type was proliferative endometrium in five and hyperplastic endometrium in five. Saline infusion sonohysterography was technically inadequate in two patients, who subsequently underwent hysteroscopy with curettage. Undirected office biopsy alone, without imaging, might have missed the diagnosis of focal lesions such as polyps, submucosal myomas, and focal hyperplasia in up to 80 patients (18%).

Sonohysterography in Infertility

Endometrial Evaluation

Submucosal myomas may be a source of decreased fertility or increased risk for pregnancy loss. Endometrial polyps are more common in patients with fertility problems.[9] Fluid-enhanced sonohysterography facilitates differentiation of these entities. Intrauterine adhesions after previous pregnancy-associated curettage can also be detected with saline infusion sonohysterography (Fig. 15–15).[8] Sonohysterography can consistently diagnose intra- and pericavitary lesions in infertile women.[24] Saline infusion sonohysterography is widely used to diagnose the shape of the uterine cavity in cases of suspected uterine malformation (see Chapter 7).

Tubal Evaluation

Although fluid in the cul-de-sac (Fig. 15–16) is often seen with sonohysterography (proving tubal patency), an outline of the fallopian tubes, such as that obtained with radiographic hysterosalpingography, cannot be seen. Future studies with experimental ultrasound contrast materials or the addition of

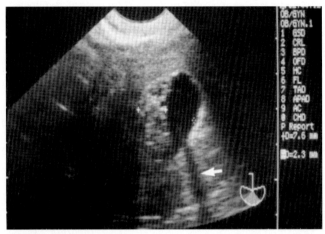

Figure 15–10. Sonohysterogram revealing a thickened, "fluffy," heterogeneous collection of tissue along the anterior wall, which measures 7.6 mm *(calipers)*. The posterior wall has thin endometrium, with a maximum thickness of 2.3 mm *(calipers)*. The acoustic shadow is caused by the catheter *(arrow)*. Because of the focal nature of this patient's pathology, she underwent formal dilation and curettage with hysteroscopy; biopsy of the affected area revealed hyperplasia.

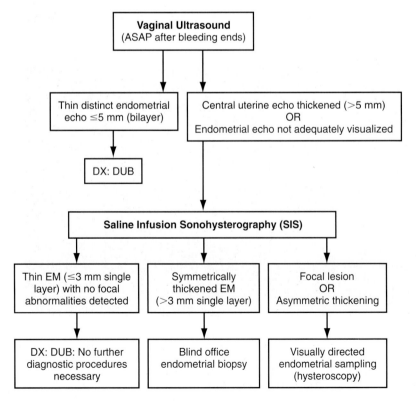

Figure 15–11. Clinical algorithm for an ultrasound-based approach in perimenopausal patients with abnormal uterine bleeding. ASAP, as soon as possible; DUB, dysfunctional uterine bleeding; DX, diagnosis; EM, endometrium.

color-flow Doppler ultrasound equipment may prove helpful in this regard.

Sonohysterography for Revealing Submucosal Involvement

In the pilot study saline infusion sonohysterography was performed in 21 women with abnormal perimenopausal uterine bleeding.[13] Although 9 of the 21 patients had obvious ultrasound and clinical evidence of fibroids, only 3 had a submucosal component. Six of 21 had intramural-subserosal myomas (Fig. 15–17) coexisting with dysfunctional uterine bleeding. This was also true in the large prospective study cited earlier[23]; although 148 of 433 women had myomas, only 22 had a submucosal component.

Sonohysterography for Distinguishing Myoma versus Polyp

Usually, polyps are clearly discernible (see Fig. 15–6), as are submucosal myomas. However, sometimes a broad-based polyp is difficult to distinguish from a submucosal myoma (see Fig. 15–7). This may be important for preoperative planning, because a truly pedunculated submucosal myoma behaves more like a polyp in terms of the skill and equipment required for its removal in the operating room, whereas a broad-based polyp may be more like a myoma and require resectoscopic capability. Also, whereas a non–fluid-enhanced sonogram may demonstrate a definite myoma that appears to be submucosal, sonohysterography may show that it is intramural and merely distorting the endometrial cavity, with a normal layer of endometrium (Fig. 15–18).

Sonohysterography and Three-Dimensional Reconstruction

A reliable ultrasound assessment requires that the endometrial echo be homogeneous, surrounded by an intact hypoechoic junctional zone, and that the operator keep in mind that the endometrial cavity is a 3D structure. Dijkhuizen et al.[25] had four cases that supposedly measured less than 10 mm (some as little as 2 mm), yet polyps were found at hysteroscopy. Such cases underscore the importance of considering the 3D character of the endometrial cavity. One cannot obtain a limited number of two-dimensional views and assume that these represent the entire endometrial cavity. Any one "frozen" ultrasound image is nothing more than a two-dimensional "snapshot," and failure to meticulously re-create 3D anatomy will result in error.

New 3D ultrasound equipment is discussed extensively in Chapter 19. When used with saline infusion sonohysterography, it can eliminate operator errors that may occur from the

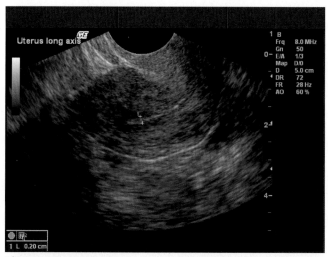

Figure 15–12. Long-axis view in a perimenopausal patient with abnormal bleeding. The study was performed in the early proliferative phase. The endometrial echo here measures 2 mm. This picture is compatible with a diagnosis of dysfunctional anovulatory bleeding; no further diagnostic procedure is necessary.

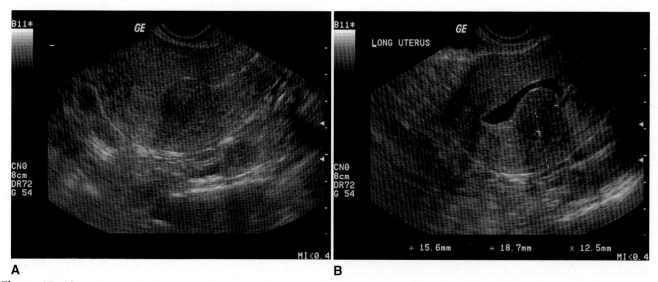

A   **B**

Figure 15–13. **A,** Long-axis view in a perimenopausal patient with abnormal uterine bleeding. Although the endometrial echo appears to be distorted in the midportion, the cause is unclear. **B,** The same patient after the introduction of sterile saline. One can clearly see a submucosal myoma measuring 15.6 by 18.7 mm. It extrudes approximately 60% into the cavity. Perhaps as important, there is 12.5 mm of myometrium from the back of the myoma to the serosa. This patient is an excellent candidate for resection.

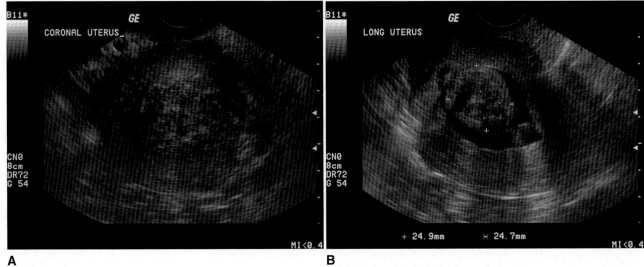

A   **B**

Figure 15–14. **A,** Coronal view in a perimenopausal patient with abnormal uterine bleeding. The central uterine echo is heterogeneous and unclear. **B,** The same patient after the introduction of sterile saline. There is a large polypoid mass extending from the lower uterine segment along the anterior wall. It measures 24.9 by 24.7 mm *(calipers)*. Such polyps are benign tumors arising from the endometrium itself and are easily removed at the time of dilation and curettage.

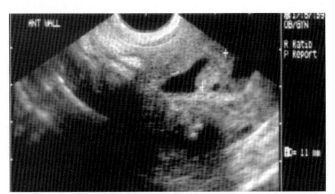

Figure 15–15. Long-axis sonohysterographic view of the uterus clearly depicting thick adhesions bridging from the anterior to the posterior wall in this patient with infertility.

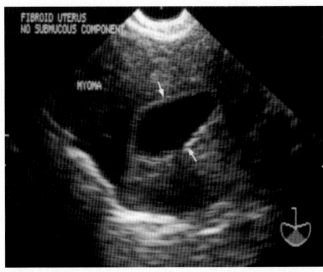

Figure 15–17. Saline infusion sonohysterogram shows intramural-subserosal myomas in a patient who had obvious clinical and sonographic evidence of fibroid changes. However, there is no submucosal component, and the endometrium surrounding the fluid is thin throughout *(arrows)*. Biopsy revealed early proliferative changes. This patient had dysfunctional uterine bleeding coexisting with intramural-subserosal myomas.

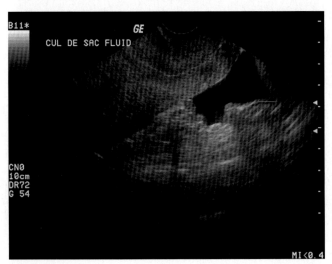

Figure 15–16. Transvaginal pelvic sonogram at the time of saline infusion sonohysterography reveals fluid in the cul-de-sac. This proves tubal patency (at least on one side). Note how low the cul-de-sac is relative to the cervix posteriorly.

failure to re-create 3D anatomy. The 3D technique usually requires a balloon catheter to prevent the run-back of fluid. This causes cramping and discomfort for the patient. Using 3D volume acquisition at the time of saline infusion sonohysterography shortens the examination time and therefore minimizes patient discomfort. Off-line analysis of the volume enables one to obtain measurements of the coronal plane of the uterus.

The use of color-flow or power Doppler to identify a central feeder vessel—pathognomonic of an endometrial polyp—is an alternative to sonohysterography for the diagnosis of

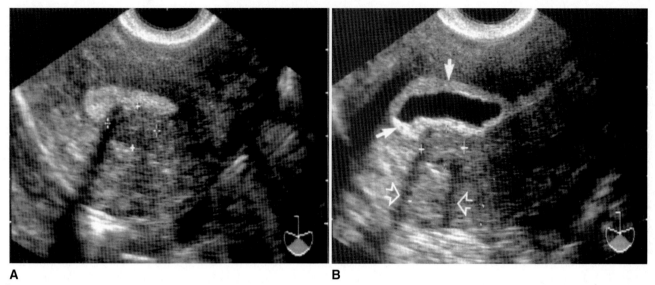

A   **B**

Figure 15–18. **A,** Long-axis view of the uterus reveals a fibroid in the midposterior region measuring 1.2 by 0.9 cm *(calipers)* and distorting the endometrium. Without fluid enhancement, this gives the impression of being significantly submucosal. **B,** Saline infusion sonohysterogram of the same patient clearly shows that this myoma is predominantly intramural. It is covered entirely by symmetrically appearing endometrium *(white arrows)*. Note the typical acoustic shadow caused by the fibroid *(open arrows)*.

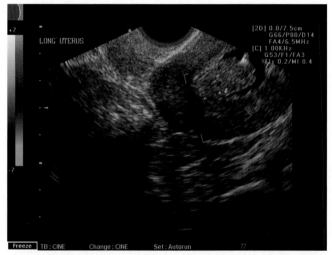

Figure 15–19. Transvaginal color Doppler scan in a patient with abnormal uterine bleeding. A polypoid lesion is clearly seen, and the central pedicle artery to the polyp is clearly visualized with color-flow Doppler.

polyps (Fig. 15–19). This had a positive predictive value of 81.3% in the study by Timmerman and associates.[26]

Sonohysterography for Revealing Unusual Ultrasound Appearance of the Uterus in Patients Taking Tamoxifen

Tamoxifen is a nonsteroidal antiestrogen that binds to the estrogen receptor and therefore has both agonistic (estrogenic) and antagonistic (antiestrogenic) actions. It has been widely used clinically as adjunctive therapy for women with breast cancer, and it is an excellent antiestrogen for breast tissue. Indeed, an overview of 61 randomized trials involving almost 29,000 women showed a significant improvement in both recurrence-free survival and overall survival in postmenopausal women with breast cancer treated with tamoxifen.[27] It is the most widely prescribed antineoplastic drug worldwide. It has more than 12 million use-years in women with breast cancer.

The first report of tamoxifen's association with endometrial neoplasia appeared in 1985.[28] Numerous letters and case reports followed.[29,30] The first prospective data, done without baseline endometrial assessment, reported a 7.5-fold increased risk of endometrial carcinoma (average annual hazard rate of 0.2 per 1000 for placebo versus 1.6 per 1000 for tamoxifen).[31] The first prospective study with baseline uterine evaluation of 16 patients revealed a 6% incidence of carcinoma, a 25% incidence of polyp formation, and a 44% incidence of proliferation after 3 years of use.[32] Only 50% of these postmenopausal patients maintained inactive atrophic endometrium while on tamoxifen therapy. Other investigators found an 18% incidence of hyperplasia in 37 women with just a 12-month duration of treatment.[33] These early studies were done with either hysteroscopy[32] or blind endometrial sampling.[33]

In the late 1980s and early 1990s, TVS was introduced to evaluate postmenopausal women with uterine bleeding,[34] and numerous patients taking tamoxifen were evaluated with this technique.[35] With the introduction of saline infusion sonohysterography came the first reports of microcystic changes on ultrasound.[36] These changes represent glandular cystic atrophy and can be present in the basalis of the endometrium, in the proximal myometrium, or even within polyps. Similar findings were reported after just 3 months of treatment with idoxifene,[37] which, like tamoxifen, is a triphenylethylene derivative. In an observational study of 44 asymptomatic, postmenopausal breast cancer patients on tamoxifen, there was a 4% incidence of carcinoma, a 9% incidence of proliferation or hyperplasia, and a 27% incidence of endometrial polyps.[38] Further, only 25% of tamoxifen patients maintained a thin, linear endometrial echo, predictive of inactive atrophic endometrium; however, with saline infusion sonohysterography,

59% of those patients ultimately demonstrated inactive surface epithelium (Figs. 15–20 to 15–24).

Controversy exists regarding which, if any, method of endometrial surveillance is appropriate for patients receiving tamoxifen therapy. In February 1996 the American College of Obstetricians and Gynecologists (ACOG) simply recommended an annual pelvic examination and Pap smear in the absence of abnormal bleeding.[39] However, ACOG warned practitioners to be alert to the increased incidence of endometrial malignancy in women taking tamoxifen and to use screening procedures and diagnostic tests at their discretion. The ACOG document further stated, "given [that] up to 39% of postmenopausal women taking tamoxifen have abnormal endometria and the annualized risk of endometrial cancer is 2-3/1000 it is apparent that hyperplastic lesions seldom evolve into invasive cancers." This is a bold statement, considering that the cited study by Kedar et al.[40] involved only 55 women on tamoxifen, and only for a median time of 2 years. Ten patients (18%) developed atypical hyperplasia,

but there were no cancers. The placebo group had no cancer and no hyperplasia. This is less than one would expect in the general population, further attesting to the small number of patients and the relatively short observation period. In April 2000 ACOG updated its committee opinion on tamoxifen and endometrial cancer, stating, "Because screening tests have not been effective in increasing the early detection of endometrial cancer in women using tamoxifen and may lead to more invasive and costly diagnostic procedures, they are not recommended."[41]

The only data on the endometrial effects of tamoxifen in healthy women (i.e., those without a diagnosis of breast cancer) come from the Breast Cancer Prevention Trial conducted by the National Surgical Adjuvant Breast and Bowel Project. This trial involved more than 13,000 women with a median follow-up of 44 months.[42] In women younger than 50 years (presumably premenopausal), there was no statistical difference in the development of endometrial carcinoma between those taking tamoxifen and those taking placebo; in women older than 50 years (presumably menopausal), the relative risk of endometrial carcinoma was 4.01 (95% confidence interval 1.70 to 10.90). The rate of endometrial carcinoma per 1000 women was 0.76 for placebo and 3.05 for tamoxifen. Because the study design lacked entry or exit data, there was no way to capture the incidence of benign endometrial changes (either proliferative endometrium or polyps) or atypical hyperplasia. The incidence of vaginal discharge that was moderately bothersome or worse was 29% in the tamoxifen group and 13% in the placebo group (no statistical analysis provided).

More recent data from Berliere et al.[43,44] suggest that low-risk and high-risk groups of patients can be identified before the initiation of tamoxifen therapy for breast cancer. They reported on the pretreatment screening of 575 postmenopausal patients with breast cancer. Baseline benign endometrial polyps were present in 16.6% before tamoxifen therapy. In two of these patients, the lesions were atypical hyperplasia that was ultimately treated with hysterectomy. The remaining patients had their polyps removed and were then followed separately from those patients without initial lesions.

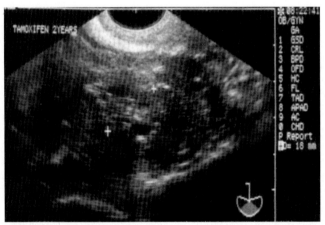

Figure 15–20. Long-axis view in a patient whose endometrial echo appears heterogeneous and irregular in texture. The endometrium surrounding the fluid appears to be thin throughout the cavity, with a maximum thickness of 1.9 mm *(calipers)*.

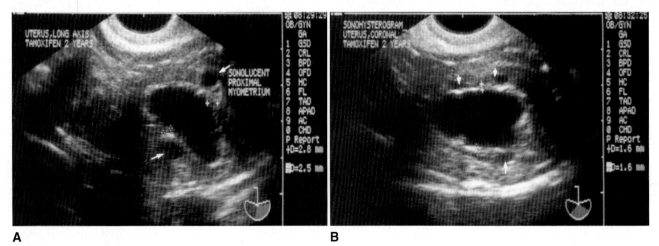

A   **B**

Figure 15–21. Long-axis (**A**) and coronal (**B**) views in the patient in Figure 15–20 after saline infusion sonohysterography with approximately 3 to 10 mL of sterile saline infused through an intrauterine insemination catheter. Note that the endometrium is thin, with a maximum thickness of 2.8 mm. At hysteroscopy, it appeared pale and atrophic, and there was scant inactive tissue on histopathology. Note the sonolucent areas in the proximal myometrium *(arrows)*, representing foci of reactivation of adenomyosis.

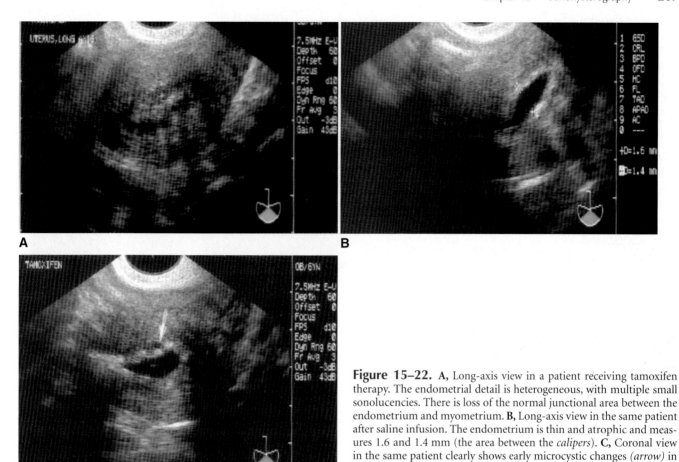

Figure 15–22. A, Long-axis view in a patient receiving tamoxifen therapy. The endometrial detail is heterogeneous, with multiple small sonolucencies. There is loss of the normal junctional area between the endometrium and myometrium. **B,** Long-axis view in the same patient after saline infusion. The endometrium is thin and atrophic and measures 1.6 and 1.4 mm (the area between the *calipers*). **C,** Coronal view in the same patient clearly shows early microcystic changes *(arrow)* in the proximal myometrium.

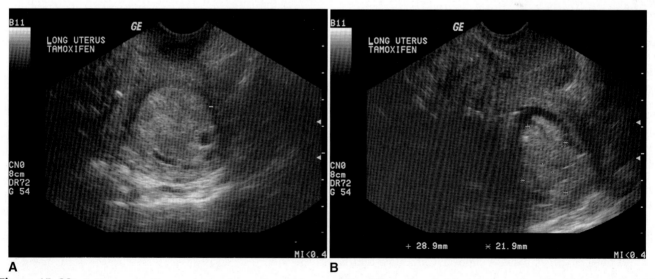

Figure 15–23. A, Transvaginal long-axis view in a patient taking tamoxifen who presented with vaginal spotting. There is a centrally thick uterine echo. **B,** The same patient after the instillation of saline. A large endometrial polyp measuring 28.9 by 21.9 mm *(calipers)* is seen. There are some microcystic changes within the polyp as well.

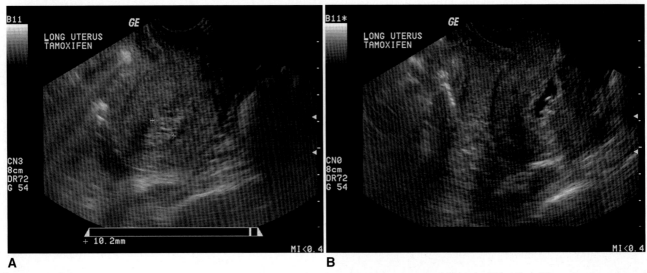

Figure 15–24. A, Long-axis view in a patient receiving tamoxifen therapy who presented with vaginal bleeding. The central uterine echo is thickened, measuring 10.2 mm *(calipers).* **B,** The same patient after the introduction of sterile saline. Note that the endometrium is thickened and somewhat shaggy and irregular. Dilation and curettage hysteroscopy revealed complex hyperplasia with atypia.

The duration of follow-up ranged from 1 to 5 years. In the group with no initial lesions, the incidence of polyps and atypical hyperplasia was 12.9% and 0.7%, respectively. In the group with initial lesions, the incidence of polyps and atypical hyperplasia was 17.6% and 11.7%, respectively. Thus, the high-risk group had 17 times the incidence of atypical hyperplasia and 1.4 times the incidence of polyp formation compared with the low-risk group.

The implication of this study is that there are distinct high- and low-risk groups for the development of endometrial hyperplasia, based on whether there is any underlying abnormality before instituting tamoxifen therapy. Therefore, it is appropriate to screen women before beginning tamoxifen therapy. In those with a "clean" uterus, the risk for subsequent abnormality is low (<1% based on the Berliere[43,44] data); no further evaluation of the endometrium is necessary, and the ACOG guidelines can be followed. If screening reveals any lesion, it should be evaluated before therapy and then subjected to ongoing surveillance. The best methods of such ongoing surveillance have been debated, with the shortcomings of both blind endometrial sampling[45] and unenhanced transvaginal ultrasound[44] being noted. The study by Barakat et al.[45] underscored the shortcomings of blind sampling. Using this technique, they found only a 3.6% incidence of polyps (4 of 111), whereas other investigators using sonohysterography or hysteroscopy found an incidence of 25% to 27%.[32,38] Love et al.[46] found a high false-positive rate using unenhanced endometrial thickness on transvaginal ultrasound as a screening parameter. This is because tamoxifen produces central uterine echoes that are thickened and can be mistaken for endometrium; in reality, this represents loss of the normal junctional zone between endometrium and proximal myometrium and microcystic changes.[36,38] Sonohysterography enhances endometrial anatomy and aids in the diagnosis of endometrial abnormalities.[47] In another study,[48] sonohysterography also added sensitivity and specificity to transvaginal ultrasound, whereas Doppler flow studies did not. An algorithm for uterine surveillance using transvaginal ultra-sound and saline infusion sonohysterography has been proposed (Fig. 15–25).

Potential Pitfalls and Concerns

Anesthesia and Analgesia

Anesthesia or analgesia is not required during sonohysterography. In more than 1000 cases, I have seen only 3 cases of a vasovagal response, reminiscent of the response seen with the insertion of a plastic intrauterine device in a nulliparous patient. The Goldstein catheter is 1.8 mm in diameter, and the procedure is extremely well tolerated. The overwhelming majority of patients experience no pain; only a few complain of minimal cramping.

Risk of Infection

Sonohysterography should be handled similarly to traditional hysterosalpingography. The decision whether to obtain gonorrhea or chlamydia cultures and whether to administer prophylactic antibiotics depends on the patient population. I do not routinely obtain cultures for sexually transmitted diseases or use prophylactic antibiotics. In more than 1000 cases, I have not experienced any infectious morbidity. Among the 1153 procedures performed,[49] the incidence of infectious complications that required surgical resolution was 0.7%, which is similar to that of diagnostic hysteroscopy[50] but less than that of hysterosalpingography.[51]

Inability to Thread the Catheter

Occasionally, it is difficult to thread the catheter into its desired position. Using the other hand to change the position of the speculum often modifies the angle of the cervix in relation to the fundus, allowing successful completion. Use of a tenaculum is a last resort. A cervical stabilizer is less painful and less traumatic and does not cause bleeding from the cervix (Fig. 15–26).

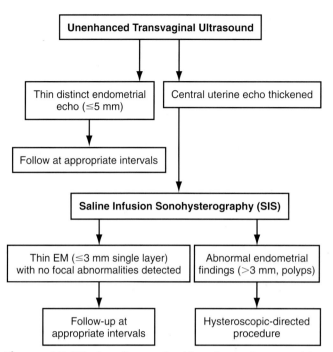

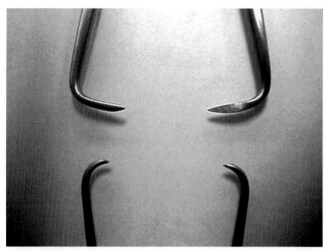

Figure 15–26. Conventional single-toothed tenaculum *(top)* and cervical stabilizer *(bottom)*. The latter has a much finer and smaller point and a simple, single ratchet. It is atraumatic and results in virtually no bleeding, yet it enables the operator to stabilize the cervix so that a sonohysterography catheter can be inserted more easily.

Figure 15–25. Surveillance algorithm for patients receiving tamoxifen therapy. EM, endometrium.

Inadequate Distention of the Cavity

In some patients, a patulous cervix results in a great deal of fluid running out transcervically. Other patients have fluid exiting through the fallopian tubes, even with slow injection and minimal pressure. As in hysteroscopy, some cavities are more difficult to distend than others. The clinician should check the position of the catheter, looking for its acoustic shadow most of the way to the uterine fundus. However, unlike hysteroscopy (which requires distention for visualization), sonohysterography requires very little fluid to outline the cavity. Even a small ribbon of fluid is sufficient to distinguish anterior and posterior endometrial surfaces and outline endometrial pathology (Fig. 15–27).

Spread of Adenocarcinoma to the Peritoneal Cavity

When there is concern about the spread of adenocarcinoma, the question is whether the benefit of the procedure outweighs any theoretical risk. It is no longer standard practice to tie the fallopian tubes with silk before a total abdominal hysterectomy and bilateral salpingo-oophorectomy for endometrial carcinoma. Further, hysteroscopy with saline or other distending media would give rise to the same theoretical concern. Among patients with endometrial carcinoma who underwent standard hysterosalpingography, survival rates were no different between those with intraperitoneal spill of the contrast medium and those without.[52] Alcazar et al.[53] performed sonohysterography on 14 consecutive patients with stage I adenocarcinoma of the endometrium. It was done during laparotomy, just after the abdomen was opened but before the start of the surgical procedure. In all 14 patients, saline readily spilled from the fallopian tubes; this fluid was analyzed, as were cell washings. Only one patient (7%) had malignant cells in the spilled fluid, causing the

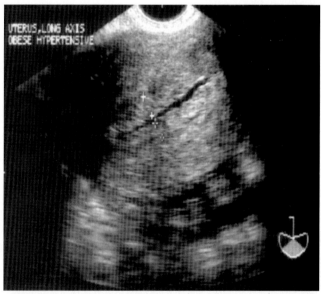

Figure 15–27. Saline infusion sonohysterogram in an obese, hypertensive patient with a thickened endometrial echo. There is virtually no uterine distention, but even this small sonolucent ribbon of fluid allows the accurate depiction of hyperplasia along the anterior and posterior walls, which measure 6.2 and 4.8 mm *(calipers)*, respectively.

authors to conclude that the risk of malignant cell dissemination exists but is small.

Timing of the Procedure

The uterus may be subjected to multiple procedures, including dilation and curettage, childbirth, myomectomy, cesarean section, and abortion. As the endometrium proliferates, it does not remain a smooth, homogeneous layer. Thus, sonohysterography is best performed as soon possible after the bleeding cycle has ended, when the endometrium is as thin as

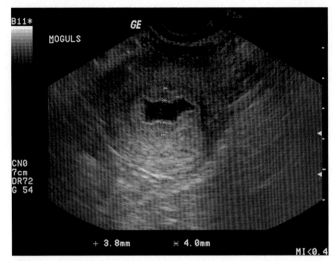

Figure 15–28. Saline infusion sonohysterogram in a patient whose last bleeding episode was 20 days ago. The endometrium is thickened and measures 3.8 and 4.0 mm (the area between the *calipers*). Also note the irregular, undulating appearance of the endometrial surface. These undulations, called "moguls," may be difficult to interpret.

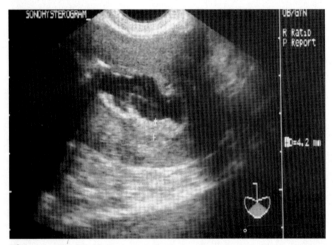

Figure 15–29. Saline infusion sonohysterogram in a patient whose last bleeding episode was 18 days ago. Note the irregular surface of the endometrium. The posterior endometrium measures 4.2 mm *(calipers)*. These undulations ("moguls") present a diagnostic difficulty. Are there areas of focal hyperplasia or small polyps? In fact, this is normal endometrium that is neither homogeneous nor smooth. This interpretive problem can be avoided by timing the procedure appropriately, during the early proliferative phase.

it is going to be all month. Otherwise, focal irregularities in the contour of the endometrium may be mistaken for small polyps or focal areas of endometrial hyperplasia (Figs. 15–28 and 15–29). This was supported in a prospective, blinded study by Wolman et al.,[54] in which there was a 27% false-positive rate when sonohysterography was performed from days 16 to 28 of the menstrual cycle but 0 false-positives when the procedure was performed before day 10.

Sometimes a patient has such irregular bleeding that she cannot tell what is the actual menses. It may be helpful in such cases to use an empirical course of a progestagen, such as medroxyprogesterone acetate 10 mg daily for 10 days, as "medical curettage" and then time the ultrasound examination to the withdrawal bleed.

Summary

Saline infusion sonohysterography enhances transvaginal ultrasound examination of the uterine cavity. It is easily and rapidly performed at minimal cost. It is extremely well tolerated by patients and virtually devoid of complications. It can obviate the need for further invasive diagnostic procedures in some patients and optimize the preoperative planning process for those who require therapeutic intervention.

REFERENCES

1. Goldstein SR: Incorporating endovaginal ultrasonography into the overall gynecologic examination. Am J Obstet Gynecol 1990;162:625-632.
2. Goldstein SR, Nachtigall M, Snyder JR, Nachtigall L: Endometrial assessment by vaginal ultrasonography before endometrial sampling in patients with postmenopausal bleeding. Am J Obstet Gynecol 1990;163:119-123.
3. Goldstein RB, Bree RL, Benson CB, et al: Evaluation of the woman with postmenopausal bleeding: Society of Radiologists in Ultrasound-Sponsored Consensus Conference statement. J Ultrasound Med 2001;20:1025-1036.
4. Langer RD, Pierce JJ, O'Hanlan KA, et al: Transvaginal ultrasonography compared with endometrial biopsy for the detection of endometrial disease: Postmenopausal Estrogen/Progestin Interventions Trial. N Engl J Med 1997;337:1792-1798.
5. Ferrazzi E, Leone FP: Investigating abnormal bleeding on HRT or tamoxifen: The role of ultrasonography. Best Pract Res Clin Obstet Gynaecol 2004;18:145-156.
6. Randolph JR, Ying YK, Maier DB, et al: Comparison of realtime ultrasonography, hysterosalpingography, and laparoscopy/hysteroscopy in evaluation of uterine abnormalities and tubal patency. Fertil Steril 1986;46:828-832.
7. Lewit N, Thaler I, Rottem S: The uterus: A new look with transvaginal sonography. J Clin Ultrasound 1990;18:331-336.
8. Parson AK, Lense JJ: Sonohysterography for endometrial abnormalities: Preliminary results. J Clin Ultrasound 1993;21:87-95.
9. Syrop C, Sahakian V: Transvaginal sonographic detection of endometrial polyps with fluid contrast augmentation. Obstet Gynecol 1992;79:1041-1043.
10. Breckenridge JW, Kurta A, Ritchie W, Macht E: Postmenopausal uterine fluid collection: Indicator of carcinoma. AJR Am J Roentgenol 1982;139:529-534.
11. Goldstein SR: Postmenopausal endometrial fluid collections revisited: Look at the doughnut not at the hole. Obstet Gynecol 1994;83:738-740.
12. Dessole S, Farina M, Capobianco G, et al: Determining the best catheter for sonohysterography. Fertil Steril 2001;76:605-609.
13. Goldstein SR: Use of ultrasonohysterography for triage of perimenopausal patients with unexplained uterine bleeding. Am J Obstet Gynecol 1994;170:565-570.
14. Ricci JV: Gynaecologic surgery and instruments of the nineteenth century prior to the antiseptic age. In The Development of Gynaecological Surgery and Instruments. Philadelphia, Blakiston, 1949, pp 326-328.
15. Word B, Gravlee LC, Widemon GL: The fallacy of simple uterine curettage. Obstet Gynecol 1958;12:642-645.
16. Stock RJ, Kanbour A: Prehysterectomy curettage. Obstet Gynecol 1975;45:537-541.
17. Vuopala S: Diagnostic accuracy and clinical applicability of cytological and histological methods for investigating endometrial carcinoma. Acta Obstet Gynecol Scand Suppl 1997;70:1.
18. Kaunitz AM, Masciello AS, Ostrowsky M, Rovvira EZ: Comparison of endometrial Pipelle and Vabra aspirator. J Reprod Med 1988;33:427-431.
19. Rodriguez MJ, Platt LD, Medearis AL, et al: The use of transvaginal sonography for evaluation of postmenopausal size and morphology. Am J Obstet Gynecol 1988;159:810-814.
20. Stovall TG, Photopulos GJ, Poston WM, et al: Pipelle endometrial sampling in patients with known endometrial cancer. Obstet Gynecol 1991;77:954-956.
21. Goldchmit R, Katz A, Blickstein I, et al: The accuracy of endometrial Pipelle sampling with and without sonographic measurement of endometrial thickness. Obstet Gynecol 1993;82:727-730.

22. Guido RS, Kanbour A, Ruhn M, Christopherson WA: Pipelle endometrial sampling sensitivity in the detection of endometrial cancer. J Reprod Med 1995;40:553-555.
23. Goldstein SR, Zelzter I, Horan CK, et al: Ultrasonography-based triage for perimenopausal patients with abnormal uterine bleeding. Am J Obstet Gynecol 1997;177:102-108.
24. Ando H, Toda S, Harada M, et al: Which infertile women should be indicated for sonohysterography? Ultrasound Obstet Gynecol 2004;24:566-571.
25. Dijkhuizen FP, Brolmann HA, Potters AE, et al: The accuracy of transvaginal ultrasonography in the diagnosis of endometrial abnormalities. Obstet Gynecol 1996;87:345-349.
26. Timmerman D, Verguts J, Konstantinovic ML, et al: The pedicle artery sign based on sonography with color Doppler imaging can replace second-stage tests in women with abnormal vaginal bleeding. Ultrasound Obstet Gynecol 2003;22:166-171.
27. Early Breast Cancer Trialists Collaborative Group: Effects of adjuvant tamoxifen and of cytotoxic therapy on mortality in early breast cancer: An overview of 61 randomized trials among 28,896 women. N Engl J Med 1988;319:1681.
28. Killackey MA, Hakes TB, Pierce VK: Endometrial adenocarcinoma in breast cancer patients receiving antiestrogens. Cancer Treat Rep 1985;69:237-238.
29. Jordan VC. Tamoxifen and endometrial cancer [letter]. Lancet 1989;2:117-120.
30. Atlanta G, Pozzi M, Vincenzoni C, Vocaturo G: Four case reports presenting new acquisitions on the association between breast and endometrial carcinoma. Gynecol Oncol 1990;37:378-380.
31. Fornander T, Rutqvist LE, Cedermark B, et al: Adjuvant tamoxifen in early breast cancer. Occurrence of new primary cancers. Lancet 1989;1:117-120.
32. Neven P, De Muylder X, Van Belle Y, et al: Hysteroscopic follow-up during tamoxifen treatment. Eur J Obstet Gynecol Reprod Biol 1990;35:235-238.
33. Gal D, Kopel S, Bashevkin M, et al: Oncogenic potential of tamoxifen on endometria of postmenopausal women with breast cancer—preliminary report. Gynecol Oncol 1991;42:120-123.
34. Goldstein SR, Nachtigall M, Snyder JR, Nachtigall L: Endometrial assessment by vaginal ultrasonography before endometrial sampling in patients with postmenopausal bleeding. Am J Obstet Gynecol 1990;163:119-123.
35. Anteby E, Yagel S, Zacut D, et al: False sonographic appearance of endometrial neoplasia in postmenopausal women treated with tamoxifen. Lancet 1992;340:433.
36. Goldstein SR: Unusual ultrasonographic appearance of the uterus in patients receiving tamoxifen. Obstet Gynecol 1994;170:447-451.
37. Fleischer AC, Wheeler JE, Kravitz B, et al: Sonographic assessment of the endometrium in osteopenic postmenopausal women treated with idoxifene. J Ultrasound Med 1999;18:503-512.
38. Schwartz LB, Snyder J, Horan C, et al: The use of transvaginal ultrasound and saline infusion sonohysterography for the evaluation of asymptomatic postmenopausal breast cancer patients on tamoxifen. Ultrasound Obstet Gynecol 1998;11:48-53.
39. American College of Obstetricians and Gynecologists (ACOG) committee opinion #169, February 1996. Tamoxifen and Endometrial Cancer.
40. Kedar RP, Bourne TH, Powles TJ, et al: Effects of tamoxifen on uterus and ovaries of postmenopausal women in a randomized breast cancer prevention trial. Lancet 1994;343:1318-1321.
41. American College of Obstetricians and Gynecologists (ACOG) committee opinion #232, April 2000. Tamoxifen and Endometrial Cancer.
42. Fisher B, Costantino JP, Wickerham DL, et al: Tamoxifen for prevention of breast cancer: Report of the National Surgical Adjuvant Breast and Bowel Project P-1 Study. J Natl Cancer Inst 1998;90:1371-1388.
43. Berliere M, Charles A, Galant C, Donnez J: Uterine side effects of tamoxifen: A need for systematic pretreatment screening. Obstet Gynecol 1998;91:40-44.
44. Berliere M, Radikov G, Galant C, et al: Identification of women at high risk of developing endometrial cancer on tamoxifen. Eur J Cancer 2000;36:S35-S36.
45. Barakat RR, Gilewski TA, Almadrones L, et al: Effect of adjuvant tamoxifen on the endometrium in women with breast cancer: A prospective study using office endometrial biopsy. J Clinical Oncol 2000;18:3459-3463.
46. Love CD, Muir BB, Scrimgeour JB, et al: Investigation of endometrial abnormalities in asymptomatic women treated with tamoxifen and an evaluation of the role of endometrial screening. J Clin Oncol 1999;17:2050-2054.
47. Markovitch O, Tepper R, Aviram R, et al: The value of sonohysterography in the prediction of endometrial pathologies in asymptomatic postmenopausal breast cancer tamoxifen-treated patients. Gynecol Oncol 2004;94:754-759.
48. Develioglu OH, Omak M, Bilgin T, et al: The endometrium in asymptomatic breast cancer patients on tamoxifen: Value of transvaginal ultrasonography with saline infusion and Doppler flow. Gynecol Oncol 2004;93:328-335.
49. Dessole S, Farina M, Rubattu G, et al: Side effects and complications of sonohysterosalpingography. Fertil Steril 2003;80:620-624.
50. Cooper JM, Brady RM: Intraoperative and early postoperative complications of operative hysteroscopy. Obstet Gynecol Clin North Am 2000;27:347-366.
51. Tuveng JM, Vold I, Jerve F, et al: Hysterosalpingography: Value in estimating tubal function, and risk of infectious complications. Acta Eur Fertl 1985;16:125-128.
52. DeVore GR, Schwartz PE, Morris J: Hysterography: A 5-year follow-up in patients with endometrial carcinoma. Obstet Gynecol 1982;60:369-372.
53. Alcazar JL, Errasti R, Zornoza A: Saline infusion sonohysterography in endometrial cancer: Assessment of malignant cells dissemination risk. Acta Obstet Gynecol Scand 2000;79:321-322.
54. Wolman I, Groutz A, Gordon D, et al: Timing of sonohysterography in menstruating women. Gynecol Obstet Invest 1999;48:254-258.

Chapter 16

Ultrasound-Guided Procedures in Gynecology

Jodi P. Lerner and Ana Monteagudo

Background

The history of ultrasound-guided procedures has come full circle. Initially, ultrasound-guided puncture procedures were performed exclusively using transabdominal sonography in both diagnostic and therapeutic roles. As transvaginal ultrasound equipment improved, especially with the advent of high-frequency probes, many procedures became the domain of transvaginal technique. However, beginning in the late 1990s, a new generation of transabdominal transducers was introduced, and therefore some procedures are once again performed transabdominally. Currently, the route of the procedure (transabdominal vs. transvaginal) is decided based on several factors—namely, patient's body habitus, location of the target structure, need to circumvent interposed structures (i.e., a vessel or bowel), and, most important, the physician's experience and familiarity with the procedure.

The percutaneous aspiration of intra-abdominal abscesses was first described by Smith and Bartrum[1] in 1974, and soon afterward, Gerzof et al.[2] used a percutaneous abdominal catheter to drain pus collections. Since its development, transvaginal sonography (TVS) has proved useful not only for imaging but for invasive diagnostic techniques and therapeutic procedures. This chapter presents the various puncture procedures and local injections performed under ultrasound guidance and discusses the experience gained using transvaginal probes.

The goal of any ultrasound-guided puncture procedure is to use the newest clinical techniques while subjecting the patient to the least invasive or traumatic method possible. Puncture procedures may be performed for diagnostic, palliative, or therapeutic reasons, although in many cases a combination of these reasons applies. The multiple advantages of ultrasound-guided puncture procedures over traditional methods include their ease of technical mastery, accurate needle placement, little (rare or no) injury to adjacent organs, versatility (portability), low cost, and speed of administration. Possible complications, although rare, include bleeding, infection, inadvertent puncture of adjacent organs, and in the case of multifetal reductions, miscarriage.

Puncture procedures are performed in three dimensions, not in the two-dimensional view of an ultrasound monitor. Because of the physical properties of sound, the third dimension is thinnest at the focal range of the probe, its thickness being inversely proportional to the operating frequency of the transducer crystal. The term *slice thickness artifact* refers to this concept and requires that the operator take the third dimension of the image into account while performing puncture procedures. At times, the tip of the needle used for the procedure may appear to be within the structure at which it is aimed, but in reality it is slightly in front of or slightly behind the structure imaged.

Transabdominal needle guides were used at the inception of the puncture technique experience. However, with increasing experience, a free-hand approach has been successfully used by many operators. The mobility of the needle within the scanning plane made this technique easy to perform. However, the free-hand technique may sometimes image only the transverse section of the needle and not the tip. With transabdominal sonography, the scanning plane may be quickly readjusted to find the needle tip. This readjustment technique is not available with the transvaginal approach because of the minimal mobility of the probe and the needle. This limitation has made the free-hand needle approach somewhat cumbersome in transvaginally guided punctures. A needle guide attached to the shaft of the probe enables the operator to keep the entire length of the needle within the scanning plane and have control over the needle tip, as well as freeing the operator's second hand to perform other tasks.

When needed, our group uses an automated puncture device (APD; Labotect, Göttingen, Germany) for transvaginal procedures. This device is a spring-loaded instrument mated to the vaginal probe (Fig. 16–1). The APD was first used for ovum pickup in assisted reproduction programs,[3] but its usefulness was limited by the need to reload and reshoot each time a new follicle had to be aspirated, and the technique was abandoned by most. We find the APD to be indispensable when extreme accuracy and precision are necessary for needle placement under transvaginal guidance.[4-9] We tested the accuracy of needle placement in vitro and found it to be ±1 to

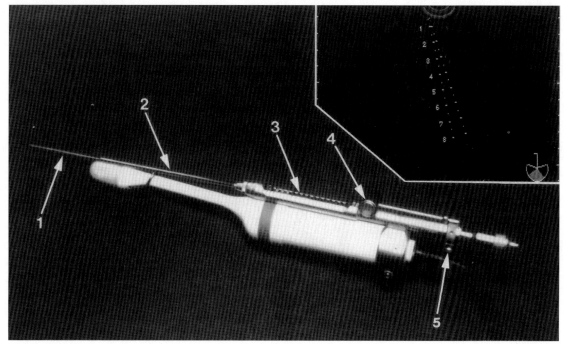

Figure 16–1. Automated puncture device attached to vaginal probe: 1, needle; 2, needle guide; 3, depth gauge; 4, trigger; 5, safety knob. *Inset,* Biopsy guide with centimeter scale.

2 mm. No anesthesia or local analgesia is needed; the procedure is virtually painless because of the needle's high-velocity entry. This is in contrast to the manual needle technique, in which the relatively slower forward motion of the needle necessitates analgesia.

Puncture Procedures

A general description of the more commonly performed transvaginally directed puncture procedures is presented. The indications and specific attributes for each of these procedures are addressed:

- Punctures of ovarian cysts
- Treatment of ectopic pregnancies
- Drainage of pelvic (fluid) contents
- Diagnostic culdocentesis
- Multifetal pregnancy reductions (if the transabdominal route is not feasible)
- Transvaginal chorionic villus sampling

Technique

Transvaginal Approach

Punctures are usually performed with the guidance of the 5- to 7.5-MHz vaginal transducer probe through a needle guide attached to the probe's shaft. A software-generated, fixed double-dotted line or biopsy guide, displayed on the ultrasound screen, marks the path of the penetrating needle. Most of these provide the operator with a centimeter scale to measure needle depth. Needles ranging from 21- to 14-gauge are used; the thinnest possible needle able to perform the desired task should be used.

When the procedure is performed by manual needle insertion, analgesia and local anesthesia may be provided by intra-venous meperidine (25 to 50 mg) combined with diazepam (5 to 10 mg). A local injection of 1 to 2 mL 1% lidocaine through the needle guide into the vaginal mucosa at the puncture site is needed if protracted manipulation is anticipated. The sequence of events using the APD is essentially the same as with the manual technique, but as previously stated, neither analgesia nor local anesthesia is necessary.

Patients should be informed about the procedure, risks, and benefits and asked to sign the informed consent form. Specifically worded consent forms are usually used in procedures such as puncture of ectopic pregnancies. The procedure should be documented by still images or videotape recordings. A detailed report describing the procedure should be written promptly and a copy sent to the referring clinician. After withdrawal of the needle, the pelvic structures and the cul-de-sac must be observed for approximately 10 minutes, or as needed, to detect any possible bleeding from the puncture site. Patients are usually rescanned after a 2- to 3-hour observation period for possible late complications.

Transabdominal Approach

Transabdominal procedures are mostly done using a free-hand approach. As with transvaginal procedures, patients should be informed about the procedure, risks, and benefits and asked to sign the informed consent form. During a transabdominal puncture procedure, the patient's abdomen is prepared with an antiseptic solution and draped, similar to the preparation for an amniocentesis. The procedure should be documented by still images or videotape recordings. A detailed report describing the procedure should be written promptly and a copy sent to the referring clinician. After withdrawal of the needle, the target structure must be observed for approximately 5 to 10 minutes, or as needed, to detect any possible bleeding from the puncture site. Depending on the puncture procedure performed, the patients are rescanned either immediately or after $1^1/_2$ to 2 hours. For example, after transabdominal chorionic villus sampling, the patient is rescanned immediately, but after a multifetal pregnancy reduction, a repeat scan is performed $1^1/_2$ to 2 hours later for possible late complications.

Puncture of Ovarian Cysts

The first transvaginal puncture procedure performed was for oocyte retrieval, after transabdominally guided transvesical follicle aspiration was already well established.[10-12] Later, transurethral–transvesical ovum pickups were used.[13] However, as transvaginal needle puncture proved to be safe and accurate, it rapidly became the technique of choice worldwide. This technique relies on a needle guide attached to the vaginal probe, which enables guided needle placement under real-time observation,[14,15] although several infertility programs perform retrievals by using the automated spring-loaded puncture device attached to the shaft of the vaginal probe.[3]

Puncture of Cysts with Simple Architecture

One of the most common indications for this technique is the puncture of ovarian cysts with simple architecture. *Simple architecture* refers to cyst morphology characterized by a smooth and thin wall, sonolucent (anechoic)–appearing fluid, no irregularities on the inner wall, and no septations or solid components. This procedure is probably the simplest of all puncture procedures to master technically. Essentially the same technique is used in the most commonly performed puncture procedure, TVS-guided follicular aspiration. The technique is shown in Figure 16–2.

In the puncture of an ovarian or parovarian cyst, the center of the cyst is targeted, and the needle inserted (Fig. 16–3) and maintained in the middle of the shrinking sonolucency throughout the aspiration. Ovarian cysts and benign, symptomatic, cystic pelvic lesions have been punctured successfully by several different groups[16-19]; for example, Ron-El et al.[19]

performed 23 punctures of ovarian cysts without complications. Concern over cell spillage into the abdominal cavity from a potentially malignant ovarian cyst prevents many clinicians from using the procedure more frequently. The aspirated fluid is usually submitted for cytologic evaluation, but a negative cytologic examination may, in fact, represent a false-negative result.[20]

Certainly, one of the primary goals of ovarian cyst puncture is to intervene in a less aggressive and invasive manner than in the traditional therapies of laparotomy and laparoscopy. Bonilla-Musoles et al.[21] studied 108 small (<7 cm) ovarian masses in perimenopausal or early post-menopausal women. These masses had been evaluated sonographically by both TVS and color Doppler sonography; because 7 of the 108 were perceived to be malignant preaspiration, the goal with this subset was to obtain a preoperative cytologic diagnosis and avoid leakage at the time of laparotomy. The goal for the remaining 101 was the avoidance of surgery altogether. The recurrence rate of punctured benign cysts was 25% by 1 year of follow-up; no difference in the recurrence rate was noted between the premenopausal and postmenopausal cases.

One of the most important questions is whether it is clinically important to puncture simple ovarian cysts—or, more precisely, ovarian or adnexal cysts with simple architecture. Many articles in the literature describe these simple adnexal cysts. However, we discuss here a review article that deals with the natural history of simple adnexal cysts in postmenopausal women.[22] Transabdominal sonography and TVS were performed in 184 asymptomatic postmenopausal women to determine the frequency and natural history of simple adnexal cysts and their relationship to hormone replacement therapy. Forty-nine women with 72 cysts were reevaluated with subsequent ultrasound scanning over 3 to 23 months. Thirty-eight of the 72 cysts (53%) disappeared completely, 20 cysts (28%) remained constant in size, 8 cysts (11%) enlarged by 3 mm or more, 2 cysts (3%) decreased in size by 3 mm or more, and 4 cysts (6%) both increased and decreased in size on repeated examinations. No statistical relationship was found in this study between the presence of the cysts or cyst activity with

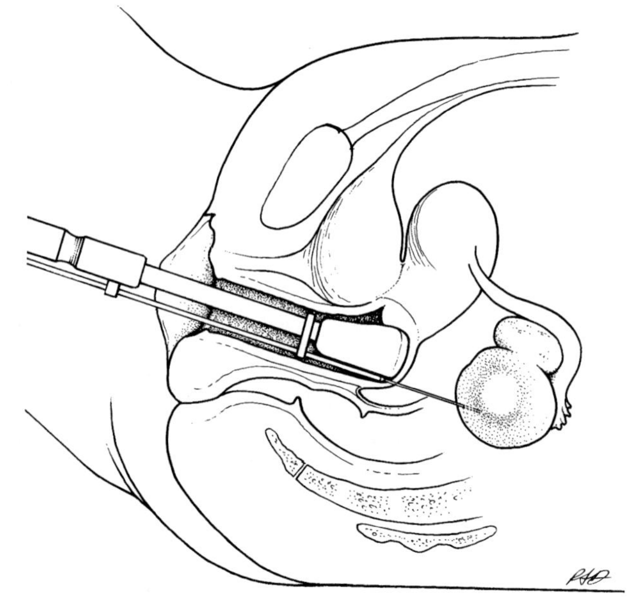

Figure 16–2. Schematic representation of the orientation of the puncture device and vaginal probe for ovarian cyst puncture.

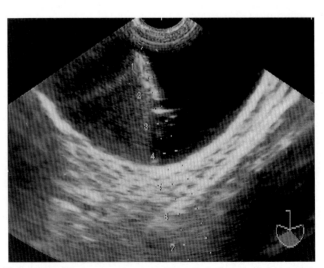

Figure 16–3. Ovarian cyst puncture. The needle is located in the center of a unilocular cyst for aspiration of cyst contents.

respect to type of hormone replacement or length of time since the onset of menopause. The authors concluded that in postmenopausal women, simple adnexal cysts that are less than 3 cm and have normal Doppler flow studies and normal CA-125 levels are most likely benign and may be conservatively managed and followed safely with ultrasound.

In another review article, Goldstein[23] evaluated the conservative approach to management of small postmenopausal cystic masses. He concluded that simple cysts are more common in postmenopausal patients than was previously thought. These cysts are unlikely to be malignant and are certainly capable of being followed conservatively. The puncture of ovarian cysts less than 3 cm in a postmenopausal patient should rarely, if ever, be an option in the management algorithm.

Aspiration of Persistent or Recurrent Ovarian Cysts

The utility of transvaginal aspiration of persistent or recurrent ovarian cysts is highly debated, as evidenced by several articles in the literature. Ron-El et al. followed their previously quoted study[19] with an investigation of 35 women between the ages of 17 and 76 years.[24] In this study, the patients were evaluated not only by gray-scale TVS but by color-flow Doppler mapping of the ovaries containing the cysts, to search for neovascularization. All 35 patients were rescanned vaginally 1, 3, 6, and 12 months after the last aspiration. A second aspiration was performed after 3 months in 14 women for cyst recurrence. Three parameters proved important in predicting the outcome of aspiration: the age of the woman, the maximum diameter of the cyst, and the location of the cysts. The older the patient and the larger the cyst encountered, the poorer the prognosis. They concluded that aspiration of large ovarian cysts should be avoided in older women.[24]

Bret et al.[25,26] published two papers describing their experience using TVS in the aspiration of ovarian cysts. They reported a 48% recurrence rate after cyst aspiration in premenopausal women and an 80% recurrence rate in postmenopausal women. This group attempted to prevent cyst recurrence by injecting alcohol immediately after cyst aspiration, but this procedure was successful in only four of seven patients.[25,26]

Andolf et al.[27] investigated the concentration of gonadal steroids and fibrinolytic indices in fluid from 96 aspirated benign ovarian cysts in an attempt to discriminate between functional and neoplastic cysts and therefore predict recurrence. The goal was to assay for these components and minimize surgery on functional cysts. Components of the plasminogen activating system (PAS), which are known to be increased in ovarian neoplasia, and gonadal steroids, which are found in higher concentrations in functional cysts, were the biochemical characteristics studied in the cyst fluid. Concentrations of estradiol (E_2) and progesterone were higher in cysts that did not recur than in those that did; a high concentration of E_2 in the fluid was the single best predictor of no recurrence. In contrast, the cyst fluid E_2 was low in all postmenopausal women analyzed because follicular cysts would not be expected to be present after menopause. Sixteen of 18 cysts in postmenopausal women recurred in this study. It has been established that several components of the PAS are increased in the peripheral blood of patients with benign ovarian tumors, and all components of the PAS are increased

in malignant ovarian tumors. In the study by Andolf et al.,[27] PAS component activity was higher in neoplastic than in functional cysts, although the difference varied based on which component was interrogated. Higher levels of urokinase plasminogen activator and lower levels of plasminogen activator inhibitor-1 were found in cysts that recurred; the conclusion supports the premise that neoplastic cysts accounted for the vast majority of the cysts that recurred and were subsequently removed at surgery.[27]

Aspiration of Cysts in Pregnant Patients

Ultrasound-guided puncture of ovarian cysts detected in pregnancy is another aspect of this topic that is frequently encountered and debated. The widespread use of ultrasound during pregnancy led to a dramatic increase in the frequency of diagnosing ovarian cysts, both symptomatic and asymptomatic. Although the great majority of these cysts are asymptomatic and presumably benign, resolving spontaneously by 16 weeks,[28] there is a subset of persistent ovarian cysts that, because of anatomic, hormonal, or vascular changes, are associated with an increased incidence of torsion, rupture, and infection in pregnant patients.[29-32] Guariglia et al.[33] report on the outcome of nine transabdominally guided ovarian cyst punctures and drainage procedures, performed from 7 to 17 weeks of gestation and yielding aspirated volumes of 60 to 520 mL. Three of the nine cysts recurred and necessitated a second puncture procedure. No procedure-related complications were noted.

Aboulghar et al.[34] transvaginally aspirated simple-appearing large ovarian cysts in three pregnant patients without complications or the need for operative intervention.

Combination of Aspiration and Cytologic Diagnosis

Yee and colleagues[35] combined the ultrasound-guided puncture of cystic adnexal masses with cytologic evaluation of the aspirates in an attempt to improve differentiation between benign and malignant ovarian and adnexal masses as a means of preventing or at least limiting surgical intervention. Forty-three ovarian cysts that were evaluated sonographically and then aspirated were studied. The Sassone morphologic scoring system was used to evaluate the ovarian cysts sonographically.[36] Thirty-six benign cysts had TVS scores ranging from 4 to 12 (median, 7). All 25 cysts that were benign by TVS or histologic study were also cytologically benign, as well as an additional 11 cysts that were not resected (TVS scores, 4 to 9). Seven cytologically and histologically malignant cysts had high TVS scores of 10 to 14 (median, 12). The combination of TVS and needle aspiration cytology was considered valuable by this group, particularly in the management of cysts with low or intermediate TVS scores and benign results on cytology.

Another group performed puncture and aspiration of seven sonographically established malignant tumors to establish the cytologic diagnosis before surgery. No significant differences were observed between cytologic and histopathologic findings in cases that went to surgery, and no evidence of leakage was noted at the time of surgery.[21]

Many experienced gynecologists oppose any kind of ovarian cyst puncture,[37] concerned that the spread of ovarian cancer from a rare, potentially malignant cyst might occur. Although their procedure was laparoscopic puncture and aspiration, Trimbos and Hacker[37] reported on two cases of a malignant ovarian cyst in which disseminated ovarian cancer was encountered 8 weeks later at laparotomy. An interesting study was described in 1996 by a Brazilian group whereby ovarian cysts were punctured within a saline-filled container to determine whether leakage of ovarian cyst cells occurs.[38] The cyst was excised at the time of laparotomy and immersed in a container with saline. The cyst was punctured and its contents aspirated through the wall of the container; the material obtained was centrifuged, and slides of the precipitate were prepared for cytology. Leakage of the cyst fluid was confirmed both by the unaided eye (visualization of a trickle leaking through the puncture site) and by examination of the slides, which confirmed the presence of cyst fluid in 27% of cases.

Aspiration of Endometriomas and Endometriotic Cysts

The aspiration of endometriomas and endometriotic cysts is considered to be relatively contraindicated, although several groups have performed these punctures. De Crespigny et al.[39] punctured 28 ovarian cysts, 6 of which appeared to be endometriomas. Aboulghar and colleagues[40] studied 21 patients in whom TVS-guided aspiration of pelvic and endometriotic cysts was performed. Reaccumulation occurred in only 6 of 17 cases of endometrioma during a 12-month follow-up, yet symptoms improved only temporarily in most of the cases. These investigators concluded that puncture and aspiration of endometriomas was inefficient for therapeutic purposes. Potential indications for aspirating endometriotic cysts include preventing the adverse effects of ovarian cysts on folliculogenesis,[41] improving ultrasound follow-up of the follicles, enabling easier retrieval technique for all follicular sites,[42] and, finally, relief of symptoms often caused by larger endometriotic cysts and adhesions. Certainly, the aspiration of endometriotic cysts is technically simple; however, its overall benefit and safety are inconclusive owing to the lack of experience with larger series. It may, in fact, be an effective technique in the treatment of selected cases, such as before ovarian stimulation for in vitro fertilization (IVF).

Conclusion

The final verdict on the widespread use of ovarian cyst puncture has not been firmly established. Certainly, the consensus, as described in an excellent 1996 editorial by Osmers,[43] is that puncture of ovarian tumors as a therapeutic approach is not appropriate for tumors of unclear etiology. Continued research and evaluation of the growing clinical experience are needed.

Treatment of Ectopic Pregnancies

Classically, the patient with an ectopic pregnancy (EP) was managed surgically by excision of the diseased tube, ovary, or cornual region of the uterus. Since the mid-1990s, however, conservative or nonsurgical approaches have been described that usually involve the use of systemic methotrexate or RU 486 (mifepristone). This chemotherapeutic agent acts as a trophoblast growth inhibitor by inhibiting DNA synthesis.[44] Systemic methotrexate treatment has been shown to be particularly useful in cases of early, unruptured tubal EPs, with a reported success rate of approximately 90%.[45-47] However, in cases of live tubal EPs, a failure rate of 30% has been reported using systemic methotrexate alone.[45]

Another nonsurgical management option for EPs is local injection of methotrexate, potassium chloride (KCl), or prostaglandins under laparoscopic or ultrasound guidance.[48,49] This option can be applied to all the various kinds of live EP but is most useful for dealing with cervical and cornual (interstitial) pregnancies. It is also an important option when the EP is part of a heterotopic pregnancy in which the intrauterine pregnancy is wanted. Insertion of a needle into an ectopic embryo under TVS guidance is similar to the combination of oocyte aspiration and multifetal pregnancy reduction. It indeed seems logical to use a puncture procedure to treat an EP, thus saving the patient from a more invasive surgical procedure. This section concentrates on the TVS-guided local injection of KCl or methotrexate.

It is not by chance that the first TVS-guided puncture procedure to treat tubal EP by injecting local methotrexate was developed by a group proficient in IVF and reproductive technologies. This group took the skills acquired performing ovum aspiration and applied them to the nonsurgical treatment of EP.[50,51] Three kinds of ectopic gestations and their puncture treatment are discussed: tubal, cornual, and cervical pregnancies.

Tubal Ectopic Pregnancies

The diagnosis of a tubal EP is made when a patient presents with a positive β-human chorionic gonadotropin (β-hCG) level and has an empty uterus by TVS. In the adnexa, the typical adnexal ring, sometimes referred to as the *bagel sign* (S. Rottem, personal communication), is evident. Live tubal EPs may be present in up to one third of all ectopic gestations. Based on our experience, cases of tubal EP must meet several criteria to be considered for TVS-guided puncture: the ectopic gestational sac must contain a live embryo/fetus with a postmenstrual age of less than 8 weeks 4 days, and the tubal diameter should not exceed 2.5 to 3 cm.

The reported complication rates for direct tubal puncture (salpingocentesis) are approximately 15% to 19%. However, it is hard to compare the success rates between different groups because there is no agreed-on basis for comparison: different kinds of EPs, nonviable and viable, with different gestational ages and different sizes, have been treated by injection. Careful evaluation of the published results reveals that because of a lack of understanding of the natural course of the disease after the injection, some of the reported cases indeed do not match the strict definition of a failed treatment. Some of the authors, including our group, were quick to consider a case a failure and institute additional treatment because of findings that now are considered part of the natural sequence of events after injection.[47] Only recently have these sequences been elucidated. The most important signs and symptoms of the postpuncture convalescent period include the following:

1. A *relatively slow decrease in serum β-hCG levels.* The slope of the decay curve for serum β-hCG levels after salpingocentesis depends on which chemical (KCl or methotrexate) was injected during the procedure. When KCl is injected at the time of salpingocentesis, between 30 and 80 days are needed for the β-hCG to become negative.[4] However, when methotrexate is injected, the β-hCG levels fall more abruptly, taking only 10 to 35 days to reach nonpregnant levels.[4,50-55]

2. *Lower abdominal cramping or pain.* Between 3 and 7 days postpuncture, the patient may experience lower abdominal pain or cramping.[47] The possible explanations for this are either uterine contractions (as the decidual cast is expelled from the uterus) or tubal abortion, with varying degrees of intra-abdominal bleeding. If the patient's vital signs and the amount of free fluid (blood in the pelvis) are not significant, the patient may be followed conservatively.
3. *TVS and color Doppler findings.* These include increasing distention of the hematosalpinx, increasing vascularity by color Doppler, and increasing venous spaces.[55] All may be signs of the normal process of resolution.

Usually, puncture is performed only after the patient has been informed and extensively counseled about her treatment options. During the risk–benefit counseling session, the procedure, the risks and complications, and the nature of the postprocedure follow-up are described. As with other puncture or local injection procedures, the patient is asked to sign an informed consent form. Before describing the technique, we stress that treatment of EPs with this procedure is still not considered the standard of care, and it requires the signing of the aforementioned informed consent form (as with any procedure).

Before the needle is inserted, the location of the uterine artery and vessels of the adnexa should be carefully established, and care should be taken not to puncture these vessels during insertion of the needle (Fig. 16–4).

The puncture technique is similar to that described previously for ovarian cysts. A 5- to 7.5-MHz transvaginal probe covered with a sterile plastic sheath is used. A needle guide should be used to ensure accurate and steady placement of the needle. We prefer to use the previously described APD; however, other needle guides mated to the vaginal probe serve the same function. The thinnest possible needle should be used; usually, a 21-gauge needle is used. The patient is placed in the lithotomy position, and the perineum is cleaned with povidone–iodine (Betadine) or a soap solution. A speculum is placed in the vagina, and the vagina and cervix are thoroughly cleaned using Betadine or a soap solution. Sterile drapes are used to create a sterile field; sterile gel is used for good sonic contact.

As described earlier, a software-generated fixed line is displayed on the monitor by which the exact depth of the EP is located (Fig. 16–5A). If the APD is used, the depth of needle penetration is controlled by the centimeter marks on the shaft of the APD. The patient is asked to hold her breath to prevent any movement during normal inspiration/expiration, and the needle is released (Fig. 16–5B). If a standard needle guide is used, the needle should be inserted rapidly; otherwise, the EP may be pushed away from the field of view rather than penetrated. The target area is located near the fetal heart, and either methotrexate or KCl is injected to stop cardiac activity. As the needle is withdrawn, methotrexate may also be injected in the area of the placental bed. Care must be exercised not to overdistend the already compromised fallopian tube.

It is important to observe the pelvic structures and the cul-de-sac after withdrawal of the needle. Patients are rescanned after 2 to 3 hours for possible complications. Complications we have encountered during such puncture procedures include immediate bleeding from the puncture site as soon as the needle is withdrawn and hematomas that slowly enlarge over several hours.

Nazac et al.[56] investigated the predictors of successful methotrexate treatment in women with unruptured tubal pregnancies. They found that when methotrexate was administered locally the success rate was better, with an odds ratio of 9.7 (95% confidence interval 3.1 to 30). In addition, they found that the success rate was poorer when the β-hCG level was 1000 mIU/mL or more. Since 2000, we have treated four nonruptured, live tubal EPs with local injection of methotrexate guided by ultrasound. All patients had some contraindication to surgery. The gestational ages of the pregnancies were between 5 weeks and 6 weeks 2 days. All patients were successfully treated by the single injection and did not require additional intramuscular injection of methotrexate.[57]

Cornual/Interstitial Ectopic Pregnancies

Approximately 2% to 4% of all tubal EPs are located in the cornual/interstitial area of the uterus (Fig. 16–6A). The rupture of a cornual pregnancy causes severe hemorrhage and exposes the patient to significant morbidity; the maternal mortality rate approaches 2.5%.[55] Historically, the procedure of choice to treat these patients has been cornual resection, which is technically feasible in more than 50% of the cases. However, in the remainder of patients, hysterectomy is unavoidable.[55]

Using TVS, the diagnosis of a cornual EP is made when the patient presents with a positive β-hCG; an empty uterine cavity; an eccentrically placed or very lateral chorionic sac seen separately and at least 1 cm from the most lateral edge of the uterine cavity; thin myometrium covering the gestational sac; myometrium present between the sac and uterine cavity (Fig. 16–6B); and no gestational sac visible above the level of the internal os in the longitudinal plane of the uterus.[7,58] Another useful sonographic sign is the interstitial line described by Ackerman et al.,[59] which is a thin echogenic line extending directly to the center of the interstitial gestational sac. In their hands, the presence of this line had 80% sensitivity, 98% specificity, and a 96% positive predictive value for

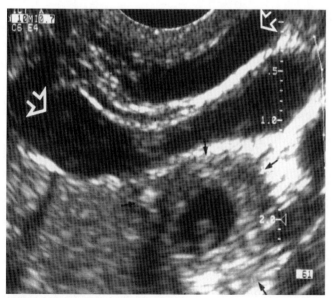

Figure 16–4. A large vessel *(open arrows)* is interposed between the transducer and the ectopic pregnancy *(black arrows).*

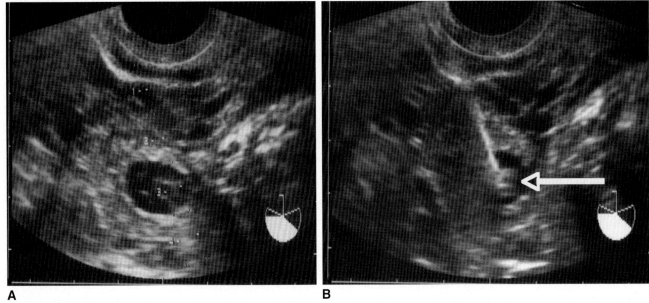

Figure 16–5. Puncture and injection of a tubal ectopic pregnancy (EP). **A,** The cross section of a live tubal EP is targeted by the software-generated centimeter display. **B,** The needle tip *(arrow)* penetrates 3 cm, to the center of the tubal gestation.

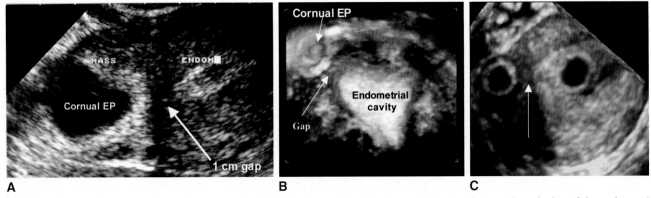

Figure 16–6. The cornual ectopic pregnancy (EP). **A,** Note the approximately 1-cm gap between the most lateral edge of the endometrial echo and the ring of the cornual EP. **B,** Three-dimensional thick-slice image of a right cornual EP. The endometrial cavity appears hyperechoic. Note the distance between the cavity and the sac *(arrow)*. **C,** A three-dimensional thick-slice image clearly shows the EP in the cornual/interstitial position *(arrow)*.

detection of an interstitial pregnancy. Care must be taken not to mistake a bicornuate or incomplete septate uterus for a cornual EP. We currently use three-dimensional ultrasound to help diagnose cornual pregnancies. This imaging technique has proven useful in cases in which a uterine malformation, such as bicornuate uterus, was not previously detected and there was uncertainty over the exact location of the gestational sac (Fig. 16–6B and C).

Karsdorp et al.[60] reported on the successful treatment of five interstitial pregnancies using methotrexate. One of the five interstitial EPs initially was punctured transvaginally and the contents aspirated and subsequently injected with methotrexate and leucovorin. Doubilet et al.[61] recently published their experience with sonographically guided injection of unusual EPs. In their series, there were six cases of cornual EPs with gestational ages ranging from 5 weeks 5 days to 10 weeks. One of the six pregnancies ruptured approximately 13 days after successful injection of KCl; this pregnancy was at 7 weeks' ges-

tation the day of the treatment. In our most recent series of puncture injections of live EPs, we had four cornual pregnancies. The gestational age of the pregnancies ranged from 5 weeks 6 days to 7 weeks 4 days, and they were injected with either methotrexate or KCl. One patient (gestational age, 7 weeks 4 days) required a second dose of methotrexate and subsequently needed surgery for rupture of her cornual EP.[57]

We have described a safe puncture route to avoid rupturing the sac of the interstitial/cornual pregnancy during needle insertion.[62] The safe route calls for inserting the needle from a medial to lateral direction, traversing myometrium first before reaching the ectopic sac (Fig. 16–7). Thus, the distended sac is not punctured through its lateral, thin wall, preventing its rupture. We believe that puncture injection of cornual EPs by TVS guidance is a valid alternative to a more extensive surgical procedure, and to be candidates for TVS-guided puncture, cases of cornual EP must be viable with a gestational age of less than 12 weeks[62] (Fig. 16–8).

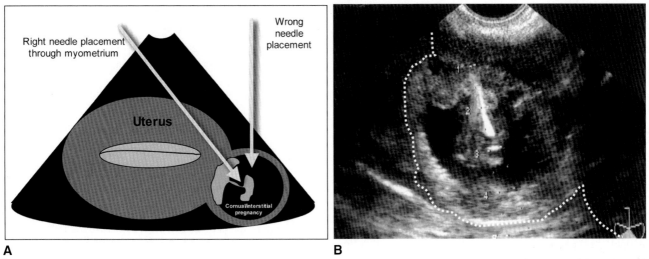

Figure 16–7. The safest puncture route to inject a cornual/interstitial ectopic pregnancy (EP). **A,** Schematic depiction of the correct and wrong directions to puncture an EP. The correct path traverses the myometrium to avoid bursting the sac. **B,** An actual puncture of a cornual pregnancy using the safe route.

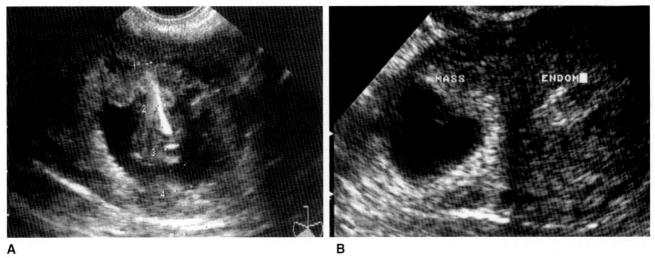

Figure 16–8. Cornual pregnancy. **A,** A transvaginal sonographic view of a cornual pregnancy with the needle in place for the injection of KCl or methotrexate. **B,** A higher-magnification view of the same fetal pole 3 weeks after the puncture; no cardiac activity was seen.

It is important to emphasize that a nonviable cornual EP with stable or declining β-hCG can often be followed by TVS, with or without parenteral methotrexate treatment. There is no need to inject such patients or take them to the operating room for cornual resection, and the long-term nonsurgical follow-up of a nonviable cornual/interstitial pregnancy can be done using serial β-hCG levels and TVS evaluation.[7,63]

Because of the limited number of live cornual EPs treated by TVS-guided puncture, the postinjection complication rates for these procedures have not been elucidated. As with salpingocentesis, the most feared complication would probably be bleeding from the site of the puncture or rupture, as seen with our case.

Based on current data, some preliminary postpuncture convalescent information is available:

1. The serum level of β-hCG returns to nonpregnant levels slowly (and initially may even increase). For cornual EPs treated with methotrexate, as in treatment of tubal EPs with salpingocentesis, the β-hCG returns more quickly to nonpregnant levels (12 weeks) than when KCl is used (15 weeks) or when the EP is followed expectantly without treatment (23 weeks).

2. Most important, the ultrasound "lesion" and its rich vascular supply, as imaged with color Doppler, persist for a prolonged period.[7,60] In our original report, in two patients who returned for follow-up 64 weeks after puncture, the ultrasound lesion (the chorionic cavity) was still evident and measured more than 1 cm.

More information is desired; however, these observations point toward the possibility of treating selected cases of cornual EP using transvaginal puncture and local injection of KCl or methotrexate. The technique for this kind of puncture procedure is identical to the one described previously for injection of tubal EP, with the aforementioned caveat: a lateral approach should be avoided to prevent rupturing the thin-walled sac.

Cervical Ectopic Pregnancies

The rarity of cervical EP is matched only by the severity of its complications. Because of under-reporting, the true incidence of cervical pregnancy is unknown. There is usually severe bleeding followed by improvised, unplanned emergency treatment. These sometimes unorthodox treatment regimens have given rise to a significant body of short communications in the medical literature. However, a consensus has not yet developed regarding the detection of these pregnancies and prevention of the sometimes unavoidable hysterectomies.[64]

We evaluated the feasibility of transvaginal methotrexate injection of viable cervical pregnancies to avoid complications of the more classic surgical procedures and to preserve fertility.[8] The first task of the obstetrician faced with the possibility of cervical pregnancy is to rule out the possibility of a nonviable intrauterine pregnancy that is in the process of passing through the cervix from the uterine cavity. Only viable cervical pregnancies should be considered for direct injection. Also, our group suggests the following ultrasound diagnostic criteria for a cervical pregnancy:

1. The placenta and the entire chorionic sac containing the live fetus should be below the internal os (Fig. 16–9). The level of the internal os on a coronal view is considered to be at the level of the approach of the uterine arteries to the cervix using Doppler or color Doppler sonography[8] (Fig. 16–10).
2. The uterine cavity is empty.
3. The cervical canal is barrel shaped and significantly dilated.

In 1994, we published our initial experience with five viable cervical pregnancies treated by transvaginal injection of methotrexate.[8] In three, the APD was used. All five cases had successful outcomes. No complications were noted, and the more extensive surgical procedure was avoided. Another group[65] has reported on 12 cases of cervical pregnancy, of which 9 were viable (the latest gestational age being 7 weeks 1 day) and 6 were injected with KCl. These were also successful outcomes. KCl injection should be considered as an additional therapeutic modality when cervical pregnancies are diagnosed early in gestation. Centini et al.[66] published a case report of a cervical pregnancy diagnosed by TVS and successfully treated at 6 weeks 4 days by needle aspiration of the products of conception and curettage of the cervical canal and uterus. Doubilet et al.[61] published their experience with a sonographically guided minimally invasive procedure for treatment of EPs. In their series, 12 of the 18 cases of cervical pregnancy were live pregnancies, all of which were successfully treated with local transvaginal injection of KCl. The gestational age of the pregnancies ranged from 5 weeks to 8 weeks 3 days. They concluded that local injection is a safe and effective alternative treatment to surgical and systemic medical therapy.

We recently injected 10 live cervical pregnancies ranging in age from 5 weeks 6 days to 10 weeks 1 day. Only one patient required additional invasive treatment; this patient was the furthest along in her pregnancy (10 weeks 1 day), and she required uterine artery embolization with blood transfusion.[57] The upper gestational age limit in which cervical pregnancies can be successfully treated with local injection has not yet been elucidated.

The technique of puncture for cervical EP is similar to that described for tubal EP. Recently, if technically possible, we began injecting one half of the methotrexate into the embryo itself and the remainder into the tiny placenta (Fig. 16–11). The most feared complication in this group of patients is bleeding either at the time of puncture or several days after the procedure. A slow and continuous brown discharge (old blood) with small amounts of tissue has been observed over the first 2 weeks postprocedure.

We occasionally encounter cases of a heterotopic cervical pregnancy with an additional live intrauterine gestation. In

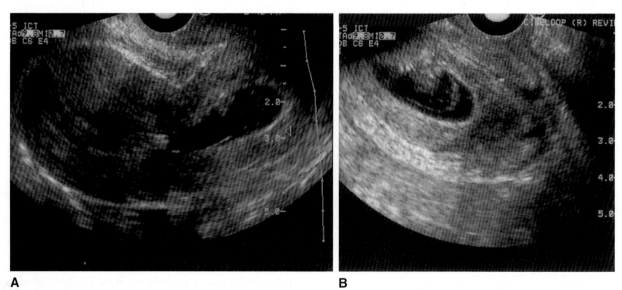

A   **B**

Figure 16–9. Cervical pregnancy. **A,** Appearance of a cervical pregnancy by transvaginal sonography. The pregnancy is located below the internal os of the cervix; the cervix appears barrel-shaped. **B,** Transverse view of the same cervical pregnancy after puncture.

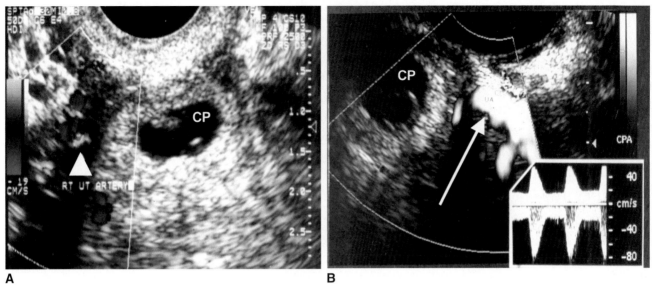

Figure 16–10. To ascertain the diagnosis of a live cervical pregnancy, color (or power) Doppler should be used. The ectopic sac in the cervix is at the level of the uterine artery's approach to the uterus. **A,** On this transverse section, the uterine artery is marked with an *arrowhead*. **B,** On a tilted plane, the approach of the uterine artery is seen *(arrow).* The *inset* depicts the typical uterine artery waveform.

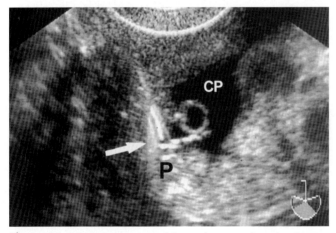

Figure 16–11. Injecting part of the methotrexate into the placenta in a case of cervical pregnancy. CP, cervical pregnancy; P, placenta.

this case, the cervical pregnancy should be injected with KCl. Extra attention should be directed toward frequent ultrasound follow-up of the injected sac and the developing intrauterine fetus (Fig. 16–12).

An interesting subset of cervical EPs is the gestation implanted in the scar of a low cervical incision for a cesarean section. This is also termed *pregnancy in the scar* (Fig. 16–13). These EPs may develop into complicated cases of pathologically adherent placental accreta or may assume the clinical picture of cervical pregnancies.

Drainage Procedures

Pelvic drainage using ultrasound guidance has been performed for many years. This procedure was first performed by inserting a needle or a drainage catheter through the vagina, guided by a transabdominal transducer.[42,67] Because of the proximity of the pelvis to the tip of the probe, TVS imaging

of the cul-de-sac is ideal for detecting pathologic conditions. Just as easily, a needle can be directed along the shaft of the vaginal transducer into fluid collections. Under continuous observation, the needle is kept in place and the fluid safely aspirated (Fig. 16–14). Septations and loculated fluid can be imaged accurately, the needle can be serially aimed and replaced in the various loculations, and the fluid collections aspirated sequentially.

The term *peritoneal inclusion cyst* is often used to describe the presence of a large, multiloculated fluid and adhesion collection in the pelvis. Other terms that have been used to describe this finding are *benign cystic mesothelioma, ovarian pseudocyst,* and *postoperative peritoneal cyst.* Patients often present with pelvic pain or the presence of a pelvic mass. These cysts are often misdiagnosed as ovarian neoplasms and are probably more common than previously thought. Several authors have theorized that peritoneal inclusion cysts are due to a reactive proliferation of mesothelium as a result of previous abdominal surgery, pelvic inflammatory disease, or endometriosis.[68]

There are two basic methods for the aspiration or drainage of pelvic fluid using transvaginal or transabdominal ultrasound guidance. The first and simplest technique is simple aspiration of the contents. Extraction of the needle at the end of the aspiration completes the procedure. The second modality is transvaginal aspiration of the pelvic fluid initially, followed by placement of a plastic catheter that is left in place for several days to ensure continuous drainage. This is particularly useful in the treatment of pelvic abscesses. The abscess is first drained using a 14-gauge needle, then a flexible guide wire is introduced through the needle. The wire is left in place, and the needle is extracted. A plastic catheter with multiple perforations is then slid over the guide wire. Finally, the guide wire is pulled and the indwelling pelvic catheter fixed to the thigh. The patient is usually rescanned 2 and 4 days after the procedure and the tube extracted if there is no further drainage of fluid or no pelvic fluid appears on the scan.

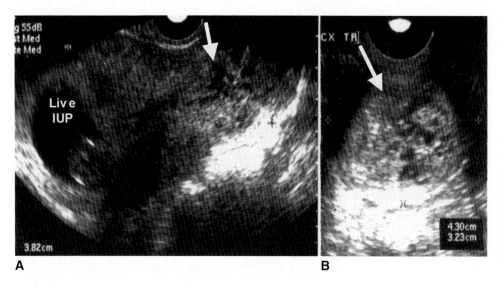

Figure 16–12. Sagittal (**A**) and transverse (**B**) follow-up ultrasound images of a cervical heterotopic pregnancy 2 weeks after injection of the cervical ectopic pregnancy. Note the disorganized tissue in the cervix (*arrows*).

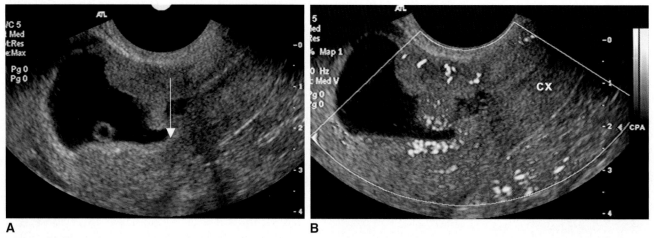

Figure 16–13. Ectopic pregnancy in a scar of a previous cesarean section. **A,** The *arrow* points to the insertion of the placenta on the scar. **B,** Color Doppler image of the same area depicted in **A.**

Twenty-seven drainage procedures have been performed by our group: 3 simple needle insertions and drainage of inflammatory pelvic collections, 5 drainage catheter placements for pelvic abscesses as a result of pelvic inflammatory processes, 1 evacuation of a postoperative pelvic hematoma, and 18 aspirations for postoperative pelvic peritoneal inclusion cysts. Six of the 12 inclusion cysts reaccumulated, but to a much smaller size, and became asymptomatic. Patients with catheter placements for drainage were discharged in 5 to 9 days with no need for additional treatment after a follow-up scan confirmed the efficacy of the procedure. No complications were encountered. In two patients, the puncture site had to be widened by a #11 surgical blade at the time of the procedure to accommodate the catheter.

Although the peritoneal inclusion cyst is a benign lesion, recurrence rates are high, and patients often experience return of symptoms. Recurrence rates have been reported to be as high as 50%,[69] and investigators have been searching for a tool to decrease this high rate. Sclerotherapy at the time of puncture and drainage has been attempted to decrease the recurrence rate of inclusion cysts. Kairaluoma et al.[70] reported on

the successful use of aspiration and sclerotherapy for symptomatic perihepatic inclusion cysts, but they conceded that the procedure was most successful when the sclerosant was in contact with the entire mucosal surface of the cyst, and because the majority of these cysts have septations, this was difficult to achieve.[70] Jeong and Kim[71] instilled sclerosant into seven patients with known symptomatic peritoneal inclusion cysts: Betadine and ethanol were used either singly or in combination. All seven procedures were technically feasible, and five of the seven patients immediately felt an improvement in their abdominal pain. During the follow-up period of 4 to 60 months (mean, 24.7 months), the symptoms of abdominal pain disappeared in all patients and follow-up sonography revealed that the size of all the cystic lesions decreased by more than 50%, and the lesions disappeared completely in four of the seven patients. No long-term complications or clinically relevant recurrences were noted in the follow-up period.[71]

Drainage of a pelvic fluid collection of any etiology is a technically easy procedure with little morbidity and high patient tolerance. If no catheter is left in place, it may be per-

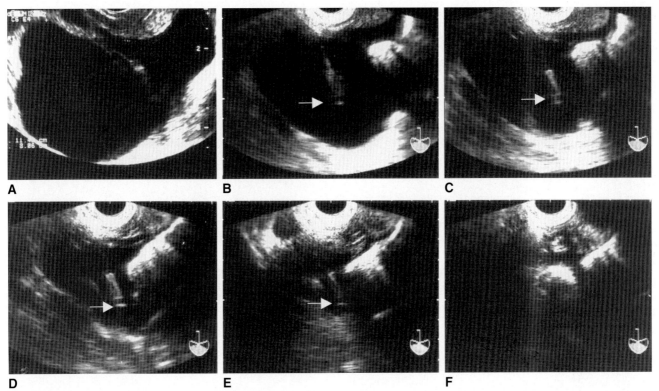

Figure 16–14. Several images (**A** to **F**) of an aspiration procedure to drain a pelvic peritoneal inclusion cyst. The tip of the needle must be kept in the center of the sonolucent fluid *(arrows)*.

formed in an office or emergency department setting (Fig. 16–15).

Diagnostic Culdocentesis

Before the advent of sonography, blind culdocentesis was the gold-standard diagnostic test for identification of a ruptured EP. Although transabdominal sonography somewhat increased the rate of correct ultrasound diagnosis relative to blind culdocentesis, culdocentesis continued to play a key role in the diagnosis of tubal pregnancy as recently as the early 1980s. Now, with the increasing availability of TVS and its high sensitivity for imaging the cul-de-sac and any fluid it may contain, the indications to perform a blind diagnostic culdocentesis have significantly decreased. In many institutions, the indications to perform culdocentesis have changed, and its use in the diagnosis of a ruptured EP is declining rapidly. Stovall and Ling[72] delineate a diagnostic and therapeutic algorithm that minimizes surgical intervention for EP; in this algorithm, culdocentesis is eliminated.

Recent developments in diagnostic and treatment modalities require reevaluation of the importance and role of a blind and often painful procedure such as culdocentesis. Noninvasive techniques such as a rapid β-hCG test or TVS have contributed to rapid and accurate diagnoses without the use of culdocentesis. Laparoscopy has recently become widely incorporated into the diagnostic and therapeutic armamentarium in the management of EP.[66,73] Patients in whom ectopic gestation cannot be ruled out by sonography and pregnancy testing are probably best managed by laparoscopy rather than culdocentesis. In a recent study, Vermesh et al.[74] concluded that culdocentesis is an invasive and painful procedure with very little

value in a clinical setting where TVS and rapid pregnancy testing are available. Chen et al.[75] studied the correlation between ultrasound detection of echogenic pelvic fluid and culdocentesis in the evaluation of EP and prediction of hemoperitoneum: the goal was to determine whether there is any role for culdocentesis. As predicted, TVS performed much better than culdocentesis in patients with EP. The sensitivity and specificity of echogenic fluid for establishing hemoperitoneum were 100% and 100%, respectively, compared with 66% and 80%, respectively, for culdocentesis. These authors concur with other groups in stating that culdocentesis should play no role in the diagnosis of EP except in the unusual circumstance in which high-resolution sonography cannot be readily performed.

TVS can readily detect the smallest amounts of pelvic fluid and even, at times, distinguish between completely sonolucent pelvic contents (normal pelvic fluid) and fluid containing particulate matter (blood or pus) in the pelvis. If there still is a need for direct analysis of pelvic fluid, the use of a sonographically directed transvaginal puncture is strongly suggested. This enables accurate needle placement and avoids dry taps or inadvertent needle insertion into structures such as dilated blood vessels.

Transvaginal culdocentesis is performed under real-time ultrasound guidance, in direct contrast to blind culdocentesis. A needle guide or the APD can be used to optimize needle placement. The technique of TVS-guided culdocentesis is similar to that described for pelvic fluid drainage. Important differences between the traditional (blind) technique and TVS-guided culdocentesis are that there is no need to place a tenaculum, the needle is introduced under real-time

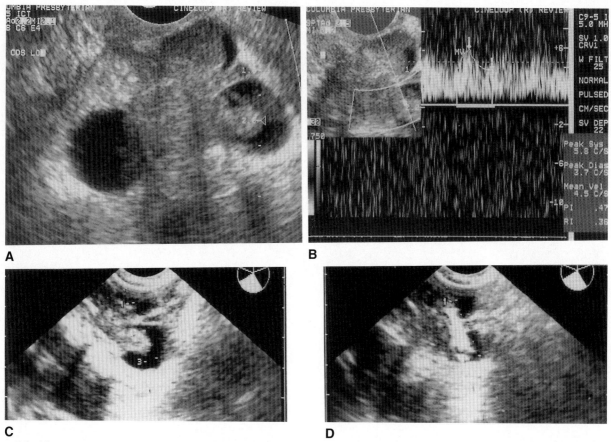

Figure 16–15. Drainage of a pelvic collection. **A,** Transvaginal sonographic view of complex collection in a patient with a history of fully treated ovarian cancer. **B,** Color Doppler study reveals high diastolic flow with low pulsatility index (PI) and resistance index (RI). **C,** The needle guide is superimposed on the monitor screen over the area of the collection to be punctured. **D,** The needle is seen within the pelvic collection, and fluid is aspirated and sent to cytology for analysis.

sonography, the fluid pocket can be very precisely targeted, no air is injected into the abdominal cavity, and, finally, all the fluid can be removed (this is important if the indication for culdocentesis was drainage of a peritoneal inclusion cyst).

Raziel et al.[76] used TVS-guided culdocentesis in the diagnosis of ruptured corpus luteum cysts. Aspiration of blood from the peritoneal cavity assisted in the presumptive diagnosis of ruptured corpus luteum cyst in patients with abdominal pain and a negative pregnancy test result. However, the availability of a high-resolution ultrasound machine with a vaginal probe has led to routine TVS assessment of peritoneal fluid; therefore, the Raziel group no longer performs culdocentesis for this purpose.[76]

Lincoln et al.[77] describe a combination of techniques, including transvaginal culdocentesis, in the outpatient treatment of ovarian hyperstimulation syndrome (OHSS). Forty-eight women were treated with outpatient transvaginal culdocentesis during their IVF cycle. Inclusion criteria included the presence of abdominal ascites on ultrasound and clinical symptoms of shortness of breath, abdominal distention, or discomfort; all patients were classified as having moderate to severe OHSS. After confirming the presence of abdominal ascites, ultrasound-guided transvaginal culdocentesis was performed through the posterior cul-de-sac in a manner similar to oocyte retrieval for IVF. Intravenous rehydration with crystalloid solution and albumin was part of the

protocol. The quantity of fluid removed ranged from 500 to 3000 mL in the donor IVF group and 122 to 4000 mL in the nondonor IVF group. Outpatient treatment of OHSS in this study was successful in over 90% of cases, with no complications directly attributable to outpatient culdocentesis.

It is reasonable to assume that the presence of a clinician sufficiently trained in TVS and a readily available vaginal probe will decrease or perhaps eliminate the need for diagnostic culdocentesis for cases such as those discussed previously. It is also important to equip all emergency departments with ultrasound machines with a transvaginal probe because most culdocentesis procedures are performed in this setting.

Multifetal Pregnancy Reduction

Multifetal pregnancy reduction (MFPR) is a puncture procedure that is not in the portfolio of every practicing obstetrician/gynecologist. The procedure is briefly discussed here to provide general information for the interested reader. References are provided to facilitate further research.

Since the early 1990s, the increased use of ovulation-inducing drugs as well as the increasing number of programs using reproductive technologies have resulted in an inordinately large number of high-order multifetal pregnancies. It is logical to assume—and it also has been proved—that as the number of fetuses in any given pregnancy increases, so does the risk of complications during the pregnancy. The probability of achieving a term pregnancy with healthy neonates is inversely proportional to the number of fetuses.[78-84]

After sonography was introduced for imaging and assessing the early pregnancy, the concept of "reducing" the number of fetuses in utero to a desired lower number was ready to be implemented. The transcervical ultrasound–guided suction procedure was introduced for selectively reducing the number of multifetal gestations.[80] The transabdominal ultrasound–guided technique was first presented by French physicians[76,85] and adopted by others.[77,86-92] The development of TVS guidance for IVF ovum aspiration and embryo transfer led to the successful application of these techniques to multifetal reduction procedures.[5,6,9,93-97]

Currently, we perform almost all of our MFPRs transabdominally between the 11th and 12th postmenstrual weeks of gestation (Fig. 16–16A). This timing is ideal because the nuchal translucency can be measured and an early anatomic survey can be performed. Occasionally, it is practically impossible to perform this procedure transabdominally. Reasons for performing MFPR transvaginally include maternal body habitus, abdominal scarring, myomatous uterus, or position of the fetus to be reduced. Briefly, the technique for trans-

vaginal MFPR is very similar to the transabdominal procedure. After a detailed risk–benefit counseling session, a baseline mapping of the chorionic sacs is obtained (before the puncture). Subsequently, the nuchal translucency is measured and an early anatomic survey is performed. If any of the fetuses in the pregnancy have either a thick nuchal translucency (2.5 mm) or a cystic hygroma, these are the ones targeted for reduction; otherwise, the fetuses that are the easiest to reach are selected. The area of the heartbeats of the targeted fetus is sought (Fig. 16–16B), and after the needle tip is placed, 0.5 to 1 mL of 2 mEq/mL KCl solution is injected through the needle to stop the heart. The heartbeat for each injected fetus is observed for approximately 3 to 5 minutes to confirm cessation. The patients are rescanned 1 hour later and then 1 week after the procedure for follow-up. All of our patients are started on oral prophylactic antibiotics (cephalexin, 2 g/day) the day before the procedure and continue to take the antibiotics to complete a 10-day course. If the procedure is to be performed transvaginally, negative vaginal cultures are required.

We recently reported on the outcome of 290 consecutive cases of MFPRs.[98] The pregnancy outcomes, namely, pregnancy loss before 24 weeks, were evaluated for transabdominal

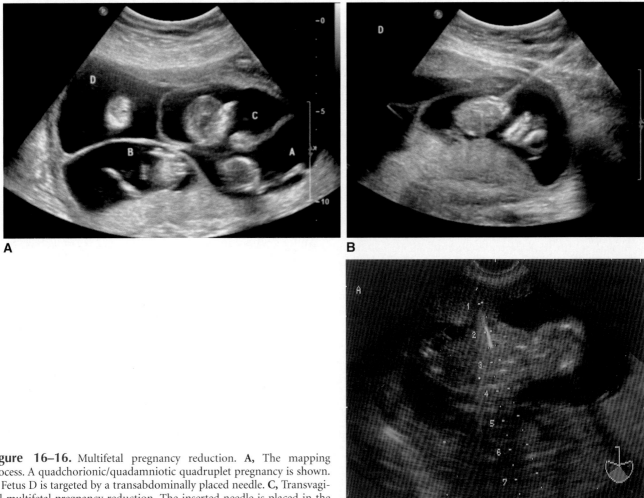

Figure 16–16. Multifetal pregnancy reduction. **A,** The mapping process. A quadchorionic/quadamniotic quadruplet pregnancy is shown. **B,** Fetus D is targeted by a transabdominally placed needle. **C,** Transvaginal multifetal pregnancy reduction. The inserted needle is placed in the area of the fetal heart.

Table 16–1	Pregnancy Losses before 24 Weeks by Starting Number of Fetuses			
	Losses/Procedures (%)			
Starting Numbers	Total*	Transabdominal Route	Transvaginal Route	P Value
2	2/42 (4.8%)	0/32 (0%)	2/10 (20%)	.08
3	10/152 (6.6%)	3/110 (2.7%)	7/42 (16.7%)	.006
4	1/56 (1.8%)	1/42 (2.4%)	0/14 (0%)	.56
5	3/21 (14.3%)	2/13 (15.4%)	1/8 (12.5%)	.65
≥6	1/7 (14.3%)	1/6 (16.7%)	0/1 (0%)	.27
Total	17/278 (6.1%)	7/203 (3.45%)	10/75 (13.3 %)	.004

*Twelve patients with both transabdominal and transvaginal procedures were not included.
Data from Timor-Tritsch IE, Bashiri A, Monteagudo A, et al: Two hundred ninety consecutive cases of multifetal pregnancy reduction: Comparison of the transabdominal versus the transvaginal approach. Am J Obstet Gynecol 2004;191:2085-2099.

versus transvaginal procedures. The results demonstrated that the overall pregnancy loss rate for the transabdominal procedure was 3.45%, and that for the transvaginal procedure, 13.3%. Table 16–1 shows the results of this study in greater detail.

In conclusion, MFPR is a safe clinical procedure that can be offered to women with a high-order multifetal pregnancy. The procedure can be performed either transabdominally or transvaginally in the late first or very early second trimester. However, because of the higher rate of pregnancy loss before 24 weeks' gestation, the transvaginal route should be limited to cases in which the transabdominal procedure is not feasible. The recent trend in most IVF centers to place a maximum of two or three embryos has resulted in a drastically decreased number of high multiple pregnancies due to IVF; however, medical treatments still result in high multiple pregnancies.

Chorionic Villus Sampling

With the increased acceptance of first-trimester screening for fetal aneuploidies using nuchal translucency, chorionic villus sampling (CVS) is becoming the test of choice for many patients who have an abnormal result on the first-trimester screen. The advantage of CVS is that it can be performed after the 10th postmenstrual week, ideally between 11 weeks and 12 weeks 6 days. CVS performed before the 10th week of pregnancy is associated with an increased risk of transverse limb abnormalities; the risk decreases with advancing gestational age, and beyond the 11th week, the risk is similar to the background rate.[99] The indications for the procedure are (1) to obtain a fetal karyotype as a result of increased maternal age, abnormal first-trimester screening result, or abnormal first-trimester ultrasound; (2) to perform genetic testing, such as for cystic fibrosis; and (3) to test the fetus in the context of familial biochemical disorders.

The procedure can be performed either transabdominally or transcervically. During the transabdominal procedure, the patient is prepared and draped as for an amniocentesis. The placenta is identified by ultrasound and the needle (20 gauge) is inserted into the placenta along its long axis. For the transcervical procedure, the patient is advised to have vaginal cultures performed before the procedure (a negative result is a prerequisite) as well as to come for the procedure with a full bladder. The full bladder aids in the visualization of the placenta and straightens an anteverted uterus. The patient is then placed in the lithotomy position and prepared and draped, and a sterile speculum is placed in the vagina. The procedure

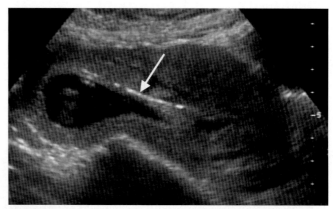

Figure 16–17. Transcervical chorionic villus sampling. The *arrow* points to the catheter within the placenta.

is performed using a long plastic catheter containing a flexible guide wire. The uterus is imaged in the long axis and the catheter is inserted the full length of the placenta (Fig. 16–17). As the catheter is slowly withdrawn, suction is applied using the attached syringe.

Pregnancy loss rates after CVS seem to be somewhat higher compared with loss rates after amniocentesis. The risk of pregnancy loss after CVS is approximately 0.5% to 1.0%, and that after amniocentesis is approximately 0.25% to 0.5%.[100] Spotting after CVS is more commonly seen after the transcervical than the transabdominal procedure (3.2% vs. 1.5%), and bleeding is also more common after transcervical CVS (2.5% vs. 0.2%).[101]

Transvaginal Sonography–Assisted Intrauterine Procedures

Traditionally, most gynecologic interventions in the uterine cavity, except those performed under hysteroscopic guidance, use the "blind" technique. Among these procedures are dilation, curettage, termination of pregnancy, insertion and removal of intrauterine devices, myomectomies, and polypectomies. Complications sometimes accompany these blind procedures, including perforation of the uterine wall and leaving behind products of conception.

Transabdominal sonography–guided intrauterine procedures were described by Goldenberg et al.,[102] Hornstein et al.,[103] Shalev and Zuckerman,[104] and many others.[105-113] However, this

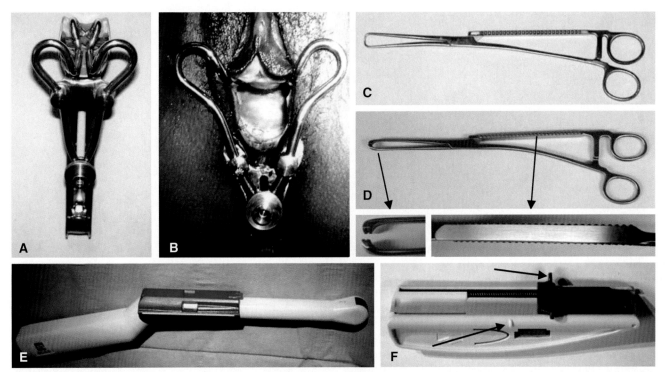

Figure 16–18. Device attached to the transvaginal sonography (TVS) probe for TVS-assisted gynecologic surgery. **A** and **B,** A special speculum enables the placement of the transvaginal probe. **C** and **D,** Specially modified vulsellum (tenaculum) with serrated handle to accommodate the adaptor. *Insets* show closer views of the tip *(left)* and handle *(right)*. **E,** A plastic bracket wraps around the ultrasound probe to attach the adaptor. **F,** The adaptor. *Arrows* indicate the points to be aligned for proper functioning.

technique requires a second operator to hold the transabdominal transducer. The bladder must be filled to provide an acoustic window for better imaging. If the traditionally used transabdominal probe could be replaced by a high-frequency probe attached to the tenaculum holding the cervix, a significantly better image would be obtained continuously on the monitor. In addition, a single operator (i.e., the surgeon) could accomplish both tasks—imaging and operating—simultaneously.

Such a system was described by Timor-Tritsch et al.[114] The system (Ron-Tech Medical, Ltd., Herzelya, Israel) includes a special vaginal speculum (Fig. 16–18A and B) and a modified vulsellum (tenaculum) (Fig. 16–18C and D).

A plastic coupling bracket is snapped on the midshaft of a vaginal transducer (Fig. 16–18E). An adapter (Fig. 16–18F) is equipped with two sensitive springs that enable an effortless sliding of the probe (attached to it by the bracket) while the tenaculum (attached to the other side of it) is moved, without putting strain on the cervix or losing contact between the tip of the probe and the anterior vaginal fornix. The assembled unit (Fig. 16–19) can be operated by the surgeon holding it in one hand (Fig. 16–20), just as he or she would hold a tenaculum alone, and the surgical procedure can be performed in the usual fashion.

With the transvaginal probe in place, the operator can follow the intrauterine procedure in real time on the ultrasound machine monitor placed beside the operating table (Fig. 16–21).

To study the performance of this device, 45 patients underwent intrauterine surgical procedures.[114] Forty had pregnancy terminations, three had curettages for early pregnancy complications, one patient had polypectomy, and one patient had

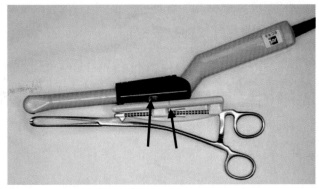

Figure 16–19. The assembled transducer, adaptor, and tenaculum system. *Left arrow* indicates the attachment to the probe; *right arrow* indicates the attachment to the tenaculum.

myomectomy. Five attending physicians performed 26 procedures, and 19 procedures were performed by residents.

All the procedures were completed, as expected, without complications. Safety was thought to be increased by 80% of the operators. The exact end point of the procedure could be detected more accurately. Only 12% of the operators (mostly the attendings who were used to performing these procedures without such devices placed in the vagina) felt that the device interfered with the performance of the procedure.

The authors concluded that the high-resolution images of the cervical canal and uterine cavity provided during all stages of the surgery were a significant aid in providing real-time information. More important, the end point of the procedure

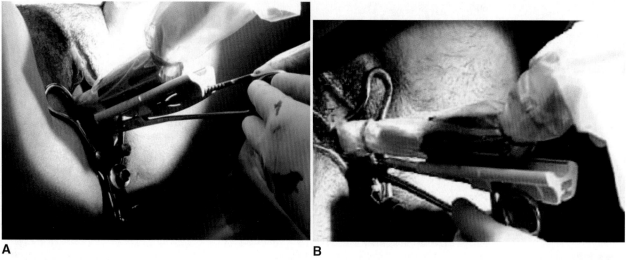

Figure 16–20. The entire transducer–adaptor–tenaculum in place during a procedure. **A,** The tenaculum, manipulated by the operator's left hand, is holding the transducer, which is superior. **B,** A close-up look at the system.

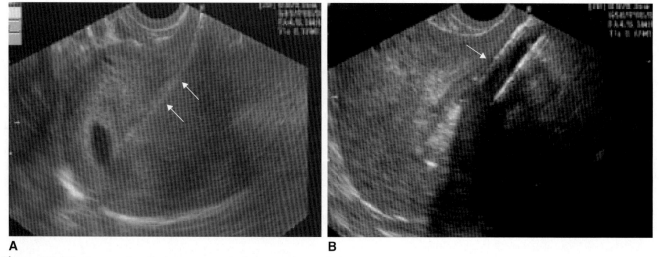

Figure 16–21. Images taken during a transvaginal sonography–guided intrauterine procedure. **A,** A dilator is placed in the cervix *(arrows)*. **B,** The suction canula is inserted *(arrow)*.

could be seen clearly. The device inspired a sense of increased safety in the users.

This device appears to provide an improved alternative to transabdominal ultrasound guidance for intrauterine surgical procedures.

Summary

This chapter describes, evaluates, and summarizes most of the transvaginally performed puncture procedures. Such procedures are minimally invasive, they save time for physician and patient alike, they are simple and relatively easy to perform under real-time imaging, they do not require anesthesia or hospitalization, they are cost-effective and have a low incidence of procedure-related complications, and they are preferable in patients who have undergone multiple abdominal surgeries.

There are also some disadvantages, however rare or minor. Some of the procedures require advanced ultrasound training and experience, and a few are not definitive treatments and require lengthy or frequent follow-up scans. Puncture procedures remain less popular than traditional surgical approaches, for various reasons: Puncture procedures are rarely used in teaching hospitals where laparoscopy is taught; a referring provider may lose income if, instead of personally performing the surgery, he or she refers the patient for puncture to an ultrasound laboratory; and pelvic drainages are traditionally performed in radiology departments. The acquired experience, however, encourages consideration of this treatment modality in individually evaluated cases. Some of them can be performed in an office or emergency department setting, others only in hospitals under carefully monitored protocols.

We have found the APD to be indispensable. Its extreme accuracy and high patient tolerance have revolutionized our ability to care for our patients who require these procedures.

Finally, the possibility of adding TVS guidance to gynecologic surgery opens new avenues to avoid relatively blind intracavitary uterine interventions, thus increasing patient safety.

REFERENCES

1. Smith EH, Bartrum RJ Jr: Ultrasonically guided percutaneous aspiration of abscesses. AJR Am J Roentgenol Radium Ther Nucl Med 1974;122:308-312.
2. Gerzof SG, Johnson WC, Robbins AH, Nabseth DC: Expanded criteria for percutaneous abscess drainage. Arch Surg 1985;120:227-232.
3. Kemeter P, Feichtinger W: Trans-vaginal oocyte retrieval using a trans-vaginal sector scan probe combined with an automated puncture device. Hum Reprod 1986;1:21-24.
4. Timor-Tritsch I, Baxi L, Peisner DB: Transvaginal salpingocentesis: A new technique for treating ectopic pregnancy. Am J Obstet Gynecol 1989;160:459-461.
5. Timor-Tritsch IE, Peisner DB, Monteagudo A: Puncture procedures utilizing transvaginal ultrasonic guidance. Ultrasound Obstet Gynecol 1991;1:144-150.
6. Timor-Tritsch IE, Peisner DB, Monteagudo A, et al: Multifetal pregnancy reduction by transvaginal puncture: Evaluation of the technique used in 134 cases. Am J Obstet Gynecol 1993;168:799-804.
7. Timor-Tritsch IE, Monteagudo A, Matera C, Veit CR: Sonographic evolution of cornual pregnancies treated without surgery. Obstet Gynecol 1992;79:1044-1049.
8. Timor-Tritsch IE, Monteagudo A, Mandeville EO, et al: Successful management of viable cervical pregnancy by local injection of methotrexate guided by transvaginal ultrasonography. Am J Obstet Gynecol 1994;170:737-739.
9. Timor-Tritsch IE, Monteagudo A: Puncture procedures using the transvaginal probe in obstetrics and gynecology. Ultrasound Q 1993;11:41-57.
10. Lenz S, Lauritsen JG: Ultrasonically guided percutaneous aspiration of human follicles under local anesthesia: A new method of collecting oocytes for in vitro fertilization. Fertil Steril 1982;38:673-677.
11. Lenz S, Lauritsen JG, Kjellow M: Collection of human oocytes for in vitro fertilisation by ultrasonically guided follicular puncture. Lancet 1981;1:1163-1164.
12. Wikland M, Nilsson L, Hansson R, et al: Collection of human oocytes by the use of sonography. Fertil Steril 1983;39:603-608.
13. Parsons J, Riddle A, Booker M, et al: Oocyte retrieval for in-vitro fertilisation by ultrasonically guided needle aspiration via the urethra. Lancet 1985;1:1076-1077.
14. Dellenbach P, Nisand I, Moreau L, et al: Transvaginal, sonographically controlled ovarian follicle puncture for egg retrieval. Lancet 1984;1:1467.
15. Gleicher N, Friberg J, Fullan N, et al: EGG retrieval for in vitro fertilisation by sonographically controlled vaginal culdocentesis. Lancet 1983;2:508-509.
16. Schwimmer S, Marik J, Lebovic J: Percutaneous ovarian cyst aspiration using continuous transvaginal ultrasonographic monitoring. J Ultrasound Med 1985;4:259-260.
17. Fornage BD, O'Keeffe F: Ultrasound-guided transvaginal biopsy of malignant cystic pelvic mass. J Ultrasound Med 1990;9:53-55.
18. Granberg S, Crona N, Enk L, et al: Ultrasound-guided puncture of cystic tumors in the lower pelvis of young women. J Clin Ultrasound 1989;17:107-111.
19. Ron-El R, Herman A, Weinraub Z, et al: Clear ovarian cyst aspiration guided by vaginal ultrasonography. Eur J Obstet Gynecol Reprod Biol 1991;42:43-47.
20. Buckley CH: Is needle aspiration of ovarian cysts adequate for diagnosis? Br J Obstet Gynaecol 1989;96:1021-1023.
21. Bonilla-Musoles F, Ballester MJ, Simon C, et al: Is avoidance of surgery possible in patients with perimenopausal ovarian tumors using transvaginal ultrasound and duplex color Doppler sonography? J Ultrasound Med 1993;12:33-39.
22. Levine D, Gosink BB, Wolf SI, et al: Simple adnexal cysts: The natural history in postmenopausal women. Radiology 1992;184:653-659.
23. Goldstein SR: Conservative management of small postmenopausal cystic masses. Clin Obstet Gynecol 1993;36:395-401.
24. Weinraub Z, Avrech O, Fuchs C, et al: Transvaginal aspiration of ovarian cysts: Prognosis based on outcome over a 12-month period. J Ultrasound Med 1994;13:275-279.
25. Bret PM, Atri M, Guibaud L, et al: Ovarian cysts in postmenopausal women: Preliminary results with transvaginal alcohol sclerosis. Work in progress. Radiology 1992;184:661-663.
26. Bret PM, Guibaud L, Atri M, et al: Transvaginal US-guided aspiration of ovarian cysts and solid pelvic masses. Radiology 1992;185:377-380.
27. Andolf E, Casslen B, Jorgensen C, et al: Fluid characteristics of benign ovarian cysts: Correlation with recurrence after puncture. Obstet Gynecol 1995;86:529-535.
28. Nelson MJ, Cavalieri R, Graham D, Sanders RC: Cysts in pregnancy discovered by sonography. J Clin Ultrasound 1986;14:509-512.
29. Buttery BW, Beischer NA, Fortune DW, Macafee CA: Ovarian tumours in pregnancy. Med J Aust 1973;1:345-349.
30. Ballard CA: Ovarian tumors associated with pregnancy termination patients. Am J Obstet Gynecol 1984;149:384-387.
31. Hess LW, Peaceman A, O'Brien WF, et al: Adnexal mass occurring with intrauterine pregnancy: Report of fifty-four patients requiring laparotomy for definitive management. Am J Obstet Gynecol 1988;158:1029-1034.
32. Lee CH, Raman S, Sivanesaratnam V: Torsion of ovarian tumors: A clinicopathological study. Int J Gynaecol Obstet 1989;28:21-25.
33. Guariglia L, Conte M, Are P, Rosati P: Ultrasound-guided fine needle aspiration of ovarian cysts during pregnancy. Eur J Obstet Gynecol Reprod Biol 1999;82:5-9.
34. Aboulghar M, Mansour R, Serour G: Ovarian cysts during pregnancy: The role of ultrasonically guided transvaginal aspiration. Ultrasound Obstet Gynecol 1992;2:349-351.
35. Yee H, Greenebaum E, Lerner J, et al: Transvaginal sonographic characterization combined with cytologic evaluation in the diagnosis of ovarian and adnexal cysts. Diagn Cytopathol 1994;10:107-112.
36. Sassone AM, Timor-Tritsch IE, Artner A, et al: Transvaginal sonographic characterization of ovarian disease: Evaluation of a new scoring system to predict ovarian malignancy. Obstet Gynecol 1991;78:70-76.
37. Trimbos JB, Hacker NF: The case against aspirating ovarian cysts. Cancer 1993;72:828-831.
38. Matthes AC, Moreira de Andrade JM, Bighetti S: Selection of criteria for the treatment of ovarian cysts on the bases of ultrasound and cytology. Gynecol Obstet Invest 1996;42:244-248.
39. De Crespigny LC, Robinson HP, Davoren RA, Fortune D: The 'simple' ovarian cyst: Aspirate or operate? Br J Obstet Gynaecol 1989;96:1035-1039.
40. Aboulghar MA, Mansour RT, Serour GI, Rizk B: Ultrasonic transvaginal aspiration of endometriotic cysts: An optional line of treatment in selected cases of endometriosis. Hum Reprod 1991;6:1408-1410.
41. Thatcher SS, Jones E, Decherney AH: Ovarian cysts decrease the success of controlled ovarian stimulation and in vitro fertilization. Fertil Steril 1989;52:812-816.
42. Nosher JL, Winchman HK, Needell GS: Transvaginal pelvic abscess drainage with US guidance. Radiology 1987;165:872-873.
43. Osmers R: Sonographic evaluation of ovarian masses and its therapeutical implications. Ultrasound Obstet Gynecol 1996;8:217-222.
44. Sand PK, Stubblefield PA, Ory SJ: Methotrexate inhibition of normal trophoblasts in vitro. Am J Obstet Gynecol 1986;155:324-329.
45. Lipscomb GH, McCord ML, Stovall TG, et al: Predictors of success of methotrexate treatment in women with tubal ectopic pregnancies. N Engl J Med 1999;341:1974-1978.
46. Ory SJ, Villanueva AL, Sand PK, Tamura RK: Conservative treatment of ectopic pregnancy with methotrexate. Am J Obstet Gynecol 1986;154:1299-1306.
47. Carson SA, Buster JE: Ectopic pregnancy [comments]. N Engl J Med 1993;329:1174-1181.
48. Pansky M, Golan A, Bukovsky I, Caspi E: Nonsurgical management of tubal pregnancy: Necessity in view of the changing clinical appearance. Am J Obstet Gynecol 1991;164:888-895.
49. Kooi S, Kock HC: A review of the literature on nonsurgical treatment in tubal pregnancies. Obstet Gynecol Surv 1992;47:739-749.
50. Feichtinger W, Kemeter P: Conservative treatment of ectopic pregnancy by transvaginal aspiration under sonographic control and methotrexate injection [letter]. Lancet 1987;1:381-382.
51. Feichtinger W, Kemeter P: Treatment of unruptured ectopic pregnancy by needling of sac and injection of methotrexate or PG E$_2$ under transvaginal sonography control: Report of 10 cases. Arch Gynecol Obstet 1989;246:85-89.
52. Popp LW, Mettler L, Weisner D, et al: Ectopic pregnancy treatment using pelviscopic or vaginosonographically-guided intrachorionic injection of methotrexate and POR 8. Ultrasound Obstet Gynecol 1991;1:136-143.
53. Shalev E, Zalel Y, Bustan M, Weiner E: Ectopic pregnancy: Sonographically-guided transvaginal reduction. Ultrasound Obstet Gynecol 1991;1:127-131.

54. Venezia R, Zangara C, Comparetto G, Cittadini E: Conservative treatment of ectopic pregnancies using a single echo-guided injection of methotrexate into the gestational sac. Ultrasound Obstet Gynecol 1991;1:132-135.

55. Atri M, Bret PM, Tulandi T, Senterman MK: Ectopic pregnancy: Evolution after treatment with transvaginal methotrexate. Radiology 1992;185:749-753.

56. Nazac A, Gervaise A, Bouyer J, et al: Predictors of success in methotrexate treatment of women with unruptured tubal pregnancies. Ultrasound Obstet Gynecol 2003;21:181-185.

57. Monteagudo A, Minor V, Stephenson C, et al: Non-surgical management of live ectopic pregnancy with ultrasound-guided local injection: A case series. Ultrasound Obstet Gynecol 2005;25:282-288.

58. De Boer CN, Van Dongen PW, Willemsen WN, Klapwijk CW: Ultrasound diagnosis of interstitial pregnancy. Eur J Obstet Gynecol Reprod Biol 1992;47:164-166.

59. Ackerman TE, Levi CS, Dashefsky SM, et al: Interstitial line: Sonographic finding in interstitial (cornual) ectopic pregnancy. Radiology 1993;189:83-87.

60. Karsdorp VH, Van Der Veen F, Schats R, et al: Successful treatment with methotrexate of five vital interstitial pregnancies. Hum Reprod 1992;7:1164-1169.

61. Doubilet PM, Benson CB, Frates MC, Ginsburg E: Sonographically guided minimally invasive treatment of unusual ectopic pregnancies. J Ultrasound Med 2004;23:359-370.

62. Timor-Tritsch IE, Monteagudo A, Lerner JP: A "potentially safer" route for puncture and injection of cornual ectopic pregnancies. Ultrasound Obstet Gynecol 1996;7:353-355.

63. Zalel Y, Caspi B, Insler V: Expectant management of interstitial pregnancy. Ultrasound Obstet Gynecol 1994;4:238-240.

64. Yankowitz J, Leake J, Huggins G, et al: Cervical ectopic pregnancy: Review of the literature and report of a case treated by single-dose methotrexate therapy. Obstet Gynecol Surv 1990;45:405-414.

65. Frates MC, Benson CB, Doubilet PM, et al: Cervical ectopic pregnancy: Results of conservative treatment. Radiology 1994;191:773-775.

66. Centini G, Rosignoli L, Severi FM: A case of cervical pregnancy. Am J Obstet Gynecol 1994;171:272-273.

67. McArdle CR, Simon L, Kiejna C: Vaginal drainage of posthysterectomy abscess under direct ultrasonic guidance. Obstet Gynecol 1984;63:90S-92S.

68. Weiss SW, Tavassoli FA: Multicystic mesothelioma: An analysis of pathologic findings and biologic behavior in 37 cases. Am J Surg Pathol 1988;12:737-746.

69. Ross MJ, Welch WR, Scully RE: Multilocular peritoneal inclusion cysts (so-called cystic mesotheliomas). Cancer 1989;64:1336-1346.

70. Kairaluoma MI, Leinonen A, Stahlberg M, et al: Percutaneous aspiration and alcohol sclerotherapy for symptomatic hepatic cysts: An alternative to surgical intervention. Ann Surg 1989;210:208-215.

71. Jeong JY, Kim SH: Sclerotherapy of peritoneal inclusion cysts: Preliminary results in seven patients. Korean J Radiol 2001;2:164-170.

72. Stovall TG, Ling FW: Ectopic pregnancy: Diagnostic and therapeutic algorithms minimizing surgical intervention. J Reprod Med 1993;38:807-812.

73. Pouly JL, Mahnes H, Mage G, et al: Conservative laparoscopic treatment of 321 ectopic pregnancies. Fertil Steril 1986;46:1093-1097.

74. Vermesh M, Graczykowski JW, Sauer MV: Reevaluation of the role of culdocentesis in the management of ectopic pregnancy. Am J Obstet Gynecol 1990;162:411-413.

75. Chen PC, Sickler GK, Dubinsky TJ, et al: Sonographic detection of echogenic fluid and correlation with culdocentesis in the evaluation of ectopic pregnancy. AJR Am J Roentgenol 1998;170:1299-1302.

76. Raziel A, Ron-El R, Pansky M, et al: Current management of ruptured corpus luteum. Eur J Obstet Gynecol Reprod Biol 1993;50:77-81.

77. Lincoln SR, Opsahl MS, Blauer KL, et al: Aggressive outpatient treatment of ovarian hyperstimulation syndrome with ascites using transvaginal culdocentesis and intravenous albumin minimizes hospitalization. J Assist Reprod Genet 2002;19:159-163.

78. Walker EM, Patel NB: Mortality and morbidity in infants born between 20 and 28 weeks gestation. Br J Obstet Gynaecol 1987;94:670-674.

79. Caspi E, Ronen J, Schreyer P, Goldberg MD: The outcome of pregnancy after gonadotrophin therapy. Br J Obstet Gynaecol 1976;83:967-973.

80. Syrop CH, Varner MW: Triplet gestation: maternal and neonatal implications. Acta Genet Med Gemellol (Roma) 1985;34:81-88.

81. Botting BJ, Davies IM, Macfarlane AJ: Recent trends in the incidence of multiple births and associated mortality. Arch Dis Child 1987;62:941-950.

82. Mckeown T, Record RG: Observations on foetal growth in multiple pregnancy in man. J Endocrinol 1952;8:386-401.

83. Levene MI: Grand multiple pregnancies and demand for neonatal intensive care. Lancet 1986;2:347-348.

84. Gonen R, Heyman E, Asztalos EV, et al: The outcome of triplet, quadruplet, and quintuplet pregnancies managed in a perinatal unit: Obstetric, neonatal, and follow-up data. Am J Obstet Gynecol 1990;162:454-459.

85. Dumez Y, Oury JF: Method for first trimester selective abortion in multiple pregnancy. Contrib Gynecol Obstet 1986;15:50-53.

86. Birnholz JC, Dmowski WP, Binor Z, Radwanska E: Selective continuation in gonadotropin-induced multiple pregnancy. Fertil Steril 1987;48:873-876.

87. Brandes JM, Itskovitz J, Timor-Tritsch IE, et al: Reduction of the number of embryos in a multiple pregnancy: Quintuplet to triplet. Fertil Steril 1987;48:326-327.

88. Berkowitz RL, Lynch L, Chitkara U, et al: Selective reduction of multifetal pregnancies in the first trimester. N Engl J Med 1988;318:1043-1047.

89. Evans MI, Fletcher JC, Zador IE, et al: Selective first-trimester termination in octuplet and quadruplet pregnancies: Clinical and ethical issues. Obstet Gynecol 1988;71:289-296.

90. Farquharson DF, Wittmann BK, Hansmann M, et al: Management of quintuplet pregnancy by selective embryocide. Am J Obstet Gynecol 1988;158:413-416.

91. Tabsh KM: Transabdominal multifetal pregnancy reduction: Report of 40 cases. Obstet Gynecol 1990;75:739-741.

92. Lynch L, Berkowitz RL, Chitkara U, Alvarez M: First-trimester transabdominal multifetal pregnancy reduction: A report of 85 cases. Obstet Gynecol 1990;75:735-738.

93. Itskovitz J, Boldes R, Thaler I, et al: First trimester selective reduction in multiple pregnancy guided by transvaginal sonography. J Clin Ultrasound 1990;18:323-327.

94. Itskovitz J, Boldes R, Thaler I, et al: Transvaginal ultrasonography-guided aspiration of gestational sacs for selective abortion in multiple pregnancy. Am J Obstet Gynecol 1989;160:215-217.

95. Shalev J, Frenkel Y, Goldenberg M, et al: Selective reduction in multiple gestations: Pregnancy outcome after transvaginal and transabdominal needle-guided procedures. Fertil Steril 1989;52:416-420.

96. Gonen Y, Blankier J, Casper RF: Transvaginal ultrasound in selective embryo reduction for multiple pregnancy. Obstet Gynecol 1990;75:720-722.

97. Monteagudo A, Timor-Tritsch IE: Transvaginal multifetal pregnancy reduction: Which? When? How many? Ann Med 1993;25:275-278.

98. Timor-Tritsch IE, Bashiri A, Monteagudo A, et al: Two hundred ninety consecutive cases of multifetal pregnancy reduction: Comparison of the transabdominal versus the transvaginal approach. Am J Obstet Gynecol 2004;191:2085-2099.

99. Firth H: Chorion villus sampling and limb deficiency: Cause or coincidence? Prenat Diagn 1997;17:1313-1330.

100. Centers for Disease Control and Prevention: Chorionic villus sampling and amniocentesis: Recommendations for prenatal counselling. MMWR Recomm Rep 1995;44:1-12.

101. Brambati B, Tului L, Cislaghi C, Alberti E: First 10,000 chorionic villus samplings performed on singleton pregnancies by a single operator. Prenat Diagn 1998;18:255-266.

102. Goldenberg RL, Davis RO, Hill D: The use of real-time ultrasound as an aid during difficult therapeutic abortion procedures. Am J Obstet Gynecol 1984;148:826-827.

103. Hornstein MD, Osathanondh R, Birnholz JC, et al: Ultrasound guidance for selected dilatation and evacuation procedures. J Reprod Med 1986;31:947-950.

104. Shalev E, Zuckerman H: Operative hysteroscopy under real-time ultrasonography. Am J Obstet Gynecol 1986;155:1360-1361.

105. Letterie GS, Case KJ: Intraoperative ultrasound guidance for hysteroscopic retrieval of intrauterine foreign bodies. Surg Endosc 1993;7:182-184.

106. Letterie GS: Ultrasound guidance during endoscopic procedures. Obstet Gynecol Clin North Am 1999;26:63-82.

107. Shalev E, Shimoni Y, Peleg D: Ultrasound controlled operative hysteroscopy. J Am Coll Surg 1994;179:70-71.

108. Shalev E: Ultrasound guidance for intrauterine surgery. Fertil Steril 1995;64:664-665.

109. Letterie GS, Kramer DJ: Intraoperative ultrasound guidance for intrauterine endoscopic surgery. Fertil Steril 1994;62:654-656.

110. Kohlenberg CF, Pardey J, Ellwood DA: Transabdominal ultrasound as an aid to advanced hysteroscopic surgery. Aust N Z J Obstet Gynaecol 1994;34:462-464.

111. Rotmensch J, Waggoner SE, Quiet C: Ultrasound guidance for placement of difficult intracavitary implants. Gynecol Oncol 1994;54:159-162.

112. Fleischer AC, Burnett LS, Jones HW 3rd, Cullinan JA: Transrectal and transperineal sonography during guided intrauterine procedures. J Ultrasound Med 1995;14:135-138.

113. Ohl J, Bettahar-Lebugle K: Ultrasound-guided transcervical resection of uterine septa: 7 years' experience. Ultrasound Obstet Gynecol 1996;7:328-334.

114. Timor-Tritsch IE, Masch RJ, Goldstein SR, et al: Transvaginal ultrasound-assisted gynecologic surgery: Evaluation of a new device to improve safety of intrauterine surgery. Am J Obstet Gynecol 2003;189:1074-1079.

Chapter 17

Color Doppler Mapping in Gynecology

Ilan E. Timor-Tritsch

The use of color mapping to display moving targets, such as blood flow, is increasing, even as we continue to gather information about its clinical usefulness. The role of color and power Doppler sonography in obstetric and gynecologic practice has grown, but even greater applicability is likely in the future.

Background

It is important to place the technical evolution of color-coded flow examinations in a historical perspective. The history of color Doppler sonography is relatively short. In 1959, Satomura[1] reported on the use of Doppler frequency shifts to detect flow in blood vessels. This technology was applied to obstetrics at the end of the 1970s by Fitzgerald and Drumm[2] and McCallum et al.[3] In the mid-1980s, Taylor et al.[4] described the flow-velocity waveforms of the ovarian and uterine arteries. The superposition of Doppler signal information onto a real-time ultrasound image and the color coding of different velocities and flow directions started with the description by Namekawa at al.[5] in 1982. It took several years to perfect the technique and to develop the first transvaginal ultrasound probes capable of performing color Doppler sonography and then make them commercially available. By the late 1980s and early 1990s, pioneering research in the gynecologic applications of color Doppler was being published by Kurjak, Hata, Bourne, and Fleischer and their respective colleagues,[6-10] among a few others. These reports stimulated many other groups and researchers, and as a result, an abundance of research and clinical observations appeared in the scientific journals.

Doppler Technique

Chapter 2 discusses the physics and the background knowledge needed to understand the Doppler phenomenon on which clinical ultrasound technology is based. Interested readers can also consult several textbooks on the subject.[11-20] Here, only the necessary background related to color Doppler technology is summarized.

Stationary targets within tissues scanned by ultrasound reflect the echoes received from the oscillating transducer crystal source back to the transducer with no change in frequency. However, when sound waves are reflected back from moving structures (e.g., erythrocytes), there is a change in frequency called the frequency shift or Doppler shift. This shift is proportional to the velocity of the moving target:

$$\Delta F = v \ (2f \cos \theta / c),$$

where F is the Doppler shift, v is the velocity of the flow, f is the frequency of the emitted pulses, θ is the angle between the incident sound wave and the direction of the flow, and c is the velocity of sound in the tissue. This equation is the basis for blood velocity measurements using Doppler equipment (Fig. 17–1). Because red blood cells moving within a vessel do so at different velocities, the Doppler signal received by the transducer contains a spectrum of Doppler shifts. Such a flow-velocity waveform therefore displays an array of different frequencies, called the blood flow profile. These pulsatile flow profiles not only can be seen on the monitor but also can be heard by the observer, because the difference in the frequency shifts is within the audible sound range. A number of clinical applications were based on this audible signal, including the widespread pocket instruments to listen to the fetal heartbeat and sound-directed Doppler waveform analyzers. The latter gave way to more sophisticated image-guided Doppler equipment. When the Doppler technique was combined with the use of higher-frequency transvaginal probes placed near the pelvic blood vessels, the result was superior resolution and increased knowledge about the circulatory physiology of the reproductive organs.[21]

Color Doppler

Color Doppler sonography consists of mapping the whole ultrasound image for Doppler signals. The blood flow within a scanning "slice" (or any other moving structures) yields a host of velocities superimposed onto the gray-scale image. Structures (i.e., blood cells) approaching the transducer are assigned one color (usually red). Targets moving away from the transducer are assigned a different color (usually blue) (Fig. 17–2). The brightness or intensity of the color is proportional to the velocity of the target (i.e., blood flow). The Doppler shift is not only velocity dependent but also angle dependent. Either color

232

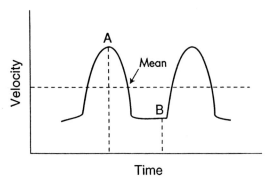

Figure 17–1. Resistance to flow as measured by the different equations applied to the Doppler velocity waveforms.

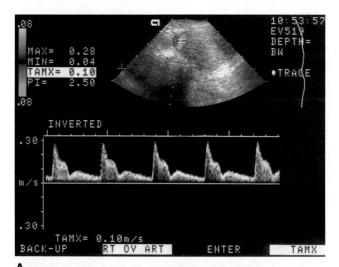

A

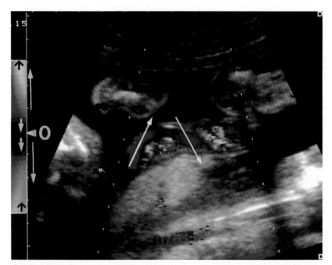

Figure 17–2. A free loop of the umbilical cord is interspaced by color-coded Doppler sonography and used as an example to explain the color display of the flow. Flow toward the transducer is red, and flow away from the transducer is blue. Higher velocities show brighter colors (see the color bar on the left). Because the velocity is angle dependent, the sharper the angle between the flow and the transducer, the brighter the color. Flow "seen" by the transducer at a 90-degree angle is not color-coded and therefore appears black (*white arrows* pointing at the direction of blood flow in the cord and *arrowhead with 0* pointing at the color bar).

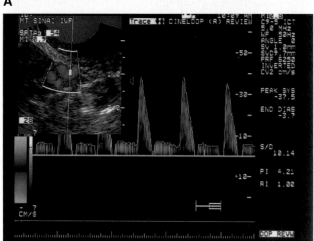

B

Figure 17–3. Uterine artery Doppler flow measurements in a patient with a low (favorable) pulsatility index (**A**) and one with a high (unfavorable) pulsatility index (**B**). (See also Chapter 13.)

is brighter if the blood flow matches the axis of the sound waves. A significant number of transvaginal probes are now equipped with color Doppler capability. This makes the identification of individual vessels or a mesh of smaller capillaries contained in an area of interest feasible.

Once a vessel is identified, its qualitative and quantitative interrogation is possible. The qualitative evaluation is as simple as activating the appropriate controls on the control panel. The quality of blood flow within vessels or organs is informative because the direction of flow (in the fetal vessels and the heart) and the presence or absence and abundance of color have clinical implications (e.g., vascular tumors, corpus luteum, ectopic pregnancy, adnexal torsion). The precise quantitative evaluation of flow velocity has some obstacles. This value is dependent on the insonation angle and vessel diameter. Thus, velocities in tortuous or irregular vessels (with changing diameters) are hard or impossible to obtain. To obtain optimal results, the Doppler angle should be 15 to 50

degrees to the axis of the interrogated vessel. To pick up even the lowest flow velocities, the wall filter should be kept at the lowest possible value. Ideally, the angle between the incidental beam and the direction of the flow should be 0.

A practical surrogate for the true velocity measurement is the calculation of different flow indices (Fig. 17–3), such as the impedance indices that express the distal resistance to flow. Several such indices have been developed:

- Pulsatility index (PI)[22]
- Pourcelot resistance index (RI)[23]
- S/D ratio[24] (systolic/diastolic ratio)
- D/A ratio[25] (diastolic/average* ratio)

Several clinical entities and diagnoses are based on assumptions derived from this semiqualitative analysis of the downstream flow within organs or tumors.

Power Doppler

Power Doppler examination was introduced into clinical practice around 1990. The Doppler signal has three dimensions:

*A is the temporal average of the peak frequency shift over one cycle.

frequency (based on the velocity of blood flow), which is the basis for color mapping; *amplitude,* or intensity of the reflected signal (proportional to the number of red blood cells scattering the ultrasound beam); and the *time* it takes for the changes in frequency and amplitude of the signals to develop. It took several years to overcome the technical challenges and clinically apply the amplitude-based information obtained from analyzing and displaying this energy of the Doppler signal. As opposed to the spectral analysis of Doppler signals, the Doppler energy or power display is angle independent and does not indicate the direction of blood flow relative to transducer placement. The amplitude, however, is affected by the wall filter. The high-pass filter removes high-amplitude, low-frequency signals generated by adjacent tissue movement (e.g., bowel). For optimal imaging, an appropriate wall filter setting is required. Amplitude mapping is helpful in displaying low-volume or low-velocity blood flow situations. In these cases, a low-threshold wall filter is necessary. Power Doppler imaging is also influenced by the power gain. Increasing the gain increases the sensitivity for detecting slow-velocity blood vessels. Unfortunately, in these cases, undesirable artifactual signals are generated by the movement of surrounding organs or tissues.[26]

If directional flow information is not important (and this is the case in most gynecologic pathologies), it is reasonable to start the color mapping examination by turning on the power Doppler mode. In most gynecologic (as well as most obstetric) cases, power Doppler is the first-line method of evaluating blood flow. An advantage of power Doppler over color Doppler is its higher sensitivity to low flow velocities (e.g., suspected adnexal torsion, pathologic blood flow in ovaries).

More recent developments in power Doppler technology allow one to obtain additional information about the blood supply to organs by means of three-dimensional (3D) power Doppler angiography. At present, the main beneficiary of 3D power Doppler angiography is the human fetus. However, gynecologic applications of this technique may eventually add significant clinical information to the classic gray-scale and color Doppler ultrasound examination. Chapter 19 provides additional information on the use of 3D power Doppler evaluation in gynecology.

Color Doppler in Early Pregnancy

There is still some debate whether it is safe to perform color Doppler studies during early pregnancy,[11] and several papers have been published on the subject.[17] The presence or the absence of an embryonic heartbeat can be adequately addressed by real-time gray-scale transvaginal sonography (TVS). Thus, I believe that there is little need to use color or power Doppler sonography to evaluate an early pregnancy (up to 10 to 12 weeks). If, however, the use of color or power Doppler is specifically indicated for diagnostic work-up, it should be used judiciously (Fig. 17–4).

In one case, color Doppler sonography proved to be important in diagnosing a patient with subchorionic bleeding (Fig. 17–5A to C). Fetal heartbeats were present; however, the color flow clearly showed a good placental blood supply, and the placenta's attachment to the uterine wall was normal (Fig. 17–5D and E).

Color and Power Doppler in Ectopic Pregnancy

Chapter 13 discusses the ultrasound evaluation of ectopic pregnancy. In the vast majority of cases, ectopic pregnancy can be detected using the gray-scale pictures obtained with high-frequency transvaginal ultrasound probes.[27-32] Here, only the specific applications of color and power Doppler sonography are discussed.

The physiologic changes in the vascular supply during a normal intrauterine pregnancy are those of a progressively low-impedance and high-velocity flow to the developing placenta. This is the same Doppler signal profile seen in tubal ectopic pregnancies. Although it was expected that color Doppler technology would yield better results than simple gray-scale methods, it proved to be superior only in expeditiously finding the blood vessels around the ectopic pregnancy and then allowing an evaluation of the blood flow profile with

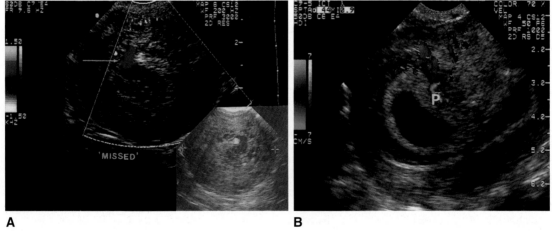

A   **B**

Figure 17–4. A, Early pregnancy failure detected several weeks after embryonic demise. The lacunar blood flow *(arrow)* is typical of these so-called missed abortion cases. The *inset* is the gray-scale image of the same case. **B,** Patient with a bleeding but live 6-week 3-day intrauterine pregnancy. Note the large semicircular subchorionic hematoma surrounding the chorionic sac from below. The placenta (P) is firmly attached to the uterine wall and is well supplied by blood flow.

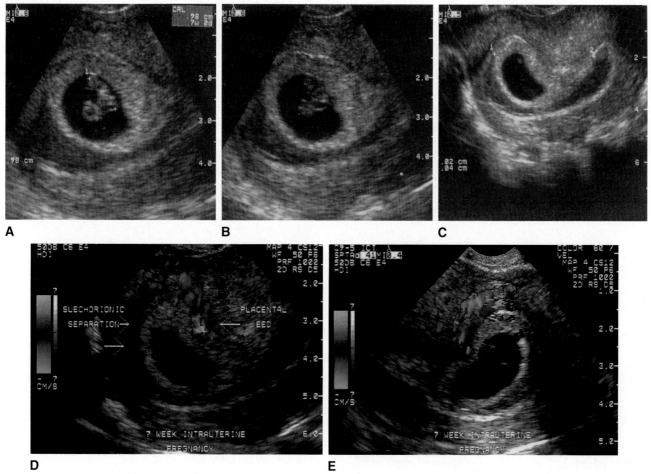

Figure 17–5. Subchorionic hematoma (separation of the chorion) in a live 6.5-week intrauterine pregnancy. **A** and **B,** Coronal views of the uterus. **C,** Sagittal view of the uterus. **D** and **E,** Color-flow images showing the normal blood supply of the firmly attached anterior placenta.

semiquantitative measurement methods. Thus, color-flow capabilities may enable a faster diagnosis, but they increase the sensitivity of the test only incrementally.

Intracavitary and Pericavitary Findings

If the presence of an intrauterine pregnancy can be established, an ectopic gestation can be ruled out. It is therefore important to make a distinction between a physiologic, normal blood flow to an intrauterine pregnancy (or, more precisely, to the early placenta) and an abnormal blood flow. Even if the ultrasound signs of a normal pregnancy are not yet visible, the abundant color around the endometrium close to the future site of the early placenta can be seen as early as 36 days after the last menstrual period (Fig. 17–6).[33] A velocity cut-off value of 21 cm/second has been suggested to distinguish an intrauterine pregnancy from a pseudogestational sac. In the case of a pseudogestational sac, typical placental flow is not seen.[34]

Detection of Blood Flow to the Ovaries

To better distinguish between a corpus luteum and an ectopic pregnancy in the tube or the ovary, scrutinize the typical color Doppler scan of the ovary containing the corpus luteum. With a corpus luteum, a rich ringlike color can be detected within the ovary (Fig. 17–7). If resistance to flow is measured, usually

a low PI and RI can be demonstrated in the vessels around the corpus luteum (Fig. 17–8).

In normal and spontaneous cycles, only one corpus luteum can be seen at the appropriate time. It is therefore extremely important to scrutinize the ipsilateral side for a coexisting ectopic gestation. Pellerito et al.[35] found that 86% of ectopic pregnancies were on the same side as the corpus luteum. However, in patients undergoing ovarian hyperstimulation, multiple or superovulation is the case, and several "color rings" may coexist around the many emptied follicles. In this case, detection of an ectopic pregnancy may have to rely on its gray-scale characteristics (see Chapter 14).

With gray-scale sonography, only the tubal ring (if it is detected) is more echogenic than the corpus luteum, which, in the overwhelming majority of cases, appears much less echogenic.[36] If color is "applied" to the corpus luteum, this demonstrates a relatively dense lace of "bright" blood vessels that appear to be an integral part of its wall (Fig. 17–9). In contrast, the blood flow of the tubal ring containing the early placenta and an ectopic pregnancy displays color *around* but not within the hyperechoic wall of the structure (Fig. 17–10).

Color-Flow Study of Ectopic Pregnancy

An intact tubal ectopic pregnancy demonstrates blood flow around the trophoblast or the early placenta within the tube.

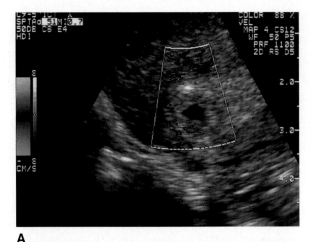

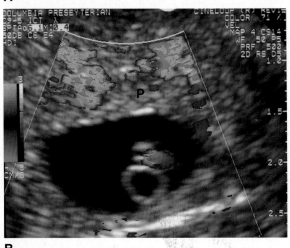

Figure 17–6. A, Circular color flow is depicted in this 5-week normal intrauterine pregnancy. The hyperechoic layer surrounding the sonolucent center is usually devoid of detectable flow. **B,** This 6-week 1-day normal intrauterine pregnancy shows the normal blood supply to the tiny placenta (P).

Sometimes, in very early or relatively small ectopic pregnancies, gray-scale (TVS) cannot pinpoint the lesion. Color-coded flow reinforces the fact that the structure in question is an ectopic gestation (see Fig. 17–10).

Trials to evaluate patients with presumed ectopic pregnancies have used semiquantitative methods of measuring resistance to flow. Kurjak et al.[37] suggested an RI of 0.40 or less as the cut-off to make a diagnosis of an ectopic pregnancy. Others followed suit, and soon a scientific discussion ensued about the value of Doppler evaluation and color Doppler studies in ectopic pregnancies. Although it is difficult to compare Doppler flow studies with regard to their efficacy in the work-up of ectopic pregnancies, Table 17–1 summarizes some of the literature on the subject.[17]

Relying on studies done in abnormal intrauterine pregnancies,[38,39] other Doppler studies support the observations that the impedance to flow is lower and the subjective appearance of color abundance is higher on the side of a tubal ectopic pregnancy.[40-42]

In another study, Tekay and Jouppila[43] evaluated the subjective appearance of color flow in ectopic pregnancies with different levels of β-human chorionic gonadotropin (β-hCG). It was evident that ectopic pregnancies associated with a higher serum β-hCG level demonstrated a lower resistance to flow, whereas those with a relatively lower hormone level showed much less color and a higher resistance to flow.

Megier and Desroches[44] studied 100 cases of tubal ectopic pregnancy and found that color Doppler facilitated the diagnosis of tubal ectopic pregnancies smaller than 1 cm in diameter and echogenic lesions (nonviable or bleeding ectopic pregnancies) smaller than 2 cm.

The Doppler indices of blood flow in the uterine and spiral arteries and the corpus luteum in ectopic and intrauterine pregnancies were studied by Jurkovic et al.[45] Their results showed that blood flow impedance in the uterine and spiral arteries and the corpus luteum is similar in intrauterine and ectopic pregnancies. Peak velocity in the uterine artery reflects a decreased blood supply to the ectopic pregnancy. Atri[46] was able to discriminate between a corpus luteum and an ectopic pregnancy based on Doppler flow indices.

It is clear that color Doppler sonography in patients with suspected ectopic pregnancy can complement the traditional high-frequency transvaginal ultrasound examination. With color Doppler, the diagnosis can probably be established or ruled out faster and with marginally higher accuracy. However, the correct diagnosis can reliably be made based on clinical information, serum β-hCG levels, and TVS, without the necessity of color Doppler scanning.[47,48] Interested readers are referred to an exchange of letters on the pros and cons of color Doppler sonography in ectopic pregnancies.[49-51]

Cornual and Interstitial Pregnancies

There are only a few articles about the use of color Doppler to evaluate cornual or interstitial pregnancies.[52,53] Based on personal experience in the conservative management of cornual pregnancies,[54] I consider color Doppler sonography to be of limited use in the diagnostic process but extremely valuable for follow-up. Localizing the site of the lesion over the long-term follow-up period is helpful (Fig. 17–11). In cases treated with minimally invasive local potassium chloride or methotrexate injections in live embryos or ultrasound follow-up of nonlive cornual gestations, color Doppler scanning enabled visualization of the lesion for 1 year or longer. In fact, there is a similarity between the natural evolution of an injected or conservatively managed cornual pregnancy and a "missed" intrauterine pregnancy. Blood flow around the chorionic sac and within the decidua demonstrates comparable patterns.

Cervical and Cesarean Scar Pregnancies

The diagnosis of a cervical pregnancy relies on several diagnostic criteria—some sonographic, and some histologic. Sonographically, a live pregnancy must be seen below the level of the internal os. Anatomically, the uterine artery approaches the uterus at the level of the internal os, so identifying the uterine artery with color Doppler sonography (see Fig. 17–10) and localizing the cervical position of the pregnancy at the level of this artery facilitate the diagnosis. Thus, the simultaneous imaging of the uterine artery and a viable pregnancy on the same coronal (transverse) picture is proposed as a new ultrasound criterion to establish the diagnosis of cervical pregnancy.[55] In the remainder of the diagnostic process, as in

Figure 17–7. Corpus luteum. **A,** The typical circular flow pattern of a corpus luteum by color Doppler. **B,** Gray-scale ultrasound could barely depict this fresh corpus luteum. **C,** Color Doppler sonography was able to reveal the abundant mesh of blood vessels around it. **D,** Power Doppler is probably the most effective method.

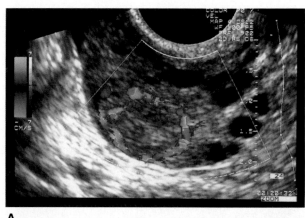

A

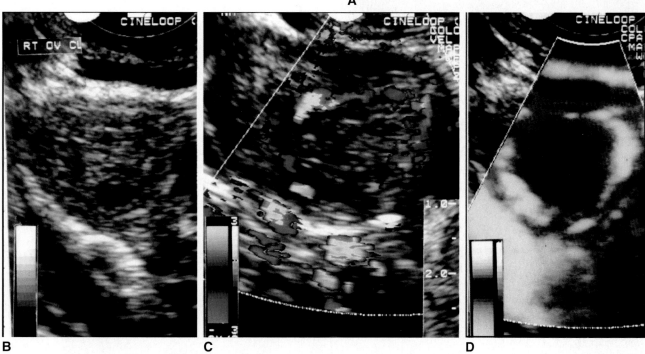

B   C   D

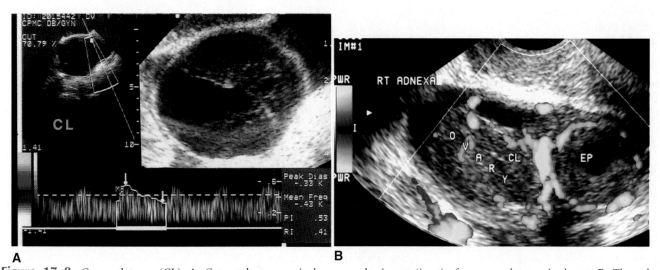

A   B

Figure 17–8. Corpus luteum (CL). **A,** Gray-scale transvaginal sonography image *(inset)* of a corpus luteum is shown. **B,** The color Doppler–directed sample volume reveals a high diastolic blood flow with a low pulsatility index (0.53) and resistance index (0.41). EP, ectopic pregnancy.

other types of ectopic pregnancy, color Doppler scanning is helpful but not necessary. Power Doppler (two-dimensional as well as 3D) assessment of cervical pregnancies has been addressed by several authors.[56,57] Roussis et al.[58] used color Doppler to monitor the conservative treatment of a cervical pregnancy. Many consider a pregnancy in the scar of a previous cesarean section a subset of cervical pregnancy. Accurate localization of this rare ectopic pregnancy may be facilitated by color or power Doppler interrogation of the suspicious area.[59,60]

Conclusion

In conclusion, the most important advance in the diagnosis of ectopic pregnancy was TVS. The addition of color and power Doppler is secondary, although its use may indirectly increase the sensitivity and specificity of the diagnostic process by examining the uterus, endometrial cavity, ovaries, corpus luteum, and suspected location of the ectopic gestation. Color and power Doppler are of greater importance for follow-up in cases in which conservative management or puncture injection treatment was chosen.

Color and Power Doppler in Diagnosis of Adnexal Masses

The most useful application of color Doppler is in the diagnostic work-up of patients with pelvic masses. Because these masses are potentially malignant, increasing the sensitivity and specificity of the ultrasound examination is of utmost importance. Gray-scale TVS can achieve high diagnostic precision by determining the morphologic attributes of these masses.[61-67] Transvaginal color Doppler sonography can

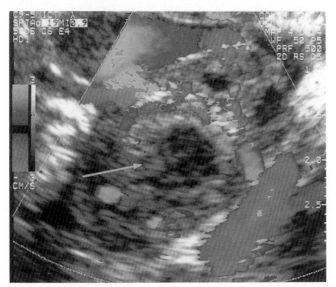

Figure 17–9. Ringlike blood supply of a corpus luteum *(long arrow)* in the left ovary.

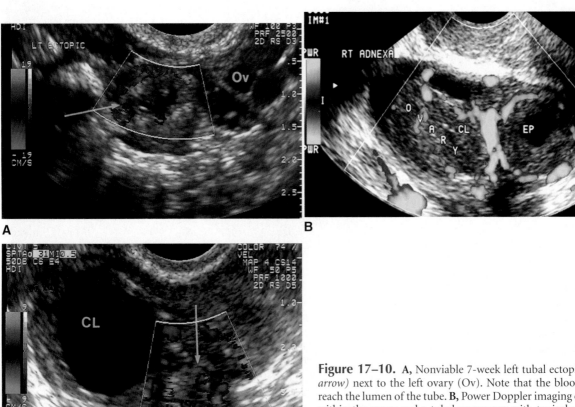

Figure 17–10. A, Nonviable 7-week left tubal ectopic pregnancy *(long arrow)* next to the left ovary (Ov). Note that the blood supply does not reach the lumen of the tube. **B,** Power Doppler imaging of a corpus luteum within the ovary and a tubal pregnancy with typical subserosal, peripheral blood vessels. **C,** Right-sided 7-week nonviable ectopic (tubal) pregnancy *(long arrow)* demonstrates rich blood flow to the tubal gestation. An ipsilateral corpus luteum (CL) is also imaged. EP, ectopic pregnancy.

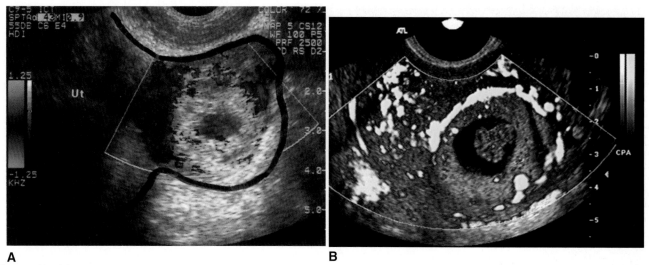

A   **B**

Figure 17–11. Cornual pregnancy. **A,** Color-coded flow around the hyperechoic trophoblast of a viable cornual pregnancy of 6.5 weeks. The bulging lesion is outlined *(black line)*. **B,** Power Doppler image of a live cornual pregnancy. Circular blood flow is still evident around the ectopic gestational sac. Ut, uterus.

Table 17–1	Summary of Doppler Flow Studies in the Work-up of Ectopic Pregnancy					
Author	Year	Number	Sensitivity (%)*	Specificity (%)*	Positive Predictive Value (%)	Negative Predictive Value (%)
Taylor et al.[38]	1989	70	73 (53)	—	85	81
Kurjak et al.[37]	1991	73	88	97	97	89
Taylor & Meyer[39]	1991	23	96 (17)	93	—	—
Pellerito et al.[35]	1992	65	95 (54)	98 (98)	97	—
Emerson et al.[40]	1992	—	87 (71)	100 (99)	—	—

*Percentages in parentheses represent transvaginal sonographic evaluations only.
Adapted from Kurjak A (ed): An Atlas of Transvaginal Color Doppler: The Current State of the Art. London, Parthenon Publishing Group, 1993.

further refine the diagnosis by providing complementary path physiologic information. As previously mentioned, 3D power Doppler angiography may be a useful technique to increase the diagnostic effectiveness of ultrasound.[68]

The detection of adnexal tumors relies on demonstrating increased vascularity or an abundance of vascular patterns and by measuring high-velocity flow and low vascular impedance in the suspicious mass (Fig. 17–12). Both the qualitative and the semiquantitative properties of tumors are based on neovascularization or angiogenesis.

Neovascularization in tumors consists of pathologic tortuous, dilated, or sometimes saccular vessels (lakes) with changing calibers (Fig. 17–13) that do not maintain the classic organization of arterioles, venules, and capillaries. At times, pathologic anastomoses appear between arteries and veins. These newly formed vessels lack the muscular layer, which maintains a relatively high resistance to flow (RI and PI) in normal tissues. Because this regulatory function is lacking, these vessels may demonstrate a continuous high diastolic flow, a smaller difference between systolic and diastolic peaks, and low pulsatility. Because the relatively fast-growing tumor tissue has increased blood flow needs, flow velocity is greater. Owing to the multiple arteriovenous communications, a highly vascularized area is seen (see Figs. 17–12 and 17–13).

Interested readers are referred to other work on the subject of tumor neovascularity.[69-73]

Malignant tumors show low RI and PI. Flow can be detected in the center of the tumor or, if tumor necrosis occurs, adjacent to the necrotic area (Fig.17–14). Systolic velocities are somewhat higher, and the diastolic notch is usually absent (present in a normal arterial flow pattern between the systolic and diastolic components of the waves). Flow can also be appreciated in the septum, if such a structure exists (Figs. 17–15 and 17–16), or in a papilla (Fig. 17–17).

Benign masses demonstrate higher impedance to flow, a more peripherally located vessel pattern, and lower maximal systolic velocities (Figs. 17–18 and 17–19).

Researchers used to agree on the basic color Doppler blood flow characteristics of benign and malignant ovarian tumors.[6-10,74-90] However, doubts were raised as to the value of color Doppler velocity and resistance-to-flow assessments as predictors of malignant changes. One article by Tekay and Jouppila[91] criticized the value of Doppler assessment of ovarian tumors. They found a significant overlap between the ranges of PI and of RI values obtained from benign and malignant ovarian tumors. The RI values were below the cut-off point, considered to be 0.40, in a disturbing 43% of benign ovarian tumors and in 25% of normal ovaries.

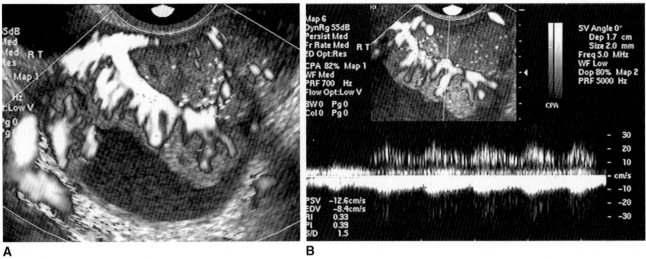

A   **B**

Figure 17–12. Vascular supply to ovarian cancer. **A,** Richly vascularized solid area of the ovary is highlighted by power Doppler interrogation. **B,** There is high diastolic flow (resistance index, 0.33; pulsatility index, 0.39) and a relatively high peak systolic velocity of 12.6 cm/second.

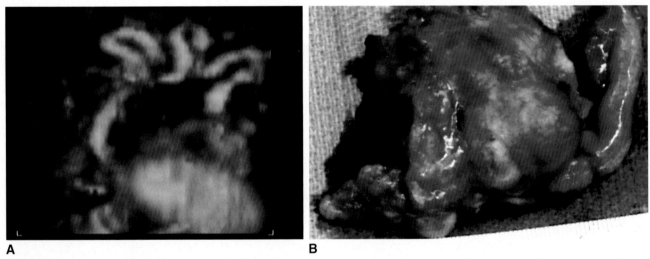

A   **B**

Figure 17–13. Aberrant, pathologic vessels of ovarian cancer. **A,** Three-dimensional power Doppler angiogram demonstrates pathologic, tortuous blood vessels. **B,** Pathologic specimen of the ovary.

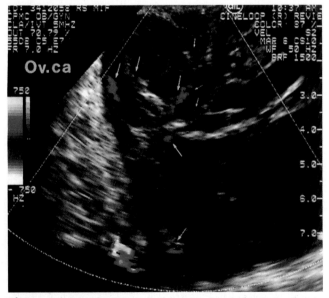

Figure 17–14. The bizarre and profuse shape of the color flow in this histologically proven ovarian cancer is marked *(arrows).*

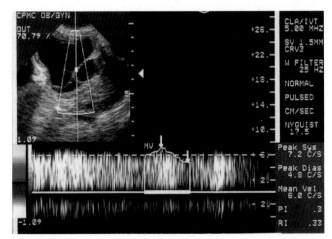

Figure 17–15. The extremely low pulsatility and resistance indices (0.3 and 0.33, respectively) of a patient with ovarian cancer. The flow was sampled from a vessel in a septum.

In most cases, the clinical value of adding color Doppler to the morphologic scanning of TVS is that it may avoid some major surgical procedures, allowing the use of less invasive interventions, such as laparoscopy. However, color Doppler sonography and power Doppler angiography should be considered in cases of nondiagnostic or questionable evaluations by TVS.[92] The mere detection of "central flow" in pathologic ovarian tissue or vascularization of a papillary projection in cases of suspected ovarian malignancy definitely warrants attention. The value of 3D color and power Doppler evaluation of ovarian tumors is still being investigated.[93-96] More on the subject of 3D Doppler for the detection of ovarian pathology can be found in Chapter 19. Early ultrasound screening for ovarian cancer is covered in Chapter 18.

Color and Power Doppler to Evaluate Adnexal Torsion

Torsion of the ovary or fallopian tube is a gynecologic emergency. With multiple areas of torsion along the pedicle, the blood supply to the adnexal organ is cut. The ovary itself receives its blood supply through the ovarian branch of the uterine artery, reaching it through the ovarian ligament and the ovarian artery directly from the aorta, which runs through the infundibulopelvic ligament laterally to the ovary. Ovarian or tubal torsion usually occurs if one of these structures is enlarged (e.g., ovarian tumor, ovarian hyperstimulation, hydrosalpinx). In some cases, no cause can be determined. About 20% of cases of adnexal torsion occur during pregnancy.

The ultrasound features of adnexal torsion are discussed in Chapter 22. These features were described mostly during transabdominal sonography[97,98]; only a few reports are based on TVS. There is no question that TVS adds to the

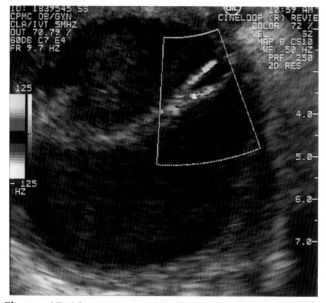

Figure 17–16. In the septum of an endometrial cyst, color Doppler sonography reveals blood flow.

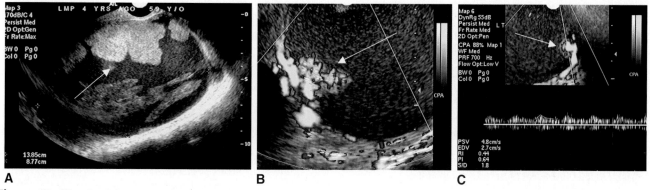

Figure 17–17. Blood flow in an ovarian papilla. **A,** Gray-scale image of papillary protrusions into an ovarian tumor *(arrow)*. **B,** Power Doppler highlights the flow in a papilla. **C,** Resistance indices may or may not show high diastolic flow; however, the presence of flow in the papilla is suspicious of malignancy.

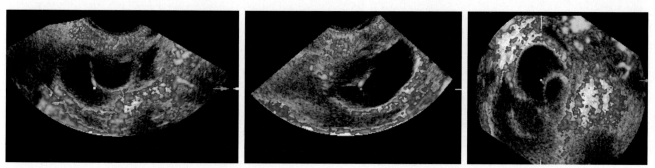

Figure 17–18. Blood flow is scarce in a proven benign serous cystadenoma of the ovary.

sensitivity and specificity of transabdominal sonography; however, even high-quality transvaginal pictures may be nonspecific and lack pathognomonic features. The following features are detectable on gray-scale TVS and indicate ovarian torsion: enlarged ovaries, sometimes with volumes well above 12 to 14 mL; peripherally pushed follicles; and a large, central (sometimes hyperechoic) hilar area devoid of follicles

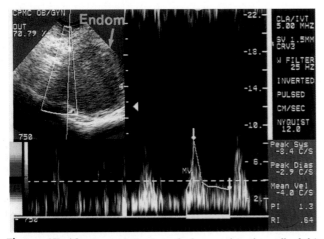

Figure 17–19. It was difficult to find a vessel in the wall of this endometrial cyst. The pulsatility index was 1.3, and the resistance index was 0.64.

(Fig. 17–20A and B). With color or power Doppler interrogation of this extensive hilar area, no blood vessel signals are obtained (Fig. 17–20C).

Unfortunately, sometimes ultrasound images are nonspecific for ovarian torsion. Figure 17–21 depicts one such case in which the diagnosis was established by an excellent clinical evaluation of the patient, leading to timely surgical management. The ultrasound visualization of twisted, hyperstimulated ovaries and the torsion of ovarian masses (benign or malignant) is the typical picture of underlying pathology leading to torsion.

TVS is an excellent "palpatory" tool in addition to its main imaging capability. In most cases, touching the detected pathology by gentle movements of the transducer probing for pain helps establish the correct diagnosis.

The main feature of adnexal torsion is the complete (at times gradual, partial, or even intermittent) cessation of blood flow to the involved organs. It is therefore logical to evaluate the blood supply to the adnexa if torsion is clinically suspected. Color Doppler sonography is the best tool to perform this examination. The fast, early, and expeditious diagnosis, in principle, should enable the administration of appropriate treatment before irreversible ischemic changes lead to gangrene and necrosis. In addition to the classic radical surgical treatment of removing the affected organ or tube, laparoscopic unwinding and preserving of the adnexa have been suggested.[99-101] Such a conservative approach definitely requires an early diagnosis.

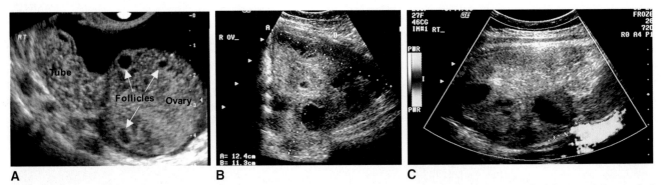

Figure 17–20. Torsion of the ovary. **A,** The ovary is enlarged, and the follicles are pushed to its periphery. **B,** The hilar area is hyperechoic. **C,** Color Doppler interrogation reveals no blood flow.

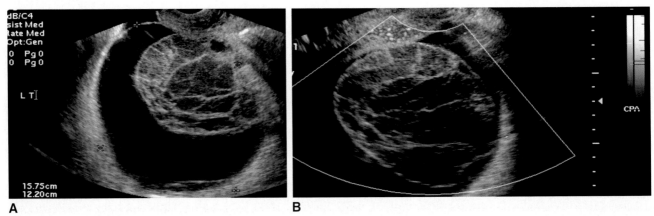

Figure 17–21. Torsion of the ovary. **A,** This twisted ovary contains a corpus luteum. **B,** Color Doppler interrogation reveals no blood flow.

Color-coded flow studies can almost always establish whether the blood supply to the organ in question is present or absent. However, only small series, but no prospective studies, have been published with regard to the sensitivity and specificity of color Doppler sonography in patients suspected of having adnexal torsion.[102-106] If the clinical signs and symptoms indicate the possibility of adnexal torsion, failure to detect blood flow using color Doppler supports the diagnosis of torsion. However, the lack of color may also be caused by physiologic states (e.g., low flow velocities) or technical problems (e.g., unfavorable vessel angle). Therefore, significant operator experience is needed to arrive at the conclusion of "no adnexal blood flow." The opposite (i.e., the detection of arterial color flow) would seemingly allow one to rule out adnexal torsion; however, blood flow was seen in three cases of surgically proven ovarian torsion.[104] It is possible that venous and lymphatic occlusion occurs first, causing the incipient clinical symptoms, after which the arterial circulation is affected, and occlusion becomes total.[107]

The possibility of selective torsion of the ovary or fallopian tube should always be entertained. Selective tubal torsion has been reported.[108,109] If only the fallopian tube twists, normal blood flow will be seen within the ovary; however an engorged, tender structure, perhaps with some sonographic signs of hydrosalpinx, will be detected (Fig. 17–22).

In a series of 12 cases, Fleischer et al.[102] reported the following findings:

- Detection of central flow was associated with viable adnexa.
- Flow was not seen within the mass but might be seen in the capsular area around the mass.
- Early diagnosis may contribute to early and conservative surgery.

Recently, an additional ultrasound sign of adnexal torsion—the pedicle sign—was described. This sign consists of color or power Doppler imaging of a spiral arrangement or coiling of the blood vessels approaching the adnexa (Fig. 17–23). This sign is not universally present, but when detected, it is a relatively sure indication of a twisted ovary or fallopian tube.[110,111]

Color Doppler to Diagnose Pelvic Congestion Syndrome

Pelvic pain in women of reproductive age is the reason for many visits to the gynecologist. Over the past 100 years, many different causes have been considered, but it is beyond the scope of this chapter to describe all these explanations and theories. Recently, however, it was suggested that the combination of dilated pelvic veins and a buildup of excess blood in the adjacent vasculature is the best explanation for this occurrence. In a series of articles, Beard et al.[112-114] explored vascular stasis as an explanation for pelvic pain. Phlebographic studies showed excessive dilation of the ovarian vein draining

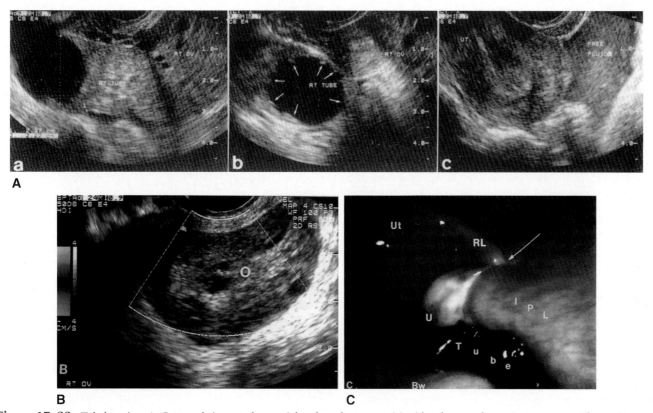

Figure 17–22. Tubal torsion. **A,** Gray-scale images show a right adnexal structure (a) with a dense and a cystic component. The cystic structure (b) shows tiny hyperechoic nodules (*small arrows*), resembling beads on a string. Some free fluid is in the pelvis (c). **B,** The color study, which shows no flow in the structure seen in **A,** depicts flow to the right ovary (O). **C,** Tubal torsion was highly suspected. The laparoscopic picture reveals selective torsion of the right tube and the normal-appearing right ovary. Bw, bowel; IPL, infundibulopelvic ligament; RL, round ligament; Ut, uterus. (Courtesy of Drs. Z. Leibovici and A. Condrea.)

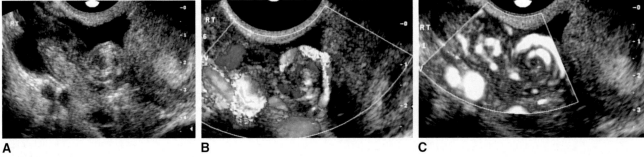

Figure 17–23. The twisted pedicle sign. If the transducer is placed at a 90-degree angle to the incoming blood vessel in the infundibulopelvic ligament, when the torsion is incomplete or intermittent, a spiraling vessel will be seen on gray scale (**A**), color Doppler (**B**), and power Doppler (**C**).

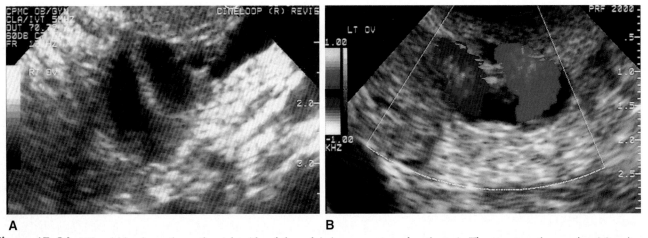

Figure 17–24. Dilated blood vessels on the right side of the pelvis in a menopausal patient. **A,** The structure (measuring 2.2 cm) was diagnosed as an ovarian cyst. **B,** Color flow reveals the nature of the cyst.

the pelvis through the infundibulopelvic ligament.[113-115] Laparoscopy has been used to confirm the reason for this syndrome,[116-118] but despite direct visualization of the pelvis, false-negative results have been obtained.

The use of transabdominal sonography in the work-up of patients with pelvic pain did not lead to significant advances in solving the problem. Transvaginal color Doppler seems to be the most definitive noninvasive diagnostic technique.[119-122] Indeed, color Doppler–directed flow velocity measurements enable the differentiation between arterial and venous flow.

Despite attempts to explain pelvic pain by the presence of vascular dilation (venous, arterial, or mixed),[123] there are no reliable studies that enable us to make a firm connection between the two. However, I have seen patients with pelvic pain and a significantly dilated vascular pattern demonstrating unilateral or bilateral dilated pelvic veins (Fig. 17–24).

The distended venous structures in the adnexa achieve a caliber greater than 4 to 5 mm with slow velocities (<3 cm/second) (AC Fleischer, personal communication). Park et al.[124] studied 32 patients with pelvic congestion syndrome using transabdominal sonography and TVS and reported the following findings: dilated left ovarian vein with reversed caudal flow, presence of varicocele, dilated arcuate veins crossing the uterine myometrium, polycystic changes of the ovary, and variable duplex waveform during Valsalva's maneuver. Combined transabdominal sonography and TVS is potentially

useful as a noninvasive screening tool to determine which patients with chronic pelvic pain may benefit from selective ovarian venography and transcatheter embolization.

Hysterosalpingography under Color Doppler Guidance

Tubal obstruction is a cause of infertility in about 15% of couples. The classic work-up to determine tubal obstruction or patency included laparoscopy and radiographic hysterosalpingography. Lately, sonographic hysterosalpingography with and without color-flow Doppler imaging has been used to diagnose blocked tubes.

Gray-scale sonography, using the transabdominal or the transvaginal route, was based on (1) detecting injected free fluid in the cul-de-sac after its passage from the cervix, through the uterine cavity and tubes, and into the pelvis, and (2) following sonographic contrast material flowing through the tube. The transabdominal method did not produce sufficiently good results because it is based on an indirect evaluation of presumed tubal patency.[125,126] After the introduction of transvaginal probes, different contrast materials were tested, including air bubbles containing normal saline,[127-130] a coated albumin compound,[130] Echovist (SHU 450),[131-137] dextran solution,[138] and other materials.[139,140] The results were variable

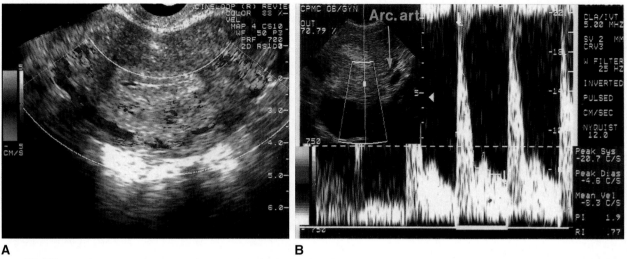

Figure 17–25. Uterine arcuate arteries and veins. **A,** Color highlights the posterior section of the arcuate vessels in a patient in the secretory phase of her menstrual cycle. **B,** High velocities and resistance indices are demonstrated: systolic peak velocity, 20.7 cm/second; pulsatility index, 1.9; resistance index, 0.77.

and ranged between 50% and 85% agreement when compared with laparoscopic chromopertubation. When color-flow Doppler became available, several groups started using this technology to display the sudden fluid jets bursting through a patent tube. The direction of the flow seen inside the uterine cavity and then passing through the tubes and into the pelvic cavity can be based on the color Doppler display, as well as on the positive or negative frequency shift.[134,141-143]

The procedure is usually performed under transvaginal ultrasound control and guidance. A catheter is placed into the uterine cavity; usually a balloon-tipped catheter is used, which prevents reflux. Saline is then injected through the catheter under transvaginal ultrasound control. Once the passage is located, a relatively "wide" sample volume color window is activated to verify the fluid passing through the area of interest. Using small jets of fluid, one can observe the color flow. A similar sample volume window can be placed in the area of the tubal fimbria and capture the flow displayed by the Doppler shifts. The correlation with laparoscopic chromopertubation is reportedly as high as 82% to 92%.[141,142] One should look for fluid in the cul-de-sac and account for the approximate amount that was injected. It is possible to verify tubal patency on each side.

Color Doppler hysterosalpingography can be performed as an office procedure, provided that the ultrasound equipment has color-flow capabilities. The color Doppler technique can also be used for transcervical tuboplasty under ultrasound guidance.

Color and Power Doppler in Evaluation of the Uterus

Knowledge of the normal blood supply of the uterus is important for the diagnosis of pathologic conditions. As a general rule, the caliber of the uterine arteries and arterial network is different from that of the venous network, which appears larger and more dilated. The arteries can also be recognized by their pulsatile nature. It is easy to locate the approach of the uterine arteries passing through the cardinal ligaments to the uterus.

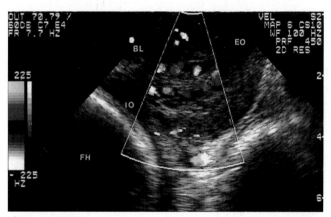

Figure 17–26. Sagittal view of the cervix in a second-trimester normal pregnancy. A certain amount of physiologic color flow is detected along the cervical canal extending from the internal os (IO) to the external os (EO). BL, bladder; FH, fetal head.

These arteries typically display a high PI and a high RI, as well as a typical diastolic notch. At times, the arcuate arteries and veins can be seen within the myometrium, assuming a circular shape at its outer two thirds. These vessels may be extremely thin; however, at times they are impressive in size, often raising the question whether this is normal. Color flow enhances the detection of these arcuate vessels (Fig. 17–25A). These arteries, much like the uterine arteries, have high peak velocity and RI and PI ratios (Fig. 17–25B). Smaller branches supplying blood to the endometrium can also be visualized. It seems obvious and natural that the blood supply to the endometrium varies during the menstrual cycle, differing before, during, and after ovulation as well as during menstruation.[144,145]

It is important to be familiar with the normal blood supply of the cervix seen on the median view (Fig. 17–26). The practical importance of this is the ability to differentiate the usually abundant blood supply to the pregnant cervix from the even richer blood supply of a placenta with low implantation (namely, in the area of the internal os) and exhibiting the

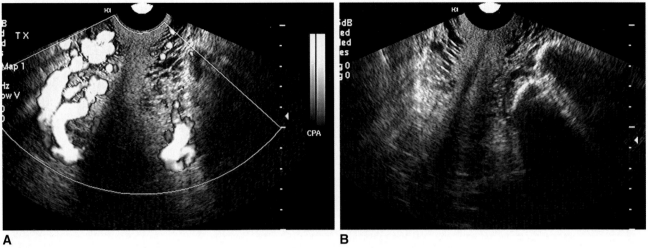

Figure 17–27. A patient with Klippel-Trénaunay-Weber syndrome has a vascular malformation in the uterus. **A,** Power Doppler image. **B,** Even without color enhancement, it is possible to see the sonolucent areas corresponding to the dilated vessels.

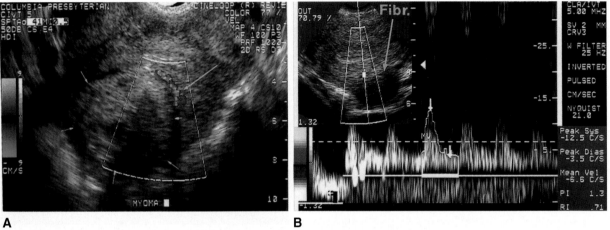

Figure 17–28. A, The feeding vessel *(long arrow)* of this uterine myoma *(small arrows)* is revealed by color Doppler sonography. **B,** Benign uterine fibroids show high resistance to flow (pulsatility index, 1.3; resistance index, 0.71).

features of placenta accreta. If the diagnosis is placenta accreta, large and impressive lacunar structures usually demonstrate visible blood flow and turbulence, as well as jetlike streams into these vascular "lakes."[146] Color Doppler is instrumental in the diagnosis and management of pathologically adherent placentas.[147-149]

Color Doppler imaging may be able to diagnose large vascular malformations of the uterus, a condition with potentially grave consequences.[150-152] A similar picture occurs in patients with Klippel-Trénaunay-Weber syndrome, in which dilated vessels nearly replace part of the myometrium (Fig. 17–27).

Uterine fibroids are an extremely prevalent disease of the uterine smooth muscle. It is usually easy to find feeding vessels for the fibroid in the uterus (Fig. 17–28). Color Doppler studies have been reported in the literature.[153-155]

One of the most clinically rewarding uses of color Doppler evaluation of the uterus is the identification of a pedunculated fibroid extending into the broad ligament or into the cul-de-sac. In this case, differentiating a fibroid from an ovarian mass is extremely important. If, by using color Doppler to identify

the vessels, a link between the uterus and the tumor can be established, one can state firmly that the structure is indeed a fibroid arising from the uterus and not an adnexal mass (Fig. 17–29).

The use of color Doppler in the diagnosis of uterine sarcoma has also been evaluated.[146,153] Eight patients with uterine sarcoma were studied, with no statistically significant differences found between the RI of the right and left uterine arteries. Abnormal blood vessels were seen in all cases within the tumor itself. There was a decrease in the RI from normal to myomatous to sarcomatous uteri. This is to be expected, because sarcoma is a fast-growing tumor requiring ample blood supply for its growth. If there are differences in the RI between the vessels feeding a normal uterus, the arteries supplying a benign fibroid, and the blood supply to a fast-growing uterine sarcoma, it may be possible to differentiate between benign and malignant conditions of the uterus. Such differentiation cannot, at this time, be made on the basis of gray-scale sonography.

The issue of endometrial polyps was discussed in Chapter 5. With the use of color mapping, it is relatively easy to detect a feeding vessel to a polyp (see Figs. 5–26 and 5–27) or a submucosal fibroid (see Figs. 5–30 and 5–31).

A large amount of research has gone into efforts to diagnose endometrial cancer in its early stages. Using TVS, endometrial pathology can be suspected if an abnormally thick, nonhomogeneous endometrium is seen. In cases of frank endometrial carcinoma, the breakup of the usually well-defined and intact endometrial–myometrial interface is detectable.[156] However, the ultimate sensitivity and specificity of these signs must still be solidified. The problem of differentiating benign hypoplasia from a malignant process has not been solved. It is therefore logical that research has focused on

the blood supply to the endometrium. Figure 17–30 depicts an example of endometrial cancer, demonstrating the abundant and pathologic blood flow to the pathologic endometrium. If tumor angiogenesis occurs with the formation of an endometrial cancer, detection of this abnormal blood flow with low impedance could be useful. Bourne et al.[157] compared 17 patients with endometrial cancer to 85 patients without endometrial pathology. A low PI was considered to predict a positive result in 94% and a negative result in 91%.

Kurjak et al.[158] addressed the same question and found lower resistance in patients with endometrial cancer as opposed to those without the disease. They evaluated 16 postmenopausal patients with abnormal uterine bleeding. Nine had endometrial carcinoma, and seven did not. No flow was detected around and within the endometrium in known cancer patients; however, in all the patients with endometrial cancer, pulsating intratumoral blood flow was seen. The conclusion of the authors was that color Doppler evaluation to detect endometrial carcinoma in postmenopausal women with abnormal uterine bleeding is feasible; it had a sensitivity and specificity of 100% in their hands. They suggested that this diagnostic tool be used to select patients who require diagnostic surgery for endometrial cancer.

Kupesic-Urek et al.[159] evaluated 276 patients with uterine tumors before hysterectomy. Neovascularization, which was detected by color Doppler sonography, was seen in 67% of the benign masses and in all the malignant masses ($n = 26$). Blood flow evaluation showed a significantly lower RI (0.37 ± -0.07) in patients with endometrial cancer than in those with benign uterine lesions (0.54 ± 0.09). In cases of endometrial cancer, central vessels tended to have a lower velocity than those found in the periphery. Hata et al.[160] studied 10 patients with

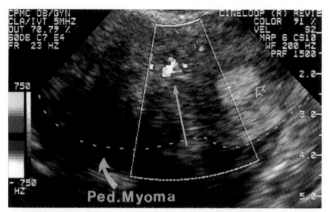

Figure 17–29. The blood vessel *(long arrow)* feeding the pedunculated myoma *(curved arrow)* arising from the right side of the uterus clearly shows the nature of the structure. The endometrium is indicated *(open arrow)*.

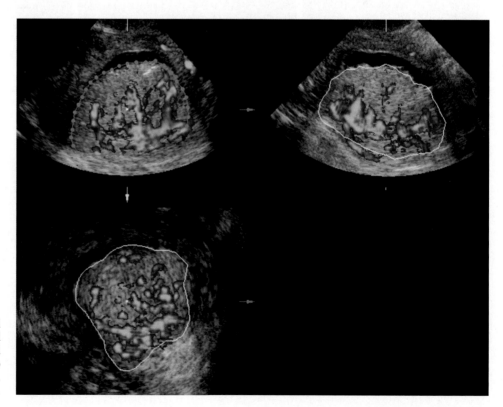

Figure 17–30. Three-dimensional power Doppler picture (orthogonal planes) of posterior wall endometrial cancer. Saline infusion was used to enhance the location of the lesion. Note the abundant vascular pattern.

endometrial cancer and found a low RI compared with that of normal uteri (0.53 versus 0.76).

The relative paucity of literature on the use of color Doppler imaging to diagnose endometrial cancer may be due to the fact that other reliable diagnostic tests are available, and this disease generally presents early enough to enable successful treatment. However, if screening programs for the early detection of ovarian cancer are developed, the opportunity to evaluate the endometrial blood supply at the same time would significantly reduce the individual costs involved.

Last, color or power Doppler interrogation may help differentiate between retained placental tissue that is detached from the wall and waiting to be expelled or extracted and a placental cotyledon that is still attached to its vascular supply (Fig. 17–31). In this case, in addition to the more echogenic placental tissue, a blood vessel with flow in it will be seen.[161]

Color Doppler in Diagnosis of Trophoblastic Disease

The literature is scarce on the use of color Doppler in diagnosing gestational trophoblastic disease. The main diagnostic issue is to reliably predict and differentiate malignant gestational trophoblastic disease (choriocarcinoma) from its benign counterpart (hydatidiform mole).

Chapter 5 discussed the appearance of hydatidiform mole using TVS (see Fig. 5–40). This is characterized by a typical gray-scale picture. Superimposing color Doppler scanning reveals the ample vascularization of the hydatidiform mole (Fig. 17–32; see also Fig. 5–42).

It appears that gray-scale sonography is insufficient to reliably diagnose invasive trophoblastic disease. Many authors[162-167] suggest that color Doppler scanning can be helpful both to diagnose invasive moles and, after successful treatment, to follow the reduction of detectable blood flow to the lesion.

Color Doppler evaluation of gestational trophoblastic disease is claimed to be useful when choriocarcinoma is a possibility.[168-170] Owing to the presence of many newly formed blood vessels, color-directed evaluation is feasible. Six cases of choriocarcinoma studied by color Doppler were reported by Kurjak et al.[171] Low impedance values inside the richly vascularized tissue of the choriocarcinoma were measured. Power Doppler evaluation clearly helped in the case of metastatic trophoblastic disease and accurately localized the lesion in the angle between the urinary bladder and the urethra (see Fig. 5–44).

Clearly, more experience is needed to reliably predict malignancy in cases of gestational trophoblastic disease; however, color Doppler sonography is an important adjunct in diagnosing the malignant variant of this disease.

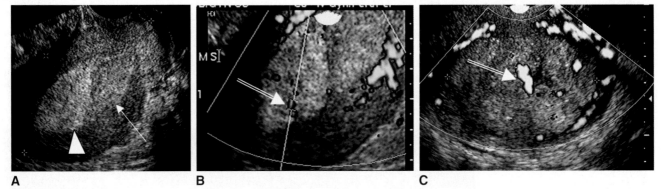

A   **B**   **C**

Figure 17–31. Retained products of conception. **A,** Gray-scale image. Note the hyperechoic portion *(arrowhead)* of the placental remnant next to the hypoechoic portion *(arrow).* **B,** The hyperechoic part has a feeding vessel; therefore, this is a perfuse ("live") "placental polyp." **C,** A clear and rather large vessel is feeding the placental remnant ("placental polyp").

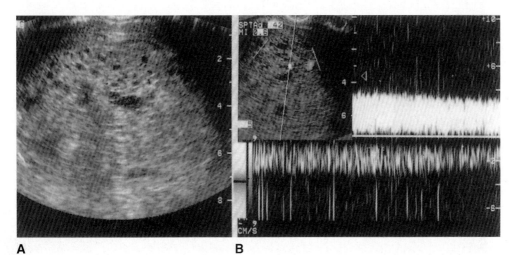

A   **B**

Figure 17–32. Views of a hydatidiform mole at 12.5 weeks of amenorrhea. **A,** Note the multiple sonolucencies of various sizes. **B,** Color Doppler–directed flow evaluation reveals continuous low-resistance flow patterns. (Courtesy of Drs. L. Baxi and A. Monteagudo.)

Summary

The initial enthusiasm surrounding the introduction of color and power Doppler sonography in gynecology is reflected in the literature published during the past 5 to 10 years. Most manufacturers developed and marketed equipment capable of displaying color flow, but the high cost of research and development meant that machines with color Doppler capability were expensive. When the efficacy of color Doppler scanning was analyzed, cost was definitely a factor. Fortunately, the price of ultrasound machines is continually decreasing, and almost all machines that provide color capabilities now have an acceptable price tag. Indeed, an ultrasound machine without color and power Doppler features is a rarity.

Almost all clinical diagnoses can be made using gray-scale ultrasound techniques. Although color and power Doppler help significantly in many clinical situations, an ultrasound laboratory without such capabilities can still perform many basic and accurate studies and refer dubious cases to centers providing this extra service. Tertiary or referral centers or even very busy private offices should have color Doppler imaging available to refine certain diagnoses and arrive at them more quickly. It is also important to devote time to research and to establish which clinical entities benefit from this additional diagnostic capability.

As with most technologic and scientific advances, it will take some time for the ultimate role of 3D color and power Doppler angiography in gynecology to be established.

REFERENCES

1. Satomura A: Study of the flow pattern in peripheral arteries by ultrasonics. J Acoust Soc Jpn 1959;15:151-158.
2. Fitzgerald DA, Drumm JE: Noninvasive measurement of human fetal circulation using ultrasound: A new method. BJM 1977;2:1450-1454.
3. McCallum WD, William CS, Napel S, Daigle RE: Fetal blood velocity waveform. Am J Obstet Gynecol 1978;132:425-429.
4. Taylor KJW, Burns PN, Wells PNT, et al: Ultrasound Doppler flow studies of the ovarian and uterine arteries. Br J Obstet Gynaecol 1985;92:240-246.
5. Namekawa K, Kasai C, Tsukamoto M, Koyano A: Imaging of blood flow using autocorrelation. Ultrasound Med Biol 1982;8:138-142.
6. Kurjak A, Zalud I, Jurkovic D, et al: Transvaginal color Doppler for the assessment of pelvic circulation. Acta Obstet Gynecol Scand 1989;68:1231-1235.
7. Hata T, Hata K, Senoh D, et al: Doppler ultrasound assessment of tumor vascularity in gynecologic disorders. J Ultrasound Med 1989;8:309-314.
8. Bourne T, Campbell S, Steer C, et al: Transvaginal colour flow imaging: A possible new screening technique for ovarian cancer. BMJ 1989;299:1367-1370.
9. Fleischer AC, Rogers WH, Rao BK, et al: Transvaginal color Doppler sonography of ovarian masses with pathological correlation. Ultrasound Obstet Gynecol 1991;1:275-278.
10. Fleischer AC, Rodgers WH, Rao BK, et al: Assessment of ovarian tumor vascularity with transvaginal color Doppler sonography. J Ultrasound Med 1991;10:563-568.
11. Kremkau FW: Diagnostic Ultrasound: Principles and Instruments, 4th ed. Philadelphia, WB Saunders, 1993.
12. McDicken WN: Diagnostic Ultrasonics: Principles and Use of Instruments, 3rd ed. Edinburgh, Churchill Livingstone, 1991.
13. Timor-Tritsch IE, Rottem S (eds): Transvaginal Ultrasound, 2nd ed. New York, Chapman & Hall, 1991.
14. Hykes DL, Hedrick WR, Starchman DE: Ultrasound Physics and Instrumentation, 2nd ed. Chicago, Mosby-Year Book, 1992.
15. Chervenak FA, Isaacson GC, Campbell S (eds): Ultrasound in Obstetrics and Gynaecology. Boston, Little, Brown, 1993.
16. Jaffe R, Warsof SL: Color Doppler Imaging in Obstetrics and Gynecology. New York, McGraw-Hill, 1992.
17. Kurjak A (ed): An Atlas of Transvaginal Color Doppler: The Current State of the Art. London, Parthenon Publishing Group, 1993.
18. Copel JA, Reed KL (eds): Doppler Ultrasound in Obstetrics and Gynecology. New York, Raven Press, 1994.
19. Sladkevicius P: Doppler ultrasound studies in gynecology [thesis]. Malmo, Sweden, University of Lund, 1994.
20. Jaffe R, Pierson RA, Abramawowicz JS (eds): Imaging in Infertility and Reproductive Endocrinology. Philadelphia, JB Lippincott, 1994.
21. Thaler I, Manor D, Brandes J, et al: Basic principles and clinical applications of the transvaginal Doppler duplex system in reproductive medicine. J In Vitro Fert Embryo Transf 1990;7:74-85.
22. Gosling RG, King DH: Ultrasonic angiology. In Harens AW, Adamson L (eds): Arteries and Veins. Edinburgh, Churchill Livingstone, 1975, p 61.
23. Pourcelot L: Applications clinique de l'examen Doppler transcutane. In Peronneau P (ed): Velocimetric Ultrasonore Doppler. Paris, Inserm, 1974, p 213.
24. Stuart B, Drumm J, Fitzgerald DE, Duignan N: Fetal blood velocity waveforms in normal pregnancy. Br J Obstet Gynaecol 1980;87:780-785.
25. Maulik D, Saini VD, Nanda NC, Rosenzeig MS: Doppler evaluation of fetal hemodynamics. Ultrasound Med Biol 1982;8:705-710.
26. Maulik D: Sonographic color flow mapping: Basic principles. In Maulik D (ed): Doppler Ultrasound in Obstetrics and Gynecology, 2nd ed. Heidelberg, Germany, Springer Verlag, 2005.
27. de Crespigny LC: Demonstration of ectopic pregnancy by transvaginal ultrasound. Br J Obstet Gynaecol 1988;95:1253-1256.
28. Nyberg DA, Mack LA, Jeffrey RB, Laing FC: Endovaginal sonographic evaluation of ectopic pregnancy: A prospective study. AJR Am J Roentgenol 1987;149:1181-1186.
29. Dashefsky SM, Lyons EA, Levi CS, et al: Suspected ectopic pregnancy: Endovaginal and transvesical US. Radiology 1988;169:181-184.
30. Rempen A: Vaginal sonography in ectopic pregnancy: Prospective evaluation. J Ultrasound Med 1988;7:381-387.
31. Cacciatore B, Stenman U-H, Ylostalo P: Comparison of abdominal and vaginal sonography in suspected ectopic pregnancy. Obstet Gynecol 1989;73:770-774.
32. Timor-Tritsch IE, Yeh MN, Peisner DB, et al: The use of transvaginal ultrasonography in the diagnosis of ectopic pregnancy. Am J Obstet Gynecol 1989;161:157-161.
33. Dillon EH, Feyock AL, Taylor KJW: Pseudogestational sacs: Doppler US differentiation from normal or abnormal intrauterine pregnancies. Radiology 1990;176:359-364.
34. Pellerito JS, Taylor KJW: Ectopic pregnancy. In Copel JA, Reed KL (eds): Doppler Ultrasound in Obstetrics and Gynecology. New York, Raven Press, 1995, p 41.
35. Pellerito JS, Taylor KJW, Quedens-Case C, et al: Ectopic pregnancy: Evaluation with endovaginal color flow imaging. Radiology 1992; 183:407-411.
36. Rottem S, Timor-Tritsch IE: Think ectopic. In Timor-Tritsch IE, Rottem S (eds): Transvaginal Sonography, 2nd ed. New York, Chapman & Hall, 1991, p 373.
37. Kurjak A, Zalud I, Schulman H: Ectopic pregnancy: Transvaginal color Doppler of trophoblastic flow in questionable adnexa. J Ultrasound Med 1991;10:685-689.
38. Taylor KJW, Ramos IM, Feyock AL, et al: Ectopic pregnancy: Duplex Doppler evaluation. Radiology 1989;173:93-96.
39. Taylor KJW, Meyer WR: New techniques in the diagnosis of ectopic pregnancy. Obstet Gynecol Clin North Am 1991;18:39-54.
40. Emerson DS, Cartier MS, Altieri LA, et al: Diagnostic efficacy of endovaginal color Doppler flow imaging in an ectopic pregnancy screening program. Radiology 1992;183:413-420.
41. Jaffe R, Warsof SL: Color Doppler imaging in the assesssment of uteroplacental blood flow in abnormal first trimester intrauterine pregnancy: An attempt to define etiologic mechanisms. J Ultrasound Med 1992;11:42.
42. Kirchler HC, Kolle D, Schwegel P: Changes in tubal blood flow in evaluating ectopic pregnancy. Ultrasound Obstet Gynecol 1992;2:283-288.
43. Tekay A, Jouppila P: Color Doppler flow as an indicator of trophoblastic activity in tubal pregnancies detected by transvaginal ultrasound. Obstet Gynecol 1992;80:995-999.
44. Megier P, Desroches A: Color and pulsed Doppler ultrasonography imaging of tubal ectopic pregnancy: Study of 100 cases. J Radiol 2003;84:1753-1756.
45. Jurkovic D, Bourne TH, Jauniaux E, et al: Transvaginal color Doppler study of blood flow in ectopic pregnancies. Fertil Steril 1992;57:68-73.
46. Atri M: Ectopic pregnancy versus corpus luteum cyst revisited: Best Doppler predictors. J Ultrasound Med 2003;22:1181-1184.
47. Szabo I, Csabay L, Belics Z, et al: Assessment of uterine circulation in ectopic pregnancy by transvaginal color Doppler. Eur J Obstet Gynecol Reprod Biol 2003;106:203-208.

48. Stein MW, Ricci ZJ, Novak L, et al: Sonographic comparison of the tubal ring of ectopic pregnancy with the corpus luteum. J Ultrasound Med 2004;23:57-62.

49. Atri M: Ectopic pregnancy: Evaluation with endovaginal color Doppler flow imaging. Radiology 1993;187:19.

50. Brown DL: Diagnosis of ectopic pregnancy with endovaginal color Doppler US. Radiology 1993;187:20-24.

51. Pellerito JS, Taylor KJW: Ectopic pregnancy: Evaluation with endovaginal color Doppler flow imaging-response. Radiology 1993;187:21-27.

52. Bernardini L, Valenzano M, Foglia G: Spontaneous interstitial pregnancy on a tubal stump after unilateral adenectomy followed by transvaginal colour Doppler ultrasound. Hum Reprod 1998;13:1723-1726.

53. Vicino M, Loverro G, Resta L, et al: Laparoscopic cornual excision in a viable large interstitial pregnancy without blood flow detected by color Doppler ultrasonography. Fertil Steril 2000;74:407-409.

54. Timor-Tritsch IE, Monteagudo A, Matera C, Veit RC: Sonographic evaluation of cornual pregnancies treated without surgery. Obstet Gynecol 1992;79:1044-1049.

55. Timor-Tritsch IE, Monteagudo A, Mandeville ED, et al: Successful management of viable cervical pregnancy by local injection of methotrexate guided by transvaginal sonography. Am J Obstet Gynecol 1994;170:737-739.

56. Su YN, Shih JC, Chiu WH, et al: Cervical pregnancy: Assessment with three-dimensional power Doppler imaging and successful management with selective uterine artery embolization. Ultrasound Obstet Gynecol 1999;14:284-287.

57. Monteagudo A, Minior VK, Stephenson C, et al: Non-surgical management of live ectopic pregnancy with ultrasound-guided local injection: A case series. Ultrasound Obstet Gynecol 2005;25:282-288.

58. Roussis P, Ball RH, Fleischer AC, Herbert CM: Cervical pregnancy: A case report. J Reprod Med 1992;37:479-481.

59. Chou MM, Hwang JI, Tseng JJ, et al: Cesarean scar pregnancy: Quantitative assessment of uterine neovascularization with 3-dimensional color power Doppler imaging and successful treatment with uterine artery embolization. Am J Obstet Gynecol 2004;190:866-868.

60. Seow KM, Huang LW, Lin YH, et al: Cesarean scar pregnancy: Issues in management. Ultrasound Obstet Gynecol 2004;23:247-253.

61. Granberg S, Wikland M, Jansson I: Macroscopic characterization of ovarian tumors and the relation to the histological diagnosis: Criteria to be used for ultrasound evaluation. Gynecol Oncol 1989;35:139-144.

62. Granberg S, Norstrom A, Wikland M: Tumors in the lower pelvis as imaged by vaginal sonography. Gynecol Oncol 1990;37:224-229.

63. Sassone AM, Timor-Tritsch IE, Artner A, et al: Transvaginal sonographic characterization of ovarian disease: Evaluation of a new scoring system to predict ovarian malignancy. Obstet Gynecol 1991;78:70-76.

64. Ferrazzi E, Zanetta G, Dordoni D, et al: Transvaginal ultrasonographic characterization of ovarian masses: Comparison of five scoring systems in a multicenter study. Ultrasound Obstet Gynecol 1997;10:192-197.

65. Timmerman D, Schwarzler P, Collins WP, et al: Subjective assessment of adnexal masses with the use of ultrasonography: An analysis of interobserver variability and experience. Ultrasound Obstet Gynecol 1999;13:11-16.

66. Timmerman D, Verrelst H, Bourne TH, et al: Artificial neural network models for the preoperative discrimination between malignant and benign adnexal masses. Ultrasound Obstet Gynecol 1999;13:17-25.

67. Timmerman D, Valentin L, Bourne TH, et al: Terms, definitions and measurements to describe the sonographic features of adnexal tumors: A consensus opinion from the International Ovarian Tumor Analysis (IOTA) Group. Ultrasound Obstet Gynecol 2000;16:500-505.

68. Strickland B: The value of arteriography in the diagnosis of bone tumors. Br J Radiol 1959;32:705-709.

69. Folkman J, Merler E, Abernathy C, Williams G: Isolation of a tumor factor responsible for angiogenesis. J Exp Med 1971;133:275-288.

70. Folkman J: Tumor angiogenesis. Adv Cancer Res 1985;43:175-200.

71. Shubick P: Vascularization of tumors: A review. J Cancer Res Clin Oncol 1982;103:211-216.

72. Jain RK, Ward-Harley K: Tumor blood flow-characterization, modifications and role in hyperthermia. Trans Sonics Ultrasonics 1984;31:504-509.

73. Jain RK: Determination of tumor blood flow: A review. Cancer Res 1988;48:2641-2646.

74. Hata K, Hata T, Seoh O, et al: Transition of ovarian arterial compliance during the human menstrual cycle, assessed by Doppler ultrasound-correlation with serum hormone levels. Nippon Sanka Fujinka Gakkai Zasshi 1990;42:662-666.

75. Hata K, Hata T, Senoh D, et al: Change in ovarian arterial compliance during the human menstrual cycle assessed by Doppler ultrasound. Br J Obstet Gynaecol 1990;97:163-166.

76. Kurjak A, Zalud I, Alfirevic A: Evaluation of adnexal masses with transvaginal color ultrasound. J Ultrasound Med 1991;10:295-297.

77. Hata K, Makihara K, Hata T, et al: Transvaginal color Doppler imaging for hemodynamic assessment of reproductive tract tumors. Int J Gynaecol Obstet 1991;36:301-308.

78. Bourne TH, Campbell S, Steer CV, et al: Detection of endometrial cancer by transvaginal ultrasonography with color flow imaging and blood flow analysis: A preliminary report. Gynecol Oncol 1991;40:253-259.

79. Bourne TH, Jurkovic D, Waterstone J, et al: Intrafollicular blood flow during human ovulation. Ultrasound Obstet Gynecol 1991;1:53-59.

80. Kurjak A: Ultrasound and ovarian cancer [editorial]. Ultrasound Obstet Gynecol 1991;1:231-233.

81. Hata K, Hata T, Manabe A, Kitao M: Ovarian tumors of low malignant potential: Transvaginal Doppler ultrasound features. Gynecol Oncol 1992;45:259-264.

82. Weiner Z, Thaler I, Beck D, et al: Differentiating malignant from benign ovarian tumors with transvaginal color flow imaging. Obstet Gynecol 1992;79:159-162.

83. Hata K, Hata T, Manabe A, et al: A critical evaluation of transvaginal Doppler studies, transvaginal sonography, magnetic resonance imaging, and CA 125 in detecting ovarian cancer. Obstet Gynecol 1992;80:922-926.

84. Hata K, Hata T, Manabe A, et al: New pelvic sonoangiography for detection of endometrial carcinoma: A preliminary report. Gynecol Oncol 1992;45:179-184.

85. Kawai M, Kano T, Kikkawa F, et al: Transvaginal Doppler ultrasound with color flow imaging in the diagnosis of ovarian cancer. Obstet Gynecol 1992;79:163-167.

86. Natori M, Kouno H, Nozawa S: Flow velocity waveform analysis for the detection of ovarian cancer. Med Rev 1992;40:45-50.

87. Kurjak A, Kupesic-Urek S: Transvaginal color Doppler in early detection of ovarian cancer. J Eur Med Ultrasound 1992;12:15-17.

88. Timor-Tritsch IE, Lerner JP, Monteagudo A, Santos R: Transvaginal ultrasonographic characterization of ovarian masses by means of color flow-directed Doppler measurements and a morphologic scoring system. Am J Obstet Gynecol 1993;168:909-913.

89. Kurjak A, Schulman H, Sosic A, et al: Transvaginal ultrasound, color flow and Doppler waveform of the postmenopausal adnexal mass. Obstet Gynecol 1993;80:917-921.

90. Bourne TH, Campbell S, Reynolds KM, et al: Screening for early familial ovarian cancer with transvaginal ultrasonography and colour blood flow imaging. BMJ 1993;306:1025-1029.

91. Tekay A, Jouppila P: Intraobserver variation in transvaginal Doppler blood flow measurements in benign ovarian tumors. Ultrasound Obstet Gynecol 1997;9:120-124.

92. Guerriero S, Alcazar JL, Ajossa S, et al: Comparison of conventional color Doppler imaging and power Doppler imaging for the diagnosis of ovarian cancer: Results of a European study. Gynecol Oncol 2001;83:299-304.

93. Kurjak A, Kupesic S, Sparac V, Kosuta D: Three-dimensional ultrasonographic and power Doppler characterization of ovarian lesions. Ultrasound Obstet Gynecol 2000;16:365-371.

94. Raine-Fenning NJ, Campbell BK, Clewes JS, et al: The reliability of virtual organ computer-aided analysis (VOCAL) for the semiquantification of ovarian, endometrial and subendometrial perfusion. Ultrasound Obstet Gynecol 2003;22:633-639.

95. Kurjak A, Kupesic S, Sparac V, et al: The detection of stage I ovarian cancer by three-dimensional sonography and power Doppler. Gynecol Oncol 2003;90:258-264.

96. Cohen LS, Escobar PF, Scharm C, et al: Three-dimensional power Doppler ultrasound improves the diagnostic accuracy for ovarian cancer prediction. Gynecol Oncol 2001;82:40-48.

97. Graif M, Shalev J, Strauss S, et al: Torsion of the ovary: Sonographic features. AJR Am J Roentgenol 1984;143:1331-1334.

98. Warner M, Fleischer AC, Edell SL, et al: Uterine adnexal torsion: Sonographic findings. Radiology 1985;154:773-775.

99. Bider D, Ben-Rafael Z, Goldenberg M, et al: Outcome of pregnancy after unwinding of ischaemic-haemorrhagic adnexa. Br J Obstet Gynaecol 1989;96:428-430.

100. Ben-Rafael Z, Bider D, Mashiach S: Unwinding of ischaemic haemorrhagic adnexum via laparoscopy. Fertil Steril 1990;53:569-571.

101. Gordon JD, Hopkins KL, Jeffrey RB, Giudice LC: Adnexal torsion: Color Doppler diagnosis and laparoscopic treatment. Fertil Steril 1994;61:383-385.

102. Fleischer AC, Stein SM, Cullinan JA, Warner MA: Color Doppler sonography of adnexal torsion. Paper presented at the 39th Annual Convention of AIUM, March 26-29, 1995, San Francisco.
103. Van Voorhis BJ, Schwaiger J, Syrop CH, Chapter FK: Early diagnosis of ovarian torsion by color Doppler ultrasonography. Fertil Steril 1992;58:215-217.
104. Rosado W, Trambert M, Gosink B, Pretorius D: Adnexal torsion: Diagnosis by using Doppler sonography. Am J Radiol 1992;159:1251-1253.
105. Schiller VL, Grant EG: Doppler ultrasonography of the pelvis. Radiol Clin North Am 1992;30:735-742.
106. Fleischer AC, Kepple DM: Transvaginal color Doppler sonography: Clinical potentials and limitations. Semin Ultrasound CT MR 1992;13:69-80.
107. Nichols D, Julian P: Torsion of the adnexa. Clin Obstet Gynecol 1985;28:375-380.
108. Elchalad U, Caspi B, Schachter M: Isolated tubal torsion: Clinical and ultrasonographic features. J Ultrasound Med 1993;2:115-117.
109. Sherer DM, Liberto L, Abramovicz JS, Words JR: Endovaginal sonographic features associated with isolated torsion of the fallopian tube. J Ultrasound Med 1991;10:107-109.
110. Auslender R, Lavie O, Kaufman Y: Coiling of the ovarian vessels: A color Doppler sign for adnexal torsion without strangulation. Ultrasound Obstet Gynecol 2002;20:96-97.
111. Lee EJ, Kwon HC, Joo HJ: Diagnosis of ovarian torsion with color Doppler sonography: Depiction of twisted vascular pedicle. J Ultrasound Med 1998;17:83-89.
112. Beard RW, Reginald PW, Pearce S: Pelvic pain in women: BMJ 1986;293:1160-1162.
113. Beard RW, Reginald PW, Wadsworth J: Clinical features of women with chronic lower abdominal pain and pelvic congestion. Br J Obstet Gynaecol 1988;95:153-161.
114. Reginald PW, Pearce S, Beard R: Pelvic pain due to venous congestion. Prog Obstet Gynecol 1990;13:275-292.
115. Kaupila A: Uterine phlebography with venous compression: A clinical and roentgenological study. Acta Obstet Gynecol Scand 1970;49:33-34.
116. Beard RW, Belsey EM, Liberman BA, Wilkinson JCM: Pelvic pain in women. Am J Obstet Gynecol 1977;128:566-570.
117. Sterns HC, Sneeden UD: Observations on the clinical and pathological aspects of the pelvic congestion syndrome. Am J Obstet Gynecol 1966;94:718-732.
118. Renaer M: Chronic pelvic pain without obvious pathology. In Chronic Pelvic Pain in Women. New York, Springer, 1981, p 162.
119. Juhasz B, Kurjak A, Lampe LG: Pelvic varices simulating bilateral adnexal masses: Differential diagnosis by vaginal color Doppler. J Clin Ultrasound 1992;20:81-84.
120. Berger RB, Taylor KJW, Rosenfield AT: Pelvic varices simulating cystic ovaries: Differentiation by pulsed Doppler. J Clin Ultrasound 1992;10:186-189.
121. Jain KA, Jeffrey RB, Sommer FG: Gynaecologic vascular abnormalities: Diagnosis with Doppler US. Radiology 1991;178:549-551.
122. Bonilla-Musoles F, Ballester MJ: Transvaginal color Doppler in the diagnosis of pelvic congestion syndrome. In Kurjak A (ed): An Atlas of Transvaginal Color Doppler. London, Parthenon Publishing Group, 1994, p 207.
123. Hobbs JT: The pelvic congestion syndrome. Br J Hosp Med 1990;43:200-206.
124. Park SJ, Lim JW, Ko YT, et al: Diagnosis of pelvic congestion syndrome using transabdominal and transvaginal sonography. AJR Am J Roentgenol 2004;182:683-688.
125. Randolph RJ, Kang Ying Y, Maier DB, et al: Comparison of real-time ultrasonography, hysterosalpingography and laparoscopy/hysteroscopy in the evaluation of uterine abnormalities and tubal patency. Fertil Steril 1986;46:828-832.
126. Richman TS, Viscomi CN, de Cherney A, et al: Fallopian tubal patency assessed by ultrasound following fluid injection. Radiology 1984;152:507-510.
127. Volpi E, De-Gradis T, Sismondi P, et al: Transvaginal salpingosonography (TSSG) in the evaluation of tubal patency. Acta Curr Fertil 1991;22:2325-2328.
128. Mitri FF, Andronikou AD, Perpinyal S, et al: A clinical comparison of sonographic hydrotubation and hysterosalpingography. Br J Obstet Gynaecol 1991;98:1031-1036.
129. Allahbadia GN, Nalawade YV, Patkar VD, et al: The Sion test. Aust N Z J Obstet Gynecol 1992;32:67-70.
130. Tufekci EC, Girit S, Gayirli E, et al: Evaluation of tubal patency by transvaginal sonosalpingography. Fertil Steril 1992;57:336-340.
131. Hotel J, Rassmunsen C, Morris H: First clinical experience with sonicated albumin (Albunex) as an intrafallopian ultrasound contrast medium. Ultrasound Obstet Gynecol 1993;3:106.
132. Deichert V, Schlief R, Sandt H, Juhnke I: Transvaginal hysterosalpingo-contrast sonography (HyCoSy) compared with conventional tubal diagnostics. Hum Reprod 1989;4:418-424.
133. Schlief R, Deichert U: Hysterosalpingo-contrast sonography of the uterus and fallopian tubes: Results of a clinical trial of a new contrast medium in 120 patients. Radiology 1991;178:213-215.
134. Fobbe F, Becker R, Koch HC, et al: The demonstration of the patency of the uterine tubes with color-coded duplex sonography in combination with ultrasonic contrast media. Rofo Fortschr Geb Rontgenstr Neuen Bildgeb Verfahr 1991;154:349-353.
135. Venezia R, Zangara C: Echohysterosalpingography: New diagnostic possibilities with SHU 450 Echovist. Acta Eur Fertil 1991;22:279-282.
136. Deichert U, Schlief R, van de Sandt M, Daume E: Transvaginal hysterosalpingo-contrast sonography for the assessment of tubal patency with gray scale imaging and additional use of pulsed wave Doppler. Fertil Steril 1992;57:62-67.
137. Balen FG, Allen CM, Siddle NC, Lees WR: Ultrasound contrast hysterosalpingography—evaluation as an outpatient procedure. Br J Radiol 1993;66:592-599.
138. Bonilla-Musoles F, Simon C, Serra V, et al: An assessment of hysterosalpingosonography (HSSG) as a diagnostic tool for uterine cavity defects and tubal patency. J Clin Ultrasound 1992;20:175-181.
139. Crequat J, Pennehouat G, Cornier E, et al: Evaluation of intrauterine pathology and tubal patency by contrast echography. Contracept Fertil Sex 1993;21:861-864.
140. Friberg B, Joergensen C: Tubal patency studied by ultrasonography: A pilot study. Acta Obstet Gynecol Scand 1994;73:53-55.
141. Stern J, Peters AJ, Coulam CB: Color Doppler ultrasonography assessment of tubal patency: A comparison study with traditional techniques. Fertil Steril 1992;58:897-900.
142. Allahbadia GN: Fallopian tube patency using color Doppler. Int J Gynaecol Obstet 1993;40:241-244.
143. Peters AJ, Coulam CB: Hysterosalpingography with color Doppler ultrasonography. Am J Obstet Gynecol 1991;164:1530-1534.
144. Sladkevicius P, Valentin L, Marsal K: Blood flow velocity in the uterine artery and ovarian arteries during the normal menstrual cycle. Ultrasound Obstet Gynecol 1993;3:199-208.
145. Sladkevicus P, Valentin L, Marsal K: Blood flow velocity in the uterine and ovarian arteries during menstruation. Ultrasound Obstet Gynecol 1994;4:421-427.
146. Guy GP, Peisner DB, Timor-Tritsch IE: Ultrasound evaluation of uteroplacental blood flow patterns of abnormally located and adherent placentas. Am J Obstet Gynecol 1990;163:723-727.
147. Comstock CH, Lee W, Vettraino IM, et al: The early sonographic appearance of placenta accreta. J Ultrasound Med 2003;22:19-23.
148. Comstock CH, Love JJ Jr, Bronsteen RA, et al: Sonographic detection of placenta accreta in the second and third trimesters of pregnancy. Am J Obstet Gynecol 2004;190:1135-1140.
149. Taipale P, Orden MR, Berg M, et al: Prenatal diagnosis of placenta accreta and percreta with ultrasonography, color Doppler, and magnetic resonance imaging. Obstet Gynecol 2004;104:537-540.
150. Deckner C, Schiesser M, Bastert G: Diagnosis of uterine vascular malformation using Doppler ultrasound. Ultraschall Med 2004;25:141-143.
151. Kelly SM, Belli AM, Campbell S: Arteriovenous malformation of the uterus associated with secondary postpartum hemorrhage. Ultrasound Obstet Gynecol 2003;21:602-605.
152. Timmerman D, Wauters J, Van Calenbergh S, et al: Color Doppler imaging is a valuable tool for the diagnosis and management of uterine vascular malformations. Ultrasound Obstet Gynecol 2003;21:570-577.
153. Kurjak A, Kupesic-Urek S, Miric D: The assessment of benign uterine tumors by transvaginal color Doppler. Ultrasound Med Biol 1992;18:645-649.
154. Carter J, Perrone T, Carson L, et al: Uterine malignancy predicted by transvaginal sonography and color flow Doppler ultrasonography. J Clin Ultrasound 1993;21:405-408.
155. Fleischer AC, Kepple DM: Benign conditions of the uterus, cervix and endometrium. In Nyberg DA, Hill LM, Bohm-Velez M, Mendelson EB (eds): Transvaginal Ultrasound. St Louis, Mosby-Year Book, 1992, p 38.
156. Fleischer AC, Gordon AN, Entman SS: Transvaginal scanning of the endometrium. J Clin Ultrasound 1990;18:337-349.
157. Bourne TH, Reynold KMM, Campbell S: Screening for ovarian and uterine carcinoma. In Nyberg DA, Hill LM, Bohm-Velez M, Mendelson

EB (eds): Transvaginal Ultrasound. St Louis, Mosby-Year Book, 1992, p 267.

158. Kurjak A, Shalan H, Sosic A, et al: Endometrial carcinoma in post-menopausal women: Evaluation by transvaginal color Doppler sonography. Am J Obstet Gynecol 1993;169:1597-1603.

159. Kupesic-Urek S, Shalan H, Kurjak A: Early detection of endometrial cancer by transvaginal color Doppler. Eur J Obstet Gynecol 1993;49:46-49.

160. Hata K, Hata T, Manabe A, et al: New pelvic sonoangiography for detection of endometrial carcinoma: A preliminary report. Gynecol Oncol 1992;45:179-184.

161. Tal J, Timor-Tritsch I, Degani S: Accurate diagnosis of postabortal placental remnant by sonohysterography and color Doppler sonographic studies. Gynecol Obstet Invest 1997;43:131-134.

162. Shimamoto K, Sakuma S, Ishigaki T, Makino N: Intratumoral blood flow: Evaluating with color Doppler echography. Radiology 1987;165:683-685.

163. Aoki S, Hata H, Hata K, et al: Doppler color flow mapping on an invasive mole. Gynecol Obstet Invest 1989;27:52-54.

164. Flam F: Colour flow Doppler for gestational trophoblastic neoplasia. Eur J Gynaecol Oncol 1994;15:443-448.

165. Hsieh FJ, Wu CC, Lee CN, et al: Vascular patterns of gestational trophoblastic tumors by color Doppler ultrasound. Cancer 1994;74:2361-2365.

166. Oguz S, Sargin A, Aytan H, et al: Doppler study of myometrium in invasive gestational trophoblastic disease. Int J Gynecol Cancer 2004;14:972-979.

167. Tsukihara S, Harada T, Terakawa N: Ultrasound-guided local injection of methotrexate to treat an invasive hydatidiform mole. J Obstet Gynaceol Res 2004;30:202-204.

168. Desai RK, Desberg AL: Diagnosis of gestational trophoblastic disease: Value of endovaginal color flow Doppler. Am J Radiol 1991;157:787-788.

169. Matijevic R, Kurjak A, Shalan H: New approach to diagnose gestational trophoblastic disease by transvaginal color Doppler sonography. Ultrasound Obstet Gynecol 1991;2:133.

170. Matijevic R, Kurjak A, Shalan H: Predicting malignancy in gestational trophoblastic disease by transvaginal color and pulsed Doppler sonography. Ultrasound Obstet Gynecol 1992;1:133.

171. Kurjak A, Matijevic R, Kupesic S, Malda K: Gestational trophoblastic disease. In Kurjak A (ed): An Atlas of Transvaginal Color Doppler. London, Parthenon Publishing Group, 1994, p 125.

Chapter 18

Transvaginal Sonography and Ovarian Cancer

Leeber Cohen and David A. Fishman

There is little doubt that transvaginal sonography (TVS) is an imaging modality that every practitioner of obstetrics and gynecology should be able to perform and interpret. It is difficult to contemplate the management of threatened abortion in early pregnancy or the evaluation of suspected ectopic pregnancy without this powerful tool. It also has become abundantly clear that bimanual examination is very inaccurate in the identification of adnexal masses. A study by Padilla et al.[1] clearly demonstrated that even under general anesthesia, more than two thirds of adnexal masses were missed. Furthermore, residents and attending physicians identified such masses only marginally better than medical students. Goldstein[2] made a powerful argument that TVS should be incorporated into routine gynecologic visits even in asymptomatic women. Others disagree, arguing that the costs, unnecessary surgical interventions, and lack of evidence that ovarian cancer deaths would be decreased speak against routine transvaginal screening at annual visits in asymptomatic women.[3]

It is critical that the gynecologic practitioner understand the cyclic nature of ovarian activity as well as the protocols for avoiding operating unnecessarily on follicular and hemorrhagic cysts. The propensity of hydrosalpinges and peritoneal inflammatory processes to masquerade as ovarian neoplasms must also be understood. A knowledge of the most common ovarian tumor types and their echo characteristics is also required.

Epidemiology

Ovarian cancer is the fifth leading cause of cancer death in women, after cancer of the lung, breast, colon, and pancreas. In 2002 there were 23,300 new cases with 13,900 deaths. At 45 years of age a low-risk woman has a 1/2500 annual risk for development of ovarian cancer, with a 1.6% lifetime risk. Risk factors include nulliparity, decreased fertility, early onset of menses, and late menopause. High-risk women include those with personal history or strong family history of breast, ovarian, and colon cancer. Other high-risk women include those with known *BRCA* mutations and Lynch-type syn-

dromes. Ninety percent of women are diagnosed at 45 years of age and older. The great majority of these cases are of epithelial origin, with 70% to 75% diagnosed at stage III to IV. The 5-year survival rate for advanced-stage disease is only 10% to 15%, even with the use of aggressive surgical debulking and newer chemotherapy regimens.[4-6]

Interpretation of adnexal sonography is complicated by the constantly changing appearance of the ovary as it responds to cyclic hormonal fluctuation. Cysts greater than 2.5 cm in diameter are not uncommon in asymptomatic premenopausal women. Borgfeldt and Andolf[7] identified a cyst greater than 2.5 cm in 6% of women aged 25 to 40 years. Schulman et al.[8] identified cystic masses greater than 2.5 cm in 13% of premenopausal women. The series of Osmers et al.[9] included 1072 premenopausal ovarian masses, of which 570 were functional cysts and corpora lutea, 264 were endometriotic cysts, 192 were benign neoplasms, and 46 were malignancies. Surgery was avoided in 90% of the functional cysts and corpora lutea by rescanning in 6 weeks and placing the patients on birth control medication if the cyst was not resolved, and then rescanning 6 weeks later.[9] These findings are similar to those of Pinotti et al.,[10] who found that 61% of cystic ovarian masses resolved spontaneously.

The role of birth control pills in the treatment of persistent cysts is unclear. A paper by Spanos[11] popularized the preoperative hormonal therapy of cystic adnexal masses. In his series, 81 of 286 cystic masses persisted after hormonal treatment for 6 weeks. A small, randomized series by Steinkampf et al.[12] from 1990 of 48 patients with functional cysts failed to demonstrate a benefit of hormonal suppression by birth control pills versus expectant management without hormonal suppression (Figs. 18–1 through 18–10).

The appearance of the corpus luteum and resorbing hemorrhagic cyst can easily be misinterpreted by the inexperienced sonologist. The endosalpingeal folds in a hydrosalpinx as well as the small, excrescence-like structures seen with these hydrosalpinges can also be mistaken for neoplasia. Multiloculated, fluid-filled peritoneal inclusion cysts that appear after pelvic inflammatory processes, myomectomy, surgery for endometriosis, bowel surgery, or transplantation can be

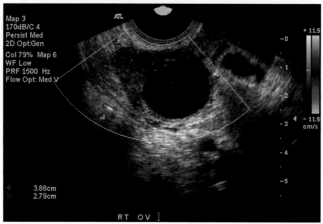

Figure 18–1. A typical follicular cyst in a 28-year-old woman. This follicular cyst measures approximately 2 cm in mean diameter. It is thin walled. No excrescences or mural nodules are noted. Peripheral vascular flow in this example is not unusual. Rescan of the patient two menstrual cycles later revealed spontaneous resolution of the cyst. Patients are normally scheduled for scanning on days 5 to 10 of the menstrual cycle to avoid new follicles and ovulation. Follicular cysts are usually less than 5 cm in mean diameter. However, persistent follicular cysts as large as 8 cm can be encountered. Spontaneous resolution usually occurs within 2 months but may take up to 4 months. The role of birth control pills for treating persistent simple cystic masses thought to be follicular cysts remains controversial. When these cysts fail to resolve, the most commonly found lesion is cystadenoma.

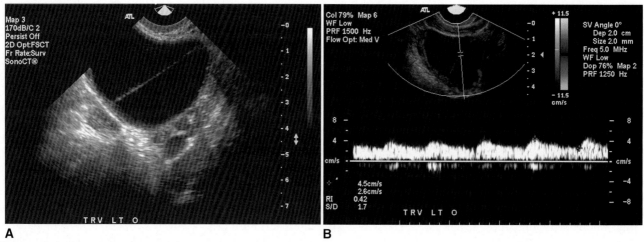

A   **B**

Figure 18–2. **A,** A follicular cyst in a 30-year-old patient. The mean diameter is 2.5 cm. The cyst wall is thin. No excrescences or mural nodules are noted. The septation is thin (<2 mm). Single or multiple thin septations can be seen within follicular cysts. **B,** Color Doppler reveals intermediate-resistance flow (resistance index, 0.42) within the septation. Peripheral flow is noted in the cyst wall. Peripheral flow and flow in thin septations are not uncommon features of physiologic follicular cysts. This cyst spontaneously resolved. Even if the RI had been low (≤0.4), expectant management would still have been followed in this case.

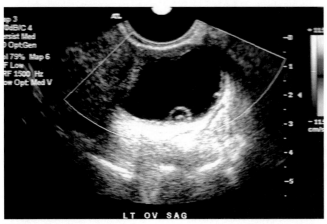

Figure 18–3. A follicular cyst. Subcysts are another feature that can be seen in physiologic follicular cysts. This cyst also resolved spontaneously.

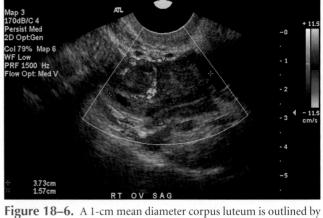

Figure 18–6. A 1-cm mean diameter corpus luteum is outlined by peripheral vascular flow. Typically, the corpus luteum is hypoechoic compared with surrounding ovarian tissue.

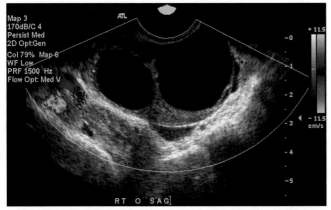

Figure 18–4. Multiple follicular cysts with or without peripheral flow are a common finding in perimenopausal women, as in this 52-year-old women with irregular menses. This patient was rescanned in 2 months, with resolution of these cysts and new ones on the left ovary.

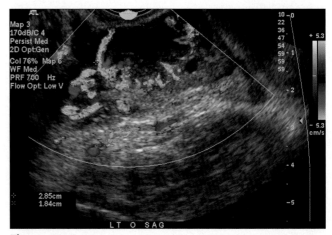

Figure 18–7. This 1.5-cm mean diameter corpus luteum displays circumferential peripheral flow as well as tangential vessels entering the stroma of the corpus luteum. Pulsed Doppler typically reveals low-resistance vessels. To inexperienced eyes, these vessels can be confused with the neovascularization seen in some malignant masses.

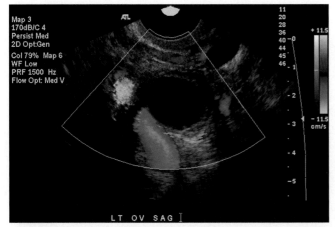

Figure 18–5. A simple 2-cm mean diameter cyst in a postmenopausal women. No solid elements are noted inside the cyst wall and color Doppler is unremarkable. These patients are normally rescanned at 3 months, at 6 months, and at yearly intervals to ensure stability.

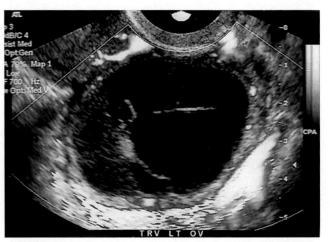

Figure 18–8. This 3.5-cm mean diameter corpus luteum cyst displays the typical appearance of a retracting hemorrhagic clot.

easily confused with adnexal neoplasia (Figs. 18–11 through 18–13).

Excluding functional cysts, hemorrhagic cysts, hydrosalpinges, peritoneal adhesive disease, and paratubal cysts, the most commonly encountered adnexal masses in premenopausal women are endometriomas, cystic teratomas, serous cystadenomas, and mucinous cystadenomas. In the series of Koonings et al.,[13] at 20 to 29 years of age, cystic teratomas, serous cystadenomas, and mucinous cystadenomas are responsible for 72% , 15%, and 11% of benign ovarian neoplasms, respectively. By 40 to 49 years of age, cystic teratomas, serous cystadenomas, and mucinous cystadenomas are responsible for 43%, 46%, and 8% of the benign ovarian neoplasms, respectively. At 60 to 69 years of age, cystic teratomas have decreased to 16% of benign neoplasms, serous cystadenomas have increased to 59%, and mucinous cystadenomas have increased to 11%[13] (Figs. 18–14 through 18–21).

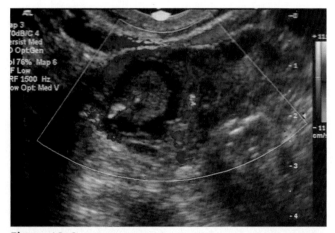

Figure 18–9. This 32-year-old patient had a complex mass with a central mural nodule and central vascular flow that at first glance appeared suspicious for malignancy. Because the patient had a negative follicular study 3 weeks earlier, it was thought unlikely that this represented the onset of a malignant ovarian neoplasm. The patient was rescanned 2 weeks later, after the onset of her menses, and the mass had resolved.

Tamoxifen-stimulated cysts in premenopausal women can be confused with both unilocular and multilocular cystadenomas. These patients can also present with large hemorrhagic cysts and hemoperitoneum (Figs. 18–22 and 18–23).

In the series by Koonings et al.,[13] the risk of an ovarian neoplasm's being frankly malignant is 4% at age 20 to 29 years, 14% at 30 to 39 years, 35% at 40 to 49 years, and 46% at 50 to 59 years. The chances of the neoplasm's being borderline in the same age groups are 2.4%, 5.3%, 6.3%, and 3.9%, respectively. These percentages should not be confused with the chance at surgery that an ovarian mass is malignant, because the percentages do not include endometriomas, hydrosalpinges, and peritoneal adhesive disease, which are frequent causes for surgery.

This series also probably underestimates the number of benign cystadenomas in menopausal women. Owing to the more frequent use of computed tomography, magnetic resonance imaging, and pelvic ultrasound, we now know that 3% to 5% of menopausal women will have cystic masses identified on the ovary. This subject is reviewed later in the section on Asymptomatic Menopausal Cysts. Histologically, they are usually serous cystadenomas.

In women younger than 20 years of age, the most common malignant ovarian neoplasms are malignant germ cell tumors and granulosa cell tumors. By age 40 years, approximately 90% to 95% of malignant ovarian neoplasms are of epithelial origin. Approximately 5% are granulosa cell tumors and the occasional rare malignant germ cell tumor.

Gray-Scale Interpretation

Gray-scale ultrasound is very sensitive but not ideally specific for differentiating between benign and malignant ovarian lesions. Multiple gray-scale scoring systems have been described, but the scoring system of Sassone et al.,[14] introduced in 1991 and later modified by Lerner et al.[15] in 1994, is illustrative. The weighted scoring system assesses and scores wall structure, shadowing, septa, and internal echogenicity. A score of less than 3 was considered benign. Score means were 1.8 for benign masses, 3.9 for tumors of low malignant potential, and 5.6 for malignant tumors. The sensitivity was 96.8%,

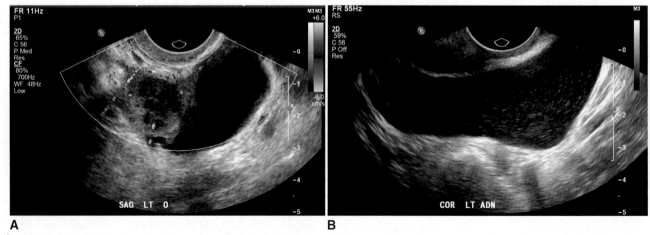

A **B**

Figure 18–10. A, This 38-year-old patient underwent left salpingo-oophorectomy for a large endometrioma. She presented with mid-cycle pain, and an ovarian remnant with central hemorrhagic clot is noted. **B,** A fluid loculation medial to the ovary is clearly displayed.

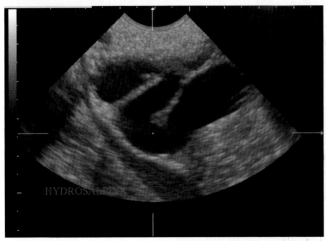

Figure 18–11. A classic two-dimensional image of a hydrosalpinx with endosalpingeal folds. An entire chapter could be dedicated to hydrosalpinges because their appearance can be quite complex. They are frequently a cause of unnecessary surgery because they are interpreted as multiseptate masses suspect for malignancy.

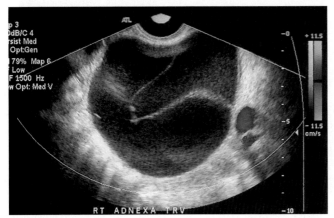

Figure 18–12. Fluid-filled peritoneal adhesive disease. These masses can be seen after subtotal hysterectomy, myomectomy, cystectomy, laser surgery for endometriosis, bowel surgery, and numerous other etiologies. Reoperation is frequently difficult and can lead to bowel perforations and obstruction. Careful history is required, as in this patient who had undergone myomectomy. If surgery is necessary, bowel preparation and a highly qualified gynecologic surgeon experienced in bowel surgery are recommended.

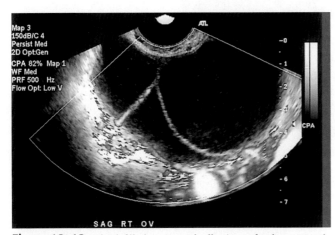

Figure 18–13. Fluid-filled peritoneal adhesions after laparoscopic cholecystectomy with spillage of bile and stones into the pelvis.

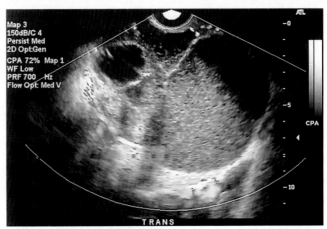

Figure 18–14. This image displays the classic appearance of a benign mucinous cystadenoma. Several locules are noted, with varying degrees of low-level echoes. The power Doppler clearly displays flow in the septations. No solid elements are noted in the locules, which made malignancy unlikely. In addition, back-to-back crowding of the cystic locules is absent.

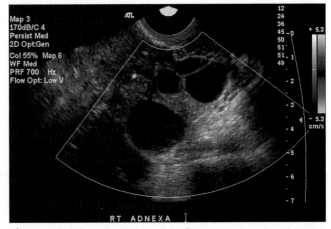

Figure 18–15. This multiloculated mass in a 60-year-old patient was a benign serous cystadenoma. No solid elements are noted within the locules, and Doppler is unremarkable.

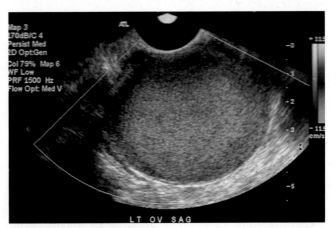

Figure 18–16. The classic appearance of an endometrioma. These masses can be unilocular or multilocular. They are typically filled with low-level uniform echoes, although speckling sometimes is noted. Color Doppler reveals no flow centrally. If recent bleeding has not occurred within the cyst, it may have varying degrees of internal echogenicity and even appear centrally anechoic. Except for physiologic cysts, endometriomas are the most common masses found on the ovary. It should be noted that acute hemorrhagic corpora lutea, mucin, and pus may have internal echogenicity similar to that of endometriomas. History and clinical examination are vital for interpreting imaging studies of the adnexa.

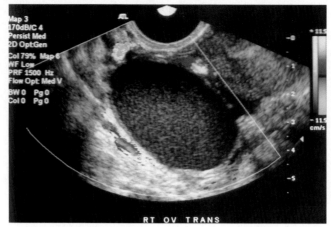

Figure 18–17. A unilocular endometrioma.

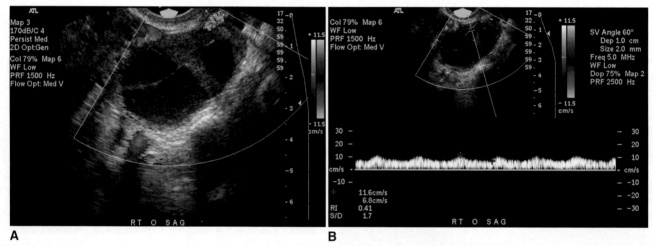

A
B

Figure 18–18. **A,** This perimenopausal 56-year-old patient presented for evaluation of leiomyomas and bleeding. Incidentally, these cystic locules filled with low-level echoes were noted. **B,** Pulsed Doppler examination of the same patient reveals an arteriole with intermediate resistance bordering on low resistance (resistance index, 0.41) on the periphery of the cysts. Pathologic study revealed benign endometriomas.

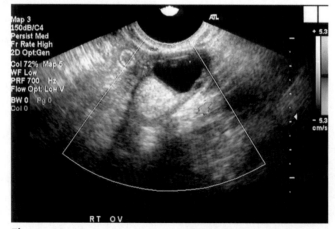

Figure 18–19. A 28-year-old patient with the classic appearance of a cystic teratoma. A 1.5-cm, well-circumscribed, densely echogenic mass with posterior shadowing is clearly seen. No flow is noted in the densely echogenic core. Flow may be noted if the cystic teratoma contains thyroid tissue (struma ovarii). Cystic teratomas are the most common benign tumor of the ovary in women aged 20 to 40 years, after which time serous cystadenomas become more common.

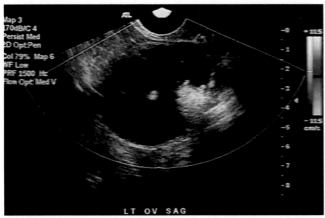

Figure 18–20. A premenopausal cystic teratoma in a 25-year-old patient. The papillary excrescence can be confused with those seen in adenofibromas, borderline tumors, and papillary serous cystadenocarcinomas. The other echogenic debris and shadowing is suggestive of a cystic teratoma or adenofibroma. The absence of blood in the papillary excrescence is suggestive of a benign process. Magnetic resonance imaging may be useful in equivocal cases because fat can clearly be identified in many cystic teratomas using this imaging modality.

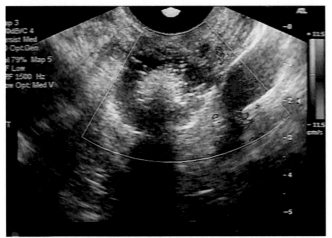

Figure 18–21. This cystic teratoma displays abundant hair with shadowing and echoes typical of sebaceous material. Some cystic teratomas may display only a few hairlike strands, and rarely they may be anechoic.

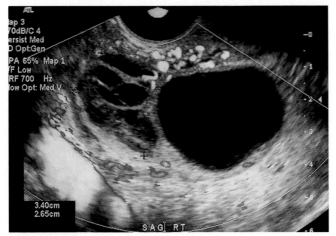

Figure 18–22. This 40-year-old woman on tamoxifen for breast cancer presented with right lower quadrant pain. This hemorrhagic cyst with retracting clot and adjacent follicle resolved spontaneously.

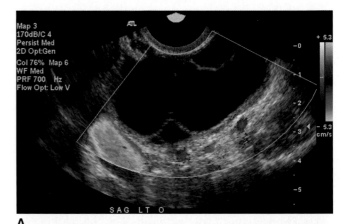

A

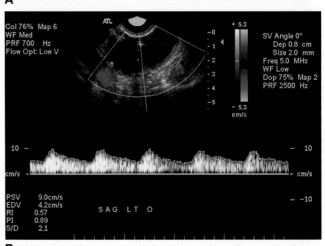

B

Figure 18–23. A, A 38-year-old patient on tamoxifen for breast cancer with a stimulated ovary with multiple follicles. **B,** The same patient as in **A.** Pulsed Doppler reveals intermediate-resistance vessels in the septations between the cysts. The exact incidence of hemorrhagic cysts and stimulated ovaries with tamoxifen is not known. Several case reports of women requiring emergent surgery for torsion or hemorrhage have been published.

specificity 77%, positive predictive value 29.4%, and negative predictive value 99.6%. The system allowed for the accurate prediction of benign cystic teratomas owing to their posterior shadowing. The authors concluded that the less-than-ideal positive predictive value was due to the complex and malignant-appearing nature of some benign tumors. The authors suggested that the addition of color Doppler may improve specificity.

A study by Ferrazzi et al.[16] looked at five different scoring systems for assessing ovarian masses by ultrasound. They developed a multicenter scoring system that was based on the previously published systems of Sassone et al.,[14] Lerner et al.,[15] Granberg et al.,[17] and DePriest et al.[18] Typical cystic teratomas were excluded from scoring. Using a cut-off value of 8, they achieved a sensitivity of 93%, with 56% specificity. Using a cut-off value of 9, the sensitivity was 87% and the specificity 67%. False-positive results for hemorrhagic corpora lutea and cystic teratomas remained a problem, as had been shown by previous authors. Although their scoring system performed better than the other four systems, the authors note "that no completely reliable differentiation of malignant masses can be obtained by sonographic imaging alone."

Guerriero et al.[19] advocated the use of histologic prediction. Masses are labeled as benign when they display ultrasound patterns typical of endometrioma, cystic teratoma, serous cystadenoma, hydrosalpinx, mucinous cystadenoma, hemorrhagic cyst, or paraovarian cyst.[19] Masses are considered malignant if they are solid, contain solid papillae greater than 3 mm, or contain thickened septa. In a combination of premenopausal and postmenopausal women, sensitivity was 100%, specificity 83%, positive predictive value 28%, and negative predictive value 100%. Positive predictive values were worse in premenopausal patients than in postmenopausal patients, 28% versus 55%. Color Doppler as an independent test performed much less optimally, but the addition of Doppler as a secondary test improved overall positive predictive values to 73%—to 50% in premenopausal patients and 84% in postmenopausal patients.

The typical appearance of cystic teratomas, endometriomas, and hemorrhagic cysts on TVS has been described in the literature.[20-25] The high accuracy of TVS for predicting these masses preoperatively has been described by Milad and Cohen.[26] Valentin[27] has stated that histology can be correctly predicted only 50% of the time.

In Europe, ovarian masses are now widely described using the criteria of the International Ovarian Tumor Analysis (IOTA) group,[28] published in 2000. The examination is considered incomplete without a Doppler examination. Masses are described as unilocular, unilocular-solid, multilocular, multilocular-solid, solid, or not classifiable. Septa, internal echogenicity, shadowing, internal wall irregularities, and ascites are described. Papillary projections must measure at least 3 mm to be considered solid elements. Dermoid plugs as seen in cystic teratomas are assigned to the "not classifiable" category.

Color Doppler

With publication of the study by Kurjak et al.[29] in 1991, there initially was a great deal of hope that a resistance index (RI) of less than 0.4 would differentiate between benign and malignant masses. In a series of 690 masses, they reported a sensitivity of 96.4%, a specificity of 99.8%, and an overall accuracy of 99.5%. A veritable flood of papers followed, but all reported less ideal results.[29-35] Fleischer et al.,[30] in a group of ovarian masses, using a pulsatility index (PI) of less than 1.0 as the cut-off, found a sensitivity of 100%, a specificity of 83%, and a positive predictive value of 73%. Timor-Tritsch et al.[31] found that cut-off values of 0.46 for RI and 0.62 for PI, combined with the Sassone scoring system,[14] could differentiate benign from malignant ovarian masses. Hata et al.[32] were able to achieve only an acceptable sensitivity using an RI cut-off of less than 0.7, yielding a sensitivity of 53% and a positive predictive value of 59%.

In 1993, Kurjak et al.[36] published another paper on the detection of stage I ovarian cancer and concluded that a Doppler RI cut-off of less than 0.4 could be used to detect ovarian cancer in normal-sized ovaries. A report by Tekay and Jouppila[37] evaluated the presence of low-resistance vessels in premenopausal ovaries. Low-resistance vessels were identified in 43% of benign tumors and 25% of normal ovaries in premenopausal women. Scanning in the follicular phase did not improve these results. Fleischer and Jones,[38] in an editorial predicting the results of future logistic regression studies, stated that the evaluation of an adnexal mass required a multiparameter approach that included age, gray-scale ultrasound, and Doppler results. A National Institutes of Health Consensus Development Panel on Ovarian Cancer[39] concluded in 1995 that color Doppler evaluation of the ovarian mass was investigational, and that its only benefit may be to improve specificity. There is no good published evidence that color or power Doppler can be used to detect ovarian cancer in either premenopausal or postmenopausal women with normal-sized ovaries.

In the mid-1990s, an attempt was made to use color Doppler energy and peak systolic velocity measurements to improve diagnostic accuracy. Tailor et al.[40] found that specificity was improved from 60% to almost 80% by using a combination of power Doppler and a temporal average maximum velocity of greater than 12 cm/second. Many investigators have found power Doppler to be too susceptible to motion artifact to use on a routine basis. In 1998, Guerriero et al.[19] suggested using power Doppler as a secondary test. Masses identified as suspicious for malignancy because of solid elements were evaluated with power Doppler. Masses with no arterial flow in the echogenic solid portion of the mass were labeled benign. Masses with arterial flow in the echogenic solid portion of the mass were labeled malignant. Among 192 masses, they found 100% sensitivity for gray-scale sonography alone, with a specificity of 86%. With the addition of power Doppler, specificity improved to 95%.

A meta-analysis by Kinkel et al.[41] in 2000 reviewed 46 published studies. Receiver operating characteristic curves revealed a significantly higher performance for the combination of morphologic gray-scale analysis and color Doppler indices than for either alone. At this time, there was no consensus regarding which Doppler technique should be used, color Doppler or power Doppler. Similarly, there was no agreement over whether it was best to use RI, PI, temporal average maximum velocity, or no indices but just to score the presence or absence of flow in solid elements. Clearly, the combination of gray-scale ultrasound and Doppler has improved specificity, but the best way to use Doppler remains unresolved.

Logistic Regression for Assessing Risk of Malignancy

Logistic regression analyses have been published by Tailor et al.,[40] Timmerman et al.,[42] Schelling et al.,[43] and Alcazar et al.[44] The three most consistent findings in logistic regression analyses have been that the most predictive elements for assessing the risk of malignancy in an ovarian mass are age, the presence of solid elements, and the presence of central arterial flow in these solid elements. Velocimetry measurements should be taken but no absolute velocimetry cut-off used (Figs. 18–24 through 18–32). In our experience, the false-negative screens for ovarian cancer occur in women who have stage I ovarian cancer without apparent morphologic changes in the ovary, in women with primary peritoneal cancer, and in some cases of borderline tumors where the excrescences (papillae) do not exhibit flow. False-positive results include thecomas and interligamentous and pedunculated leiomyomas.

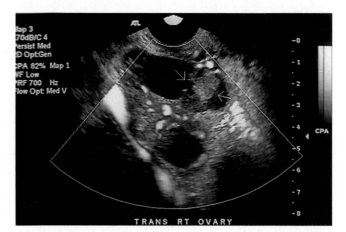

Figure 18–24. A 33-year-old patient with a stage IA serous borderline tumor. The papillary excrescence with central flow is labeled with *arrows*.

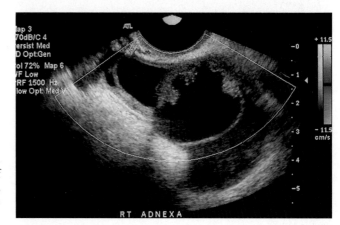

Figure 18–25. A 38-year-old patient with a stage IA serous borderline tumor. No flow is noted within the excrescences. The cytology of the surrounding fluid was negative. In our unpublished experience, approximately 25% of borderline tumors do not show flow within their papillary excrescences.

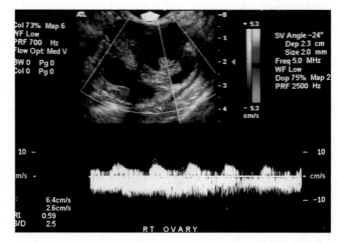

Figure 18–26. A 27-year-old patient with a stage IA serous borderline tumor. Pulsed Doppler reveals an intermediate-resistance vessel (resistance index, 0.59). Although in our laboratory we have not found absolute RI cut-offs to be useful in distinguishing benign from borderline or malignant neoplasms, it remains part of our protocol to take velocimetry measurements when pulsatile flow is detected.

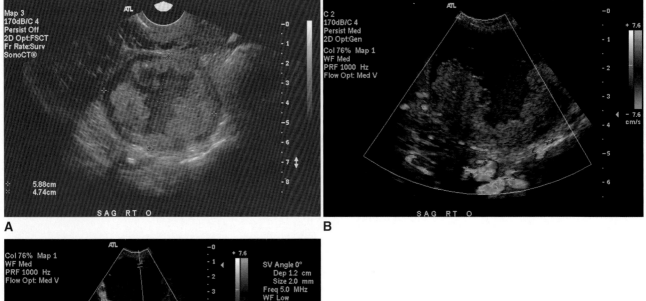

Figure 18–27. A, A 26-year-old patient at 20 weeks' gestation was referred to us for a heterogeneous mass with multiple solid elements. B, In the same patient, multiple small arterioles were noted within the solid elements. C, Pulse Doppler revealed low-resistance vessels (resistance index, 0.36). The differential diagnosis included borderline tumor, papillary adenocarcinoma, and, much less likely, luteoma with cystic degeneration. Surgery revealed a stage IA serous borderline tumor.

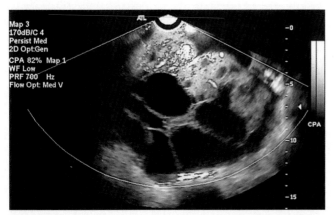

Figure 18–28. A postmenopausal stage IIIC papillary adenocarcinoma. Multiple abnormal vessels are seen in the solid elements of the tumor.

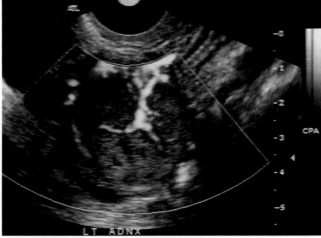

Figure 18–29. A postmenopausal, poorly differentiated stage IIIC adenocarcinoma. Abnormal blood vessels are seen entering the tumor.

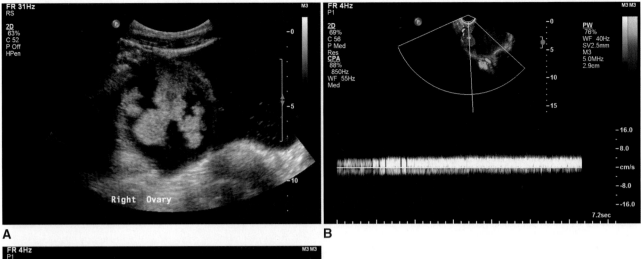

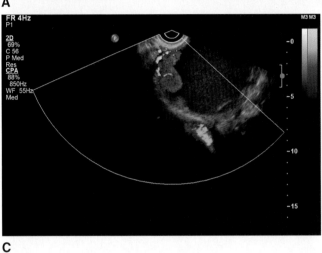

Figure 18–30. **A,** A stage III clear cell carcinoma in a 34-year-old patient. **B,** Only venous flow was detectable in the tumor's solid elements. Although pulsatile arteriolar flow is usually noted centrally within the solid elements of malignant ovarian tumors, in some cases a pulsatile arteriolar waveform cannot be obtained. In any case, the critical features are the presence or absence of solid elements, blood flow within those solid elements, and the distribution of vessels. **C,** In this image from the same patient, a blood vessel can be seen entering a solid papillary excrescence.

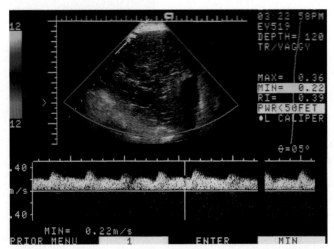

Figure 18–31. A stage I granulosa cell tumor. These tumors are not infrequently confused with endometriomas because they can be seen in women in their reproductive years. Color Doppler clearly demonstrates flow centrally within the mass.

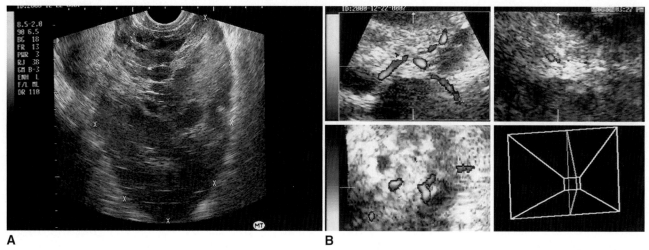

Figure 18–32. A, An abdominal scan of a 13- × 6-cm mass in a 25-year-old women. **B,** In the same patient, three-dimensional transvaginal acquisition reveals multiple blood vessels entering the solid elements of the tumor. Surgery revealed a stage I malignant germ cell tumor.

Three-Dimensional Ultrasound

Early studies by Chan et al.,[45] Bonilla-Musoles et al.,[46] and Kurjak et al.[47] explored the possibilities of three-dimensional (3D) power imaging. The technique allowed for geometric imaging of the vasculature tree of ovarian tumors. Arteriovenous shunts, stenoses, and microaneurysms could be demonstrated. The authors believed that an assessment of tumor angiogenesis using fractal mathematics would lead to a more accurate diagnosis of ovarian malignancy than use of grayscale morphology and Doppler flow indices. A study by Cohen et al.[48] found that 3D power Doppler imaging improved the diagnostic accuracy for ovarian cancer prediction. The technique improved the visualization of tumor excrescences and permitted volumes of tumor vascular architecture to be stored. Their study did not directly compare two-dimensional and 3D Doppler (Figs. 18–33 through 18–35).

Software for quantifying 3D vascular flow has been available since 1999. Parleitner et al.[49] published initial results on the use of virtual organ computer-aided analysis (VOCAL) technology (Kretztechnik; Zipf, Austria) to quantify vascular flow. A more recent study by Jarvela et al.[50] (2003) used 3D power Doppler for ovarian mass evaluation and demonstrated that intraobserver variation was less than interobserver variation for flow measurements, but that overall measurements were reproducible. Another method of 3D ultrasound quantitative analysis of gynecologic tumors has been reported by Testa et al.[51] Overall, these techniques remain investigational.

Ovarian Cancer Screening

Several major premises about ovarian cancer screening must be introduced before reviewing the literature. Ovarian cancer screening primarily is screening for epithelial ovarian cancer. Borderline epithelial ovarian cancers should not be included or should be analyzed separately because their inclusion will falsely elevate the number of frank ovarian cancers that are detected at screening. Patients who are included in ovarian cancer screening must be asymptomatic. The inclusion of women who are referred with known masses, particularly

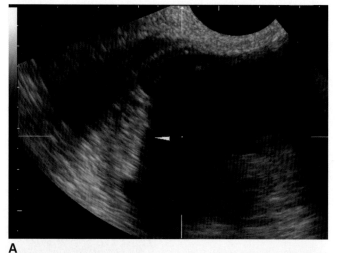

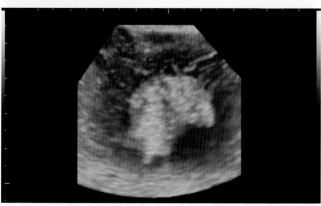

Figure 18–33. A, This malignant germ cell tumor had a thickened internal capsule with a 3.5-cm long area of excrescence. **B,** In the same patient, three-dimensional rendering of this structure reveals a mural nodule with a blood vessel entering it.

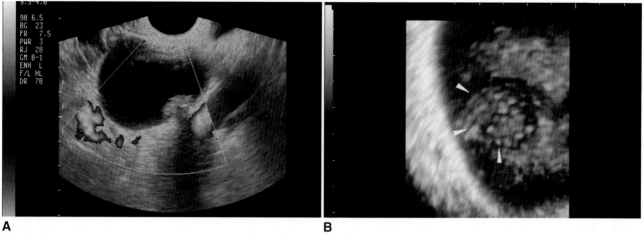

Figure 18–34. A, A complex mass with a mural nodule and excrescences. Power Doppler shows no flow within the mass. Pathologic examination revealed an adenofibroma. **B,** In the same patient, three-dimensional imaging reveals multiple excrescences on the surface of the mural nodule *(arrowheads).*

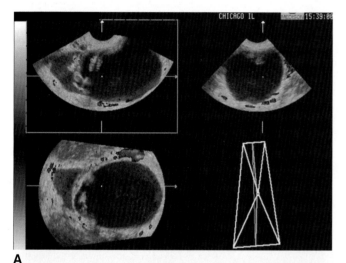

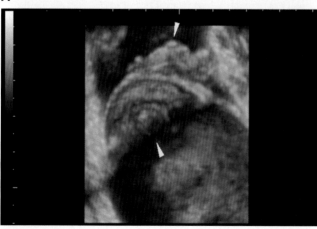

Figure 18–35. A, Three-dimensional volume acquisition of an adenofibroma with thickened septations with multiple excrescences. Power Doppler is unremarkable for flow within the septations. **B,** In the same patient, three-dimensional rendering of the septation with excrescences *(arrowheads).*

masses that should have been palpable on routine examination, is misleading.

Analysis of the published literature is best achieved by dividing studies into those that screened low-risk subjects and those that screened high-risk subjects. As shown by Bell et al.,[52] the sensitivity of sonography for the detection of stage I ovarian cancer may be very different between the two groups. In a 1998 review of the literature, they found that the sensitivity for detection of stage I ovarian cancer was 25% (95% confidence interval [CI] 3 to 65) in high-risk women. Among low-risk women, the sensitivity was 67% (95% CI 22 to 96).[52] The very wide CIs make it clear that very large screening studies are required to get a true accuracy.

The report of Bell et al. also made clear that the false-positive rate could be decreased from approximately 2% to 0.5% by the addition of Doppler to gray-scale imaging.

Van Nagell et al.[53] have been performing ovarian cancer screening on a predominantly low-risk population for nearly 15 years. Their report, published in 2000, included 14,469 women, 57,214 scans, and 25 ovarian malignancies. After eliminating borderline tumors and granulosa cell tumors, the overall sensitivity for stage I epithelial ovarian cancer was 38%. A much larger study by Sato et al.[54] of 183,034 Japanese women detected 12 of 17 cases of epithelial ovarian cancer at stage I. This did not include borderline or granulosa cell tumors.

Results in high-risk women have been highly variable. In a study of 2500 self-referred high-risk women followed with annual TVS, Tailor et al.[55] found 11 ovarian cancers. After excluding borderline tumors, three of seven tumors (42%) were stage I. Karlan and associates,[56] from the United States, in a study of 1261 subjects followed serially with annual TVS, found 10 ovarian cancers. Seven cases were stage IIIC primary peritoneal tumors, and three cases were stage I epithelial ovarian cancers. The National Ovarian Cancer Early Detection Program has reported on 4526 high-risk women with a total of serial 12,709 scans. Ninety-eight women were identified with persistent masses, of whom 49 underwent surgical evaluation. There were 37 benign ovarian masses and 12 gynecologic malignancies. The detected malignancies included four stage IIIC fallopian tube carcinomas, four stage III primary peritoneal carcinomas, two stage III epithelial ovarian cancers, and two stage IA endometrial carcinomas. All 12 patients were asymptomatic and had unremarkable scans 6 and 12 months before diagnosis. The authors concluded that screening ultrasound was of little value in the detection of early-stage disease in this high-risk population.[57]

Ongoing trials include the United Kingdom Collaborative Trial.[58] This study randomizes 200,000 postmenopausal women into a 1:1:2 grouping consisting of annual measurement of CA-125, annual transvaginal scans, and control subjects, respectively. The study is powered to demonstrate a 30% reduction in cancer deaths. The Prostate, Lung, Colorectal, and Ovarian (PLCO) cancer trial in the United States includes 148,000 men and women aged 55 to 74 years. The women undergo CA-125 measurement and TVS annually. The study is randomized and will last 13 years from the completion of randomization, which is still ongoing.

Asymptomatic Menopausal Cysts

Simple cystic masses greater than 2.5 cm have been found in 3% to 5% of menopausal women undergoing imaging studies of the pelvis. Many investigators, including Bonilla-Musoles et al.,[59] Goldstein et al.,[60] and Bailey et al.,[61] have found that there is a very low risk of malignancy if the cysts are simple without multiple or thick septations, solid elements, or ascites. This subject has recently been reviewed by Nardo et al.,[62] who advise using a 5-cm cut-off for expectant management of unilocular simple ovarian cysts, and by Modesitt et al.[63] from the University of Kentucky Ovarian Cancer Screening program, who extended the recommendation to 10 cm.

Contrast Agents in Diagnosis

Reports by Orden et al.[64] and Kupesic and Kurjak[65] in 2000 reviewed initial attempts to use contrast-enhanced sonography to distinguish benign from malignant masses. The kinetics of contrast uptake and washout were reviewed in a second report by Orden et al.[66] in 2003. In 2004, Marret et al.[67] published a series of 101 adnexal masses, 23 malignant and 78 benign, evaluated with Levovist. Time–intensity curves were obtained using power Doppler. Using receiver operating characteristic curve analysis, the area under the curve and washout times were the most accurate parameters for differentiating benign from malignant masses. Both these measures were significantly increased in malignant tumors. Sensitivity was approximately 96% (95% CI 78% to 99.9%) and specificity 95% (95% CI 87% to 99%).

Emoto et al.[68] recently reported a case of ovarian cancer in a normal-sized ovary detected by contrast-enhanced sonography. This raises the possibility that early-stage ovarian cancer may be detected using contrast agents.

REFERENCES

1. Padilla L, Radosevich DM, Milad MP: Accuracy of pelvic examination in detecting adnexal masses. Obstet Gynecol 2000;96:593-598.
2. Goldstein SR: Routine use of office gynecologic ultrasound. J Ultrasound Med 2002;21:489-492.
3. Cohen L: Should transvaginal ultrasound be performed at annual examination in asymptomatic women? Int J Fertil 2003;48:150-153.
4. Greenlee RT, Murray T, Bolden S, Wingo PA: Cancer statistics, 2000. CA Cancer J Clin 2000;50:7-33.
5. Yancik R: Ovarian cancer: Age contrasts in incidence, histology, disease stage at diagnosis, and mortality. Cancer 1993;71:517-523.
6. Yancik R, Ries LG, Yates JW: Ovarian cancer in the elderly: An analysis of Surveillance, Epidemiology, and End Results Program data. Am J Obstet Gynecol 1986;154:639-647.
7. Borgfeldt C, Andolf E: Transvaginal sonographic ovarian findings in a random sample of women 25-40 years old. Ultrasound Obstet Gynecol 1999;13:345-349.
8. Schulman H, Conway C, Zalud I, et al: Prevalence in a volunteer population of pelvic cancer detected with transvaginal ultrasound and color flow Doppler. Ultrasound Obstet Gynecol 1994;4:414-420.
9. Osmers R, Osmers M, von Maydell B, et al: Preoperative evaluation of ovarian tumors in the premenopause by transvaginosonography. Am J Obstet Gynecol 1996;175:428-434.
10. Pinotti JA, de Frazin CM, Marusi EF, Zeferino LC: Evolution of cystic and adnexal tumors identified by echography. Int J Gynaecol Obstet 1988;26:109-114.
11. Spanos WJ: Preoperative hormonal therapy of cystic adnexal masses. Am J Obstet Gynecol 1973;116:551-556.
12. Steinkampf M, Hammond K, Blackwell R: Hormonal treatment of functional ovarian cysts: A randomized, prospective study. Fertil Steril 1990;54:775-777.
13. Koonings P, Campbell K, Mishell D, Grimes D: Relative frequency of primary ovarian neoplasms: A 10 year review. Obstet Gynecol 1989;74:921-926.
14. Sassone AM, Timor-Tritsch IE, Artner A, et al: Transvaginal sonographic characterization of ovarian disease: Evaluation of a new scoring system to predict malignancy. Obstet Gynecol 1991;78:70-76.
15. Lerner JP, Timor-Tritsch IE, Federman A, Abramovich G: Transvaginal ultrasonographic characterization of ovarian masses with an improved, weighted score. Am J Obstet Gynecol 1994;170:81-85.
16. Ferrazzi E, Zanetta G, Dordoni D, et al: Transvaginal ultrasonographic characterization of ovarian masses: A comparison of five scoring systems in a multicenter trial. Ultrasound Obstet Gynecol 1997;10:192-197.
17. Granberg S, Norstrom A, Wikland M: Tumors in the lower pelvis as imaged by vaginal sonography. Gynecol Oncol 1990;37:224-229.
18. DePriest PD, Shenson D, Fried A, et al: A morphologic index based on sonographic findings in ovarian cancer. Gynecol Oncol 1993;51:7-11.
19. Guerriero S, Ajossa S, Risalvato A, et al: Diagnosis of adnexal malignancies by using color Doppler energy imaging as a secondary test in persistent masses. Ultrasound Obstet Gynecol 1998;11:277-282.
20. Cohen L, Sabbagha R: Echo patterns of benign cystic teratomas by transvaginal ultrasound. Ultrasound Obstet Gynecol 1993;3:120-123.
21. Caspi B, Appelman Z, Rabinerson D, et al: Pathognomonic echo patterns of cystic teratomas of the ovaries. Ultrasound Obstet Gynecol 1996;7:275-279.
22. Mais V, Guerriero S, Ajossa S: Transvaginal ultrasound in the diagnosis of cystic teratoma. Obstet Gynecol 1995;85:48-52.
23. Cohen L, Valle R, Sabbagha R: A comparison of preoperative ultrasound images of surgically proven endometriomas scanned by both transabdominal and transvaginal techniques. J Gynecol Surg 1995;11:27-32.
24. Kupfer MC, Schwimmer SR, Lebovic J: Transvaginal sonographic appearance of endometriomata: Spectrum of findings. J Ultrasound Med 1992;11:129-133.
25. Okai T, Kobayashi K, Ryo E, et al: Transvaginal sonographic appearance of hemorrhagic functional ovarian cysts and their spontaneous regression. Int J Gynaecol Obstet 1994;44:47-52.
26. Milad M, Cohen L: Preoperative ultrasound assessment of adnexal masses in premenopausal women. Int J Gynaecol Obstet 1999;66:137-141.
27. Valentin L: Pattern recognition of pelvic masses by gray-scale ultrasound imaging: The contribution of Doppler ultrasound. Ultrasound Obstet Gynecol 1999;14:338-347.
28. Timmerman D, Valentin L, Bourne TH, et al: Consensus statement: Terms, definitions and measurements to describe the sonographic features of adnexal tumors: A consensus opinion from the International Ovarian Tumor Analysis (IOTA) group. Ultrasound Obstet Gynecol 2000;16:500-505.
29. Kurjak A, Zalud I, Alfirevic Z: Evaluation of adnexal masses with transvaginal color ultrasound. J Ultrasound Med 1991;10:295-297.
30. Fleischer A, Rodgers W, Rao B, et al: Assessment of ovarian tumor vascularity with transvaginal color Doppler sonography. J Ultrasound Med 1991;10:563-568.
31. Timor-Tritsch I, Lerner J, Monteagudo A, et al: Transvaginal ultrasonographic characterization of ovarian masses by means of color flow-directed Doppler measurements and a morphologic scoring system. Am J Obstet Gynecol 1993;168:909-913.

32. Hata K, Hata T, Manabe A, et al: A critical evaluation of transvaginal Doppler studies, transvaginal sonography, magnetic resonance imaging, and CA125 in detecting ovarian cancer. Obstet Gynecol 1992;80:992-996.

33. Bromley B, Goodman H, Benaceraff BR: Comparison between sonographic morphology and Doppler waveform for the diagnosis of ovarian malignancy. Obstet Gynecol 1994;83:125-130.

34. Valentin L, Sladkevicius P, Marsal K: Limited contribution of Doppler velocimetry to the differential diagnosis of extrauterine pelvic tumors. Obstet Gynecol 1994;83:425-433.

35. Tekay A, Jouppila P: Validity of pulsatility and resistance indices in classification of adnexal tumors with transvaginal color Doppler ultrasound. Ultrasound Obstet Gynecol 1992;2:338-344.

36. Kurjak A, Shalan H, Matijevic R, et al: Stage I ovarian cancer by transvaginal color Doppler sonography: A report of 18 cases. Ultrasound Obstet Gynecol 1993;3:195-198.

37. Tekay A, Jouppila P: Blood flow in benign ovarian tumors and normal ovaries during the follicular phase. Obstet Gynecol 1995;86:55-59.

38. Fleischer A, Jones H: Color Doppler sonography of ovarian masses: The importance of a multiparameter approach [editorial]. Gynecol Oncol 1993;50:1-2.

39. NIH Consensus Development Panel on Ovarian Cancer: NIH consensus conference. Ovarian cancer: Screening, treatment, and follow-up. JAMA 1995;273:491-497.

40. Tailor A, Jurkovic D, Bourne T, et al: Comparison of transvaginal color Doppler imaging and color Doppler energy for assessment of intraovarian blood flow. Obstet Gynecol 1998;91:561-567.

41. Kinkel K, Hricak H, Lu Y, et al: US characterization of ovarian masses: A meta-analysis. Radiology 2000;217:803-811.

42. Timmerman D, Bourne TH, Tailor A, et al: A comparison of methods for preoperative discrimination between malignant and benign adnexal masses: The development of a new logistic regression model. Am J Obstet Gynecol 1999;181:57-65.

43. Schelling M, Braun M, Kuhn W, et al: Combined transvaginal B-mode and color Doppler sonography for differential diagnosis of ovarian tumors: Results of a multivariate logistic regression analysis. Gynecol Oncol 2000;77:78-86.

44. Alcazar J, Jurado M: Prospective evaluation of a logistic model based on sonographic morphologic and color Doppler findings developed to predict adnexal malignancy. J Ultrasound Med 1999;18:837-842.

45. Chan L, Lin S, Uerpairojkit B, et al: Evaluation of adnexal masses using three-dimensional ultrasonographic technology: Preliminary report. J Ultrasound Med 1997;16:349-354.

46. Bonilla-Musoles F, Raga F, Osborne N: Three-dimensional ultrasound evaluation of ovarian masses. Gynecol Oncol 1995;59:129-135.

47. Kurjak A, Kupesic S, Breyer B, et al: The assessment of ovarian tumor angiogenesis: What does three-dimensional power Doppler add? Ultrasound Obstet Gynecol 1998;12:136-146.

48. Cohen LS, Escobar PF, Scharm C, et al: Three-dimensional power Doppler ultrasound improves the diagnostic accuracy for ovarian cancer prediction. Gynecol Oncol 2001;82:40-48.

49. Pairleitner H, Steiner H, Hasenoehrl G, Staudach A: Three-dimensional power Doppler sonography: Imaging and quantifying blood flow and vascularization. Ultrasound Obstet Gynecol 1999;14:139-143.

50. Jaravela IY, Sladkevicius P, Tekay AH, et al: Intraobserver and interobserver variability of ovarian volume, gray-scale, and color flow indices obtained using transvaginal three-dimensional power Doppler ultrasonography. Ultrasound Obstet Gynecol 2003;21:277-282.

51. Testa AC, Mansueto D, Lorusso D, et al: Angiographic power 3-dimensional quantitative analysis in gynecologic solid tumors: Feasibility and reproducibility. J Ultrasound Med 2004;23:821-828.

52. Bell R, Petticrew M, Sheldon T: The performance of screening tests for ovarian cancer: Results of a systematic review. Br J Obstet Gynaecol 1998;105:1136-1147.

53. van Nagell JR Jr, DePriest PD, Reedy MB, et al: The efficacy of transvaginal sonographic screening in asymptomatic women at risk for ovarian cancer. Gynecol Oncol 2000;77:350-356.

54. Sato S, Yokoyama Y, Sakamoto T, et al: Usefulness of mass screening for ovarian cancer using transvaginal ultrasonography. Cancer 2000;89:582-588.

55. Tailor A, Bourne TH, Campbell S, et al: Results from an ultrasound based familial ovarian cancer screening clinic: A 10-year observational study. Ultrasound Obstet Gynecol 2003;21:378-385.

56. Karlan BY, Baldwin RL, Lopez-Leuvanos E, et al: Peritoneal serous papillary carcinoma, a phenotypic variant of familial ovarian cancer: Implications for ovarian cancer screening. Am J Obstet Gynecol 1999;180:917-928.

57. Fishman D, Cohen L, Blank S, et al: The role of ultrasound evaluation in the detection of early-stage epithelial ovarian cancer. Am J Obstet Gynecol 2005;192:1214-1221.

58. Jacobs I, Skates SJ, MacDonald N, et al: Screening for ovarian cancer: A pilot randomized trial. Lancet 1999;353:1207-1210.

59. Bonilla-Musoles F, Ballester J, Simon C, et al: Is avoidance of surgery possible in patients with perimenopausal ovarian tumors using transvaginal ultrasound and duplex color Doppler sonography? J Ultrasound Med 1993;12:33-39.

60. Goldstein S, Subramanyam B, Snyder J, et al: The postmenopausal cystic adnexal mass: The potential role of ultrasound in conservative management. Obstet Gynecol 1989;76:8-10.

61. Bailey C, Ueland F, Land G, et al: The malignant potential of small cystic ovarian tumors in women over 50 years of age. Gynecol Oncol 1998;69:3-7.

62. Nardo LG, Kroon ND, Geginald PW: Persistent unilocular ovarian cysts in a general population of postmenopausal women: Is there a place for expectant management? Obstet Gynecol 2003;102:589-593.

63. Modesitt SC, Pavlik EJ, Ueland FR, et al: Risk of malignancy in unilocular ovarian cystic tumors less than 10 cm. in diameter. Obstet Gynecol 2003;102:594-599.

64. Orden MR, Gudmundsson S, Kirkinen P: Contrast-enhanced sonography in the examination of benign and malignant adnexal masses. J Ultrasound Med 2000;19:783-788.

65. Kupesic S, Kurjak A: Contrast-enhanced, three-dimensional power Doppler sonography for differentiation of adnexal masses. Obstet Gynecol 2000;96:452-458.

66. Orden MR, Jurvelin JS, Kirkinen PP: Kinetics of a US contrast agent in benign and malignant adnexal tumors. Radiology 2003;226:405-410.

67. Marret H, Suaget S, Giraudeau B, et al: Contrast-enhanced sonography helps in discriminating benign from malignant adnexal masses. J Ultrasound in Med 2004;23:1629-1639.

68. Emoto M, Fujimitsu R, Hiwasaki H, Kawarabayashi T: Diagnostic challenges in patients with tumors: Case 3. Normal sized ovarian cancer detected by color Doppler ultrasound using microbubble contrast agent. J Clin Oncol 2003;21:3703-3705.

Chapter 19

Three-Dimensional Ultrasound in Gynecology

Ilan E. Timor-Tritsch and Ana Monteagudo

In an "opinion article" in 1994,[1] Timor-Tritsch credited the authors who had reported on three new obstetric diagnostic and therapeutic technologies based on the use of ultrasound and laser techniques.[2-4] Yet today, only one of the procedures is still practiced, after undergoing improvements and modifications.[3] It is common for therapeutic procedures that appear promising at first to fail to live up to expectations, owing perhaps to their complicated nature or cost. In the area of obstetrics and gynecology, however, we are confident that sonography in general and three-dimensional (3D) ultrasound in particular, a relative newcomer to the field, will stand the test of time.

The use of 3D ultrasound technology started in the late 1970s, and its applications have continued to grow. It first had considerable diagnostic impact in obstetrics, and it is now beginning to prove its usefulness in gynecology as well. Although the gynecologic uses of 3D ultrasound are in their infancy, we predict that this technology will enhance the diagnostic imaging of the female pelvis.

The operating system of all ultrasound machines is based on digital processing, and the heart of any ultrasound equipment is a dedicated computer. In the case of 3D ultrasound scanners, unlike with 2D ultrasound, it is not enough to only acquire the region of interest. The next step is to use data points in the 3D volume data set, reconstruct the different planes, and then manipulate them to obtain the desired image using the many rendering possibilities. All this is performed by special proprietary software that is relatively easy to use. Several companies even offer proprietary laptop versions of their volume-handling software; this makes it possible to study and manipulate the volumes off-line, without tying up the actual scanner. We generally create a CD and work on the images as time allows. The four 3D software programs currently available are 4D View (Kretztechnik-General Electric), for the 730 Voluson series; QLab (Phillips), for the IU22 and HD11 series; Sono View Pro, for Medison; and 3D Viewer, for Siemens equipment.

For technical information on 3D ultrasound, readers are referred to Chapter 2. In addition, there are several excellent textbooks available.[5-8] Although they may be heavily weighted toward obstetric uses, they provide valuable information about this powerful imaging modality.

This chapter concentrates on 3D ultrasound of the uterus, fallopian tubes, and ovaries and discusses 3D power Doppler angiography in relation to the pelvic organs.

Examination of the Uterus

It is simple to determine the volume of a moderate-sized uterus. If the uterus is large, volumes of the fundus, body, and cervix can be acquired separately. A uterine volume can be acquired with the uterus in the sagittal or the transverse plane. When displaying the orthogonal planes, the upper left box is labeled "box A," the upper right box is labeled "box B," the lower left is "box C," and the lower right, "box D," is usually the rendering box, which displays the volume in different rendering modalities. If the volume is obtained in the sagittal plane, the anteverted or retroverted uterus will be represented by the longitudinal sagittal plane (Fig. 19–1, box A); the cross-sectional (transverse) plane (Fig. 19–1, box B); and the coronal plane (Fig. 19–1, box C). By a few rotations of the x, y, and z axes, it is possible to display the true coronal plane of the uterus (Fig. 19–2, box C). In this orientation, one can visualize the longitudinal sagittal plane (Fig. 19–2, box B) and the cross-sectional (transverse) plane (Fig. 19–2, box A). By tilting and scrolling through the different planes, it is possible to scrutinize the uterine cavity, endometrium, and cervix (Fig. 19–3). The ability to study the uterus in any desired plane is of great importance. However, the most useful plane enabled by 3D reconstruction is the coronal plane, which was seldom seen by traditional two-dimensional (2D) scanning.[9-11]

The process of "navigating" (scrolling) through the different planes becomes even more important if the examination is enhanced by injecting saline (saline infusion sonohysterography [SIS]) into the cavity (Fig. 19–4). SIS-enhanced 3D ultrasound of the uterus allows a thorough examination of the uterine cavity, the endometrial lining, and any pathologies therein.

3D ultrasound is a valuable tool for diagnosing most uterine malformations.[10-15] It has a distinct advantage over 2D imaging in its ability to visualize the uterine anatomy and pathology; 3D ultrasound is as effective as magnetic resonance imaging but less costly and much faster. To correctly classify a uterine malformation, the following anatomic regions must be described: (1) the shape of the surface contours of the fundus, (2) the shape of the uterine cavity, (3) the anatomy of the cervix, and (4) the anatomy of the vagina. The first three can easily be imaged by 3D ultrasound (Fig. 19–5). The vagina must undergo bimanual palpation as well as speculum

Text continued on p. 273

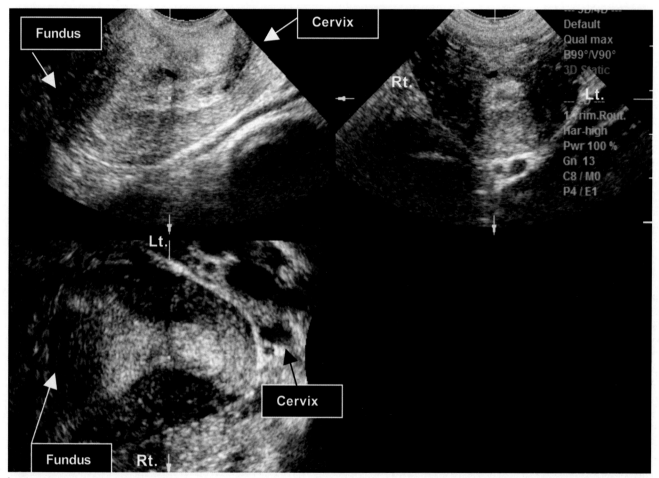

Figure 19–1. Acquisition of the volume of a normal uterus in the sagittal plane. Box A, Sagittal section of the uterus. Box B, Cross (transverse) section. Box C, Coronal plane seen tilted on its side.

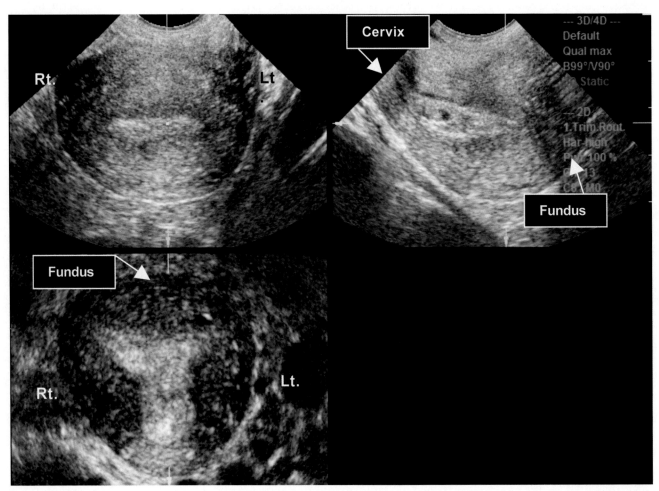

Figure 19–2. Acquisition of the volume of a normal uterus in the transverse plane. Box A, Transverse section. Box B, Sagittal section. Box C, Coronal section seen "upright."

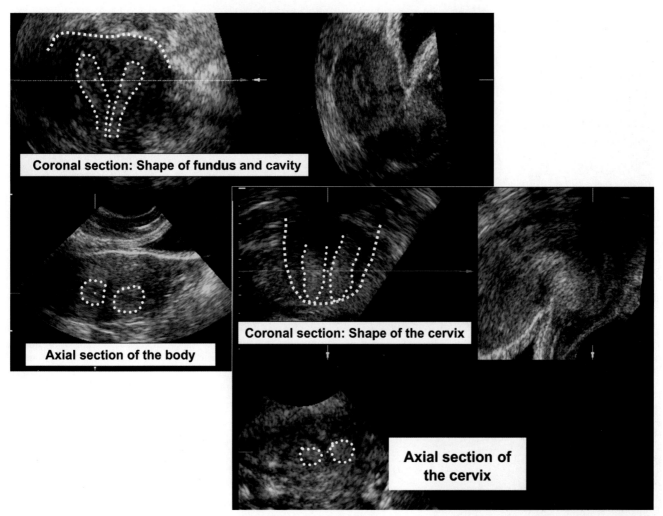

Figure 19–3. Complete septate uterus. **A,** On a coronal section (box A), the outer fundal contours are normal; two cavities are separated by a deep septum. On an axial section of the body (box C), which was obtained at the level of the horizontal line shown in the coronal section, the two cavities are seen. **B,** Here, the cervix is positioned so that it can be studied in a coronal plane (box A), revealing two cervical canals. On an axial section (box C), obtained at the level of the horizontal line shown in box A of part **B**, the two cervical canals are evident.

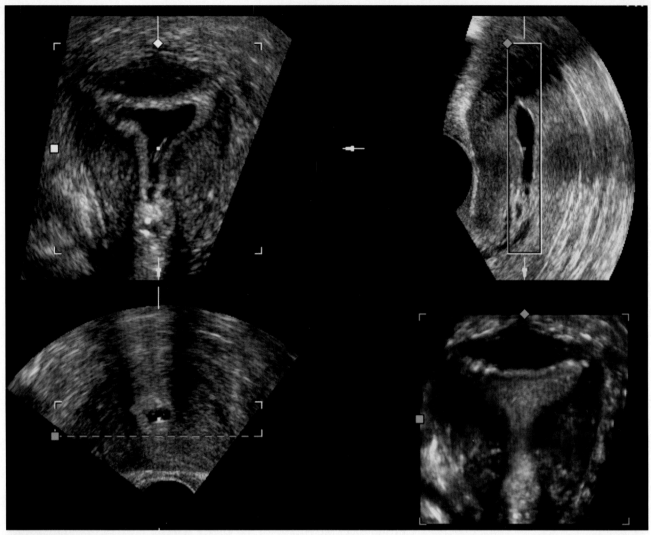

Figure 19–4. Saline infusion sonohysterography performed using 3D sonography. Regardless of the orientation at the time of the acquisition, the volume is rotated to display the coronal plane in box A. Box B contains the sagittal plane, and box C the axial plane. The rendered "thick slice" is seen in the rendered box D.

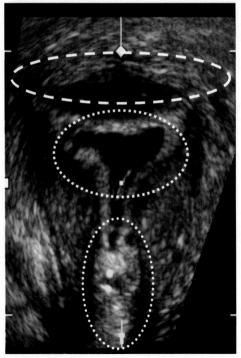

Figure 19–5. On a saline infusion sonohysterogram, with the uterus displayed in the coronal plane, it is easy to assess the shape of the fundus *(upper oval)*, the cavity *(middle oval)*, and the cervix *(lower oval)*.

examination; however, fluid in the vagina may be revealed by sonography.

Obtaining the 3D volume at the time of SIS greatly enhances the value of the information obtained about the uterine anatomy (Fig. 19–6).[16,17] In addition, owing to the fast acquisition period with 3D ultrasound, the uterus must be distended for a shorter time than when using 2D ultrasound, making the 3D technique more comfortable for the patient.

In some cases, a special technique of 3D rendering, the inversion technique, is useful.[13] A dedicated software subroutine inverts sonolucent (echo-free) voxels to transparent ones, which can then be opacified and displayed as "echogenic" structures. This technique was used to produce the "cast" of the uterine cavity seen in Figure 19–7. With this display modality, it was easy to make the diagnosis of arcuate uterus in this patient.

An additional 3D technique is the "thick-slice" display (Fig. 19–8). Several sagittal slices are "collapsed" into one plane. When these collapsed slices are rendered in the coronal plane, the echogenicity of the endometrium becomes "exaggerated," allowing better definition of the structure of the cavity. In other words, this technique increases the contrast between weakly and strongly echogenic tissues such as the myometrium and the secretory endometrium. This display mode is particularly useful to highlight the uterine cavity by using the echogenic endometrium as a natural contrast material. If a patient suspected of having a uterine anomaly presents for 3D work-up in the secretory phase of the cycle, or if SIS is not possible, the thick-slice method can be used. Another typical example of the thick-slice display is shown in Figure 19–9, representing an incomplete septate uterus.

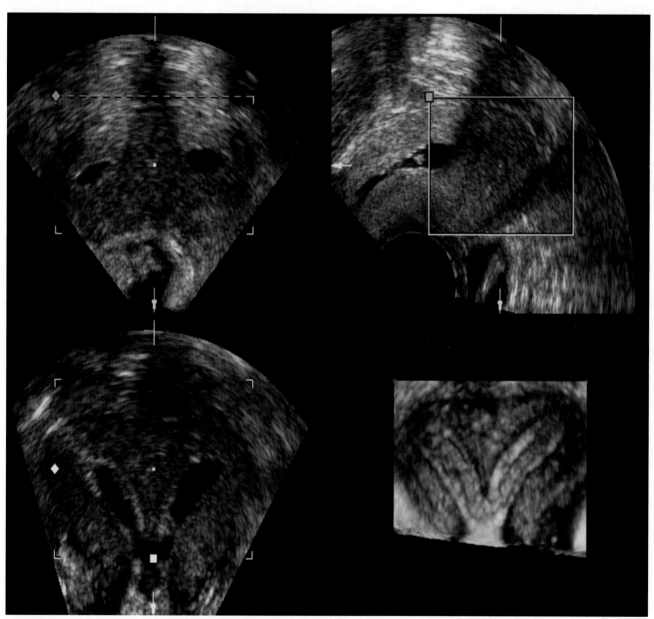

Figure 19–6. This volume was obtained while saline was infused into the cavity (saline infusion sonohysterography). The fluid enhances the image, precisely outlining the uterine cavity. Box C displays the coronal plane of the uterus. Box D represents a plane that captures the endometrium adjacent to the plane at the level of the fluid.

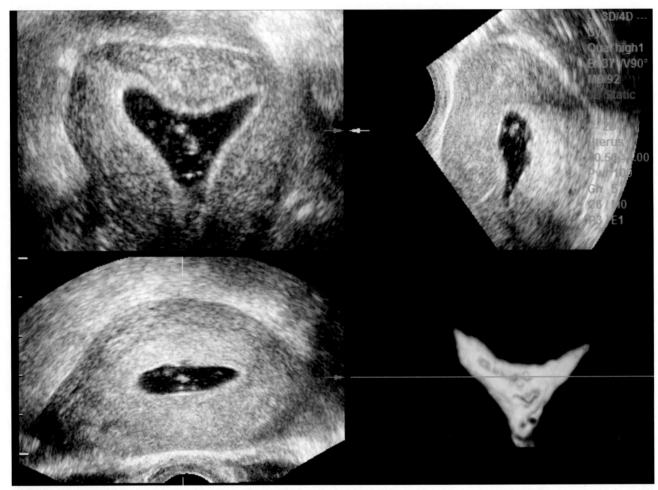

Figure 19–7. After the volume of the uterus was obtained during saline infusion sonohysterography, the 3D inversion rendering mode was used to display the "cast" of the uterine cavity in box D. This is an arcuate uterus.

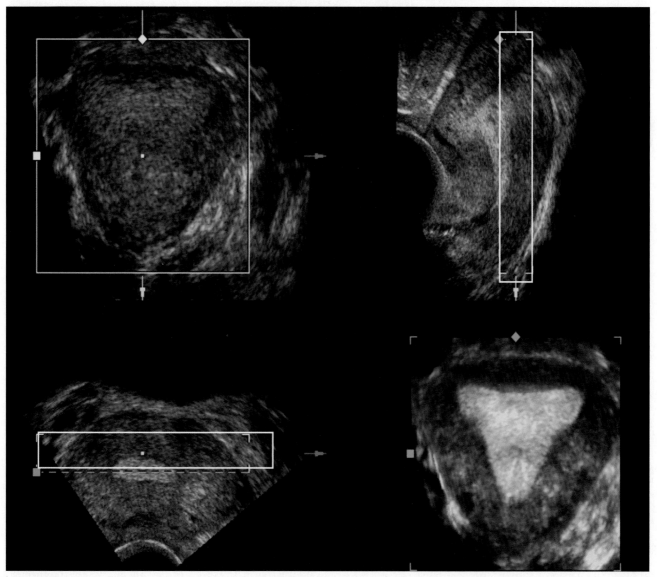

Figure 19–8. After the volume of the uterus was obtained, the region of interest to be displayed in the rendering box (box D) is defined by narrowing it, as shown in box B and box C. The thick-slice display in the rendering box (box D) emphasizes the hyperechoic endometrial cavity in the coronal plane. Box A represents the unenhanced coronal plane.

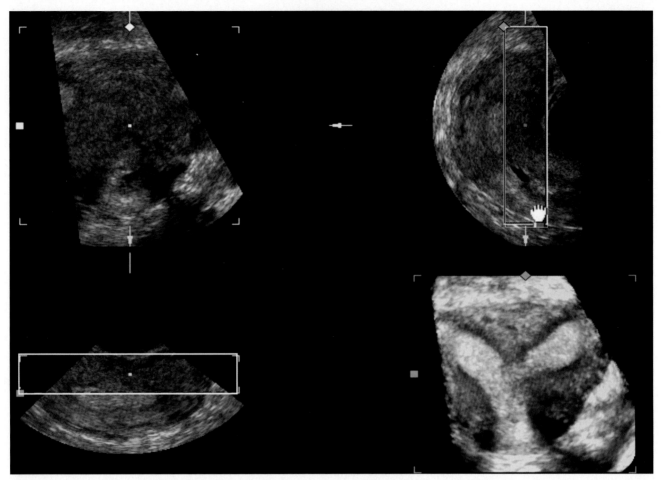

Figure 19–9. Thick-slice display of an incomplete septate uterus in box D.

3D ultrasound is useful for detecting uterine malformations in pregnancy.[18,19] If possible, this should be done in the first or early second trimester. The ability to scroll through the volume in any desired direction can be instrumental in the precise localization of sacs (mapping procedure) before multifetal pregnancy reduction is undertaken (Fig. 19–10). 3D ultrasound can also help diagnose rare cases of complicated malformations[19] (Fig. 19–11) as well as localize and define intrauterine contraceptive devices[20] (see Fig. 5–33). The reproducibility of 3D ultrasound in evaluating uterine anomalies is excellent.[21] Attempts have been made to accurately measure the volume[22] and the shape of the endometrium in ectopic pregnancies as well.[23]

Endocavitary Lesions: Polyps and Myomas

The ultrasound work-up of the uterine cavity was touched on in Chapter 7. This chapter discusses the added value of 3D ultrasound in dealing with endometrial polyps and submucosal fibroids.

An effective and time-saving way to scan for endometrial pathology is to perform SIS using 3D ultrasound. After the volume is acquired, it is possible to scroll within the volume and display the various sections using the orthogonal planes. The patient can leave the examining room while the volume is being analyzed. It is easy and takes little time to localize polyps and measure them; the vessels leading to the polyp can be seen using the power Doppler mode (Fig. 19–12). Using the inversion rendering mode at the time of SIS may enhance the ability to diagnose endometrial polyps.[13]

The protocol for the detection of submucosal myomas is the same as for localizing endometrial polyps. The sonographic differentiation between the two was discussed in Chapter 15.

Intracavitary Fluid and Other Findings

Intracavitary fluid may be hematometra, as in the case of obstructed outflow in an elderly patient with an imperforate hymen or cervical stenosis (Fig. 19–13). As discussed earlier, 3D ultrasound can be helpful in evaluating a complex combined uterine and vaginal malformation (see Fig. 19–11). Displaying the intracavitary fluid (at SIS) also helps define endometrial pathology (see Fig. 18–30). Using the inversion rendering mode is advantageous when the endometrial cavity contains significant amounts of native or injected fluid.

At times, 3D ultrasound can resolve questions about the type of intrauterine contraceptive device implanted (see Fig. 5–33). Figure 5–44 depicts the usefulness of 3D power Doppler ultrasound in diagnosing the nature, size, and proximity to the urethra and bladder of a paraurethral metastasis of trophoblastic disease.

Diagnosis of Ectopic Pregnancy

Only a few articles in the literature are devoted to the diagnosis of ectopic pregnancy by 3D ultrasound.[23,24]

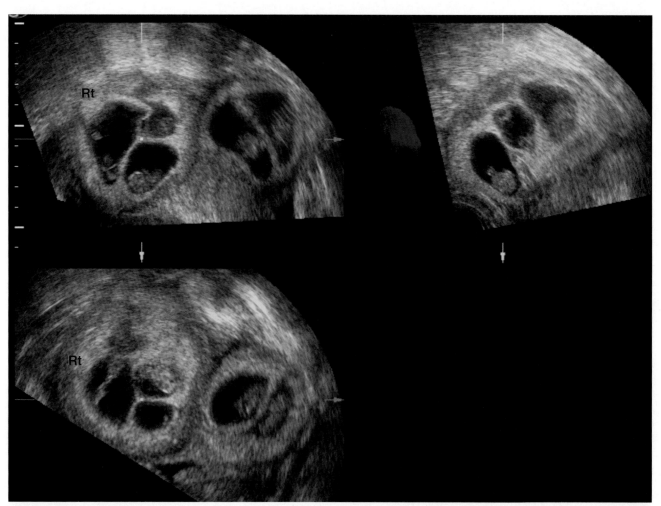

Figure 19–10. A bicornuate uterus contained sextuplets. Four embryos were in the right horn and two in the left one. Scrolling in the volume helped significantly in the precise "mapping" of the sacs before multifetal pregnancy reduction from six to two. Box A, Coronal plane. Box B, Sagittal plane. Box C, Axial plane.

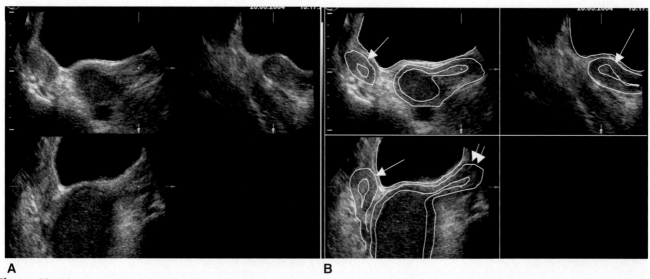

A   **B**

Figure 19–11. Intracavitary fluid. In this case, the fluid (blood) distends the vagina connected to the left uterus in a complex malformation. The *single arrow* points to the right side of the uterus, which had a normal connection to a patent right vagina. The *double arrow* marks the left side of the uterus, which was connected to a distended, blood-filled vagina that was obliterated. **A,** The three orthogonal planes. **B,** The superimposed lines explain the pathology.

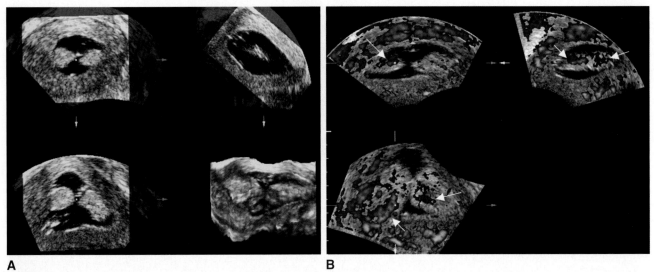

A   **B**

Figure 19–12. Endometrial polyps. **A,** Two polyps were detected on the right and left lateral walls of the cavity. Box D displays the rendered image of them. **B,** Color Doppler reveals their feeding vessels *(arrows)*.

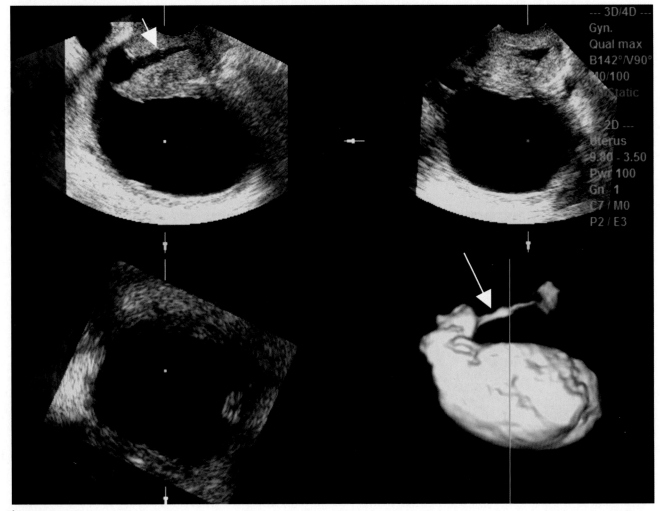

Figure 19–13. Intracavitary fluid. 3D sonography readily detects the distended, fluid-filled uterine cavity in an elderly patient with cervical stenosis. The 3D inversion rendering (box D) displays the "cast" of the fluid with the thin cervical canal *(arrow)*.

We have found the 3D technique to be useful in ascertaining the diagnosis of cornual or interstitial pregnancy. With real-time scanning, it may be difficult to make an accurate diagnosis of a cornual or interstitial pregnancy. The critical area between the eccentrically located sac and the hyperechoic decidua in the uterine cavity may be blurred, preventing an unequivocal determination. This is where 3D is of use. By displaying the coronal plane of the area of the uterus in question in the thick-slice mode, 3D ultrasound can enhance the distinct features of the cavity as well as the chorionic ring (Figs. 19–14 and 19–15). The total separation between the cavity and the ectopic sac becomes obvious, reinforcing the correct diagnosis.

3D ultrasound can also be helpful in localizing a cervical or cesarean scar pregnancy (Fig. 19–16). In these cases, it is important to get a correct impression of the sac, which has a bearing on prognosis and management.

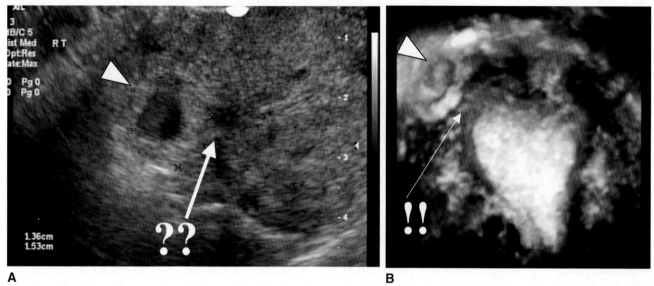

A   **B**

Figure 19–14. Cornual interstitial pregnancy. **A,** Conventional 2D sonography leaves some doubt whether the chorionic sac *(arrowhead)* is indeed in an ectopic position. The *arrow* points toward the area that should represent a discontinuous segment between the sac and the uterine cavity. **B,** On 3D sonography, there is no doubt that myometrium is interposed between the sac *(arrowhead)* and the hyperechoic cavity. The thick-slice technique was used to generate this image.

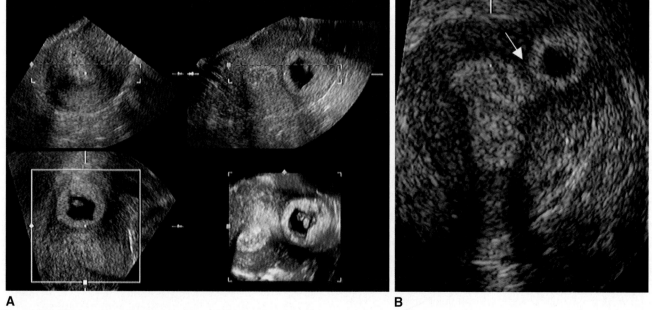

A   **B**

Figure 19–15. Cornual pregnancy of 7 weeks 4 days. **A,** The orthogonal planes pinpoint the exact location of the ectopic gestation. The rendered image (box D) emphasizes the ectopic location. **B,** In the coronal plane, the lack of continuity between the endometrium and the coronal gestational sac becomes evident. The *arrow* points to the interposing myometrium.

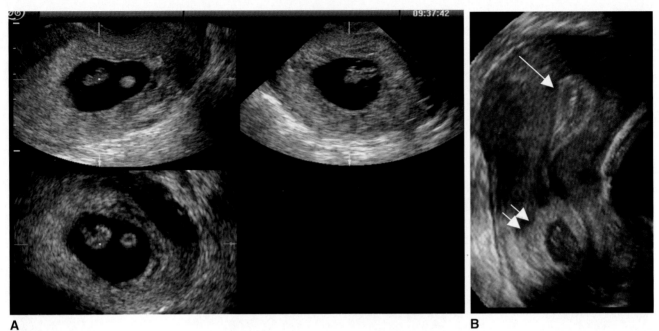

Figure 19–16. Cervical pregnancy. **A,** The orthogonal planes correctly locate the ectopic gestation within the cervix. **B,** The thick-slice panoramic view depicts the empty uterine cavity *(single arrow)* and the gestation in the cervix *(double arrows)*.

Examination of the Fallopian Tube

3D ultrasound offers a comprehensive picture of the fallopian tube if pathology is involved. The most striking results are obtained if fluid fills the tube. Hydrosalpinx is often misdiagnosed as a pelvic fluid collection or an ovarian lesion. Obtaining a volume of the target area (Fig. 19–17A) enables postprocessing and, after scrolling, turning to obtain the best plane to demonstrate the true nature of the pathology (Fig. 19–17B). Demonstration of incomplete septae leaves little doubt that hydrosalpinx is the correct diagnosis, which is more difficult to establish using only 2D ultrasound.

The usefulness of 3D in examining adnexal pathology is demonstrated in Figure 19–18. In these pictures, the initial orthogonal planes were not helpful until the inversion rendering mode was used. In both examples, a clear "cast" of the endotubal fluid outlined hydrosalpinges.

Examination of the Ovaries

The use of 3D imaging of the ovaries lagged behind imaging of other pelvic organs. The first articles in the literature approached 3D imaging of the ovaries through volume determinations.[25,26]

In 2000 Kurjak et al.[27] described the characterization of ovarian lesions using 3D power Doppler techniques. Contrast media were also studied to better define adnexal masses.[28] In a natural development, 3D ultrasound began to be used to detect ovarian cancer.[29-31] Morphologic assessment by 3D ultrasound yielded additional information (versus 2D sonography) in 58% of cases. 3D ultrasound also correctly diagnosed two cases of fallopian tube cancer.[30]

In another study by Kurjak et al.,[31] 43 stage I ovarian cancers were detected preoperatively. Morphologic analysis by 3D ultrasound alone detected 74% of the cancers. The use of 3D power Doppler evaluation of tumor vascularity predicted 41 cases of stage I ovarian cancer—a 95.4% detection rate.

Combined morphologic and 3D Doppler findings achieved even higher diagnostic accuracy—97.7%.

In the meantime, the Kretztechnik company (Zipf, Austria) developed a new technology: volume determination based on outlining the contours of a structure (e.g., the ovary) on 3D (orthogonal) planes. When the outlines are advanced in a stepwise fashion (every 3, 9, 15, or 30 degrees) and the contours are redefined on each subsequent section, the volume of a 3D structure (e.g., the ovary) can be calculated automatically. Raine-Fenning et al.[32,33] used this virtual organ computer-aided analysis (VOCAL) software in 40 endometrial and ovarian volume data sets and tested the interobserver reliability of the results. An interclass correlation coefficient of 0.9 in both organs was obtained. They concluded that 3D ultrasound can reliably be used to acquire, analyze, and define ovarian and endometrial volumes. They validated this technique first in an in vitro setting.[34] Using the sculpturing tools of 3D software, it is possible to "cut" the rendered ovary in half and inspect the cut surface for irregularities or papillations (Fig. 19-19).

In 2001 Cohen et al.[35] published a study of 71 women with known adnexal masses who were evaluated by 2D ultrasound as well as 3D power Doppler angiography. Surgical staging was also performed. Transvaginal sonography identified 40 masses suspicious for cancer. 3D orthogonal (multiplanar) studies did not significantly change this number. However, the addition of 3D power Doppler interrogation reduced the number of suspicious masses to 28. None of the proven cancers had a negative power Doppler examination. The authors concluded that 3D power Doppler evaluation defined the morphologic and vascular characteristics of ovarian lesions significantly better than 2D ultrasound alone.[35] Specificity was significantly improved by the addition of 3D power Doppler analysis.

Three-Dimensional Power Doppler Angiography

3D power Doppler angiography is a new tool made possible by the evolving volume scan technology. It is a sonographic

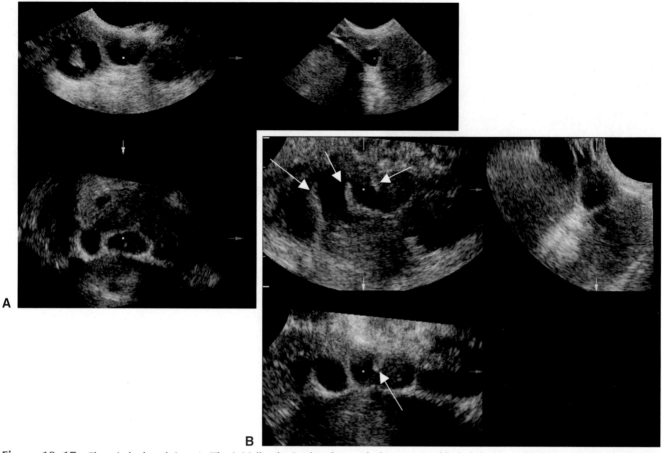

Figure 19–17. Chronic hydrosalpinx. **A,** The initially obtained orthogonal planes were of little help in establishing a diagnosis. **B,** After scrolling and turning the planes, a diagnostic picture was obtained. The incomplete septae *(arrows)* and the contiguous anechoic fluid space with the thin walls established the diagnosis of a chronic hydrosalpinx.

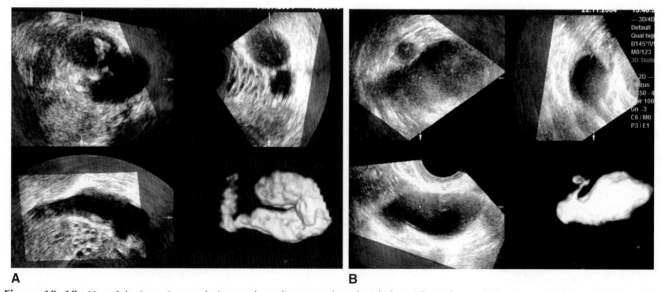

Figure 19–18. Use of the inversion rendering mode to diagnose adnexal pathology. The orthogonal planes are nondiagnostic. By rendering and inverting the volume, the diagnosis of two hydrosalpinges is clear (box D of **A** and **B**).

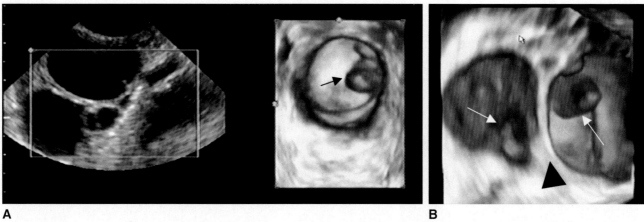

A   **B**

Figure 19–19. Papillae in an ovarian lesion. **A,** Side-by-side pictures of a cystic ovarian mass. The left is a two-dimensional image that shows only a hint of the papillae. The right picture clearly shows the 3D surface rendering of the papillae *(arrow)*. **B,** By "slicing" the volume containing the cyst with the electronic scalpel of the 3D software and rotating the cut surface, it is easy to see that both compartments of the cyst contain papillae. *Arrowhead* shows the dividing wall between the two cystic compartments.

"angiogram" created by power Doppler–based identification of blood flow of the vascular tree, where the vessel diameter is about 0.5 to 1 mm and blood velocity exceeds 2 to 3 mm/second. At this time, we use the GE Voluson Expert 730 model ultrasound machine and its laptop-based software (3D-View) to obtain the 3D angiographic picture.

The first step in 3D Doppler angiography is to evaluate the ovary with the power Doppler mode, setting the pulse repetition frequency just above the level necessary to suppress unwanted color artifacts. The wall filter is then set to levels that create the optimal visual picture. Then the 3D volume is obtained with the highest possible resolution (slowest acquisition speed). After displaying the orthogonal planes, the "render" mode is activated; by selecting the "color" option, the vessels contained in the entire volume appear on the screen (Fig. 19–20A).

Next, the VOCAL program is activated. The contour of the ovary is outlined electronically on any desired plane. By rotating the volume (9 degrees in the example in Fig. 19–20), the ovarian contours are outlined on each subsequent section. At the end of this process, the volume shell of the ovary appears in the rendering box (Fig. 19–20B). The actual measurement of the volume is also displayed.

At this point, several options are possible: (1) render the structure by the so-called glass-body appearance, in which the vasculature is seen within the "transparently rendered" ovary (Fig. 19–20C); (2) display only the vessels in the "cut-out" structure (Fig. 19–20D); or (3) activate the "histogram" option, which displays the different vascularization indices of the ovary (Fig. 19–20E). The histogram displays the values of the mean gray value (between 0 and 100), vascularization index (%), flow index (between 0 and 100), and vascularization flow index (between 0 and 100). Only the vascularization index is an absolute value expressing the amount of color-flow–containing voxels as a percentage of the ovarian volume.

The clinical relevance of this 3D ultrasound evaluation of flow to different organs, and its reliability, has yet to be tested. Pairleitner et al.[36] studied the reproducibility of this technique and concluded that reproducible information for all flow indices except the vascularization flow index can be obtained. They speculated that these indices may be used as a predictor of neoangiogenesis.

Fleischer et al.[37] addressed the ultrasound imaging of intratumoral vascularity with 3D color Doppler techniques. They studied 26 patients with ovarian masses. The finding of central intratumoral vascularity had a high positive predictive value of 90% for malignancy. Conversely, the absence of such vessels had a negative predictive value of 96%. Their conclusion was that color Doppler sonography in general and 3D color Doppler interrogation in particular are helpful in diagnosing vascular density in the ovary. This method seems to be useful in distinguishing benign from malignant ovarian masses.

It should be noted that 3D power Doppler angiography evaluates only blood vessels whose calibers exceed those of capillaries. Vascular endothelial growth factor as well as other factors renders the newly formed capillaries permeable to fluid. The micropermeability of blood vessels in ovarian cancer, for instance, is addressed by studies that use contrast media while viewing the ovary by transvaginal sonography to detect pathologic extravasation.

Ovarian Torsion

The general subjects of adnexal torsion, ovarian torsion, and selective fallopian torsion are addressed in Chapters 8 and 17. This subject was also touched on by Yaman et al.[38] This group used the vascularization indices to establish the diagnosis of torsion. Based on this study, they claimed that the diagnosis of ovarian torsion can be better achieved by 3D power Doppler than by 2D Doppler sonography.

A pathognomonic sign of ovarian torsion, consisting of a coiled pattern of vessels, can be obtained by 3D as well as 3D color and power Doppler evaluation. Figure 19–21 depicts the power Doppler–generated 3D angiographic image of a twisted pedicle leading to ovarian torsion (also seen in Fig. 18–23). These vessels, in spite of the torsion, still demonstrate some blood flow. The 3D angiogram of the coiled vessels has the appearance of a coiled telephone cord.

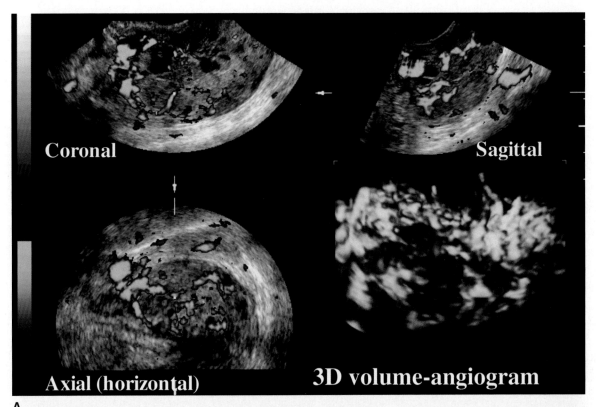

A

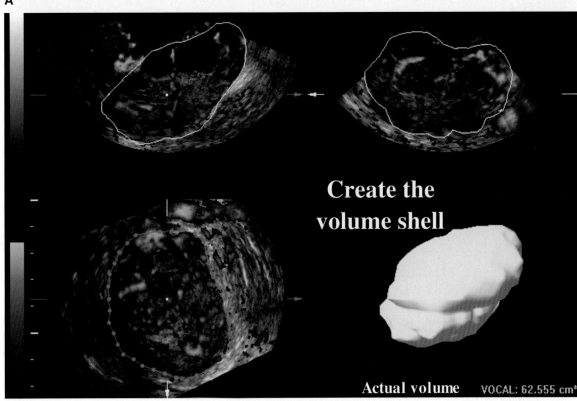

B

Figure 19–20. Evaluation of ovarian vasculature using the virtual organ computer-aided analysis (VOCAL) technique. **A,** The vasculature highlighted by power Doppler is displayed in the orthogonal planes. The rendering box is the rendered 3D power Doppler angiographic appearance of the entire volume. **B,** Using the VOCAL software, the shell of the ovary and its actual volume (in milliliters) is obtained and displayed in the rendering box (box D). *Continued*

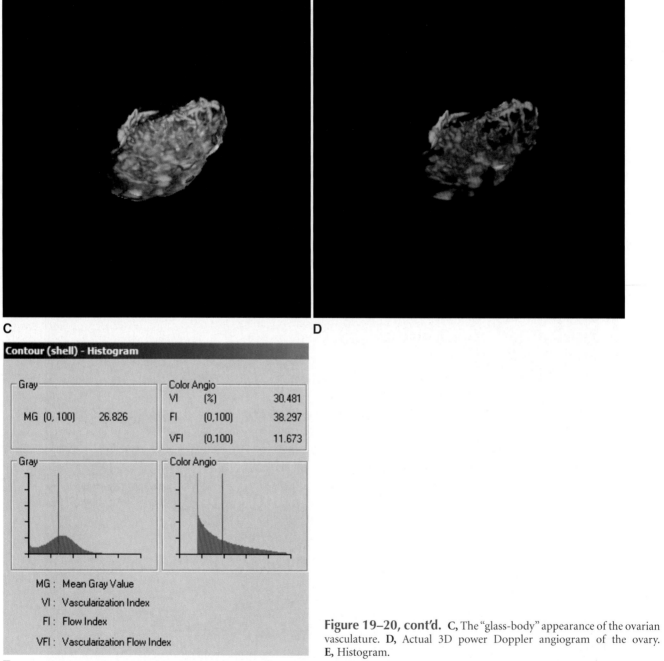

C

D

Contour (shell) - Histogram

Gray

MG (0, 100)   26.826

Color Angio

VI   (%)   30.481

FI   (0,100)   38.297

VFI   (0,100)   11.673

Gray

Color Angio

MG : Mean Gray Value

VI : Vascularization Index

FI : Flow Index

VFI : Vascularization Flow Index

E

Figure 19–20, cont'd. C, The "glass-body" appearance of the ovarian vasculature. **D,** Actual 3D power Doppler angiogram of the ovary. **E,** Histogram.

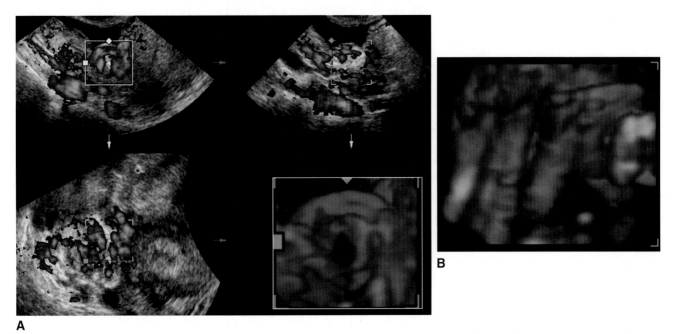

Figure 19–21. 3D power Doppler images of a twisted pedicle in a case of ovarian torsion. **A,** Color Doppler picture of the area of interest shown in the orthogonal planes. The *inset* is the 3D angiographic rendering of the twisted, coiled blood vessels (still with some blood flow) leading to the ovary. **B,** By turning the rendered 3D angiography image 90 degrees, the loops of the vessels are seen.

Summary

The application of 3D ultrasound in gynecology is a relatively new but quickly developing field. The different applications and rendering techniques are in the early stages of development; many of them have not yet been sufficiently tested to allow clinical applications. Presently, the most useful role of 3D ultrasound is in the detection of uterine malformations. We are confident, however, that 3D ultrasound will become an increasingly important and integral part of gynecologic diagnosis.

REFERENCES

 1. Timor-Tritsch IE, Condrea A: New technologies in obstetrics and gynecology: The test of time. Ultrasound Obstet Gynecol 1994;4:355-357.
 2. Lemery DJ, Vanlieferinghen P, Gasq M, et al: Fetal umbilical cord ligation under ultrasound guidance. Ultrasound Obstet Gynecol 1994;4:399-401.
 3. Ville Y, Hyett JA, Vandenbussche FP, Nicolaides KH: Endoscopic laser coagulation of umbilical cord vessels in twin reversed arterial perfusion sequence. Ultrasound Obstet Gynecol 1994;4:396-398.
 4. Giordano B, Contino B, Gippa R, et al: Use of an endolaparoscopic probe in conservative management of fallopian pregnancy. Ultrasound Obstet Gynecol 1994;4:402-405.
 5. Mertz E: 3D Ultrasound in Obstetrics and Gynecology. Philadelphia, Lippincott Williams & Wilkins, 1998.
 6. Kurjak A: Clinical Applications of 3D Sonography. New York, Parthenon Books, 2000.
 7. Nelson TR, Downey DB, Pretorius DH, Feuster A: Three-Dimensional Ultrasound. Philadelphia, Lippincott Williams & Wilkins, 1999.
 8. Kurjak A, Jackson D: An Atlas of 3D and 4D Sonography in Obstetrics and Gynecology. New York, Taylor & Francis Group, 2004.
 9. Moeglin D, Benoit B, De Ziegler D: Advantages of studying the frontal plane of the uterine cavity in 3D ultrasound. Contracept Fertil Sex 1999;27:710-720.
10. La Torre R, Prosperi Porta R, Franco C, et al: Three-dimensional sonography and hysterosalpingosonography in the diagnosis of uterine anomalies. Clin Exp Obstet Gynecol 2003;30:190-192.
11. Maymon R, Herman A, Ariely S, et al: Three-dimensional vaginal sonography in obstetrics and gynaecology. Hum Reprod Update 2000;6:475-484.
12. Kupesic S, Kurjak A, Skenderovic S, Bjelos D: Screening for uterine abnormalities by three-dimensional ultrasound improves perinatal outcome. J Perinat Med 2002;30:9-17.
13. Timor-Tritsch IE, Monteagudo A, Tsymbal T, Strok I: Three-dimensional inversion rendering: A new sonographic technique and its use in gynecology. J Ultrasound Med 2005;24:681-688.
14. Lin HH, Wu MH, Huang SC, Hsu CC: Early detection of unilateral occlusion of duplicated uterus with ipsilateral renal anomaly in young girls: Two case reports with three-dimensional sonography. Kao Hsiung J Med Sci 1999;15:244-247.
15. Salim R, Woelfer B, Backos M, et al: Reproducibility of three-dimensional ultrasound diagnosis of congenital uterine anomalies. Ultrasound Obstet Gynecol 2003;21:578-582.
16. Salim R, Lee C, Davies A, et al: A comparative study of three-dimensional saline infusion sonohysterography and diagnostic hysteroscopy for the classification of submucous fibroids. Hum Reprod 2005;20:253-257.
17. Sylvestre C, Child TJ, Tulandi T, Tan SL: A prospective study to evaluate the efficacy of two- and three-dimensional sonohysterography in women with intrauterine lesions. Fertil Steril 2003;79:1222-1225.
18. Monteagudo A, Tsymbal T: Sonographic clues to müllerian anomalies. Contemp Ob/Gyn 2005;50:62-70.
19. Monteagudo A, Strok I, Greenidge S, Timor-Tritsch IE: Quadruplet pregnancy: Two sets of twins, each occupying a horn of a septate (complete) uterus. J Ultrasound Med. 2004;23:1107-1111.
20. Hosli I, Holzgreve W, Tercanli S: Use of 3-dimensional ultrasound for assessment of intrauterine device position. Ultraschall Med 2001;22:75-80.
21. Salim R, Woelfer B, Backos M, et al: Reproducibility of three-dimensional ultrasound diagnosis of congenital uterine anomalies. Ultrasound Obstet Gynecol 2003;21:578-582.
22. Kyei-Mensah A, Maconochie N, Zaidi J, et al: Transvaginal three-dimensional ultrasound: Reproducibility of ovarian and endometrial volume measurements. Fertil Steril 1996;66:718-722.
23. Rempen A: The shape of the endometrium evaluated with three-dimensional ultrasound: An additional predictor of extrauterine pregnancy. Hum Reprod 1998;13:450-454.
24. Harika G, Gabriel R, Carre-Pigeon F, et al: Primary application of three-dimensional ultrasonography to early diagnosis of ectopic pregnancy. Eur J Obstet Gynecol Reprod Biol 1995;60:117-120.
25. Gilja OH, Hausken T, Berstad A, Odegaard S: Measurements of organ volume by ultrasonography. Proc Inst Mech Eng [H] 1999;213:247-259.

26. Schild RL, Knobloch C, Dorn C, et al: The role of ovarian volume in an in vitro fertilization programme as assessed by 3D ultrasound. Arch Gynecol Obstet 2001;265:67-72.

27. Kurjak A, Kupesic S, Sparac V, Kosuta D: Three-dimensional ultrasonographic and power Doppler characterization of ovarian lesions. Ultrasound Obstet Gynecol 2000;16:365-371.

28. Kupesic S, Kurjak A: Contrast-enhanced, three-dimensional power Doppler sonography for differentiation of adnexal masses. Obstet Gynecol 2000;96:452-458.

29. Kurjak A, Kupesic S, Jacobs I: Preoperative diagnosis of the primary fallopian tube carcinoma by three-dimensional static and power Doppler sonography. Ultrasound Obstet Gynecol 2000;15:246-251.

30. Kurjak A, Kupesic S, Sparac V, Bekavac I: Preoperative evaluation of pelvic tumors by Doppler and three-dimensional sonography. J Ultrasound Med 2001;20:829-840.

31. Kurjak A, Kupesic S, Sparac V, et al: The detection of stage I ovarian cancer by three-dimensional sonography and power Doppler. Gynecol Oncol 2003;90:258-264.

32. Raine-Fenning NJ, Campbell BK, Clewes JS, et al: The interobserver reliability of three-dimensional power Doppler data acquisition within the female pelvis. Ultrasound Obstet Gynecol 2004;23:501-508.

33. Raine-Fenning NJ, Campbell BK, Clewes JS, Johnson IR: The interobserver reliability of ovarian volume measurement is improved with three-dimensional ultrasound, but dependent upon technique. Ultrasound Med Biol 2003;29:1685-1690.

34. Raine-Fenning NJ, Clewes JS, Kendall NR, et al: The interobserver reliability and validity of volume calculation from three-dimensional ultrasound data sets in the in vitro setting. Ultrasound Obstet Gynecol 2003;21:283-291.

35. Cohen LS, Escobar PF, Scharm C, et al: Three-dimensional power Doppler ultrasound improves the diagnostic accuracy for ovarian cancer prediction. Gynecol Oncol 2001;82:40-48.

36. Pairleitner H, Steiner H, Hasenoehrl G, Staudach A: Three-dimensional power Doppler sonography: Imaging and quantifying blood flow and vascularization. Ultrasound Obstet Gynecol 1999;14:139-143.

37. Fleischer AC, Milam MR, Crispens MA, Shappell HW: Sonographic depiction of intratumoral vascularity with 2- and 3-dimensional color Doppler techniques. J Ultrasound Med 2005;24:533-537.

38. Yaman C, Ebner T, Jesacher K: Three-dimensional power Doppler in the diagnosis of ovarian torsion. Ultrasound Obstet Gynecol 2002;20:513-515.

Chapter 20

Ultrasound-Enhanced Bimanual Examination

Steven R. Goldstein

The clinical use of diagnostic ultrasound in obstetrics and gynecology has had a complicated evolution. Initially, real-time equipment had barely enough resolution to identify breech versus vertex, measure a biparietal diameter, and localize the placenta. A complete examination was extremely limited and consisted of two or three Polaroid pictures. Obstetric ultrasonography began when office nurses were sent to various short courses to learn obstetric scanning. Over time, however, obstetric scanning has become more sophisticated. The standard obstetric examination now mandates an understanding of cross-sectional body anatomy (e.g., heart, brain) that goes beyond the scope of routine training in obstetrics and gynecology.[1] Gynecologic imaging, with static arm scanners and later small-headed sector scanners, was always more involved. The equipment was large and expensive and, for the most part, remained in the domain of the imaging laboratory.

Gynecologists spend several months in the gynecologic pathology laboratory, where they routinely examine the pelvis and operate in the pelvis. (Residents in radiology, in contrast, spend 4 months rotating through neuroradiology to gain an understanding of intracranial anatomy—both normal and aberrant.) Certainly, imaging of the pelvis can and should be the domain of gynecologists. In medical school, gynecologists learned to take a history, do a directed physical examination, and then order the appropriate laboratory studies. In most people's view, sonography is a laboratory test, ordered after the history and physical examination lead to a working or differential diagnosis. I submit that transvaginal sonography can be part of the physical examination.

The bimanual examination consists of palpation to ascertain information. On the basis of thousands of examinations, many with subsequent surgical or pathologic confirmation, we mentally create an image of the anatomic findings that are in fact objective. Is the ovary enlarged? If so, is it cystic or solid? Is the uterus enlarged? Is it anteverted or retroverted? Is it irregular in contour, suggesting myomatous change? Other information is subjective and depends on the experience and interpretation of the examiner. Is there normal mobility? Is there tenderness? However, the objective component of the examination can be replaced with an image in a matter of

moments if the practitioner has the required expertise and equipment.

Further, the pelvis is a dynamic place. During the reproductive years, each month it undergoes a cycle, sometimes culminating in a pregnancy, most often culminating in menses. There should be synchrony between the ovarian findings and the endometrial response. Even in noncycling patients (postmenopausal women taking no medication and young women taking birth control pills), there are expected findings in both the ovary and the endometrium that should also be synchronous. Transvaginal sonography gives us information about the physiologic characteristics of the female pelvis; if they are aberrant, we refer to them as pathologic. This information is not otherwise available during the examination, because transvaginal sonography looks inside the ovary and uterus, allowing the clinician to function on a higher level.

An important development that facilitated gynecologic imaging was the introduction of vaginal probes. Equipment for transvaginal scanning can be used by the physician during the bimanual examination in the presence of an empty urinary bladder; the procedure requires very little time once the operator is adequately trained.

In my practice, I perform vaginal scanning only. If the clinical situation mandates full-bladder transabdominal views, I refer the patient to an imaging consultant. For some practitioners, that person will be a technician (*sonographer*) who functions as an imager elsewhere within the same practice.

Equipment Selection

For vaginal scanning in the office, the ideal situation is a dedicated small machine with one vaginal probe. The mainframe must be easily movable—flush with the examination table when in use, and then returned to the head of the table so as not to interfere with breast or abdominal palpation. The screen must be mobile enough to allow the patient to observe it with the clinician. In most cases, an abdominal transducer is not necessary to complement the vaginal probe. Because of their different applications, the machine should not be shared with an obstetric sonographer doing standard obstetric examinations in the mid-trimester. A printer or camera is mandatory. A videocassette or CD recorder is optional. Variable frequencies are very helpful. For most situations, the higher frequencies (6.5 to 7.5 MHz) are desired, but for obese patients and those with fibroids and slightly larger masses, the penetration afforded by a 5-MHz transducer may be essential.

Diagnostic Advantages

There are times when the physiologic information obtained by vaginal probe examination in the office allows an on-the-spot diagnosis, obviating the need to refer the patient for imaging, wait for the imager's report of anatomic findings, and then finalize the diagnosis and contact the patient. Consider this example: A 46-year-old P3003 patient status post–tubal ligation, usually with regular menses, presents with 8 weeks of amenorrhea. A 2-minute pregnancy test in the office is negative. Palpation reveals a normal-sized parous, anteverted uterus and a 4- to 5-cm right adnexal mass. The patient is sent for a sonogram, and the report (2 days later) reveals (1) a normal-sized uterus with thickened endometrial echo and (2) a 5.4- by 4.1-cm complex right adnexal mass, inadequately evaluated. The differential diagnosis includes endometrioma, neoplasia, and hemorrhagic cyst. Her obvious secretory endometrium (Fig. 20–1), coupled with a hemorrhagic corpus luteum showing classic clot retraction (Fig. 20–2), would have allowed the clinician to make the immediate diagnosis of delayed ovulation if the ultrasound results had been available immediately. Depending on the physician's comfort level, these findings might have been verified with a serum progesterone level, and the patient could have been told to expect a menses within a maximum of 2 weeks. Thus, an unnecessary course of progesterone for presumed anovulation (8 weeks of amenorrhea with a negative pregnancy test) could be avoided. If a normal menses does ensue, she should be re-examined in the proliferative phase of the second cycle to document the normalcy of the right ovary (Fig. 20–3). This example underscores the fact that the vaginal probe in the

hands of a gynecologist provides a gynecologic consultation, not merely objective anatomic information.[2,3]

Consider another example: The patient is a 43-year-old multipara who had a hysterectomy for postpartum hemorrhage 14 years earlier. She presents for routine gynecologic care. No masses are palpated. Enhancement of the bimanual examination with a transvaginal scan corroborates that both ovaries appear normal, but the presence of a fresh corpus luteum in the right ovary (Fig. 20–4) documents that she is still ovulatory despite the lack of a menstrual history. This also eliminates any need for serum hormonal level determinations.

Technical and Cost Considerations

Use of the vaginal probe allows higher-frequency equipment near the structures being studied, which results in excellent

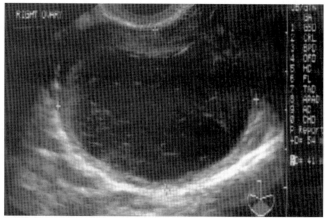

Figure 20–2. Right ovary measuring 5.4 by 4.1 cm. It is virtually replaced by a complex mass. This is the typical "cobweb" appearance of a hemorrhagic corpus luteum. Through a process of clot retraction, it will undergo maturation but may take up to two menstrual cycles to resolve.

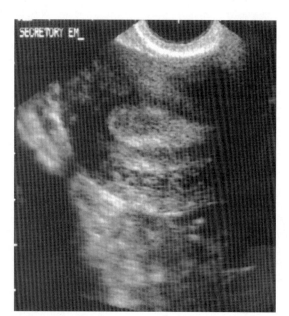

Figure 20–1. Long-axis view of the uterus reveals an obvious thickened endometrium that is homogeneous and typical of a secretory pattern.

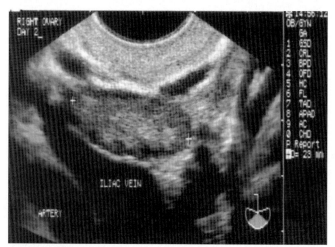

Figure 20–3. Same patient depicted in Figure 20–2. The scan should be performed after the second menses, within the first 7 to 10 days of the cycle (proliferative phase). This scan, performed on day 2, shows a totally normal right ovary in its normal anatomic location relative to the iliac vessels, with total resolution of the hemorrhagic corpus luteum.

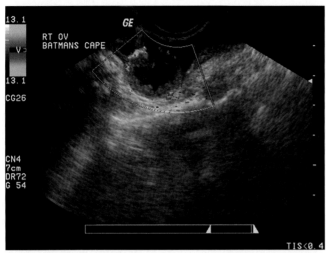

Figure 20–4. Transvaginal pelvic scan depicts a right ovary containing a fresh corpus luteum. This crenated, thick-walled structure sometimes has the classic appearance of "Batman's cape." The addition of color flow depicts a typical ring of vascularity around the fresh corpus luteum.

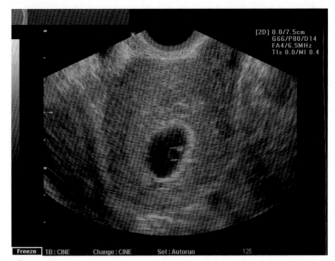

Figure 20–5. Patient at 43 days from the last menstrual period. Use of the vaginal probe was able to diagnose definitive intrauterine gestation in less than 5 seconds. The yolk sac and a 2-mm embryo attached to it are clearly visible.

resolution that is not lost with magnification. In addition, the procedure is very operator-friendly once the operator is adequately trained. The procedure is also time-efficient because it is performed with the patient still in the lithotomy position at the time of the bimanual examination. It thus adds very little time to the overall bimanual examination, and it has high patient acceptance. The drawbacks to the vaginal probe compared with traditional transabdominal scanning include a short field of view, the lack of sound enhancement provided by a filled urinary bladder, the limitations of the probe necessitated by the confines of the vagina, a new orientation for those familiar with traditional transabdominal panoramic views, and the presence of loops of bowel and the confusing echoes they generate throughout the pelvis.

In today's era of cost-consciousness, routine transvaginal sonography will probably become commonplace. There is high-quality equipment that is easy to operate. There are new devices with miniaturized ultrasonic chip technology, allowing small, lightweight equipment that can be attached to a docking station and moved from examination room to examination room. These devices are to the traditional sonography machine what the laptop is to the computer. Imaging will be available for every gynecologic examination, whether performed in the office, clinic, or emergency department. More than a decade ago, I predicted that each physician would have a personal probe, not unlike internists and their stethoscopes.[4] Though this is not yet standard, it is closer to reality.

It is less expensive for a clinician to diagnose pregnancy in a woman with amenorrhea (Fig. 20–5) by using a 22-cent condom and a vaginal probe than a $3.48 monoclonal antibody urine test for human chorionic gonadotropin. As methods of payment for health care services undergo change, physicians who shunned ultrasound-based decision making in the past will embrace it. If, instead of being paid for each dilation and curettage or laparoscopy performed, physicians had to fund those procedures out of the dollars allotted to them for their patients' health care, we would see an increased use of ultrasound to determine which patients do not need these

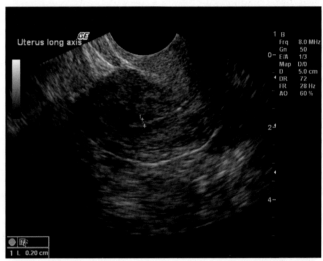

Figure 20–6. Transvaginal long-axis view of a postmenopausal patient who presented with vaginal staining. The endometrial echo was well visualized, thin, and distinct, measuring 0.2 cm (2 mm). It is clearly seen taking off from the endocervical canal and going toward the uterine fundus. Such a picture has an extremely high negative predictive value for excluding serious pathology.

invasive procedures. However, the fee charged for a visit should be increased to reflect the true cost of additional ultrasound equipment. Referral to an imaging specialist for color Doppler sonography, three-dimensional reconstructions, or consultative sonography should still be carried out when indicated. The mark of a good physician has always been knowing when to ask for help. In fact, if all gynecologists used transvaginal scanning on a routine basis, imaging specialists would be busier than ever with referrals.

The greatest contribution of gynecologic ultrasound is its high negative predictive value.[5] Ultrasound can be used to reliably predict which postmenopausal women with bleeding lack serious disease and can forgo dilation and curettage[6] (Fig. 20–6)

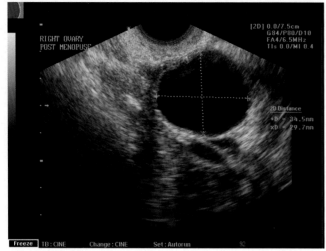

Figure 20–7. Postmenopausal patient with a cystic mass. This right ovarian cyst measures 3.5 by 3.0 cm. It is smooth walled and unilocular. Such structures are invariably benign and can be followed conservatively.

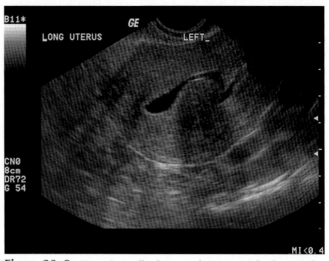

Figure 20–9. Posterior wall submucosal myoma with a large endoluminal component in a patient with significant abnormal uterine bleeding. Such a mass is most amenable to resectoscopic surgery. This type of preoperative assessment improves operative planning in terms of determining the equipment, personnel, time, and skill required.

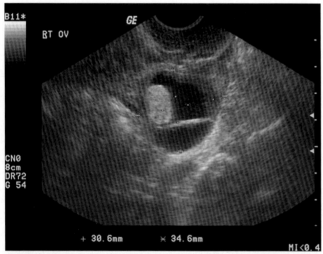

Figure 20–8. Benign cystic teratoma wholly contained within the right ovary. Overall, the ovary measures 3.5 by 3.1 cm. Note that the external contours of the ovary are not deformed. If approached laparoscopically, this ovary would appear morphologically normal from the epithelial surface. Such structures can be managed conservatively, without surgical intervention.

20–9) is diagnosed in the office with saline infusion sonohysterography, it ensures that the appropriate personnel and equipment will be available in the operating room and that enough time for resection will be allowed, because such surgery requires greater skill than simply removing a polyp.

Technique

The probe is reprocessed between patients, according to the guidelines of the American Institute of Ultrasound in Medicine.[8] For maximum safety, one should perform high-level disinfection of the probe between each use, and a probe cover or condom should be used to keep the probe clean. Ultrasound coupling gel is placed inside the condom. Outer lubricant is generally not necessary because a Pap smear and bimanual examination (with lubricant) have already been performed. The pelvic organs are imaged to confirm or deny impressions obtained during palpation. Also, physiologic information derived from the endometrial and ovarian appearance is noted. Frequent use of the abdominal hand to bring the structures closer to the probe tip improves results.

Once the probe is inserted into the vagina, it is manipulated posteriorly and anteriorly, and obliquely to the right and left, to image recognizable anatomic structures. The uterus in long-axis views (Fig. 20–10) serves as a basic anatomic landmark to orient one's eye and hand. The clinician looks for a recognizable endometrial echo surrounded by typical myometrium. The contour of the myometrial border, the homogeneity of the myometrium itself, and the character of the endometrium both subjectively and by measurement should be noted. The transducer is then turned 90 degrees to view the uterus in a semitransverse (or short-axis) plane. Moving the hand in an anteroposterior fashion allows this plane to be seen from cervix to fundus. Returning to the long-axis view, one then moves in a sagittal oblique fashion, looking for ovarian structures. These are recognized by their location in premenopausal patients immediately adjacent to the iliac

and which postmenopausal women with masses do not have cancer and can avoid surgical intervention[7] (Fig. 20–7). Transvaginal sonography allows patients with nothing more than hemorrhagic corpus luteum cysts to avoid surgery. It can result in less invasive therapies in many cases, such as a medical approach to early ectopic pregnancy, nonsurgical drug therapy for small endometriomas, or expectant management for small incidental dermoids (Fig. 20–8). When surgery is necessary, gynecologic transvaginal sonography can improve preoperative planning. For example, early recognition of a postmenopausal mass that is complex and morphologically worrisome allows a gynecologic oncologist to be consulted before surgery. When a submucosal myoma (Fig.

vessels. The iliac artery is smaller and can be seen to pulsate; the iliac vein lies above the artery, and its flow can often be seen on real-time images. In the lithotomy position, premenopausal patients without significant pelvic adhesions have ovaries that, by means of gravity, are located immediately adjacent to these vessels. Ovaries are also recognized by their appearance. They have a typical gray pattern to the stroma and contain many follicles at various stages of development, depending on which phase of the menstrual cycle the patient is in and whether she is taking oral contraceptive pills. When either ovary is found in this long-axis orientation, the transducer handle is turned 90 degrees. Assessing the ovary in two planes at right angles to each other allows three-dimensional assessment of the structure. The method of finding the contralateral ovary is the same. This imaging approach to the

uterus and the ovaries can be described as "organ-oriented" scanning, because their longitudinal and transverse planes do not match the classic planes of the body. A complete pelvic ultrasound examination should include assessment of the cul-de-sac and the region anterior to the uterus, where the bladder can often be seen to start to fill with a small amount of sonolucent urine. Characterization of the cervical region should be carried out as well.

Color-flow capability (not the resistance indices calculated with Doppler sonography) is essential for proper diagnostic imaging. It is the concept of color as morphology (Fig. 20–11). The ability to reliably distinguish blood flow within structures or to distinguish blood vessels from other anechoic structures in the pelvis that are cystic has become a necessary part of routine morphologic diagnosis.

Training and Acceptance

When a new skill is incorporated into residency training, as with fetal monitoring or laparoscopy, ultimately all graduating residents will be skilled in its use. For those physicians already in practice, postgraduate courses fill the training need. Each physician has his or her own learning curve when using a new diagnostic modality. After a physician becomes comfortable with the information derived from the vaginal probe examination, he or she can begin to factor it into overall clinical management. Until then, previous methods can be retained.

We can learn by the example of the urologic model for sonographic prostate examination. Once it was introduced, its acceptance, as with any new technology, took time. Obstetrics and gynecology has had ultrasound for more than 30 years but must always be open to new innovations. As with any new technology, there must be responsible ways of incorporating it into our routine. The greatest problem with the increased use of transvaginal scanning may be the overinterpretation of normal findings not previously imaged. This is unlike the early days of obstetric sonographic examination, when the greatest

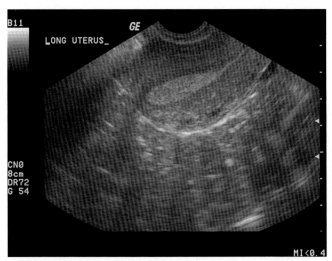

Figure 20–10. Long-axis view of the uterus in a patient with a secretory endometrium. This view provides a basic anatomic orientation for proceeding with a pelvic examination.

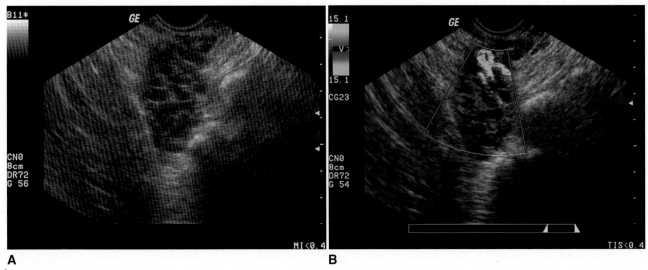

A   **B**

Figure 20–11. A, Two-dimensional pelvic scan suggesting a 4.3-cm cystic mass with internal echoes. **B,** Use of color-flow technology allows easy, rapid assessment and reveals that the sonolucent area actually represents dilated, tortuous blood vessels that were lateral to the uterus in this multiparous patient. This demonstrates the use of color to distinguish vascular from cystic structures.

fear (and rightfully so) was missing something that was present but unrecognized. With the high degree of magnification *(sonomicroscopy)*[9] that the vaginal probe allows us, conditions never before appreciated have become clinically evident. For example, the corpus luteum is not always a smooth-walled, unilocular structure; it can contain considerable debris and apppear more complex than originally thought possible.[3] Cul-de-sac fluid is shown more easily and more often with the vaginal probe. Very small, unilocular, smooth-walled postmenopausal cysts; echogenicity in postmenopausal endometria; and small, asymptomatic seedling myomas are easily seen. We need to address how to avoid overreacting to conditions that may be physiologic but previously escaped detection. This will require scientific studies to determine what of this new knowledge is important and requires intervention. An excellent example is that of endometrial fluid collections. In the 1980s, when these were viewed with transabdominal sonography, they were thought to be ominous signs of gynecologic malignancy.[10] With the vaginal probe, such collections are observed commonly, and they often represent transudate that accumulates in the endometrial cavity secondary to cervical stenosis. This naturally occurring sonohysterographic finding allows the depiction of endometrial tissue surrounding the fluid. Published observational studies clearly indicate that when the tissue surrounding the fluid is thin, it is associated with an inactive, atrophic endometrium—not the ominous finding originally described with transabdominal sonography.[11]

Current and Future Applications

Clinical practice has already been affected by vaginal probe sonography. Its most useful applications include evaluation of simple cystic, postmenopausal, adnexal masses; endometrial assessment for postmenopausal bleeding; assessment of irregular bleeding in perimenopausal patients to reduce the number of invasive diagnostic procedures and to better determine those who need surgery[12,13]; identification of early intrauterine pregnancies; the ability to diagnose and treat pregnancy failure, often before its spontaneous passage; diagnosis of extrauterine pregnancy[14]; and various aspects of infertility evaluation.[15]

The future may force us to rethink which clinical applications are appropriate for general clinicians and which should be reserved for imaging specialists. For example, in 25% of pregnancies, bleeding occurs in the first 10 weeks from the last menstrual period; in about 50% of these cases, the pregnancy will abort. The initial evaluation of these pregnancies to identify an intrauterine sac should be performed clinically. When the sac is not present or is of questionable normalcy, referral for consultative sonography is appropriate. Further, abnormal uterine bleeding accounts for 20% of gynecologic office visits. Endometrial assessment, often supplemented with saline infusion sonohysterography, is a relatively simple transvaginal sonographic maneuver that should be part of the clinician's initial approach. If the diagnosis is not easily and reliably

made, consultation should be sought. These are two common scenarios that clinicians can handle, provided that they have proper equipment, training, and interest. They can also confirm or deny the presence of masses suggested on bimanual examination, but definitive diagnosis of these masses may require more skill and training than the average clinician possesses.

Summary

An ultrasound-enhanced bimanual examination by office practitioners has tremendous assets. Diagnoses can often be made on the spot, leading to more timely therapy or, in the case of normal findings, relieving patients' anxiety. Vaginal scanning allows a more complete synthesis of the patient's gynecologic status both anatomically and physiologically at the time of the examination.

REFERENCES

1. American Institute of Ultrasound in Medicine: AIUM Practice Guideline for the Performance of an Antepartum Obstetric Ultrasound Examination. Laurel, Md, American Institute of Ultrasound in Medicine, 2003. Available at http://www.aium.org/provider/standards/obstetrical.pdf.
2. Goldstein SR: Routine use of office gynecologic ultrasound. J Ultrasound Med 2002;21:489-492.
3. Timor-Tritsch IE, Goldstein SR: The complexity of a complex mass and the simplicity of a simple cyst. J Ultrasound Med 2005;24:255-258.
4. Goldstein SR: Incorporating endovaginal ultrasonography into the overall gynecologic examination. Am J Obstet Gynecol 1990;162:625-633.
5. Langer RD, Pierce JJ, O'Hanlan KA, et al: Transvaginal ultrasonography compared with endometrial biopsy for the detection of endometrial disease: Postmenopausal Estrogen/Progestin Interventions Trial. N Engl J Med 1997;337:1792-1798.
6. Goldstein SR, Nachtigall M, Snyder JR, Nachtigall L: Endometrial assessment by vaginal ultrasonography before endometrial sampling in patients with postmenopausal bleeding. Am J Obstet Gynecol 1990;163:119-123.
7. Sassone AM, Timor-Tritsch IE, Artner A: Transvaginal sonographic characterization of ovarian disease: Evaluation of a new scoring system to predict ovarian malignancy. Obstet Gynecol 1991;78:70-77.
8. American Institute of Ultrasound in Medicine: Guidelines for cleaning and preparing endocavitary ultrasound transducers between patients. Available at http://aium.org/provider/standards/_statement selected.asp?.pdf.
9. Goldstein SR: Incorporating endovaginal ultrasound into the practitioner's routine pelvic examination. In Endovaginal Ultrasound, 2nd ed. New York, Wiley-Liss, 1991, pp 209-236.
10. Breckenridge JW, Kurtz AB, Ritchie WG, Macht EL Jr: Postmenopausal uterine fluid collection: Indicator of carcinoma. AJR Am J Roentgenol 1982;139:529-534.
11. Goldstein SR: Postmenopausal endometrial fluid collections revisited: Look at the doughnut rather than the hole. Obstet Gynecol 1994;83:738-740.
12. Goldstein SR: Menorrhagia and abnormal bleeding before the menopause. Best Pract Res Clin Obstet Gynaecol 2004;18:59-69.
13. Guven MA, Bese T, Demirkiran F: Comparison of hydrosonography and transvaginal ultrasonography in the detection of intracavitary pathologies in women with abnormal uterine bleeding. Int J Gynecol Cancer 2004;14:57-63.
14. Doubilet PM, Benson CB, Frates MC, Ginsburg E: Sonographically guided minimally invasive treatment of unusual ectopic pregnancies. J Ultrasound Med 2004;23:359-370.
15. Salim R, Jurkovic D: Assessing congenital uterine anomalies: The role of three-dimensional ultrasonography. Best Pract Res Clin Obstet Gynaecol 2004;18:29-36.

Chapter 21

Differential Diagnosis
of Inflammatory Diseases
of the Pelvis

Ilan E. Timor-Tritsch and Ana Monteagudo

In general, diagnosing tubal disease is one of the more difficult challenges in gynecologic ultrasound. The degree of difficulty increases in the presence of infected adnexa. The purpose of this chapter is twofold. First, we want to emphasize to gynecologists and sonologists the importance of understanding the natural history and manifestations of the different types and degrees of pelvic inflammatory disease (PID) through their typical ultrasound expressions. The ability to distinguish between the different types of PID is most important in the case of tubo-ovarian complex (TOC) and tubo-ovarian abscess (TOA), which carry different treatments. Second, we want to clarify the differential diagnosis between a chronic tubal disease (i.e., hydrosalpinx) and an ovarian tumor. An additional benefit from these observations is the demonstration of hydrosalpinges and infection after tubal ligation or hysterectomy.

Tubal inflammatory processes are the most common infectious diseases in the female pelvis. However, numerous entities must be considered in the differential diagnosis, including benign or malignant ovarian disease, ectopic pregnancy, pedunculated myoma, bowel disease, and fallopian tube cancer. Sometimes the diagnosis is not easy. This chapter presents the ultrasound features that will enable the clinician to distinguish among these pelvic diseases.

Tubal Inflammatory Disease

Inflammatory tubal disease can have serious consequences, sometimes leading to major surgery involving part or all of the female pelvis. More important, it may lead to infertility, ectopic pregnancy, or pelvic adhesions. It has been estimated that in the United States, approximately 10% to 15% of women in their reproductive years have at least one episode of tubal inflammatory disease, and at least 30% of infertility problems and 50% of ectopic pregnancies can be attributed to a previous infectious pelvic disease.[1,2]

Clinical Features of Tubal Disease

To understand the various pathologic states of the inflamed salpinx, the examiner must be familiar with the normal macroscopic and microscopic features of the intact organ. Figure 21–1A depicts the slender, thin, and abundant endosalpingeal folds of a normal tube on cross section under a low-power microscope. Figure 21–1B, a simplified line drawing of the tubal wall and lumen, will help clarify the pathologic states described later.

Clinical tubal inflammatory disease is almost uniformly an ascending disease. It strikes close to or during ovulation, taking advantage of the vulnerable ovarian surface and the varying amounts of blood present in the pelvis around the tubes or close to the ovaries.

The inflammation begins unilaterally, then spreads to the contralateral tube (and ovary). This sequence explains why the inflammatory processes in the two adnexa sometimes appear out of phase. Clinically, the process may heal, may become chronic, or may form an abscess. If it becomes chronic, it may result in dilated, fluid-filled tubes; hydrosalpinges or fluid may accumulate in the pelvis, forming a pelvic peritoneal inclusion cyst (Fig. 21–2).

In the *acute phase* of the disease, the acutely ill fallopian tube has a thick wall, the mucosa is edematous, and the fine, thin structure of the endosalpingeal folds disappears, replaced by thick, engorged structures (Fig. 21–3). There is some purulent exudate in the lumen that may leak through the still-patent fimbrial end into the pelvis. Later, the distal end of the tube may occlude, giving rise to a pus-filled salpinx (pyosalpinx). The ipsilateral ovary may also be involved, at first forming a TOC. After treatment this may heal or may progress to a chronic stage; if untreated, it will progress to form a TOA.

The *chronic phase* of tubal inflammatory disease is characterized by a distended, thin-walled, fluid-containing structure that tries to find a place in the pelvis. In so doing, it may kink once, twice, or even more. The inner wall structure loses most of the endosalpingeal folds, which flatten and undergo fibrosis, giving rise to solid, sonographically hyperechoic, papilla-like structures (Fig. 21–4). Adhesions may develop around the tube, and loculated pelvic fluid often accumulates in the cul-de-sac.

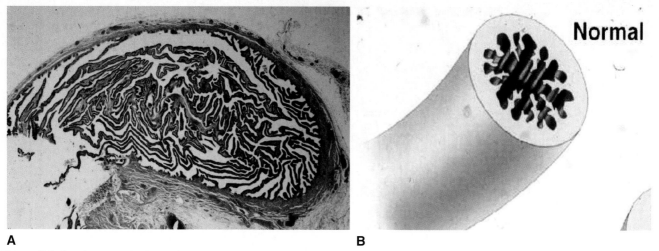

A   **B**

Figure 21–1. The normal tube. **A,** Cross section of a normal tube under a low-power microscope. Note the abundant, thin endosalpingeal folds. **B,** Line drawing of a normal tube, highlighting its cross section.

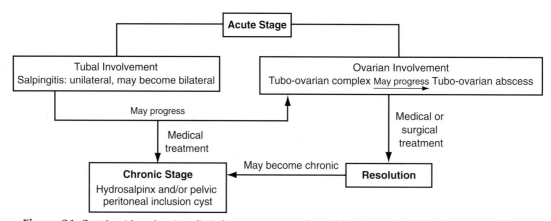

Figure 21–2. Algorithm showing clinical management and possible course of pelvic inflammatory disease.

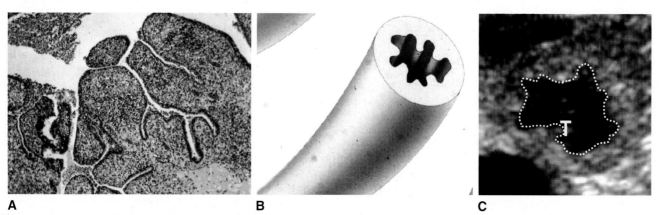

A   **B**   **C**

Figure 21–3. Acute salpingitis with some inflammatory exudate in the lumen (pyosalpinx). **A,** Histologic picture of the thick, edematous mucosa of the inflamed tube. Note the thick, richly infiltrated endosalpingeal folds. **B,** Illustration of the inflammatory process of the tube, with thick walls, edematous mucosal folds, and some fluid in the lumen, creating the cogwheel sign. **C,** Ultrasound cross section of the tube (T) with acute salpingitis; the *dotted line* traces the surface of the thick, edematous endosalpinx.

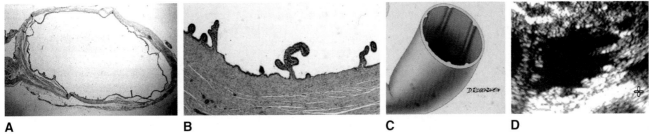

Figure 21–4. Chronic salpingitis with fluid in the tubal lumen (hydrosalpinx). **A,** Histologic appearance of the thin-walled, dilated tube under the low-power microscope. Note the total lack of endosalpingeal folds. **B,** The same tube by higher-power microscopy. Note the rudimentary, fibrosed, stunted remnants of the endosalpingeal folds. **C,** Line drawing of a dilated, thin-walled tube with mucosal nodules representing the fibrosed endosalpingeal folds. **D,** Ultrasound image of a hydrosalpinx. On cross section, hyperechoic nodules line the wall, giving it the appearance of a rosary (beads-on-a-string sign).

The power of palpatory findings, as well as the medical and surgical history, to discriminate between acute and chronic disease before ultrasound examination is disappointing. As expected, all patients with acute inflammatory tubal disease have palpatory as well as sonographic pelvic findings; however, only three fourths of patients with incidental sonographic findings have a history of PID.

Ultrasound Markers of Tubal Disease

Transvaginal sonography is the preferred route for investigating PID.

It is easier to detect a pathologic tube than a normal one. Prerequisites for visualizing a pathologic tube are fluid in the lumen, a thick wall, a tubal ectopic pregnancy, tubal torsion, or involvement by a neoplastic process.

The goal of this part of the chapter is to enable the reader to identify the different ultrasound markers of tubal disease and place them in the context of their pathogenesis. Doing so may facilitate easy recognition and proper ultrasound classification as well as guide application of the correct terminology of pelvic inflammatory processes. Correct identification of the chronic sequelae of previous inflammatory disease will enable the observer to differentiate these findings from unrelated diseases of the bowel, cystic ovarian neoplasia with papillary formations, or overt ovarian malignancy.

The examiner needs to be familiar with the ultrasound appearance of the normal fallopian tube. On transvaginal sonography, only the proximal 2 to 3 cm of a normal tube can be recognized; the slender, thin-walled, ampullary end of the normal tube is obscured by the surrounding bowel. The normal tube (and ovary) can be detected sonographically only if it is surrounded by some amount of intrapelvic fluid (Fig. 21–5).

The ultrasound appearance of tubal disease is recognizable and reproducible.[3-13] Our description[14] of the typical ultrasound appearances of inflammatory involvement of the tube and the ovary will be used in this chapter as the model for imaging this disease.

A clear grasp of the ultrasound picture in the context of the clinical setting will help to reduce the confusion surrounding the clinical diagnosis of tubal disease, which is illustrated by the large number of terms used to describe these conditions, such as PID, TOC, TOA, salpingitis, hydrosalpinx, pyosalpinx, and others. Figure 21–6 shows the clinical course

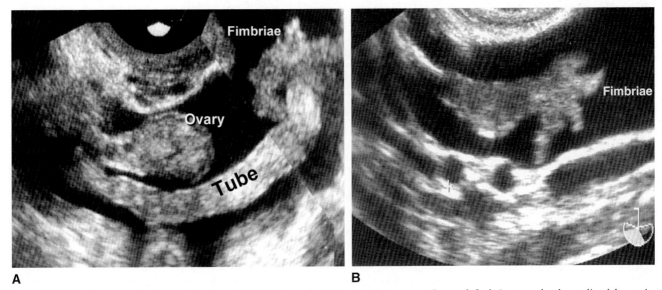

Figure 21–5. The normal tube can be imaged if fluid surrounds it. **A,** The ovary, tube, and fimbriae are clearly outlined by ascites. **B,** A normal tube with its fimbriae within pelvic fluid.

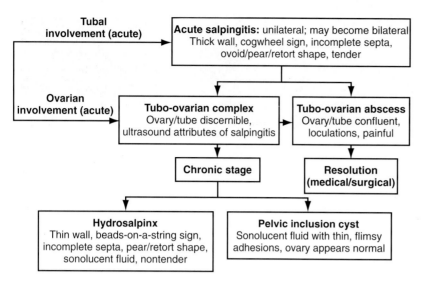

Figure 21–6. Algorithm showing the ultrasound markers of acute and chronic tubal inflammatory disease.

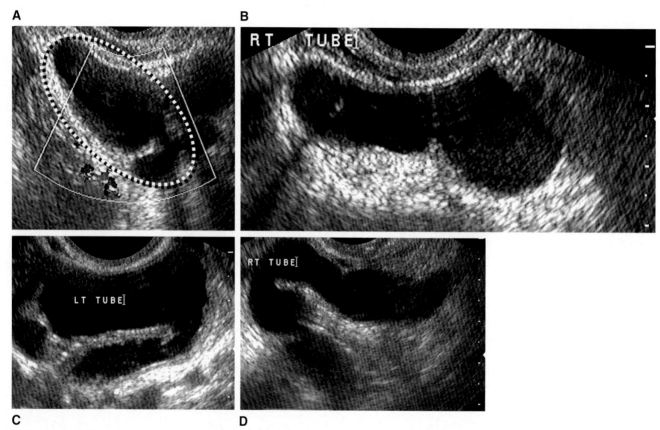

Figure 21–7. Shape as an ultrasound marker of inflammatory tubal diseases. **A,** Oval-shaped fluid-filled tube. **B,** Pear-shaped fluid-filled tube. **C,** Retort-shaped fluid-filled tube. **D,** Serpiginous fluid-filled tube.

of an ascending pelvic infection with the appropriate ultrasound expressions of the various stages of the disease, with or without ovarian involvement.

Shape

The shape of the lesion may vary, but all of the variations are recognizable and typical for the disease:

- Oval (Fig. 21–7A): this is the general shape of the lesion, which sets it apart from an ovarian lesion, which rarely if ever is oval.
- Pear shaped (Fig. 21–7B)
- Retort shaped (Fig. 21–7C): typical of a doubled-up, fluid-filled tube
- Serpiginous (Fig. 21–7D): resembles sausage links

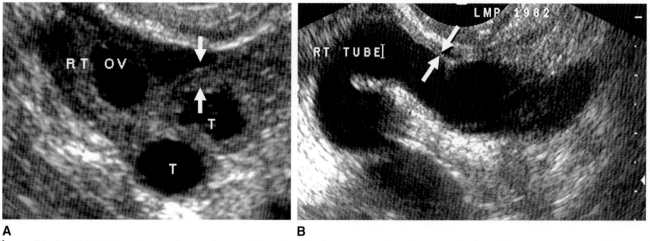

Figure 21–8. Wall thickness *(arrows)* as an ultrasound marker of inflammatory tubal disease. **A,** Thick wall (≥4 mm). **B,** Thin wall (≤3 mm).

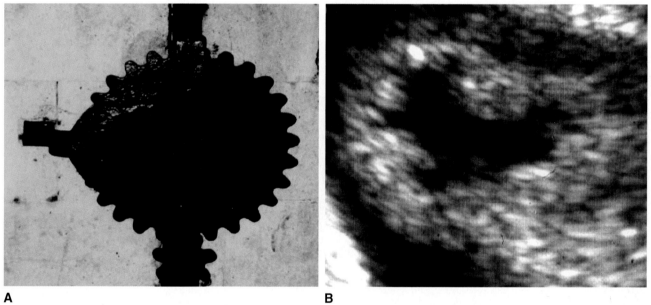

Figure 21–9. Wall structure as an ultrasound marker of inflammatory tubal disease—the cogwheel sign. **A,** A cogwheel for comparison. **B,** The cogwheel sign. A small amount of endoluminal fluid and the thickened wall give the cross section the appearance of a cogwheel.

Wall Thickness

Empirically, we call a wall thickness of 3 mm or less *thin,* and a thickness of 4 mm or more *thick* (Fig. 21–8). A thick wall is seen in the acute phase of the disease, whereas a thin wall is typical of chronic tubal disease.

Wall Structure

The ultrasound features of the diseased fallopian tube wall include the following:

- *Cogwheel sign.* The cross-sectional view of the tube reveals a thick wall, some intraluminal fluid, and thick, "edematous" endosalpingeal folds, creating the so-called cogwheel sign characteristic of the inflamed tube. This picture is usually indicative of acute tubal disease (Fig. 21–9).

- *Beads-on-a-string sign.* The walls are thin and distended by a larger amount of endoluminal fluid, and they are studded with hyperechoic nodules that show no blood flow. This cross-sectional appearance resembles a rosary (Fig. 21–10) and is typical of a chronic hydrosalpinx.
- *Incomplete septa* (Fig. 21–11). This feature results from kinking of the occluded, fluid-filled tube due to restricted space in the lesser pelvis. Sonography shows a septum of variable thickness that does not usually reach the opposite wall. Exerting pressure on the adnexa with the transducer results in a shifting of the fluid between the compartments of the tube, proving the contiguous nature of the sonolucent structures. The most probable pathogenesis of an occluded tube with incomplete septa is shown in Figure 21–12. Incomplete septa can be seen in the acute as well as the chronic stage of inflammatory tubal disease; therefore, this ultrasound

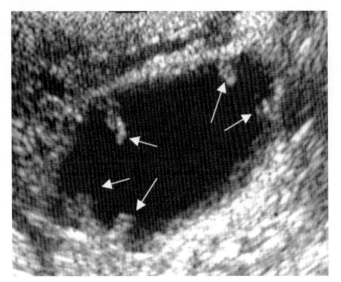

Figure 21–10. Wall structure as an ultrasound marker of inflammatory tubal disease—the beads-on-a-string sign. The *arrows* point to the hyperechoic mural nodules consistent with the fibrosed remnants of endosalpingeal folds.

sign is not a discriminatory feature between acute and chronic disease.

Fluid in the Cul-de-Sac

Large quantities of fluid in the cul-de-sac accumulate mainly in the chronic phase of PID. The fluid is usually sonolucent, and threadlike structures (adhesions) run between the pelvic organs and the wall (Fig. 21–13). This ultrasound picture is consistent with *pelvic peritoneal inclusion cyst* (or fluid).

Ovarian Involvement

In the incipient stages of PID, when the infection not only involves the tube but extends to the ovary, the ultrasound picture is easily understood. The organs appear engorged, although the tube (usually showing the typical attributes of acute infection) and the ovary can be discerned. Color Doppler shows ample flow around the involved pelvic organs. This picture is typical and should be called TOC, not TOA (Fig. 21–14).

TOA is a more advanced stage of PID in which the infection has destroyed part or all of the adnexa. Ultrasound can no longer distinguish between the ovary and the tube (Fig. 21–15A and B). Confluent fluid loculations are evident

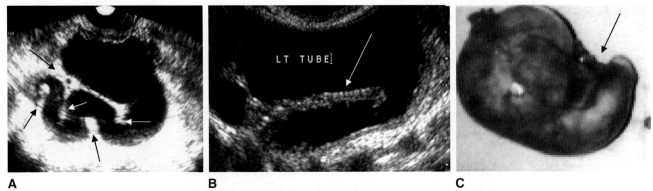

A　　　　　　　　　　**B**　　　　　　　　　　**C**

Figure 21–11. Incomplete septa as an ultrasound marker of inflammatory tubal disease. **A,** A dilated, thin-walled hydrosalpinx with convolutions demonstrating several incomplete septa *(arrows).* **B,** The *arrow* points to an incomplete septum resulting from the doubling-up of a dilated, fluid-filled tube. **C,** Postoperative specimen of a hydrosalpinx. The *arrow* points to the area where the dilated, fluid-filled tube folds, creating the sonographically detectable incomplete septum.

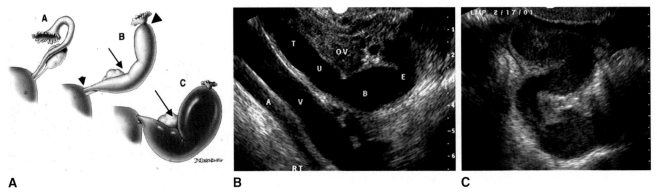

A　　　　　　　　　　**B**　　　　　　　　　　**C**

Figure 21–12. Incomplete septum. **A,** Illustration of the steps leading to the formation of an incomplete septum. A, The normal tube; B, the distal and proximal ends of the tube *(arrowheads)* occlude (the *arrow* indicates the future folding site of the tube); C, the tube fills with fluid and folds, creating the site of the incomplete septum *(arrow).* **B,** The incomplete septum is a hallmark of the chronic hydrosalpinx. A, hypogastric artery; OV, ovary; V, hypogastric vein. **C,** The incomplete septum also appears in acute salpingitis.

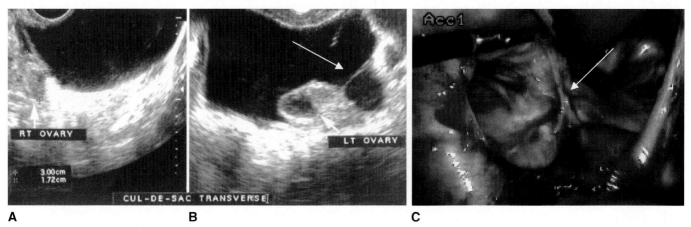

Figure 21–13. Cul-de-sac fluid as an ultrasound marker of inflammatory tubal disease. **A,** Loculated pelvic fluid within the pelvis. **B,** Thin, stringlike adhesions between the pelvic wall and pelvic organs *(arrow)*. **C,** Laparoscopic image of the sequelae of a pelvic inflammatory process. The *arrow* points to an adhesion.

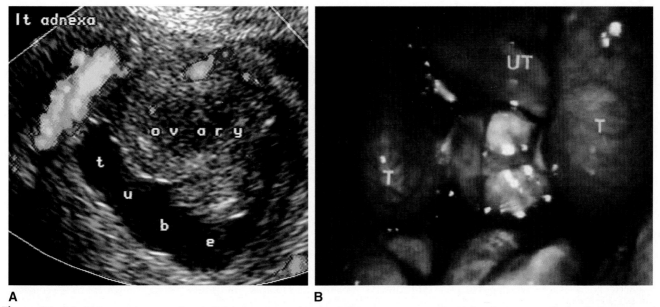

Figure 21–14. Tubo-ovarian complex. **A,** Pelvic sonogram showing inflammatory process involving the ovary and tube. **B,** Laparoscopic image in a case of tubo-ovarian complex. The ovary is covered with white fibrin deposits. The anatomy remains visible. T, tube; UT, uterus.

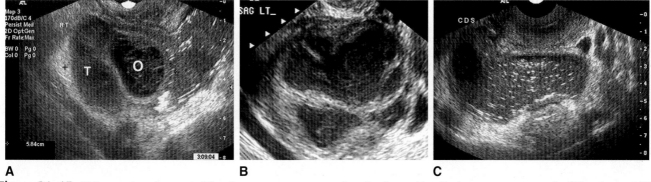

Figure 21–15. Tubo-ovarian abscess. **A,** The observer must use some imagination to identify these structures as tube (T) and ovary (O). Their ultrasound appearance is not indicative of normal anatomy. **B,** The adnexal structures are beyond recognition. **C,** Speckled fluid (pus) fills the cul-de-sac.

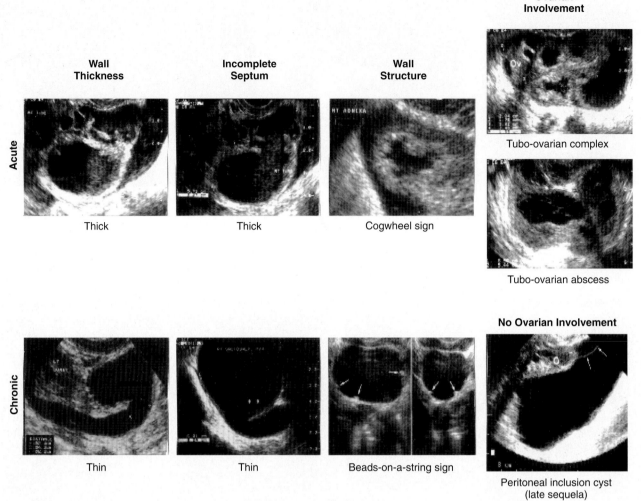

Figure 21–16. Ultrasound markers of tubal inflammatory processes in the context of the clinical course and natural history of pelvic inflammatory disease.

(Fig. 21–15C); sometimes these contain speckled fluid due to the presence of gas-producing bacteria. The abscess or abscesses may be confined within the cul-de-sac, and severe motion tenderness can be elicited by the touch of the vaginal probe. Color Doppler reveals flow only at the periphery of the lesion.

The terms *TOC* and *TOA* are used interchangeably and in a rather undefined manner in the imaging literature.[5-14] The two entities are not only sonographically but also clinically distinct and call for different therapeutic approaches. We believe this distinction can be made based on ultrasound attributes and are convinced that a TOC is an earlier stage in a process that may or may not lead to subsequent abscess formation. A TOC should therefore be diagnosed if the tubal and ovarian structures on transvaginal sonography show clear inflammatory features (e.g., thick wall, cogwheel sign). The term *TOA* should be reserved for a later phase in this acute pelvic process, when the total breakdown of adnexal structures on one or both sides is seen. Sometimes, loculated, speckled fluid above the rectum (in the cul-de-sac) can be detected sonographically. This is consistent with pus and most probably is due to debris from white blood cells and degrading tissue.

Figure 21–16 summarizes the ultrasound markers of inflammatory tubo-ovarian disease pertinent to the acute and chronic phases.

It is critical to differentiate tubal inflammatory disease from an ovarian tumor, benign or malignant. An acute inflammatory process is relatively easy to differentiate because of the acute inflammatory features. Difficulty arises when the diagnosis of chronic tubal disease demonstrating the beads-on-a-string sign and some septations has to be differentiated from that of an ovarian cystic structure with small internal papillae and septa. In the case of a chronic hydrosalpinx, the mural lesions (beads-on-a-string) are small, almost equal in size, and distributed around the thin wall, as opposed to the papillary formations of an ovarian tumor, which usually are of different sizes and located along the wall, which may itself show variable thickness. The presence of incomplete septa almost uniformly indicates the diagnosis of a fallopian tube inflammation because the true septa of ovarian tumors are seldom, if ever, incomplete.

Lately, the inversion rendering has become a useful tool in gynecologic imaging. Using this relatively simple method, a "cast" of the fluid-filled hydrosalpinx can be rendered (see Fig. 19–8). Thus, the three-dimensional display can overcome

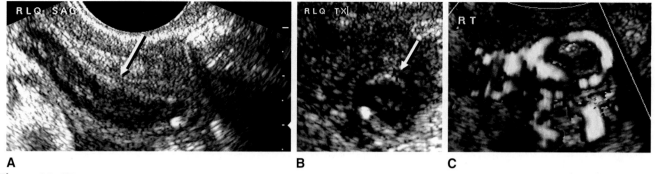

A **B** **C**

Figure 21–17. Acute appendicitis. **A,** Longitudinal section of the inflamed appendix *(arrow)*. It has a thick wall and some weakly echogenic fluid in the distended lumen. **B,** Cross section of the inflamed appendix *(arrow)*. **C,** Subserosal engorged blood vessels seen by power Doppler are typical of inflamed viscera.

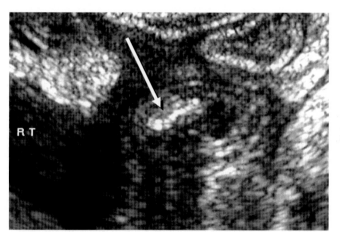

Figure 21–18. A fecalith (hyperechoic material) is seen in the lumen of the appendix *(arrow)*. Note the layered wall, typical of the ultrasound appearance of bowel.

some of the difficulties of two-dimensional imaging of a fluid-filled fallopian tube.

Other Inflammatory Processes

First and most importantly, the different pathologic processes of the bowel must be differentiated from tubal disease. Each case must be placed in the appropriate clinical context. There may be other differential diagnostic entities that we have not yet encountered.

Acute Appendicitis. The diagnosis of acute appendicitis is based on the clinical picture and simple laboratory tests such as a high white blood cell count. However, in certain cases, by using relatively high-frequency transducers, it is possible to depict the acutely inflamed appendix by ultrasound.[15-18] The first step in the ultrasound diagnosis is detecting the right ovary, thereby excluding ovarian pathology. The inflamed appendix appears as an elongated structure with a diameter of 1 cm or more, which on cross section shows two or three concentric layers, the typical hallmark of bowel on ultrasound (Fig. 21–17A and B). If color or power Doppler is applied, a richly vascularized subserosal blood flow becomes evident (Fig. 21–17C). Occasionally, a highly echogenic structure is

seen in the lumen of the appendix (Fig. 21–18). This is consistent with a fecalith (hardened stool or foreign body).

Periappendicular Abscess. Periappendicular abscess is a more advanced inflammatory process of the appendix caused by its perforation.[19,20] In this case, the local ultrasound appearance is characterized by a more severely enlarged appendix (Figs. 21–19 and 21–20) with edematous changes, abundant subserosal blood vessels on Doppler, and variable amounts of low-level echogenic fluid (pus), which sometimes can be seen in Morison's pouch (see Fig. 21–19D).

Mucocele of the Appendix. This is a rare disease of the mucosa of the appendix. In spite of a large body of literature on the subject,[21-24] the diagnosis is not readily recognized by sonographers and sonologists. Sonographic clues to this lesion include the bottle or pear shape of the affected organ, but the more typical sign is a multilayered, onion-skin appearance[24] of the appendix (Fig. 21–21). This appearance results from the hardened consecutive layers of abundant mucus produced by the goblet cells lining the lumen (see Fig. 21–21D).

Other Bowel Disease. It is important to recognize the ultrasound appearance of normal large bowel (Fig. 21–22). The more common diseases of the large bowel, such as Crohn's disease,[25-27] diverticulitis,[28-30] and Hirschsprung's disease, have generally typical ultrasound appearances (Fig. 21–23). However, the patient's history and previously diagnosed disease are frequently the main clues in imaging a specific bowel lesion.

Other Cystic Structures. Different cystic structures, such as parovarian cysts, Morgagni cysts, and mesenteric cysts, must be differentiated from chronic hydrosalpinges (Fig. 21–24).

Ovarian Torsion. Ovarian torsion is discussed in Chapter 8. However, sometimes it is difficult to diagnose this lesion by ultrasound and differentiate it from tubal inflammatory disease (Fig. 21–25).

Torsion of the Fallopian Tube. Although the tube and the ovary often undergo torsion together, the sonographer needs to be able to diagnose twisting of the tube alone.[31-33] In this case, the normal ovary with normal blood flow must be visible alongside the engorged tube, usually with some attributes of a hydrosalpinx[34] and without any detectable flow within the mass (Fig. 21–26). A parovarian cyst can also undergo torsion.[34]

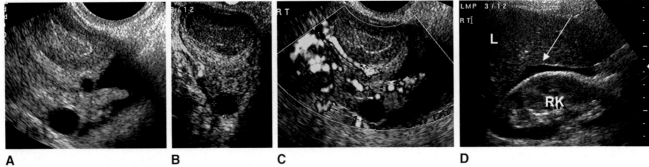

Figure 21–19. Periappendicular abscess. **A,** Cross section of the thick-walled appendix. The edematous epiploic appendix is also seen. Both are suspended in fluid (pus). **B,** Another cross section of the inflamed appendix. **C,** Power Doppler demonstrates subserosal blood vessels. **D,** Fluid is seen in Morison's pouch *(arrow)* between the liver (L) and the right kidney (RK).

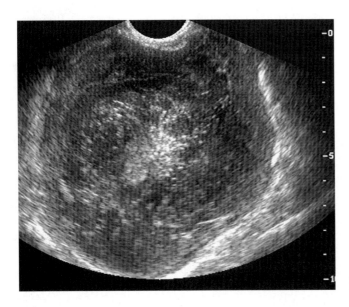

Figure 21–20. Periappendicular abscess. An inflammatory conglomerate approximately 6 cm in diameter was seen in the right lower pelvis.

Subserous, Pedunculated, or Intraligamentary Myoma. An adnexal myoma is probably the most common entity sonologists face in the differential diagnosis of tubal or ovarian disease. By detecting the contiguous feeding blood vessel connection between the uterus (usually the uterine artery) and the mass, which has the ultrasound attributes of myometrium, the diagnosis can be made relatively easily and convincingly (Fig. 21–27).

Tubal Cancer. Tubal cancer is a very rare disease, representing only approximately 1% of all gynecologic cancers. The ultrasound characteristics are a distinct adnexal mass; thick walls; solid components; occasionally the attributes of hydrosalpinx, including incomplete septa; and abundant blood flow (sometimes low resistive and pulsatile indices support the diagnosis; Fig. 21–28). In rare cases the diagnosis is made preoperatively by imaging, including ultrasound.[35-39] Otherwise it is diagnosed during exploratory surgery or in the laboratory of the pathologist.

The most common error is to misidentify tubal carcinoma as an ovarian malignancy. However, the patient must undergo surgery in either case, and most of the time it is hard to tell the two cancers apart even in the pathology laboratory.

Tubal Gestation. This extremely common differential diagnostic entity is discussed in Chapter 13 and is mentioned in several other chapters as part of their main subject, so it is not discussed further here.

Pelvic Kidney. Rarely, we have encountered an adnexal mass that was finally diagnosed as an ectopic kidney on the basis of the typical ultrasound picture of a kidney.

Summary and Conclusion

By combining the information gleaned from the patient's history with a thorough transvaginal ultrasound work-up of the pelvis, one can recognize the valuable ultrasound markers of inflammatory disease of the fallopian tubes and ovary and of their differential diagnostic entities, and can establish the appropriate diagnosis.

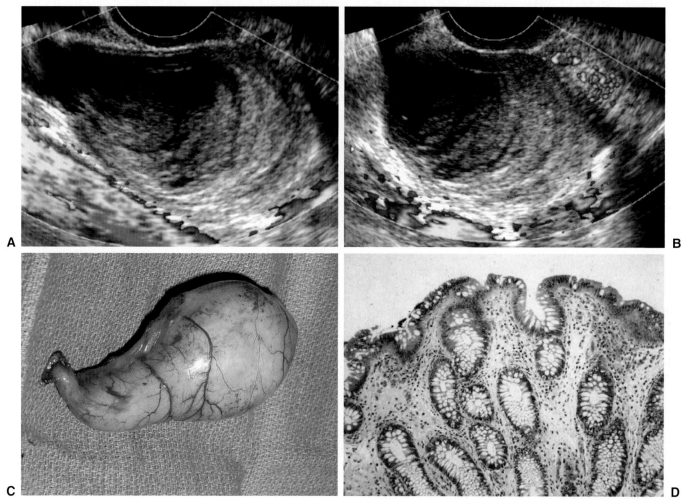

Figure 21–21. Mucocele of the appendix. **A,** Longitudinal section. Note the layered appearance of the wall (onion-skin appearance). **B,** Cross section. **C,** The pathologic specimen. **D,** The histologic picture demonstrates the large number of mucin-producing goblet cells in the wall of the mucocele.

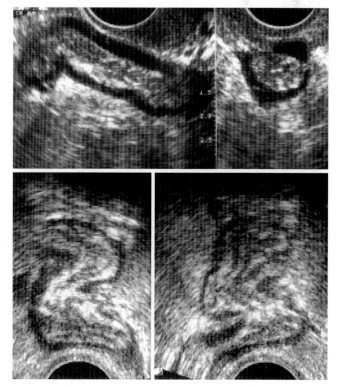

Figure 21–22. Four of the many normal ultrasound appearances of the large bowel.

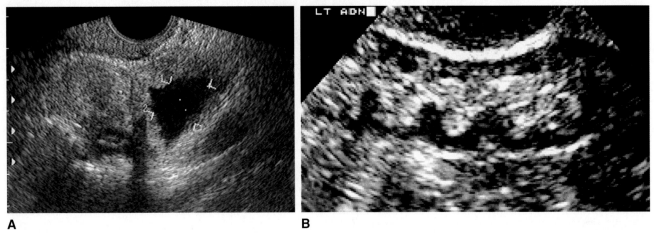

Figure 21–23. Bowel disease. **A,** Hirschsprung's disease, showing a fluid-filled large bowel. **B,** Crohn's disease. Note the multiple contractions of the wall.

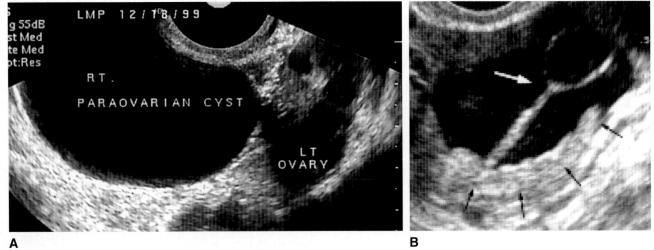

Figure 21–24. Cystic structures in the adnexa. **A,** Right parovarian cyst. The left ovary was also imaged. **B,** A Morgagni cyst *(white arrow)* attached to the tube *(small black arrows)* by a stringlike structure.

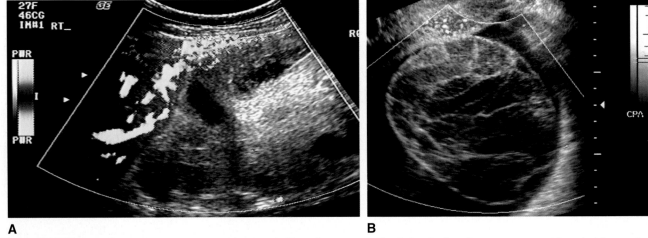

Figure 21–25. Ovarian torsion. **A,** Power Doppler was unable to demonstrate blood flow in the edematous ovary with typical hyperechoic hilus and the peripherally pushed follicles. **B,** A different case of ovarian torsion, in which it appears that a hemorrhagic corpus luteum underwent torsion. No blood vessel was seen by power Doppler interrogation.

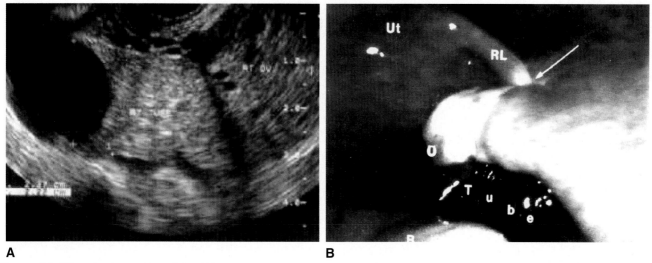

Figure 21–26. Selective torsion of the fallopian tube. **A,** On the left, the lumen and the engorged tube are seen beside a normal ovary. **B,** Laparoscopic image showing the almost black, twisted tube and the normal ovary. O, ovary; RL, round ligament; Ut, uterus. The *arrow* indicates the site of torsion.

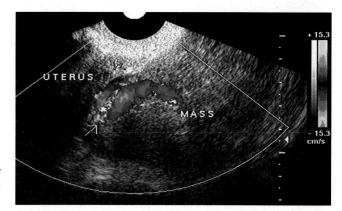

Figure 21–27. Intraligamentary myoma on the left lateral wall of the uterus. The connecting feeding vessel of the fibroid is marked by an *arrow*.

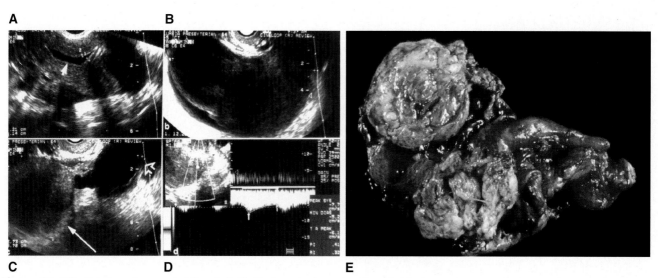

Figure 21–28. Tubal carcinoma. **A,** Dilated, fluid-filled cervix *(arrowhead)*, probably due to the typical hydrorrhea (copious watery flow through the cervix). **B** and **C,** Dilated, thickened walls of the fluid-filled tube *(arrow)*. **D,** Doppler flow velocimetry shows low resistance to flow. **E,** The surgical specimen.

REFERENCES

1. Gales W, Wasserheit JN: Genital chlamydial infections: Epidemiology and reproductive sequelae. Am J Obstet Gynecol 1991;164:1771-1781.
2. Expert Committee on Pelvic Inflammatory Disease: Research directions for the 1990s. Sex Transm Dis 1991;18:46-64.
3. Timor-Tritsch IE, Rottem S: Transvaginal ultrasonographic study of the fallopian tube. Obstet Gynecol 1987;70:424-428.
4. Timor-Tritsch IE, Bar Yam Y, Elgali S, Rottem S: The technique of transvaginal sonography with the use of a 6.5 MHz probe. Am J Obstet Gynecol 1988;158:1019-1024.
5. Tessler FN, Perrella RR, Fleischer AL, Grant EG: Endovaginal sonographic diagnosis of dilated fallopian tubes. AJR Am J Roentgenol 1989;153:523-525.
6. Bulas DI, Ahlstrom PA, Sivit CJ, et al: Pelvic inflammatory disease in the adolescent: Comparison of transabdominal and transvaginal sonographic evaluation. Radiology 1992;183:435-439.
7. Patten RM, Vincent LM, Wolner-Hanssen P, Thorpe E Jr: Pelvic inflammatory disease: Endovaginal sonography with laparoscopic correlation. J Ultrasound Med 1990;9:681-689.
8. Cacciatore B, Leminen A, Ingman-Freiberg S, et al: Transvaginal sonographic findings in ambulatory patients with suspected pelvic inflammatory disease. Obstet Gynecol 1992;80:912-916.
9. Atri M, Tran CN, Bret PM, et al: Accuracy of endovaginal sonography for the detection of fallopian tubes. AJR Am J Roentgenol 1989;153:523-525.
10. Taipale P, Tarjanne H, Ylöstalo P: Transvaginal sonography in suspected pelvic inflammatory disease. Ultrasound Obstet Gynecol 1995;6:430-434.
11. Timor-Tritsch IE, Rottem S, Lewitt N: The fallopian tube. In Timor-Tritsch IE, Rottem S (eds): Transvaginal Sonography, 2nd ed. New York, Chapman & Hall, 1991, pp 131-144.
12. Bellah RD, Rosenberg HK: Transvaginal ultrasound in a children's hospital: Is it worthwhile? Pediatr Radiol 1991;21:570-574.
13. Timor-Tritsch IE: Adnexal masses. In Goldstein SR, Timor-Tritsch IE (eds): Ultrasound in Gynecology. New York, Churchill-Livingstone, 1995, pp 103-114.
14. Timor-Tritsch IE, Lerner JP, Monteagudo A, et al: Transvaginal sonographic markers of tubal inflammatory disease. Ultrasound Obstet Gynecol 1998;12:56-66.
15. Old JL, Dusing RW, Yap W, Dirks J: Imaging for suspected appendicitis. Am Fam Physician 2005;71:71-78.
16. Rosengren D, Brown AF, Chu K: Radiological imaging to improve the emergency department diagnosis of acute appendicitis. Emerg Med Australas 2004;16:410-416.
17. Puylaert JB: Ultrasonography of the acute abdomen: Gastrointestinal conditions. Radiol Clin North Am 2003;41:1227-1242.
18. Kang WM, Lee CH, Chou YH, et al: A clinical evaluation of ultrasonography in the diagnosis of acute appendicitis. Surgery 1989;105:154-159.
19. Jaffe R, Gruber A, Abramowicz J, et al: Sonographic diagnosis of periappendicular abscess in pregnancy. Am J Obstet Gynecol 1985;153:623-624.
20. Regoly-Merei J, Ihasz M, Zaborszky A, Dubecz S: The role of real-time sonography in the differential diagnosis of acute appendicitis and in the detection of post-appendectomy complications. Orv Hetil 1989;130:827-831.
21. Kalu E, Croucher C: Appendiceal mucocele: A rare differential diagnosis of a cystic right adnexal mass. Arch Gynecol Obstet 2005;271:86-88.
22. Pitiakoudis M, Tsaroucha AK, Mimidis K, et al: Mucocele of the appendix: A report of five cases. Tech Coloproctol 2004;8:109-112.
23. Caspi B, Cassif E, Auslender R, et al: The onion skin sign: A specific sonographic marker of appendiceal mucocele. J Ultrasound Med 2004;23:117-121.
24. Degani S, Shapiro I, Leibovitz Z, Ohel G: Sonographic appearance of appendiceal mucocele. Ultrasound Obstet Gynecol 2002;19:99-101.
25. Castiglione F, de Sio I, Cozzolino A, et al: Bowel wall thickness at abdominal ultrasound and the one-year-risk of surgery in patients with Crohn's disease. Am J Gastroenterol 2004;99:1977-1983.
26. Parente F, Greco S, Molteni M, et al: Modern imaging of Crohn's disease using bowel ultrasound. Inflamm Bowel Dis 2004;10:452-461.
27. Ludwig D: Doppler sonography in inflammatory bowel disease. Z Gastroenterol 2004;42:1059-1065.
28. Farag Soliman M, Wustner M, Sturm J, et al: Primary diagnostics of acute diverticulitis of the sigmoid. Ultraschall Med 2004;25:342-347.
29. Seitz K: Sonographic diagnosis of diverticulitis: The burdensome way to acceptance. Ultraschall Med 2004;25:335-336.
30. Bruel JM: Acute colonic diverticulitis: CT or ultrasound? Eur Radiol 2003;13:2557-2559.
31. Antoniou N, Varras M, Akrivis C, et al: Isolated torsion of the fallopian tube: A case report and review of the literature. Clin Exp Obstet Gynecol 2004;31:235-238.
32. Khukla R: Isolated torsion of the hydrosalpinx: A rare presentation. Br J Radiol 2004;77:784-786.
33. Cuillier F, Harper L, Birsan A: Fallopian tube torsion: Five cases with no other element. J Gynecol Obstet Biol Reprod (Paris) 2002;31:755-764.
34. Puri M, Jain K, Negi R: Torsion of para-ovarian cyst: A cause of acute abdomen. Indian J Med Sci 2003;57:361-362.
35. Kol S, Gal D, Friedman M, et al: Preoperative diagnosis of fallopian tube carcinoma by transvaginal sonography and CA-125. Gynecol Oncol 1990;37:129-131.
36. Granberg S, Jansson I: Early detection of primary carcinoma of the fallopian tube by endovaginal ultrasound. Acta Obstet Gynecol Scand 1990;69:667-668.
37. Ajjimakorn S, Bhamarapravati Y: Transvaginal ultrasound and the diagnosis of fallopian tubal carcinoma. J Clin Ultrasound 1991;19:116-119.
38. Ekici E, Vicdan K, Danisman N, et al: Ultrasonographic appearance of fallopian tube carcinoma. Int J Gynaecol Obstet 1995;49:325-329.
39. Kurjak A, Kupesic S, Jacobs I: Preoperative diagnosis of the primary fallopian tube carcinoma by three-dimensional static and power Doppler sonography. Ultrasound Obstet Gynecol 2000;15:246-251.

Chapter 22

Pearls and Pitfalls of Transvaginal Sonography

Steven R. Goldstein

The observations in this chapter are "pearls and pitfalls" whose recognition can significantly shorten the personal learning curve, which largely reflects the clinician's experience based on the foundation of his or her understanding of the normal and abnormal obtained from initial didactic material.

Principles of Transvaginal Sonography

Patient Preparation

Although transvaginal sonography (TVS) is commonly performed by persons accustomed to imaging, it is, in reality, a specialized form of a pelvic examination. Thus, maintaining patient privacy in terms of a chaperone, draw sheet, and gown are essential. Furthermore, it is important for the patient to be able to assume the lithotomy position, preferably using a gynecologic examining table. This gives free range of motion of the probe handle in the vertical plane at the introitus. It is important for the examiner to be able to push the handle toward the floor without being blocked by a flat examining table. If a gynecologic examining table is unavailable, the patient's buttocks must be lifted with either a thick foam cushion or an inverted bedpan. The probe is reprocessed between uses according to guidelines available from the American Institute of Ultrasound in Medicine.[1] The probe is covered with a condom, the finger of an examining glove, or a sterile sheath.

Technical Considerations

Advantages

The main advantage of the vaginal probe is that it gives excellent near-field resolution despite high degrees of magnification. The effect is that of doing ultrasound through a low-power microscope, yielding a degree of magnification that is actually a form of sonomicroscopy (albeit of low power), in which we image structures that would not be discernible to the naked eye if the structure were being held at arm's length. Also, the proximity of the probe to the structure of interest allows a higher frequency to yield better resolution. Thus, whenever possible, one should use the highest-frequency probe that will give adequate penetration as well as the highest degree of magnification available once the structure of interest has been identified.

Another advantage is that TVS is performed with an empty urinary bladder, which saves time and is uniformly better accepted by patients. An empty bladder also allows for clinical correlation at the time of the pelvic examination with the patient in the lithotomy position.

Disadvantages

The pitfalls of TVS ultimately stem from the physics involved. First, the use of higher frequencies results in enhanced resolution and imaging of details not appreciated by earlier techniques. One must be careful not to overinterpret findings that may, in fact, be physiologic. Old principles cannot be applied to information obtained with new technology. Furthermore, the higher frequency of the transducer also results in limited sound penetration and a short field of view; a partially filled urinary bladder could take up an entire screen of available information. Likewise, even a mildly enlarged uterus or adnexal mass may not fit entirely in one field of view. Lacking panoramic images of the entire pelvis, we may not see structures that are out of the focal zone of the probe. Furthermore, with the vaginal probe there is a short field of vision.

A second disadvantage is that there is no sound enhancement, as seen with a full urinary bladder. Cases of pelvic ascites or polyhydramnios demonstrate how exquisite the visualization of pelvic structures (or fetal structures, in the case of polyhydramnios) is because of sound enhancement from increased transmission through fluid.

Third, transducer movement is limited by the confines of the vagina. The transducer cannot be moved in a stepwise longitudinal or transverse fashion.

Orientation

Traditionally, transabdominal pelvic scanning used multiple two-dimensional "tomograms" that allowed the examiner to mentally create a three-dimensional image of the anatomy. The Cartesian axial concepts of "longitudinal" and "transverse" are throwbacks to static arm scanners that produced images at right angles to each other at increments of 0.5 to 1 cm.

With transvaginal scanning, however, a long-axis view of the structure combined with a second view at 90 degrees to the first allows three-dimensional assessment of the organ of interest and avoids misinterpretation of images viewed in only one plane. The future availability of three-dimensional scanning may make the issue of single-plane misdiagnosis moot. With TVS, images are frozen to depict maximum recognizable anatomy. This becomes especially evident in obstetric scanning, where one locates an anatomic structure such as fetal kidney or fetal limb regardless of the transducer's orientation relative to the mother's abdomen. With the vaginal probe we look for recognizable anatomy, such as the ovary overlying the iliac vessels or the uterine fundus with its endometrial echo. Instead of longitudinal and transverse orientations, TVS uses the concept of an anatomy-derived orientation, which is a highly focused approach on the targeted organ.

Pearls and Pitfalls

Gestational Sac Location

The chorionic membrane grossly resembles a soft contact lens. Projecting from it are primary trophoblastic villi, which, as they invade maternal decidua, produce a trophoblastic decidual reaction. This is responsible for the echogenic rind surrounding the sonolucent center of the gestational sac, which corresponds to the fluid-filled chorionic cavity (see Chapter 11). The entire sonographic ensemble is called a gestational sac.[2] This appearance is not related to any double decidual sac formation.

Because pregnancy is recognized by its normality rather than by its location, definitive pregnancies when viewed with ultrasound may be located inside or outside the uterus. Furthermore, what used to be referred to as a "pseudosac" or "decidual cast" should really be thought of as nondiagnostic endometrial findings. Such pictures are compatible with decidual changes associated with ectopic pregnancy or may be associated with failing intrauterine pregnancies.

Nondiagnostic adnexal findings also may be encountered. Viewed with the vaginal probe, the corpus luteum cyst will not be a smooth-walled, unilocular structure and should not be mistaken for an extrauterine pregnancy.

Early Pregnancy Viability

Once ectopic pregnancy is ruled out, embryonic well-being should be assessed by serial ultrasound examinations rather than serial human chorionic gonadotropin determinations. Early pregnancy must be assumed to be viable (once ectopic pregnancy is definitely excluded). The early gestational sac grows approximately 1 mm/day, as does the early embryo.[3,4] Regarding viability, the question is not how early in the pregnancy cardiac activity can be assessed, but how far gestation can progress without cardiac activity's being seen on TVS before a pregnancy is *definitively* nonviable. The endothelial heart tube has folded on itself by 21 days postconception, and often cardiac activity can be perceived by M-mode sonography before an embryonic thickening along the edge of the yolk sac can actually be imaged. The ability to visualize cardiac activity will depend on the type and frequency of equipment used, the normality of the pregnancy, and the operator's visual acuity. Regardless of equipment, however, cardiac activity should be discernible on transvaginal scan by the time the embryonic length is 4 mm.[5]

Locating Ovaries

The more folliculogenesis contained within an ovary, the more likely that the ovary will be imaged by vaginal scanning techniques. It is the sonolucency of the follicles that permits easy recognition of the ovary. Thus, hormonally stimulated ovaries in women being treated for infertility are easily identified. Postmenopausal ovaries, which usually lack folliculogenesis, can be much more difficult to image. The location of the ovaries also depends on the patient's position. When a premenopausal patient assumes the lithotomy position, the ovaries, which are freely mobile, will invariably (by gravity) assume a position lateral to the uterus and can be seen immediately adjacent to the iliac vessels (Fig. 22–1). These vessels are retroperitoneal. If the patient is turned into a knee-chest position, the ovaries move slightly toward the anterior abdominal wall, but the retroperitoneal iliac vessels do not. Distantly postmenopausal ovaries or ovaries held in place by adhesions may not be seen in that location relative to the iliac vessels despite generous manipulation by the abdominal hand or subtle changes in the position of the patient (Fig. 22–2).

Bowel Gas

Gas and solid or liquid fecal material produce bizarre, complex echo patterns (Fig. 22–3) that are best recognized by their motion within the bowel (due to peristalsis). Thus, in the case of a focal ileus, loops of bowel that are not undergoing peristalsis can have a confusing and unusual appearance. When using the vaginal probe, the examiner can encounter

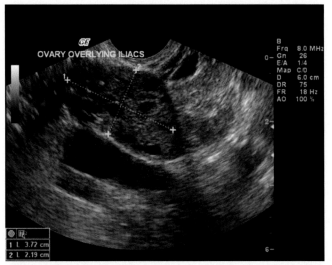

Figure 22–1. Transvaginal scan of the ovary overlying the iliac vessels. The ovary is marked by *calipers* and measures 3.7 × 2.2 cm. Numerous sonolucencies represent follicles within the ovary. When a premenopausal patient like this one assumes the lithotomy position, the ovary, if freely mobile, will invariably gravitate to a position lateral to the uterus and can be seen immediately adjacent to the iliac vessels. The ovaries are intraperitoneal, whereas the iliac vessels are retroperitoneal. If this patient were turned into a knee-chest position, the ovaries would move slightly toward the anterior abdominal wall, but the retroperitoneal iliac vessels would not.

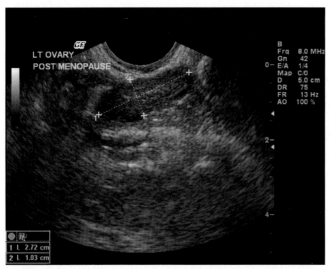

Figure 22–2. Postmenopausal ovary marked by *calipers* (2.7 × 1.0 cm). Note the lack of folliculogenesis. Note also that the postmenopausal ovary does not reach the pelvic side wall, and thus the iliac vessels are not helpful in identification.

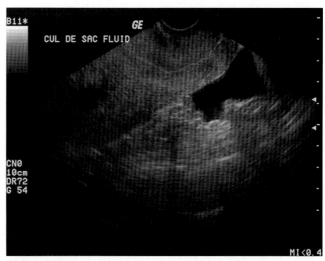

Figure 22–4. Transvaginal scan depicting a small amount of fluid in the cul-de-sac in a patient who has already ovulated this cycle. Note how low the cul-de-sac comes posterior to the uterus in reference to the cervical os. Small amounts of fluid are easily seen with the resolution provided by the vaginal probe.

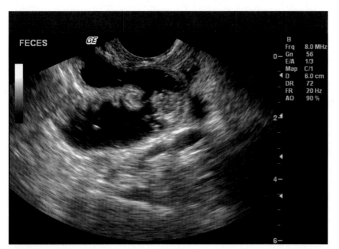

Figure 22–3. Transvaginal scan showing loops of bowel containing solid and liquid fecal material producing bizarre, complex echo patterns. These are best recognized on real-time imaging by their motion within bowel (peristalsis).

bowel gas and its resulting echoes everywhere because loops of bowel are not pushed cephalad by a filled urinary bladder, as they are in transabdominal scanning. Eventually, however, examiners learn to use this feature to their advantage in locating ovaries that are proving difficult to find, because peristaltic movement of the surrounding bowel often results in sharper delineation of the ovaries, which stand out by virtue of their static nature.

"Fluid Is Your Friend"

Fluid enhances sound transmission and creates an excellent interface with adjacent structures. Its sonolucency serves as an easily recognized marker. Thus, the fluid in an early gestational sac or in ovarian follicles, or even fluid purposely instilled into the endometrial cavity,[6] will highlight anatomic

detail. However, because fluid is so easily seen using high-frequency vaginal probes, an inexperienced examiner may mistake its physiologic presence for a pathologic process. An example is small amounts of cul-de-sac fluid (Fig. 22–4) that are often observed with TVS (it is often observed incidentally at the time of laparoscopy). The presence of this fluid, however, should be factored into the overall clinical setting. Another example is postmenopausal endometrial fluid collections[7] (see Chapter 9). With a vaginal probe, postmenopausal endometrial fluid collections are detected much more commonly than before, and the overwhelming majority represent benign transudated fluid associated with cervical stenosis.[7]

Complex Adnexal Masses

Often a mass may be appreciated on routine examination or as part of an imaging study ordered for other reasons. These are often asymptomatic but also can be associated with a range of symptoms, from mild to severe. In the past, a mass in the adnexa was described and a sonographic differential diagnosis given. For a septate or "complex" adnexal mass, the differential list included endometriosis, hemorrhagic functional cyst, and "possibly but cannot rule out" neoplasia. Depending on size, symptoms, length of time symptoms have been present, the patient's anxiety, and even the way in which the finding was presented to the patient by the physician, such cases often are subjected to "diagnostic" laparoscopy or even exploratory laparotomy. The use of TVS can often reliably distinguish between endometriomas, hemorrhagic corpora lutea, and neoplasia.[8]

Endometriomas

Transvaginal imaging of endometriomas characteristically shows low-level, diffuse, uniform internal echoes throughout (Fig. 22–5). Endometriomas may appear more sonolucent when imaged transabdominally but have a more variable appearance. An endometrioma should not be confused with a solid mass because an endometrioma will demonstrate some

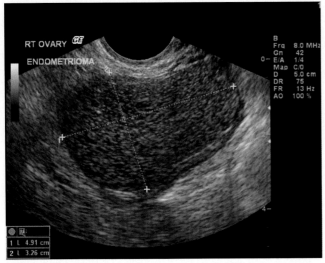

Figure 22–5. Transvaginal scan of a typical-appearing endometrioma, measuring 4.9 × 3.8 cm *(calipers)*. Note the homogeneous, ground-glass appearance typical of endometriomas.

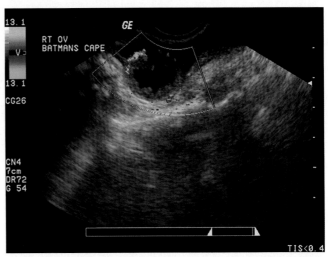

Figure 22–7. Classic example of a fresh corpus luteum within the ovary. Note the sonolucent area, which resembles the shape of Batman's cape. This image shows the typical peripheral blood flow characteristic of a corpus luteum.

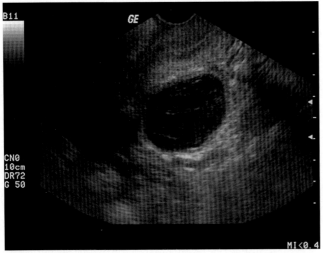

Figure 22–6. Transvaginal pelvic scan of a hemorrhagic corpus luteum. The reticular cobweb-type pattern represents clot and fibrin within this cystic structure.

posterior wall acoustic enhancement. Endometriomas are being increasingly treated by endoscopic surgery.

Corpora Lutea

Also called *hemorrhagic corpora lutea,* corpora lutea are functional cysts with fresh bleeding into the site of ovulation. The blood undergoes the same sequence of organization and clot retraction as in a test tube. Sonographically, their appearance progresses from a diffuse pattern (but more heterogeneous than an endometrioma; Fig. 22–6) to a reticular or "cobweb" pattern; by clot retraction, their final appearance may even mimic papillary projections because of bridging. Such structures (unless accompanied by some coagulation defect) are invariably self-limited and disappear. If they are so recognized, any operative intervention (diagnostic or therapeutic) can be avoided. Follow-up after the second menses in the prolifera-

tive phase of the cycle invariably shows resolution. Furthermore, a corpus luteum should never be called a *cyst,* which to many physicians denotes a pathologic structure. A normal ovary containing a corpus luteum should not be mistaken for a gestational sac (Fig. 22–7).

Malignancy

Signs of malignancy include the presence of papillary structures, irregular solid areas, and septa, as well as the presence of vascularization at color Doppler imaging. Malignancy's tendency to display certain features led to the development of morphologic scoring systems to distinguish malignant from benign disease. Various scoring systems[8,9] use vaginal probe assessment of (1) inner wall structure, (2) wall thickness (in millimeters), (3) septa (in millimeters), and (4) echogenicity to score adnexal masses. Overall, in predicting malignancy, these scoring systems have a specificity of 83%, sensitivity of 100%, positive predictive value of 37%, and negative predictive value of 100%. Such preoperative evaluation can assist the physician in making proper operative plans in terms of the expertise needed (availability of gynecologic oncologist) and the amount of operating room time expected. Ferrazzi et al.,[10] in a meta-analysis of five scoring systems, concluded that "a completely reliable differential benign from malignant masses cannot be obtained by sonographic imaging alone." Timmerman[11] compared various scoring systems with neural networks and expert sonologists. He found that on prospective testing, none of the models could outperform an expert sonologist.

Uterine Vasculature

In addition to the main uterine artery, there are rich vascular channels along the uterine borders and in the parametrium. As the transducer is angled laterally from the midsagittal long-axis view of the uterus toward the adnexa, an image of a structure resembling the ovary can often be produced (Fig. 22–8). This structure, actually consisting of uterine vessels being cut at an oblique angle by the ultrasound beam, should not be confused with the ovary itself. The use of color-flow imaging, not for Doppler assessment of resistance but simply for assess-

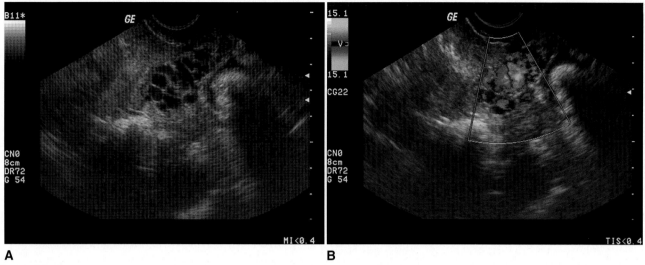

Figure 22–8. **A,** Transvaginal sonogram revealing a "multicystic" mass that could be mistaken for a complex adnexal mass. **B,** Color-flow image from same patient. What appeared to be sonolucencies actually represent vessels lateral to the uterus in this multiparous patient. They should not be confused with an adnexal mass. This is an example of "color as morphology," wherein the use of color-flow imaging was able to detect blood flow and contribute to the morphologic assessment.

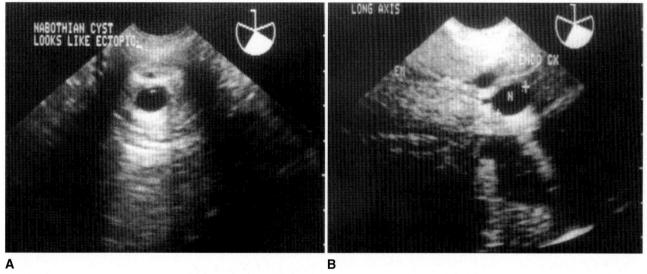

Figure 22–9. **A,** Nabothian or cervical inclusion cyst seen in coronal section. It mimics an extrauterine gestational sac. However, the increased through-transmission from the cystic structure causes the false "trophoblastic decidual reaction" to be intensified along the posterior wall instead of symmetrically surrounding the fluid-filled center. **B,** Same patient as in **A.** By viewing all structures in two planes at right angles to each other, it is clear that this cystic structure is located at the level of the internal os, and a diagnosis of cervical inclusion or nabothian cyst is easily made. EM, endometrioma; N, nabothian cyst.

ment of the presence or absence of blood flow, is important for morphologic assessment in such cases.

Nabothian and Cervical Inclusion Cysts

Small sonolucent cysts can often be seen near the region of the cervical canal. Histologically, if they are lined by squamous epithelium, they are nabothian cysts; otherwise, they are cervical inclusion cysts. Such structures seen in a coronal plane can mimic a gestational sac (Fig. 22–9A). However, invariably, what might be interpreted as the echogenic trophoblastic decidual reaction is seen only posteriorly because of enhanced through-transmission secondary to the fluid-filled center of

the cyst. A true gestational sac would be expected to show a symmetric echogenic rind around the sonolucent center. Furthermore, by imaging the structure in the corresponding long-axis plane (90 degrees to a coronal view), it is easily recognized as a cervical cyst (Fig. 22–9B). In the coronal projection alone, the examiner might not even appreciate that the structure is located in the cervix (see Fig. 22–9A).

Urinary Bladder

As it fills, the urinary bladder should be recognized by its location and the appearance of its wall. The thickness of the wall may diminish as the bladder continues to fill. Normally, it is

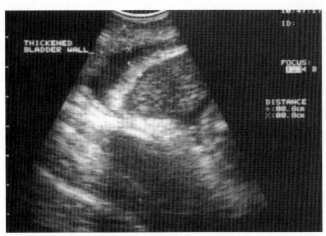

Figure 22–10. Abnormally thickened bladder wall measuring 6 and 8 mm at two positions, respectively *(calipers)*. This patient had a history of biopsy-proven interstitial cystitis. Patients with chronic urinary problems often exhibit such abnormal findings on TVS.

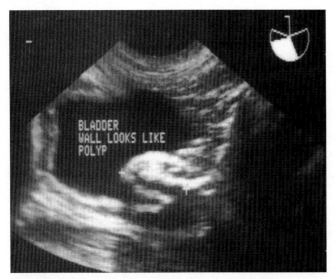

Figure 22–11. Occasionally, as the bladder fills, it is not always symmetric. An outpouching of the bladder wall depicted here, which measured 14 mm *(calipers)*, is an artifact that should not be mistaken for a bladder wall polyp. Continued observation of the bladder as it fills will show disappearance of this fold.

less than 5 mm thick. Patients with bladder dysfunction such as interstitial cystitis may present with markedly thickened, hypertrophic bladder walls (Fig. 22–10). Furthermore, the bladder does not always fill symmetrically. Small areas of bladder wall infolding should not be mistaken for polyps (Fig. 22–11). Continuous observation of the bladder as it fills will show the disappearance of such folds.

Postmenopause

Endometrium

TVS can indicate whether endometrial tissue is present in the uterine cavity; such measurements of endometrial thickness should be made on sagittal long-axis views, because coronal images may not be perpendicular to the endometrial cavity and may thus overestimate its thickness. Many studies[12] indi-

cate that in patients with vaginal bleeding, an endometrial thickness of 5 mm or less is uniformly associated with biopsy results of scant cellular material or inactive endometrium. However, an endometrial echo of 6 mm or greater in the anteroposterior dimension has been associated with virtually all histologic types. When tissue is present, the histologic diagnosis remains a function of the pathology laboratory.

Adnexa

Postmenopausal cystic adnexal masses have been studied with transabdominal sonography. Previous work[13,14] has indicated that postmenopausal unilateral and unilocular cystic masses of 5 cm or less, without ascites, have a very low incidence of malignancy. Use of the vaginal probe, however, may show small, fine septations within such masses. Morphologic scanning systems[9] (see Chapter 4) should be used to evaluate such structures. Finally, up to 18% of postmenopausal patients may exhibit small cystic structures on a routine vaginal scan.[15] New algorithms must be developed so that information obtained at such high magnification and level of detail can be applied appropriately.

Misrepresenting Three-Dimensional Anatomy

An ultrasound image frozen on the screen represents a two-dimensional slice of anatomy that the sonographer must mentally re-create as three-dimensional anatomy. This is especially important in such situations as judging the endometrial echo on a long-axis view for the purpose of measuring endometrial wall thickness in patients with postmenopausal bleeding. It is often possible to create a frozen two-dimensional image that may not be entirely representative of the three-dimensional nature of the structure. Figure 22–12A depicts a seemingly normal long-axis view of a patient who is periovulatory. This image is taken slightly to the left of center. As the transducer is moved toward the right of the midline in the long-axis view, an endometrial polyp is clearly visualized (Fig. 22–12B). The situation is analogous in the coronal plane. Figure 22–12C clearly depicts a normal-appearing periovulatory halo. By fanning the transducer down toward the cervix and up toward the fundus, one can avoid the pitfall of missing a polyp such as that depicted in Figure 22–12D.

Previous Hysterectomy

In patients with a previous hysterectomy, the vaginal cuff can appear thick and echogenic. This is especially true in patients who have had supracervical hysterectomies in whom the remaining cervix is easily seen with the vaginal probe (Fig. 22–13).

Locating the ovaries in a patient whose uterus is surgically absent may be more difficult. Often, because of adhesions, such ovaries will not be found in their usual anatomic position relative to the iliac vessels. The presence of follicles or corpora lutea will be helpful (see Fig. 20–4).

Virginal or Postmenopausal Stenotic Vaginal Introitus

In patients who are virginal with an intact hymen or in postmenopausal patients who have introital stenosis, it may be impossible to insert the vaginal probe into the vagina. In such cases, a vaginal probe with a bulbous tip (sectors) can be placed into the rectum with adequate lubrication, producing

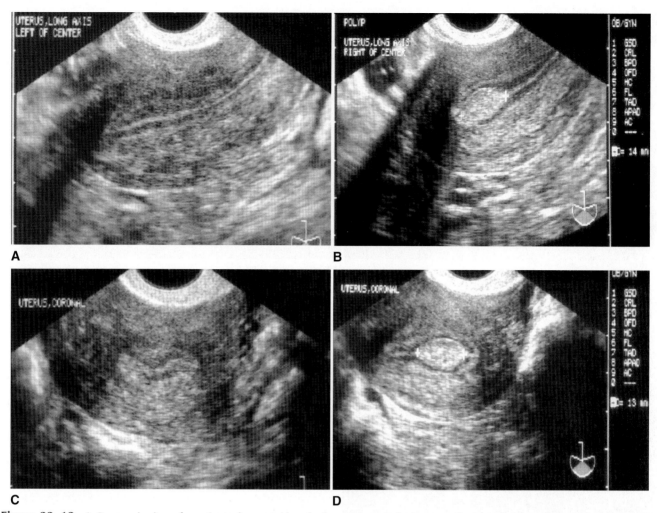

Figure 22–12. **A,** Long-axis view of a patient taken at mid-cycle that appears to show a normal periovulatory endometrial echo. **B,** Long-axis view to the right of center in the same patient. An obvious fundal polyp measuring 14 mm *(calipers)* should be noted. If only a single long-axis projection had been obtained, this polyp would have been missed. **C,** Turning into a coronal plane, this image is taken in the area of the lower uterine segment. Once again, this appears to be a normal preovulatory endometrial echo. **D,** In the same patient, as the transducer is fanned toward the fundus in a coronal plane, the polyp seen in **B** again becomes obvious. This underscores the fact that the endometrium is a three-dimensional structure and must be approached dogmatically as such, lest the examiner miss lesions that may indeed be focal, such as the polyp imaged here.

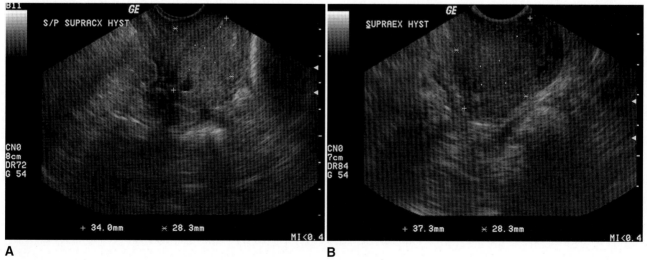

Figure 22–13. **A,** Transvaginal scan of a patient after supracervical hysterectomy. The cervix is outlined *(calipers)* and measures 3.4 × 2.8 cm. A small area of sonolucency represents endocervical mucus. **B,** Transvaginal scan of another patient after supracervical hysterectomy. Note the solid appearance of the cervix, which measures 3.7 × 2.8 cm *(calipers)*.

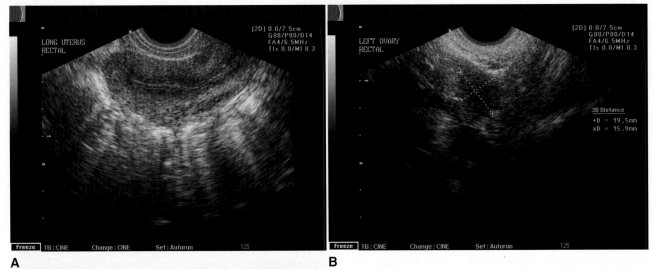

A

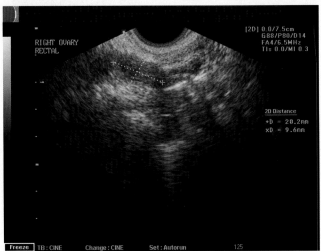

C

Figure 22–14. A, Transrectal scan of the uterus in a post-menopausal patient with a stenotic vaginal introitus. The probe can be placed easily into the rectum and can scan the uterus through the rectovaginal septum. A thin endometrial echo, compatible with inactive, atrophic endometrium, is clearly visualized. **B,** In another transrectal scan of the same patient, the left ovary measures 1.9 × 1.6 cm and lacks folliculogenesis. **C,** In the same patient, a transrectal scan shows the right ovary to measure 2.0 × 1.0 cm.

images of the pelvic structures that look virtually identical to those obtained transvaginally[16] (Fig. 22–14).

Physiologic Synchrony

The pelvis is a dynamic region. Each month, the pelvic reproductive organs undergo a cycle that most often culminates in menses, but sometimes culminates in pregnancy. On sonography, physiologic changes in the ovary should correspond to the endometrial response, or lack thereof. For instance, if a patient is on oral contraceptive pills, one would expect a thin, linear endometrial echo and ovaries that contain follicles of 10 mm or less if adequate ovarian suppression is indeed occurring. If there is a "complex-appearing mass" in the adnexa that appears to be a hemorrhagic corpus luteum, then the endometrium should also display secretory changes (Fig. 22–15). If a woman is postmenopausal and not on hormone replacement therapy, the endometrium would be expected to be inactive with an endometrial echo of less than 5 mm and a lack of folliculogenesis in the ovaries.

Terminology

Two terms are, unfortunately, misused by many imaging specialists.

1. *Complex adnexal mass.* Reporting a so-called complex mass without placing it in the temporal context that relates it to the menstrual period, and without properly describing its ultrasound characteristics (gray scale and color), presents a potential threat to the patient and confuses the referring physician. In short, the term *complex mass* should not be used if a clear diagnosis can be used.[8]

2. *Cyst.* The term *cyst* attached to the names of various structures is often used too loosely. One should not use the term *corpus luteum cyst.* The correct term is *corpus luteum.* In the rare case of a large (>4 to 5 cm) corpus luteum filled with blood or clots in a symptomatic patient, the term *hemorrhagic corpus luteum cyst* can be used. Normal follicles of the normal ovary in the reproductive years should not be called *cysts.* They are, and should be called, *follicles.*

In both cases, if the sonographer used the imprecise designation in his or her report, the patient will continue to use the misnomer, misleading her and subsequent physicians taking her gynecologic history into believing that pathologic findings were present.[8] The wording of reports has far-reaching conse-

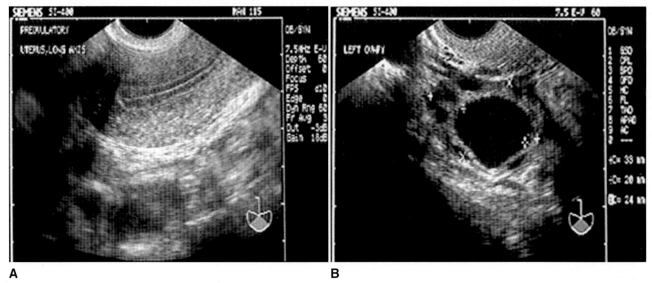

A   **B**

Figure 22–15. A, Transvaginal pelvic sonogram of the long axis of the uterus in a patient before ovulation. Note the multilayered (trilaminar) endometrium typical of the estrogen effect just before ovulation. **B,** Transvaginal pelvic scan of the left ovary in the same patient. Note the dominant follicle measuring 24 mm. Several other small follicles are seen in the periphery of the ovary. The appearance of this ovary just before ovulation is in synchrony with the endometrial findings in **A.**

quences. Correct and precise descriptions of pelvic structures cannot be replaced by terms that have a variety of meanings.

Summary

Vaginal probes, because of their high frequency and close proximity to the pelvic organs, show anatomic detail heretofore unappreciated. They require a targeted, anatomy-derived orientation that provides a less panoramic view. Thus, the sonologist must take great care to use multiple two-dimensional images in various planes to mentally re-create the true three-dimensional anatomy. Furthermore, we must be careful not to overinterpret findings that may be physiologic. Information obtained with improved, refined technology cannot simply be handled according to old established principles. New studies must be performed so that new clinical algorithms can be developed.

REFERENCES

1. American Institute of Ultrasound in Medicine: Guidelines for cleaning and preparing endocavitary ultrasound transducers between patients. Available at http://aium.org/publications/statements/_statementSelected.asp?statement=27.
2. Goldstein SR: Early pregnancy ultrasound: A new look with the endovaginal probe. Contemp Obstet Gynecol 1988;31:54.
3. Nyberg DA, Mack LA, Laing FC, Pottem RM: Distinguishing normal from abnormal gestational sac growth in early pregnancy. J Ultrasound Med 1987;6:23-27.
4. Goldstein SR, Wolfson R: Endovaginal ultrasonographic measurement of early embryonic size as a means of assessing gestational age. J Ultrasound Med 1994;13:27-31.
5. Goldstein SR: Significance of cardiac activity on endovaginal ultrasound in very early embryos. Obstet Gynecol 1992;80:670-672.
6. Goldstein SR: Use of ultrasonohysterography for triage of perimenopausal patients with unexplained uterine bleeding. Am J Obstet Gynecol 1994;170:565-570.
7. Goldstein SR: Postmenopausal endometrial fluid collections revisited: Look at the doughnut rather than the hole. Obstet Gynecol 1994;83:738-740.
8. Timor-Tritsch IE, Goldstein SR: The complexity of a "complex mass" and the simplicity of a "simple cyst." J Ultrasound Med 2005;24:255-258.
9. Lerner JP, Timor-Tritsch IE, Federman A, Abramovich G: Transvaginal sonographic characterization of ovarian masses using an improved, weighted scoring system. Am J Obstet Gynecol 1994;170:81-85.
10. Ferrazzi E, Zanetta G, Dordoni D, et al: Transvaginal ultrasonographic characterization of ovarian masses: Comparison of five scoring systems in a multicenter study. Ultrasound Obstet Gynecol 1997;10:192-197.
11. Timmerman D: The use of mathematical models to evaluate pelvic masses: Can they beat an expert operator? Best Pract Res Clin Obstet Gynaecol 2004;18:91-104.
12. Goldstein SR, Nachtigall M, Snyder JR, Nachtigall L: Endometrial assessment by vaginal ultrasonography before endometrial sampling in patients with postmenopausal bleeding. Am J Obstet Gynecol 1990;163:119-123.
13. Goldstein SR: Conservative management of small postmenopausal cystic masses. Clin Obstet Gynecol 1993;36:395-401.
14. Nardo LG, Kroon ND, Reginald PW: Persistent unilocular ovarian cysts in a general population of postmenopausal women: Is there a place for expectant management? Obstet Gynecol 2003;102:589-593.
15. Modesitt SC, Pavlik EJ, Ueland FR, et al: Risk of malignancy in unilocular ovarian cystic tumors less than 10 centimeters in diameter. Obstet Gynecol 2003;102:594-599.
16. Timor-Tritsch IE, Monteagudo A, Rebarder A, et al: Transrectal scanning: An alternative when transvaginal scanning is not feasible. Ultrasound Obstet Gynecol 2003;21:473-479.

Guidelines for Cleaning and Preparing Endocavitary Ultrasound Transducers Between Patients

Approved June 4, 2003

The purpose of this document is to provide guidance regarding the cleaning and disinfection of transvaginal and transrectal ultrasound probes.

All sterilization/disinfection represents a statistical reduction in the number of microbes present on a surface. Meticulous cleaning of the instrument is the essential key to an initial reduction of the microbial/organic load by at least 99%. This cleaning is followed by a disinfecting procedure to ensure a high degree of protection from infectious disease transmission, even if a disposable barrier covers the instrument during use.

Medical instruments fall into different categories with respect to potential for infection transmission. The most critical level of instruments are those that are intended to penetrate skin or mucous membranes. These require sterilization. Less critical instruments (often called "semi-critical" instruments) that simply come into contact with mucous membranes such as fiber optic endoscopes require high-level disinfection rather than sterilization.

   Although endocavitary ultrasound probes might be considered even less critical instruments because they are routinely protected by single use disposable probe covers, leakage rates of 0.9%-2% for condoms and 8%-81% for commercial probe covers have been observed in recent studies. For maximum safety one should therefore perform **high-level disinfection** of the probe between each use and use a probe cover or condom as an aid to keeping the probe clean.

There are four generally recognized categories of disinfection and sterilization. **Sterilization** is the complete elimination of all forms of microbial life including spores and viruses. **Disinfection,** the selective removal of microbial life, is divided into three classes:
High-Level Disinfection—Destruction/removal of all microorganisms except bacterial spores.
Mid-Level Disinfection—Inactivation of Mycobacterium Tuberculosis, bacteria, most viruses and most fungi and some bacterial spores.
Low-Level Disinfection—Destruction of most bacteria, some viruses and some fungi. Low-level disinfection will not necessarily inactivate Mycobacterium Tuberculosis or bacterial spores.

The following specific recommendations are made for the use of endocavitary ultrasound transducers. Users should also review the Centers for Disease Control and Prevention document on sterilization and disinfection of medical devices to be certain that their procedures conform to the CDC principles for disinfection of patient care equipment.

1. CLEANING—After removal of the probe cover, use running water to remove any residual gel or debris from the probe. Use a damp gauze pad or other soft cloth and a small amount of mild non-abrasive liquid soap (household dishwashing liquid is ideal) to thoroughly cleanse the transducer. Consider the use of a small brush especially for crevices and areas of angulation depending on the design of your particular transducer. Rinse the transducer thoroughly with running water, and then dry the transducer with a soft cloth or paper towel.

2. DISINFECTION—Cleaning with a detergent/water solution as described above is important as the first step in proper disinfection since chemical disinfectants act more rapidly on clean surfaces. However, the additional use of a high level liquid disinfectant will ensure further statistical reduction in microbial load. Because of the potential disruption of the barrier sheath,

additional high level disinfection with chemical agents is necessary. Examples of such high level disinfectants include but are not limited to

—2.4-3.2% glutaraldehyde products (a variety of available proprietary products including "Cidex," "Metricide," or "Procide")

—Non-glutaraldehyde agents including Cidex OPA (o-phthalaldehyde), Cidex PA (hydrogen peroxide & peroxyacetic acid)

—7.5% Hydrogen Peroxide solution

—Common household bleach (5.25% sodium hypochlorite) diluted to yield 500 parts per million chlorine (10 cc in one liter of tap water). This agent is effective but generally not recommended by probe manufacturers because it can damage metal and plastic parts.

Other agents such as quaternary ammonium compounds are not considered high level disinfectants and should not be used. Isopropanol is not a high level disinfectant when used as a wipe and probe manufacturers do generally not recommend soaking probes in the liquid.

The FDA has published a list of approved sterilants and high level disinfectants for use in processing reusable medical and dental devices. That list can be consulted to find agents that may be useful for probe disinfection.

Practitioners should consult the labels of proprietary products for specific instructions. They should also consult instrument manufacturers regarding compatibility of these agents with probes. Many of the chemical disinfectants are potentially toxic and many require adequate precautions such as proper ventilation, personal protective devices (gloves, face/eye protection, etc.) and thorough rinsing before reuse of the probe.

3. PROBE COVERS—The transducer should be covered with a barrier. If the barriers used are condoms, these should be nonlubricated and nonmedicated. Practitioners should be aware that condoms have been shown to be less prone to leakage than commercial probe covers, have a six-fold enhanced AQL (acceptable quality level) when compared to standard examination gloves. They have an AQL equal to that of surgical gloves. Users should be aware of latex-sensitivity issues and have available nonlatex-containing barriers.

4. ASEPTIC TECHNIQUE—For the protection of the patient and the health care worker, all endocavitary examinations should be performed with the operator properly gloved throughout the procedure. Gloves should be used to remove the condom or other barrier from the transducer and to wash the transducer as outlined above. As the barrier (condom) is removed, care should be taken not to contaminate the probe with secretions from the patient. At the completion of the procedure, hands should be thoroughly washed with soap and water.

Note: Obvious disruption in condom integrity does NOT require modification of this protocol. These guidelines take into account possible probe contamination due to a disruption in the barrier sheath.

In summary, routine high-level disinfection of the endocavitary probe between patients, plus the use of a probe cover or condom during each examination is required to properly protect patients from infection during endocavitary examinations. For all chemical disinfectants, precautions must be taken to protect workers and patients from the toxicity of the disinfectant.

Amis S, Ruddy M, Kibbler CC, Economides DL, MacLean AB. Assessment of condoms as probe covers for transvaginal sonography. J Clin Ultrasound 2000;28:295-8.

Rooks VJ, Yancey MK, Elg SA, Brueske L. Comparison of probe sheaths for endovaginal sonography. Obstet Gynecol 1996; 87:27-9.

Milki AA, Fisch JD. Vaginal ultrasound probe cover leakage: implications for patient care. Fertil Steril 1998;69:409-11.

Hignett M, Claman P. High rates of perforation are found in endovaginal ultrasound probe covers before and after oocyte retrieval for in vitro fertilization-embryo transfer. J Assist Reprod Genet 1995;12:606-9.

Sterilization and Disinfection of Medical Devices: General Principles. Centers for Disease Control, Division of Healthcare Quality Promotion. http://www.cdc.gov/ncidod/hip/sterile/sterilgp.htm (5-2003).

ODE Device Evaluation Information—FDA Cleared Sterilants and High Level Disinfectants with General Claims for Processing Reusable Medical and Dental Devices, March 2003. http://www.fda.gov/cdrh/ode/germlab.html (5-2003).

Courtesy of the Accreditation Council, American Institute of Ultrasound in Medicine. Available at http://www.aium.org/publications/statements/_statement
Selected.asp?statement=27. Accessed 5/8/06.

Index

Note: Page numbers followed by f indicate figures; those followed by t indicate tables.